PHYSEO

TABLE OF CONTENTS

NEUROLOGY PHARMACOLOGY....236

PSYCHIATRIC PHARMACOLOGY....278

We would like to extend a special thanks to the following contributing authors who have spent countless hours and support to make Physeo possible.

Aboozar Taiyeb Ali

Adila Reddy

Adrian Gutierrez, MD

Afshan Dhillon
MD Candidate
Saint James School of Medicine

AJ Chowdhury
MD 2024
University of Iowa

Alexandra Harding

Brian Makori Omwena Ogendi, PhD

Camelita Thrift

Genevieve Saliuk
MD Candidate 2024
UTMB School of Medicine

Jae Cheol Bae
MD Candidate, Class of 2023
St. Matthew's University of Medicine

Dr. Jabran Wasti, House Officer
Dr. Ruth K.M. Pfau Civil Hospital
Karachi, Pakistan

Janet E. Lindsley, PhD
Professor, Biochemistry
Assistant Dean, Curriculum
Adjunct Professor, Nutrition and Integrative Physiology
University of Utah School of Medicine

Julie Hansen, M.D.

Lauren Schwartz

Mohamed Elshennawy, MD

Noon Isam Eldin Hassan Hagmusa, MBBS

Richard Zhang
BMed/MD, BSc(Hons) candidate, class of 2023
University of New South Wales, Australia

Sergio R. Ortiz, MD, MPH

Tarannum Dhillon
MD Candidate
Saint James School of Medicine

FUNDAMENTALS IN PHARMACOLOGY

Fundamentals | Section 1 - Enzyme Kinetics

I. Basic premise of enzymes, substrates, and products
   A. S + E ⇄ ES ⇄ E + P

II. Michaelis-Menten Plot: Basic Principles
   A. Rate of formation of product as a function of substrate concentration
   B. More substrate → reaction velocity increases → more product
   C. Most enzymes follow a hyperbolic curve
      1. Increased rate of velocity in beginning
      2. Plateau at V_{max}

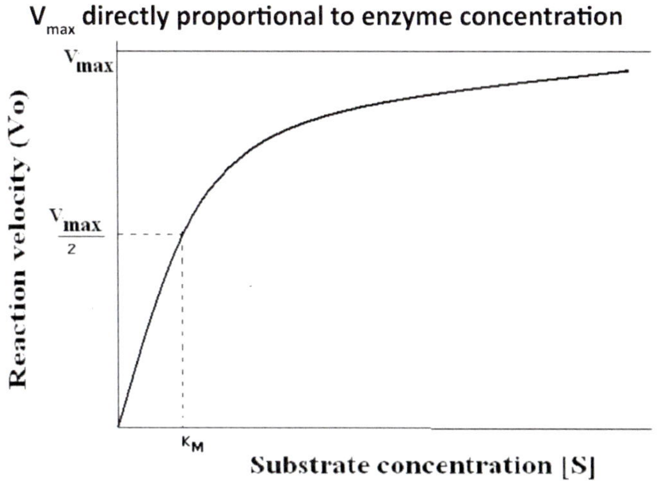

Photo Credit: Ntn024 at English Wikibooks / CC (https://creativecommons.org/licenses/by/3.0)

Figure 9.1.1 - Michaelis-Menten Plot

   D. K_m: concentration of substrate at ½ V_{max}
      1. Inversely related to affinity of enzyme for substrate
         a) Low K_m → high affinity
         b) High K_m → low affinity

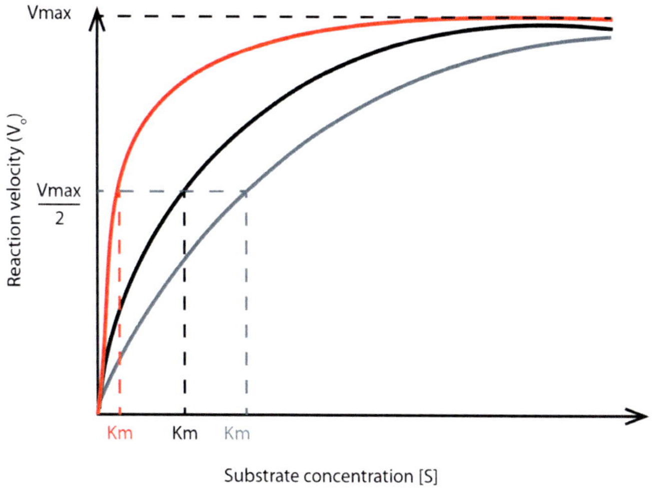

Figure 9.1.2 - Michaelis-Menten Plot of Enzymes with Various K_m

III. Lineweaver-Burk Plot
   A. Alternative to Michaelis-Menten plot
   B. Linear representation
      1. X-axis: 1/[S]
      2. Y-axis: 1/V
      3. X-intercept: -1/Km
      4. Y-intercept: 1/Vmax
   C. Higher the Vmax, the closer the y-intercept is to 0
   D. Higher the Km, the closer the x-intercept is to 0

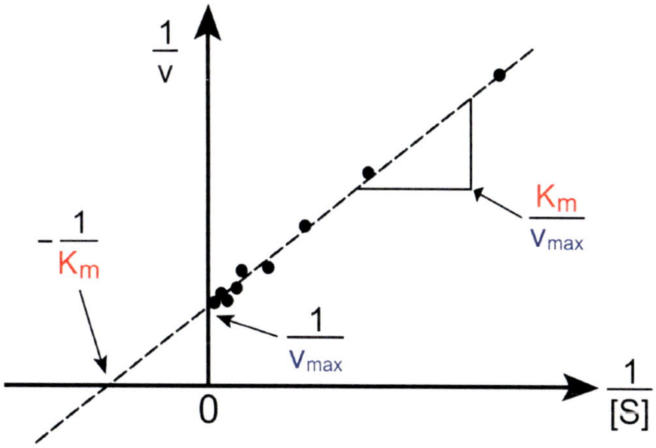

Photo Credit: Pro bug catcher at the English Wikipedia / CC BY-SA (http://creativecommons.org/licenses/by-sa/3.0/)

Figure 9.1.3 - Lineweaver-Burk Plot

	Competitive Inhibitors	Noncompetitive Inhibitors
Binding Site	- Directly compete with substrate for enzyme's active site	- Do not directly compete with substrate for enzyme's active site - Bind to allosteric site
Effect on K_m	- Increased	- Unchanged
Effect on V_{max}	- Unchanged	- Decreased
Overcome by increasing substrate concentration?	- Yes	- No

Table 9.1.1 - Table Comparing Competitive Vs Noncompetitive Inhibitors

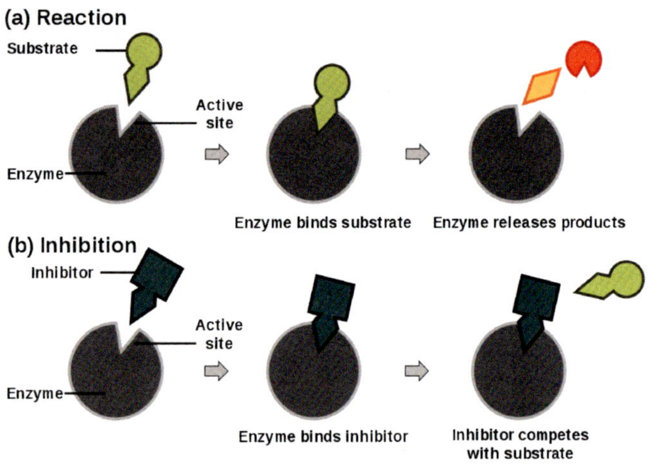

Photo Credit: Authored by Jerry Crimson Mann, modified by TimVickers, vectorized by Fvasconcellos / Public domain

Figure 9.1.4 - Mechanism of Competitive Inhibitors

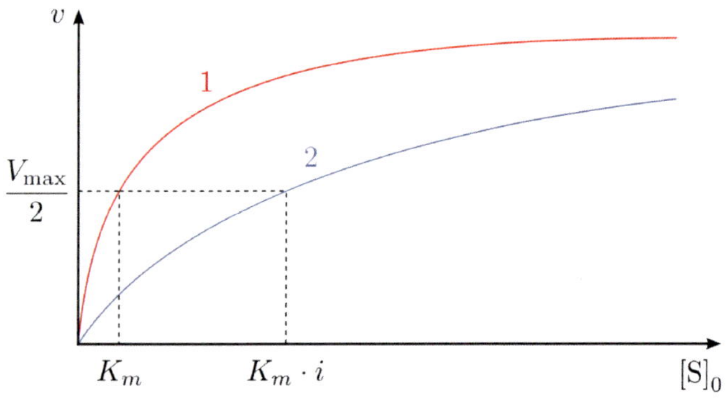

Photo Credit: Sponk (Diskussion) / Public domain

Figure 9.1.5 - Effect of Competitive Inhibitors on a Michaelis-Menten Plot

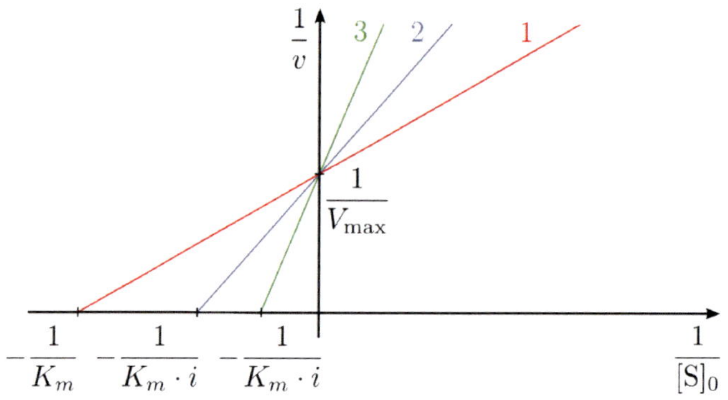

Photo Credit: Sponk / Public domain

Figure 9.1.6 - Effect of Competitive Inhibitors on a Lineweaver-Burk Plot

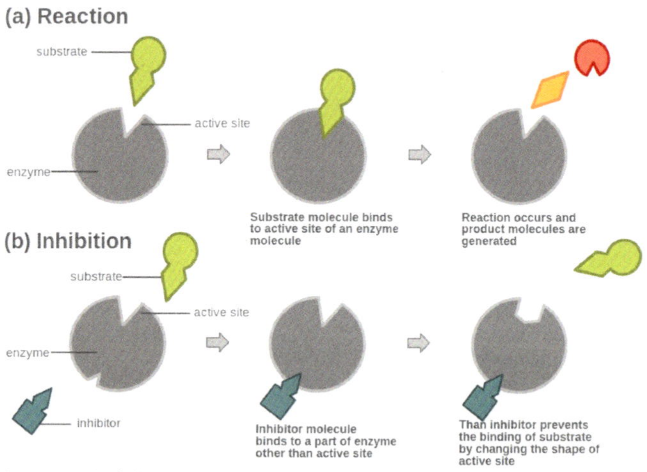

Photo Credit: srhat (talk · contribs)File:Comp_inhib.svg:SVG version:Srhat (talk · contribs)PNG version:Jerry Crimson Mann at en.wikipedia / Public domain

Figure 9.1.7 - Mechanism of Noncompetitive Inhibitors

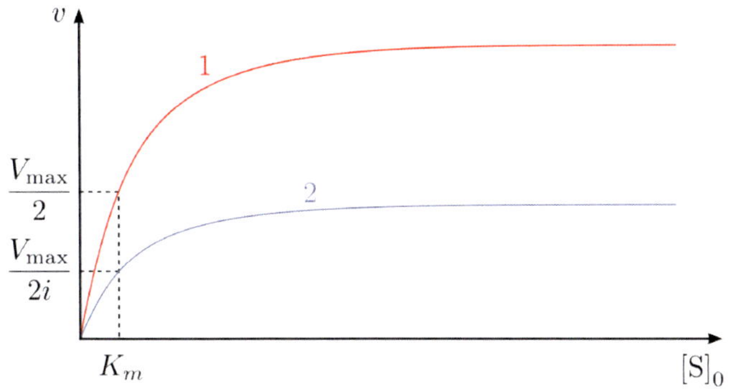

Photo Credit: Sponk / Public domain

Figure 9.1.8 - Effect of Noncompetitive Inhibitors on a Michaelis-Menten Plot

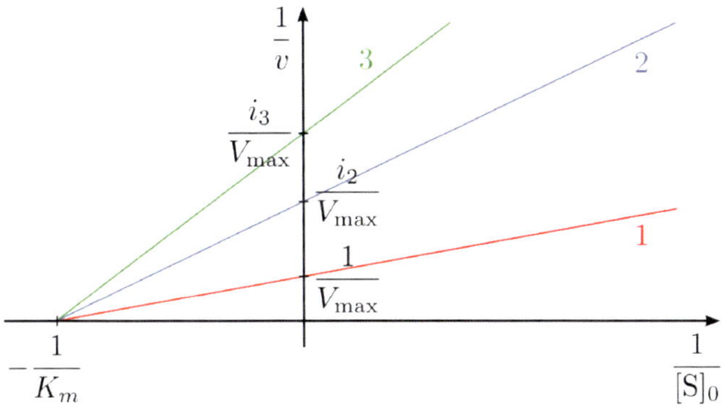

Photo Credit: Sponk / Public domain

Figure 9.1.9 - Effect of Noncompetitive Inhibitors on a Lineweaver-Burk Plot

REVIEW QUESTIONS

1. What does high Km indicate: low or high affinity?

- **High K_m would indicate low affinity of the enzyme for its substrate.**
- Km simply refers to the concentration of substrate at ½ of V_{max}. K_m is inversely related to the affinity of the enzyme for its substrate.

2. What does an x-intercept and a y-intercept indicate in Lineweaver-Burk plot?

- **In Lineweaver-Burk plot, the point where the line crosses the x-axis, also known as the x-intercept is equal to $-1/K_m$, and the point where the line crosses the y-axis, also known as the y-intercept is equal to $1/V_{max}$.**
- The Lineweaver-Burk plot is an alternative to the Michaelis-Menten plot and is a linear representation of the enzyme's kinetics.

REVIEW QUESTIONS

3. If drug X is a competitive inhibitor to drug Y, how would the values of K_m and V_{max} of drug Y change due to competitive inhibition?

- **K_m would decrease while V_{max} remains unchanged with competitive inhibition.**
- In competitive inhibition, the inhibitor directly competes with a substrate for the enzyme's active site.
- Since the competitive inhibitor, which is drug X in this case, fights for the active site along with the substrate, which is drug Y in this case, the affinity of drug Y for the enzyme gets lower. At some point, enough amount of drug X would overpower drug Y and the reaction would eventually reach V_{max}.

4. A 55-year-old male with hepatitis C is currently being treated with ribavirin, a competitive inhibitor of IMP dehydrogenase that inhibits guanine synthesis. Which of the following statements regarding the activity of ribavirin is true?

   A. The drug decreases the maximal velocity of the enzyme
   B. The drug has no effect on the maximal velocity of the enzyme
   C. The drug increases the affinity of the substrate for the enzyme
   D. The drug has no effect on the affinity of the substrate for the enzyme

- **The correct answer is B.**
- Ribavirin is a competitive inhibitor of IMP dehydrogenase. Competitive inhibitors have no effect on the maximal velocity of the enzyme or V_{max}, but decrease the affinity of the substrate for the enzyme or K_m.
- A and D are incorrect because they represent the characteristics of noncompetitive inhibitors, as noncompetitive inhibitors decrease V_{max} but have no effect on K_m.
- C is incorrect because competitive inhibitors decrease the affinity of the substrate for the enzyme, not increase.

I. Pharmacokinetics: Bioavailability (F)
   A. Fraction of administered drug that gains access to systemic circulation unchanged
      1. Oral: F < 100% due to first-pass metabolism
      2. IV: F = 100%
   B. $F = AUC_o / AUC_{iv} \times 100$

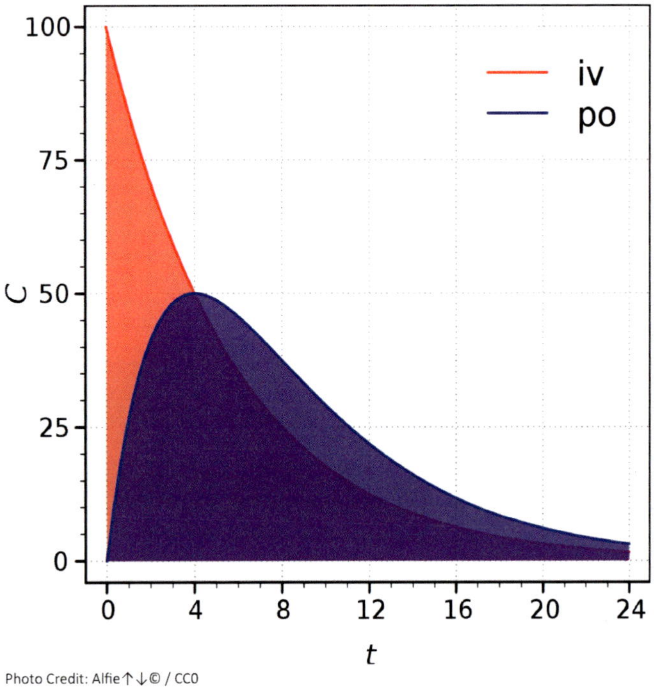

Photo Credit: Alfie↑↓© / CC0

Figure 9.1.10 - Drug Bioavailability

II. Pharmacokinetics: Volume of Distribution (V_d)
   A. Theoretical volume occupied by total amount of drug in body relative to plasma concentration
   B. V_d = Amount of drug in body / plasma drug concentration
   C. Factors affecting V_d
      1. Plasma or tissue protein bound
      2. Solubility
      3. Drug particle size

V_d	Drug Properties
Low	- Plasma protein bound - Non-lipophilic - High molecular weight
High	- Tissue protein bound - Lipophilic - Low molecular weight

Table 9.1.2 - Drug Properties and the Volume of Distribution

III. Pharmacokinetics: Clearance (CL)
   A. Volume of plasma cleared of drug per unit time
   B. CL = rate of elimination of drug / plasma drug concentration
   C. Impacted by defects in cardiac, hepatic, or renal function

IV. Pharmacokinetics: Half-life ($t_{1/2}$)
   A. Time required to reduce amount of drug in body to half of its original concentration
   B. $t_{1/2} = (0.693 \times V_d) / CL$ in first-order elimination
   C. 4-5 half lives to reach steady state concentration

V. Dosage Calculations
   A. Loading dose: initial dose given to quickly achieve target plasma concentration
   B. Dependent on V_d
   C. Maintenance dose: dose given to maintain required plasma concentration over a long period of time
   D. Renal or liver disease:
      1. Loading dose unchanged
      2. Maintenance dose decreased

VI. Equations:
   A. Loading dose (LD) = (Cp x Vd) / F
   B. Maintenance dose (MD) = (Cp x CL x τ) / F

REVIEW QUESTIONS

1. What does a low first pass metabolism indicate: a high or low bioavailability?
   - **A low first pass metabolism would indicate high bioavailability.**
   - Remember the first pass metabolism occurs mainly in the liver when the drug gets rapidly metabolized, decreasing the amount that reaches the systemic circulation in an unchanged form.
   - If a drug has a low first pass metabolism, the less it will get metabolized by the liver, and the more it would reach the systemic circulation in an unchanged form.

2. What does high Vd indicate about drug property: plasma protein bound or tissue protein bound?
   - **A high Vd indicates that the drug is tissue protein bound.**
   - Remember, if a drug is plasma protein bound, the drug will stay in the plasma and won't get absorbed into the tissue as much.
   - However, if a drug is more bound to tissue proteins, the drug will be easily distributed to the tissues, reflected by high Vd.

3. How does clearance of a drug differ in a patient with liver cirrhosis compared to a normal healthy patient?
   - **Remember that the clearance of a drug can be impacted by defects in cardiac, hepatic, or renal function.**
   - **In a patient with liver cirrhosis, the drug cannot be metabolized and cleared normally compared to a normal healthy patient and could result in the accumulation of the drug.**
   - **Therefore, the clearance would be lower in someone with liver cirrhosis compared to a normal healthy individual.**

4. How much of drug X is available after 16 hours if 100 mg of drug X is administered given that a half-life of drug X is 4 hours?
   - **6.25 mg would be available after 16 hours.**
   - Remember that half-life refers to the time required to reduce the amount of drug in the body to half of its original concentration.
   - If drug X has a half-life of 4 hours, 16 hours would mean 4 half-lives.
   - So if 100 mg of drug X was administered in the beginning, after 1 half-life, only 50 mg would be available.
   - After 2 half-life, 25 mg; 3 half-life, 12.5 mg; 4 half-life, 6.25 mg.

5. The clearance of a given drug is 50 L/h. The drug is administered by continuous IV infusion given at 200 mg/h to maintain the target plasma concentration. What is the anticipated target plasma concentration?

   A. 0.25mg/L
   B. 2mg/L
   C. 4mg/L
   D. Cannot be determined from given information

   - **The answer to the question is C.**
   - The clearance (CL) is 50L/h and the maintenance dose (MD) is 200 mg/h and the question asks about the target plasma concentration which is Cp.
     - We can use the equation, MD = (Cp x CL x) / F (write).
     - Here, the dosage interval (τ) would be 1 since the drug is administered continuously and the bioavailability (F) would be 1 since the drug is administered intravenously.
   - So we can calculate the Cp or target plasma concentration by dividing the maintenance dose, 200 mg/h, by the clearance, which is 50 L/h.

I. Metabolism
   A. Breakdown of a drug using enzymes to modify its chemical structure
      1. lipophilic → hydrophilic (more readily excreted)
   B. Rate of metabolism determines drug duration of action and side effects
   C. Split into two phases
      1. Phase I
      2. Phase II

	Reactions	Product	Notes
Phase I	- Involve CYP450: - Reduction - Oxidation - Hydrolysis	- Polar, water-soluble metabolites - May or may not be active	- Lost first in geriatric patients
Phase II	- Conjugation: - Methylation - Acetylation - Glucuronidation - Sulfation	- Highly polar, water-soluble metabolites - Usually inactive	- Renal excretion - Slow acetylators (decreased rate of metabolism) → decreased elimination → may have increased side effects

Table 9.1.3 - Phases of Drug Metabolism

II. Elimination
   A. Removal of drugs from the body
   B. 2 types
      1. Zero-order elimination
      2. First-order elimination

	Elimination Rate	Decrease in Drug Plasma Concentration	Half-Life	Examples
Zero-order elimination	- Constant amount	- Linear	- Decreases	- Phenytoin - Ethanol - Aspirin (high dose)
First-order elimination	- Constant proportion	- Exponential	- Constant	- Most drugs

Table 9.1.4 - Types of Drug Elimination

III. Urine pH
   A. Water-soluble drugs/metabolites are excreted in urine
   B. Elimination depends on metabolite charge in urine
      1. Charged metabolites are "trapped" in urine
      2. Uncharged metabolites are reabsorbed
   C. pKa: pH at which half of the drug is charged
      1. High pKa = weak acid
      2. Low pKa = weak base

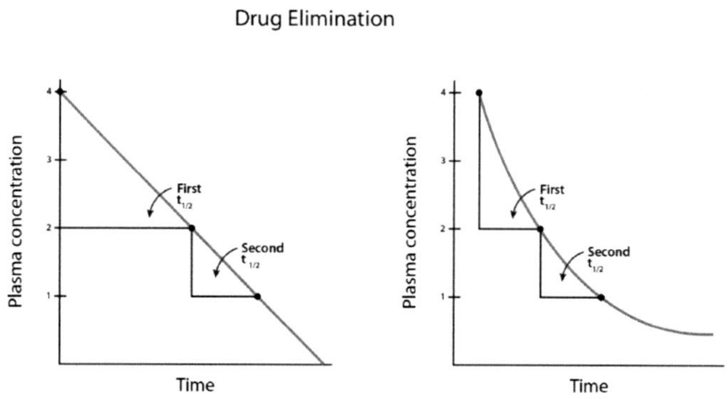

Figure 9.1.11 - Graphs Showing Drug Plasma Concentration Over Time

	Trapped In	Examples	Overdose Treatment
Weak acid	- Basic urine	- Phenobarbital - Methotrexate - Aspirin	- Alkalinize urine with sodium bicarbonate
Weak base	- Acidic urine	- Tricyclic antidepressants - Amphetamines	- Acidify urine with ammonium chloride

Table 9.1.5 - Types of Drugs Trapped in Urine

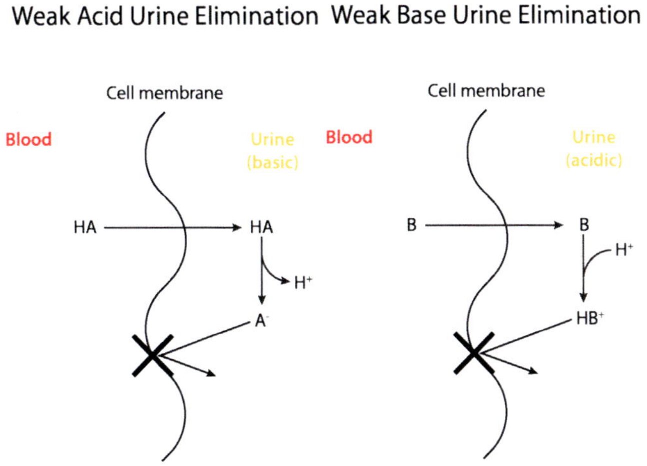

Figure 9.1.12 - Weak Acid Urine Elimination

REVIEW QUESTIONS

1. What types of drug metabolic reactions will most likely be deficient in an 85-year-old female patient?
   - **The answer is phase I reactions such as reduction, oxidation, and hydrolysis.**
   - Recall from our discussion that geriatric patients have issues with Phase I drug metabolism.
   - This means our 85-year-old patient will have issues with reactions involving CYP450, which includes reduction, oxidation, and hydrolysis.

2. For a drug undergoing first-order metabolism, how does the half-life change over time?
   - **The answer is the half-life remains constant.**
   - Elimination of drugs undergoing first-order metabolism depends on the plasma concentration of the drug.
   - Because of this, the same proportion of the drug is eliminated within a given amount of time so the half-life remains constant.

REVIEW QUESTIONS

3. If a patient overdoses on a drug that is a weak acid, what can be administered to accelerate elimination of the drug in the urine?

   A. The rate of excretion is dependent on the plasma concentration
   B. The half-life remains constant over time
   C. A constant fraction is eliminated over time
   D. The plasma concentration decreases linearly over time

   - **The correct answer is D.**
   - Weak acids become negatively charged and "trapped" in basic urine, so if we want to eliminate a weak acid in the urine we want to find a way to make the urine more basic.
   - To alkalinize the urine, we can administer sodium bicarbonate.
   - A is incorrect because the rate of excretion of phenytoin is not dependent on the plasma concentration.
   - B is incorrect because the half life will decrease overtime for drugs that following zero-order elimination.
   - C is incorrect because for drugs with zero-order elimination, a constant amount, not a constant fraction, of drug is eliminated over time.
   - All three of these statements more accurately describe drugs that follow first-order elimination.

I. Efficacy
   A. Maximum effect of drug
      1. Once maximum effect is reached, giving more drug will not result in greater effect
   B. High V_{max} = high efficacy

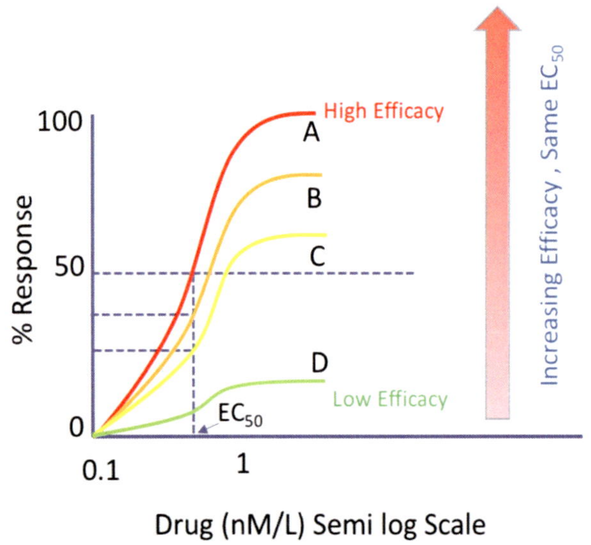

Figure 9.1.13 - Dose-Response Curve Showing the Efficacy of Various Drugs

II. Potency
   A. Amount of drug needed to produce effect
      1. Determined by receptor affinity for drug and number of receptors present
   B. Based on EC_{50}
      1. EC_{50}: concentration of drug that causes half of desired response
      2. Low EC_{50} = high potency

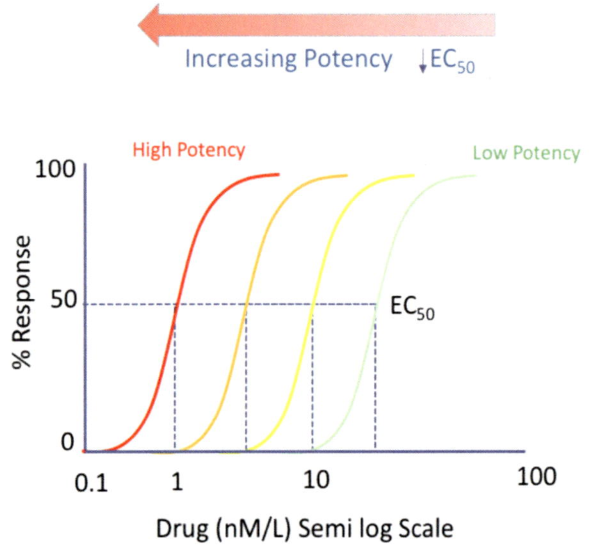

Figure 9.1.14 - Dose-Response Curve Showing the Potency of Various Drugs

III. Efficacy vs. Potency
   A. Efficacy and potency are not dependent on each other
      1. Drug can have high potency but low efficacy, and vice versa

IV. Receptor Binding
   A. Agonist: activates receptor
   B. Antagonist: inhibits receptor
   C. Full agonist: capable of producing maximal receptor response
   D. Partial agonist: produces a decreased receptor response
      1. Binds at same site as full agonist
      2. Decreased efficacy
   E. Competitive antagonist: binds at same site as agonists
      1. Decreases potency
      2. Can be overcome by adding more agonist
   F. Noncompetitive antagonist: binds at different site (allosteric) than agonists
      1. Decreases efficacy
      2. Cannot be overcome by adding more agonist

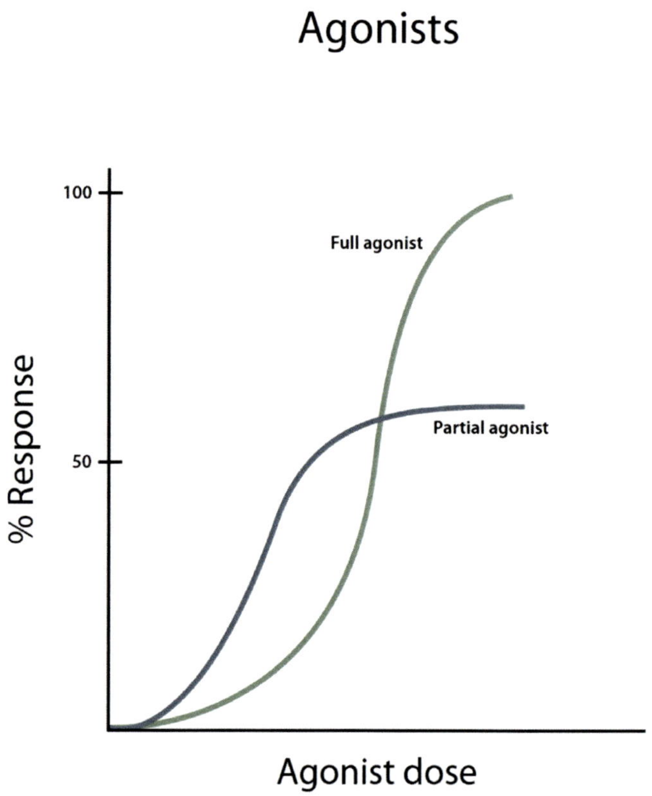

Figure 9.1.15 - Dose-Response Curves Comparing a Full and Partial Agonist

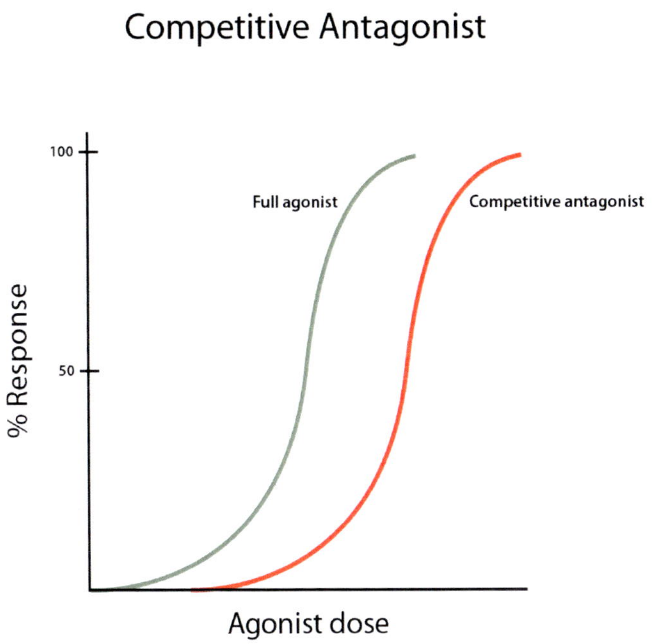

Figure 9.1.16 - Dose-Response Curves Comparing a Full and Competitive Agonist

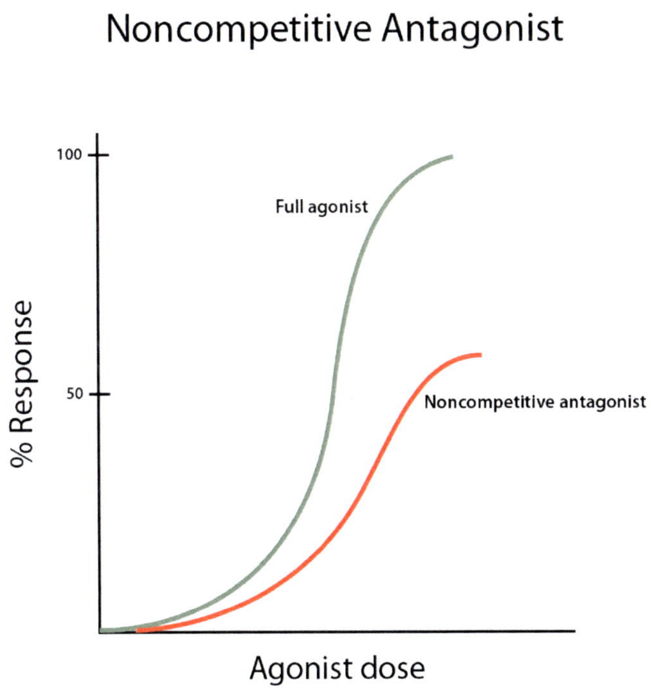

Figure 9.1.17 - Dose-Response Curves Comparing a Full and Noncompetitive Agonist

V. Therapeutic Index (TI)
  A. Used to measure safety of a drug
    1. Describes relationship between therapeutic dose and toxic dose
  B. TI = TD_{50}/ED_{50}
    1. TD_{50} = median toxic dose
  C. Replaced with LD_{50} (median lethal dose) in animal studies
    1. ED_{50} = median effective dose
  D. Safe drugs have a high TI
  E. Drugs with low TI require monitoring
    1. Examples: warfarin, lithium, digoxin, amphotericin
  F. Therapeutic window: dose range in which drug can safely and effectively treat disease
    1. Low dose to achieve therapeutic response + high dose to reach toxicity = wide therapeutic window

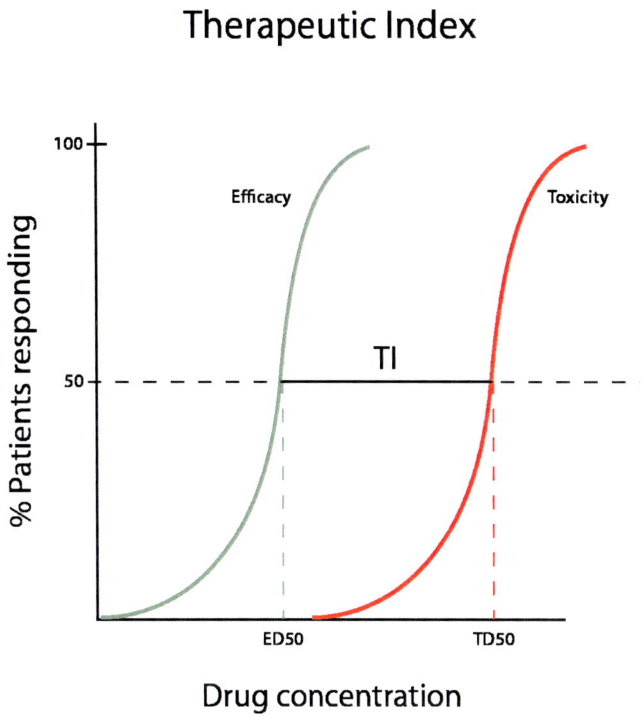

Figure 9.1.18 - Dose-Response Curve Showing the Therapeutic Index of a Drug

REVIEW QUESTIONS

1. Drug A has a higher potency that Drug B,. How would the dosage of Drug B compare to that of Drug A?
    - **A higher dosage of drug B must be administered.**
    - Potency is the amount of drug needed to produce the desired effect.
    - If Drug B has lower potency than drug A, it means more of Drug B is needed to produce the desired effect.
    - Therefore, more of drug B will need to be administered as compared to drug A.

2. Drugs A and B bind to the same receptor. When given alone, Drug A produces the maximal response, while Drug B produces half the response of Drug A. When given together, the maximal response is produced. What type of drug is Drug B?
    - **Drug B is a partial agonist.**
    - The drugs bind the same receptor, but elicit different responses.
    - Drug B's response is less than that of drug A.
    - There is no indication that drug B inhibits the activity of drug A since the maximal response is reached when the drugs are given together.
    - This means drug B must be a partial agonist, as it activates the receptor but does not produce the maximal response.

3. How is the therapeutic index calculated?
    - **TI = TD_{50}/ED_{50}**
    - Therapeutic index is used to measure the safety of a drug and describes the relationship between the therapeutic dose and the toxic dose of a drug.
    - It is calculated as the TD_{50}, or median toxic dose, divided by the ED_{50}, or the median effective dose.

4. Diazepam is an agonist at the GABA receptor. Flumazenil is a competitive antagonist at the GABA receptor that is used to treat a diazepam overdose. Which of the following best describes the effect of flumazenil on diazepam's activity at the GABA receptor?

    A. Increased efficacy
    B. Decreased efficacy
    C. Increased potency
    D. Decreased potency

    - **The answer is D.**
    - Flumazenil is a competitive antagonist, which means it competes with diazepam to bind to the GABA receptor and more diazepam would be required to reach the maximum agonist effect at the GABA receptor. Therefore, as a competitive antagonist flumazenil would result in decreased potency.
    - A is incorrect because antagonists of any type would not result in increased efficacy.
    - B is incorrect because noncompetitive antagonists result in a decrease in efficacy, while competitive antagonists do not affect efficacy.
    - C is incorrect because antagonists of any type would not result in increased potency.

Type	Definition	Example
Additive	- Effect of 2 substances together is equal to the sum of each drug used independently	- Aspirin and acetaminophen
Synergistic	- Effect of 2 drugs together is larger than the sum of each drug used independently	- Clopidogrel and aspirin
Potentiation	- Drug with no individual therapeutic effect enhances the effect of another drug	- Carbidopa and levodopa
Permissive	- Full effect of one drug requires the presence of another drug	- Cortisol and catecholamines
Antagonistic	- Effect of 2 substances together is less than the sum of each drug used independently	- Ethanol and methanol
Tachyphylactic	- Initial or repeat administration results in acute decrease of effect	- LSD, MDMA, nitrates, niacin, phenylephrine

Table 9.1.6 - Types of Drug-Drug Interactions

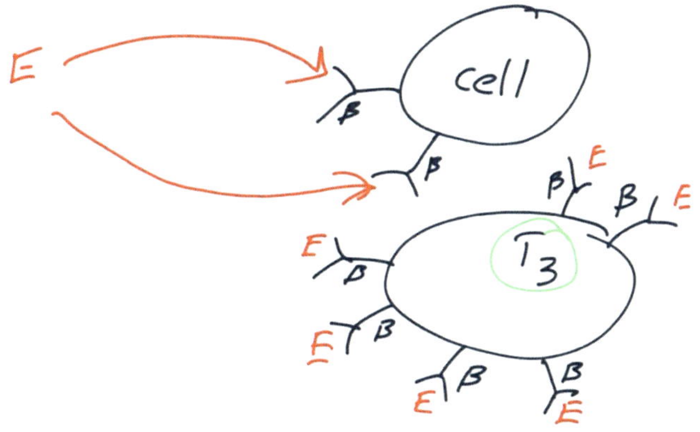

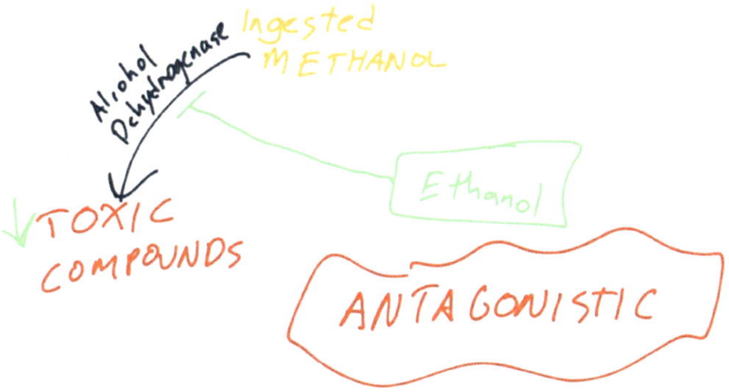

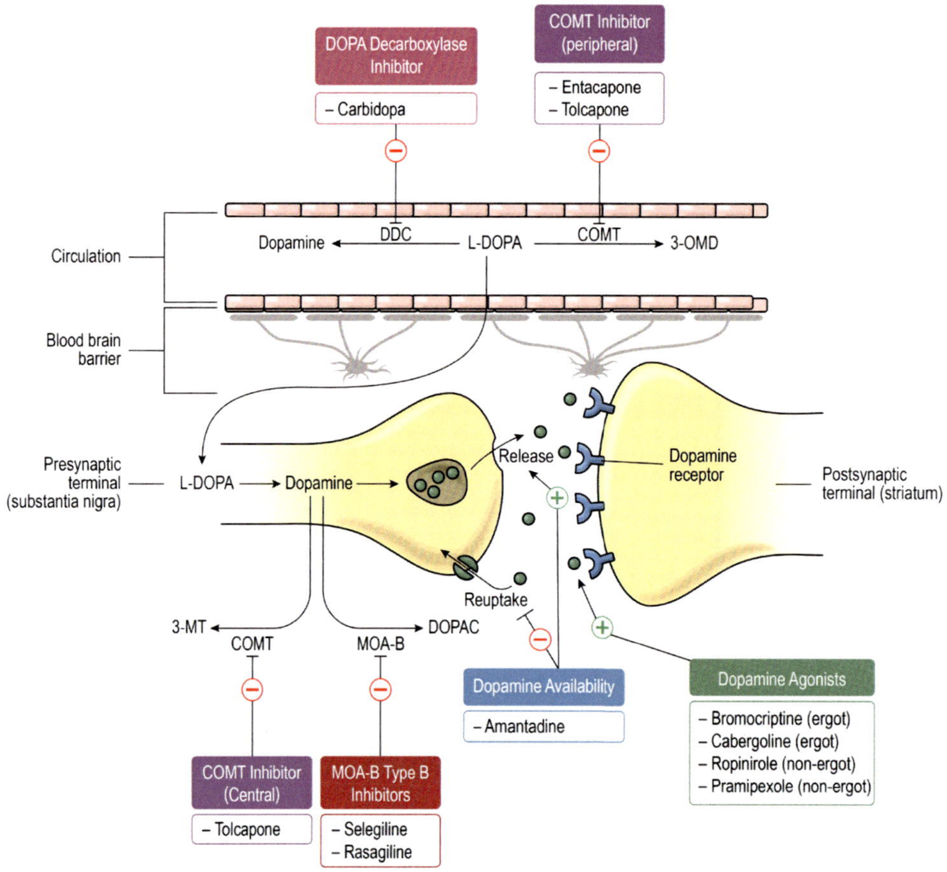

Figure 9.1.19 - Drugs that Interact with Dopamine Pathways

REVIEW QUESTIONS

1. A 67-year-old male presents to the emergency department with sudden left sided weakness of the body and face. CT scans confirm an ischemic stroke affecting branches of the right middle cerebral artery. The patient is stabilized and released with prescriptions for both clopidogrel and aspirin. Which of the following types of drug-drug interactions is the basis behind prescribing both clopidogrel and aspirin in this scenario?

   A. Additive
   B. Synergistic
   C. Permissive
   D. Potentiation

- **The answer here is B.**
- The vignette indicates that both clopidogrel and aspirin were administered to this patient after he had a stroke.
- This combination is commonly used for antiplatelet therapy in stroke prevention.
- The question asks what drug-drug interaction occurs when this combination is used.
- Since clopidogrel and aspirin have different mechanisms of action, together they exert a greater effect than if they were used individually - meaning they exhibit synergism.
- A) is incorrect because additive effects are those that add up to the sum of their parts, whereas the effect seen with clopidogrel and aspirin is greater than the sum of their parts.
- C) is incorrect because permissive effects are those in which the presence of 1 drug is required for the full effect of another.
- Both clopidogrel and aspirin can exert their maximal effects independently.
- D) is incorrect because potentiation is the use of a drug with no therapeutic effect to increase the effect of another drug.
- Both clopidogrel and aspirin have therapeutic effects on their own.

Inhibitors	Substrates	Inducers
Sodium valproate	Theophylline	Carbamazepine
Isoniazid	Anti-epileptics (except carbamazepine, phenytoin, and valproic acid)	Phenytoin
Cimetidine	Warfarin	St. John's wort
Ketoconazole	OCPs	Chronic alcohol abuse
Acute alcohol abuse	Statins (except pravastatin)	Phenobarbital
Chloramphenicol		Nevirapine
Erythromycin and clarithromycin		Rifampin
SSRIs		Griseofulvin
Verapamil		Modafinil
Sulfonamides		
Ciprofloxacin		
Omeprazole		
Metronidazole		
Amiodarone		
Ritonavir		
Grapefruit Juice		

Table 9.1.7 - Inhibitors, Substrates, and Inducers of the Cytochrome System

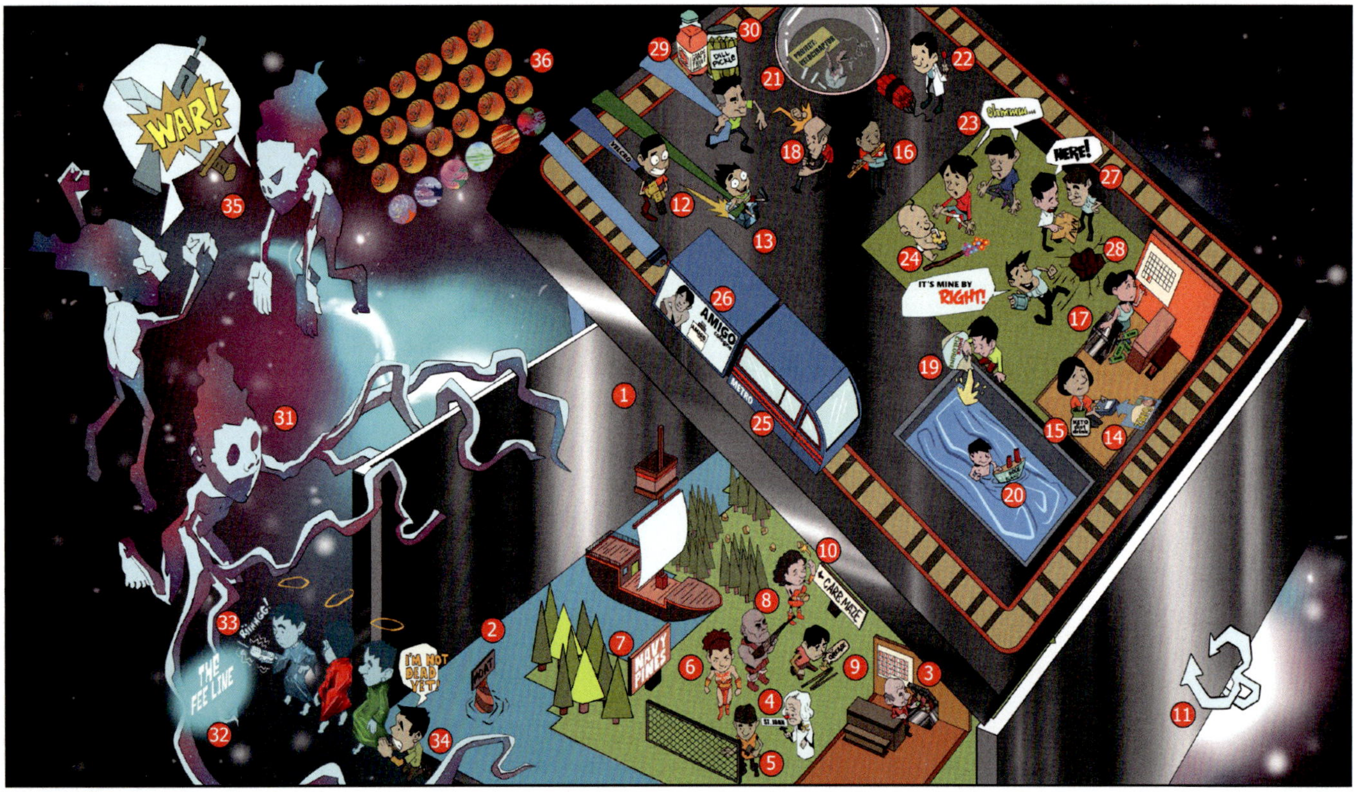

1. People living inside open chrome box: Cytochrome P-450 inducers

2. Moat inside open chrome box: modafinil induces Cytochrome P-450

3. Daily sacrifice of alcohol to gods over long time period: Chronic alcohol use causes induction of cytochrome P-450

4. St. John preaching inside chrome box: St. John's wort induces cytochrome P-450

5. Man constructing fence inside chrome box: Phenytoin induces cytochrome P-450

6. Leader of barbarian clan with phoenix war paint: Phenobarbital induces cytochrome P-450

7. Bay with ships marked with "navy pines" sign and surrounded by pine trees: Nevirapine induces cytochrome P-450

8. Barbarian holding rifle: Rifampin induces cytochrome P-450

9. Man applying grease to fence posts: Griseofulvin induces cytochrome P-450

10. Barbarina leader leaving trail of carb-rich bread crumbs through trees, marked with "carb maze" sign: Carbamazepine induces cytochrome P-450

11. Straps attached to grappling hook to pull chrome box shut: Cytochrome P450 inhibitors

12. Kid pulling velcro strap to keep box closed: Sodium valproate inhibits cytochrome P-450

13. Kid sliding down lid on ice block while pulling strap to close lid: Isoniazid inhibits cytochrome P-450

14. Woman playing Sims while sitting on top of box: Cimetidine inhibits cytochrome P-450

15. Woman drinking keto-friendly drink on top of box: Ketoconazole inhibits cytochrome P-450

16. Man wearing shawl marked "A" and playing flute on top of box: Fluconazole inhibits cytochrome P-450

17. Cute lady sacrificing alcohol to gods for first time on top of box: Acute alcohol abuse causes inhibition of cytochrome P-450

18. Man throwing ear-shaped hearing aid at clarinet player: Erythromycin and clarithromycin inhibit cytochrome P-450

19. Man pouring chlorine into pool on top of box: Chloramphenicol inhibits cytochrome P-450

20. Boy playing with "SS Rhode Island" (SSRI) boat inside pool: SSRIs inhibit cytochrome P-450

21. Scientist trying to grow colony of velociraptors on top of box: Verapamil inhibits cytochrome P-450

22. Scientist holding sulfur match near velociraptor colony: Sulfonamides inhibit cytochrome P-450

23. Meditating people chanting "ohmmm" on top of box: Omeprazole inhibits cytochrome P-450

24. Child playing with flower-shaped sippy cup next to flowery staff: Ciprofloxacin inhibits cytochrome P-450

25. Metro system on top of box: Metronidazole inhibits cytochrome P450

26. "Amigo cologne" advertisement on metro car: Amiodarone inhibits cytochrome P-450

27. Engineer pointing to NAV label on diagram while saying "here!": Ritonavir inhibits cytochrome P-450

28. Man climbing out of hole with discovered treasure saying "it's mine by right!": Ritonavir inhibits cytochrome P-450

29. Large container of grapefruit juice near strap pullers on top of box: Grapefruit juice inhibits cytochrome P-450

30. Large jar of dill pickles near strap pullers on top of box: Diltiazem inhibits cytochrome P-450

31. Eternal space gods floating outside of chrome box: Dytochrome P450 substrates

32. Deceased people waiting in "the fee line" to enter afterlife: Theophylline is metabolized by cytochrome P-450

33. Deceased person holding shaking phone: Antiepileptics are metabolized by cytochrome P-450 (except carbamazepine, phenytoin, and valproic acid)

34. Praying man in fee line wearing satins: Statins (except pravastatin) are metabolized by cytochrome P-450

35. Gods getting ready to fight while shouting "war!": Warfarin is metabolized by cytochrome P-450

36. Planetary systems arranged in rows like contraceptive pills (OCPs): OCPs are metabolized by cytochrome P-450

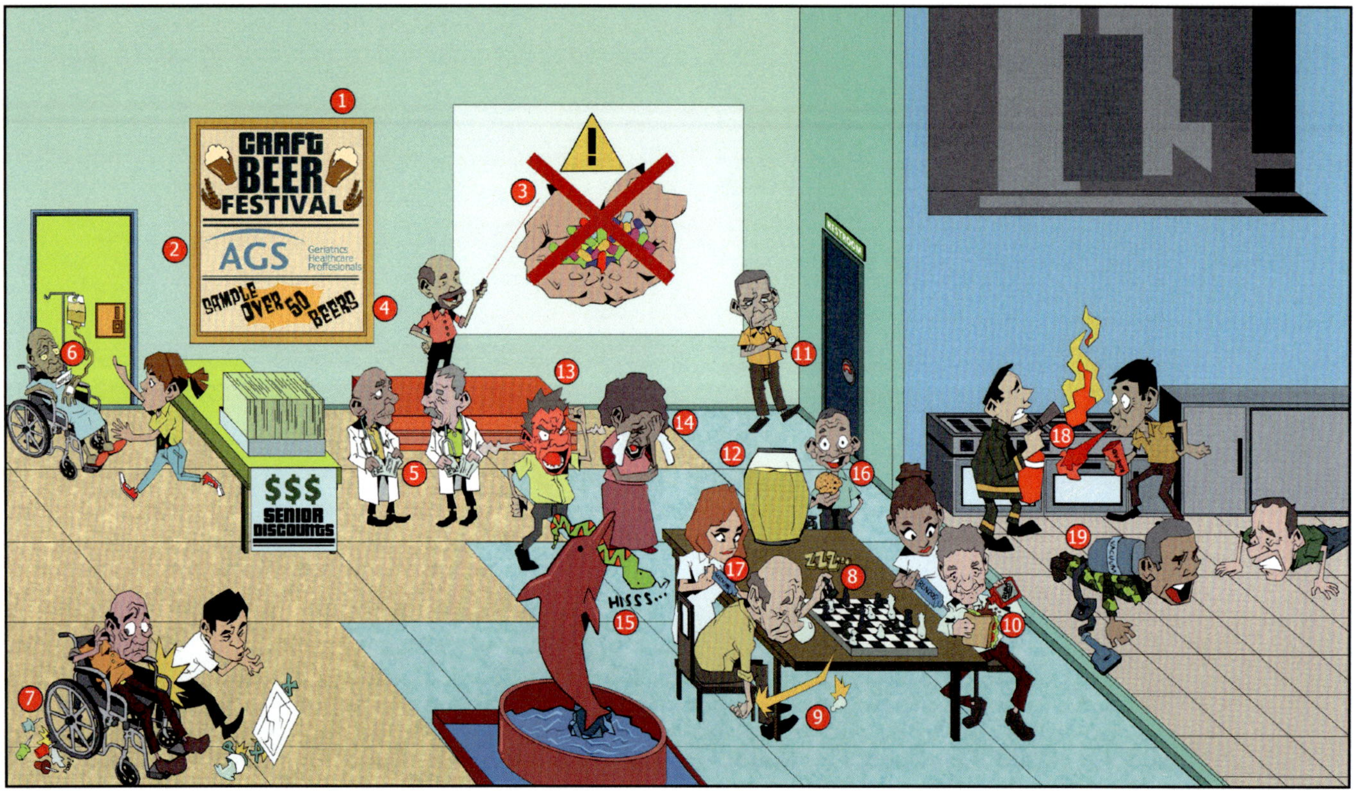

1. "Craft Beer Festival" poster in nursing home: Beers criteria

2. "American Geriatric Society" named as festival sponsor on poster: Guidelines from the American Geriatric Society (AGS)

3. Speaker at festival pointing to "no pills" presentation slide: Criteria used to reduce detrimental polypharmacy or other inappropriate medications for geriatric patients

4. "Sample over 50 beers" written on poster: A list of over 50 medications to avoid

5. Doctors convinced by speaker ripping up prescription pads: Primary target audience for the AGS Beers criteria is practicing clinicians

6. Sick, elderly palliative care patient in wheelchair unable to participate in festival: Except for palliative and hospice settings, the guidelines are intended to use in all patients 65 years and older (e.g. acute, ambulatory, institutionalized facilities)

7. Waiter dropping teacup and tray with alpha-shaped handles after bumping into man in wheelchair with deflating tire: Avoid alpha blockers due to increased risk of hypotension

8. Elderly man falling asleep: Avoid due to increased risk sedation

9. Sleeping man knocking chess piece off table: Avoid due to increased risk of falls

10. Elderly chess player pouring rum on deli sandwich: Avoid due to increased risk of delirium

11. Person taking their time in bathroom: Avoid due to increased risk of constipation

12. Bladder-shaped container with yellow lemonade on table: Avoid due to increased risk of urinary retention

13. Angry nursery home resident with red face and steam coming out of ears: Anticholinergics

14. Crying woman embarrassed by husband's tantrum: Antidepressants

15. Fountain of dolphin clutching (inhibiting) hissing snake in mouth: Antihistamines

16. Resident eating poppy seed muffin: Opioids

17. Nurses injecting two chess players with blue "benzos" syringes: Benzodiazepines also increase risk of falls, sedation and delirium

18. Firefighter holding fire extinguisher while nursing home resident spits out red drink in shock: NSAIDs can increase the risk of GI bleeding (esp. alongside other anticoagulants)

19. Drill sergeant leading difficult boot camp with vacuum pump on back: Proton pump inhibitors increase risk of *C. difficile* colitis infection

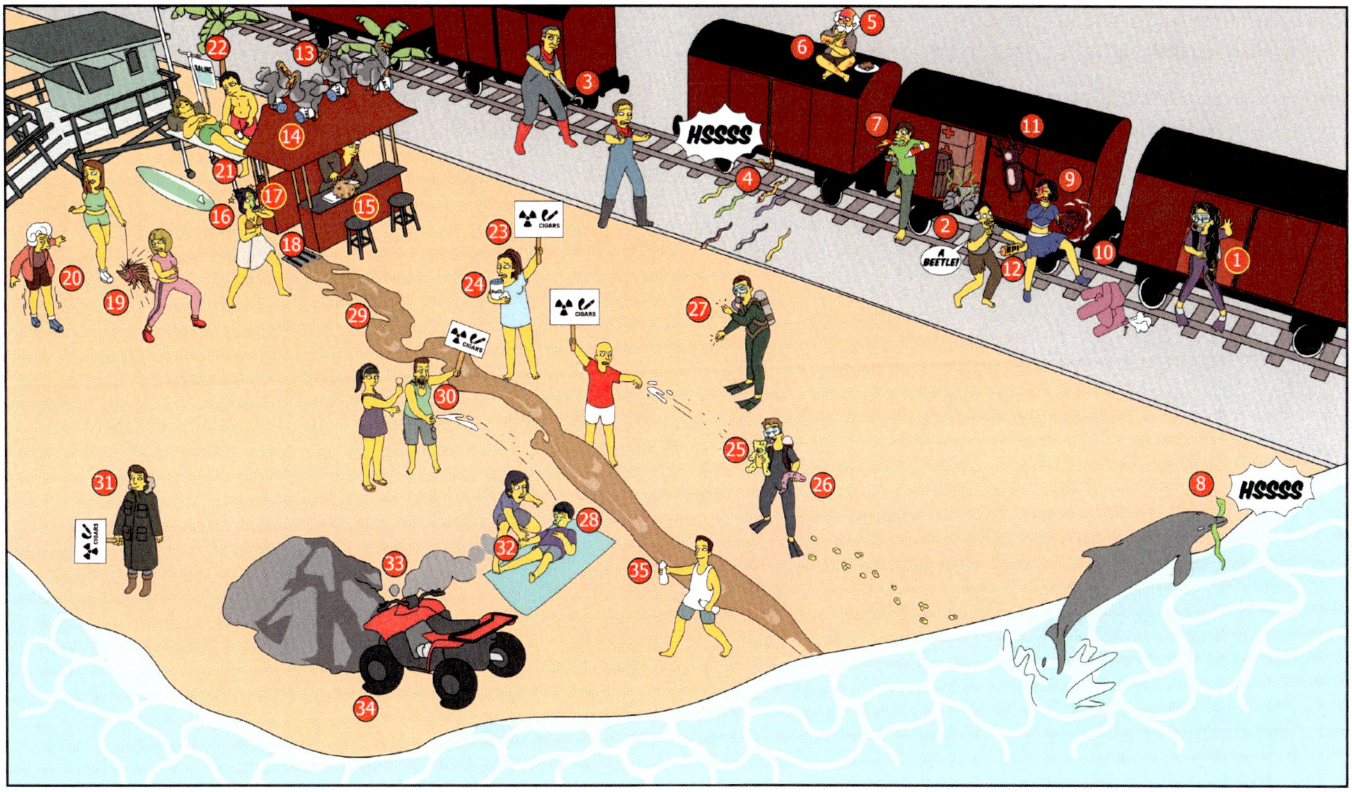

1. Girl with sea scum in braid from diving into ocean: Scombroid poisoning

2. Rotting fish with dark meat in train car: Occurs with fish with dark meat that have spoiled

3. Other train cars being disconnected from cars with rotting fish and sea scum: Scombroid poison is a bacterial decarboxylase

4. Hobo dining on top of train car while hissing snakes crawl out of train car: Decarboxylase converts histidine to histamine → high serum histamine

5. Hobo's red face due to sun exposure: Can cause flushing of face and skin redness

6. Hobo scratching hives: Can cause urticaria (hives)

7. Second hobo breathing fire after eating hot chili sauce: Can cause acute burning sensation of mouth

8. Dolphin in ocean cluting (inhibiting) hissing snake in mouth: Treat scombroid with antihistamines

9. Cheerleader hobo with swollen face choking from allergic reaction: Symptoms mimic anaphylaxis

10. Cheerleader hobo with shaking bronchial tree pom poms, swollen lips, and deflating blow-up chair: Symptoms may include bronchospasm, angioedema, and hypotension

11. Hobo pointing at large beetle on train car and exclaiming "a beetle!": Consider also providing albuterol for bronchospasm (in addition to antihistamines)

12. Hobo holding Epipen to help choking cheerleader hobo: Consider also administering epinephrine

13. Four dodo birds on pufferfish beach stand: Tetrodotoxin

14. Dodo birds holding blocked salt shakers: Binds fast voltage-gated Na^+ channels in nerve tissue, preventing depolarization

15. Pufferfish sold at stand: Tetrodotoxin comes from pufferfish

16. Dizzy woman disgusted by pufferfish stand: Tetrodotoxin can cause dizziness

17. Nauseous woman about to throw up: Tetrodotoxin can cause nausea

18. Leaky sewer allowing sewage to spill onto beach: Tetrodotoxin cna cause diarrhea

19. Beach jogger getting poked by porcupine quills: Tetrodotoxin can cause paresthesias (pins and needles)

20. Weak, elderly woman tired after walking through beach sand: Can cause weakness

21. Lifeguard hitting jellyfish sting victim's knee and unable to produce reflex response: Can cause hyporeflexia

22. IV drip for man stung by jellyfish: Supportive treatment (IV fluids)

23. Anti-smoking protester holding cigar toxin signs: Ciguatoxin

24. Anti-smoking protestor holding open salt shaker: Ciguatoxin opens Na^+ channels, causes depolarization

25. Scuba diver holding bear-shaped piece of coral from reef: Can come from barracuda (reef fish)

26. Scuba diver holding eel-shaped piece of coral from reef: Can come from moray eel (reef fish)

27. Second scuba differ snapping fingers at protestor: Can come from snapper (reef fish)

28. Nauseous child with mouthful of salt about to throw up: Can cause nausea and vomiting

29. Sewage river flowing through group of protestors: Can cause diarrhea

30. Protester with several lip piercings: Can cause perioral numbness

31. Protester wearing parka at beach: Can reverse the sensations of hot and cold

32. Father checking pulse of nauseous child laying down: Can cause bradycardia

33. ATV crashing into rock: Can cause atrioventricular (ATV) heart block

34. Deflating ATV tires: Can cause hypotension

35. Supportive man bringing water to beachgoers hit with salt by protestors: Treatment for ciguatoxin is supportive

AUTONOMICS IN PHARMACOLOGY

Autonomics | Section 1 - Adrenergic Receptors

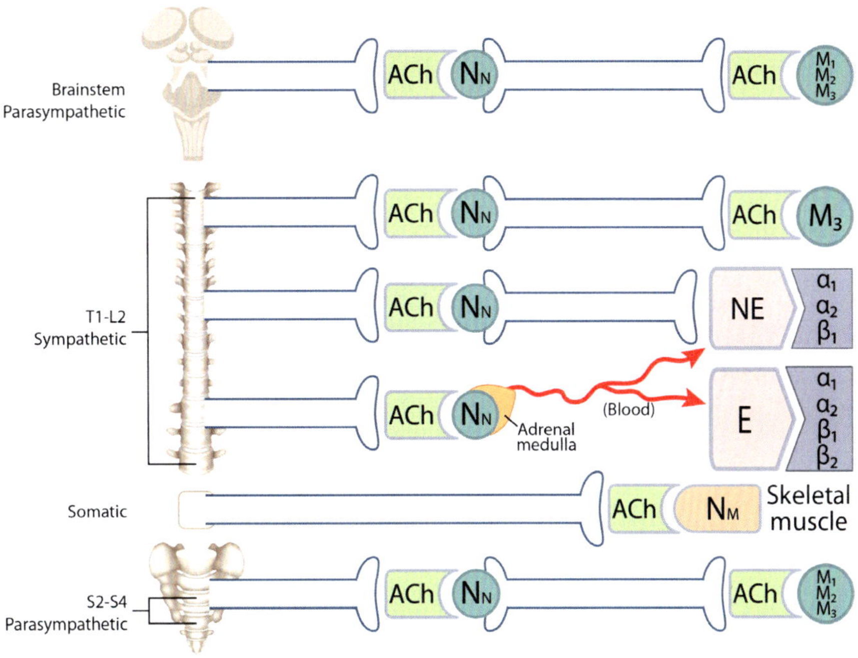

Figure 9.2.1 - Autonomic Nervous System Overview

Receptor	Actions
α_1	Mydriasis Vasoconstriction (↑ BP, ↑ VR to heart) Internal urethral sphincter contraction
α_2	↓ NE release (negative feedback) ↓ Aqueous humor production (↓ IOP) ↓ Lipolysis ↓ Insulin release ↑ Platelet aggregation
β_1	↑ Heart rate and contractility ↑ Renin release (RAAS) (↑ BP) ↑ Lipolysis
β_2	Vasodilation (skeletal muscles) Bronchodilation ↑ Aqueous humor production (↑ IOP) ↑ Insulin **release** ↑ Lipolysis
β_3	↑ Bladder capacity ↑ Thermogenesis ↑ Lipolysis

Table 9.2.1 - Adrenergic Receptors and Actions

G-Protein Pathway	Receptor and Ligand	Second Messenger
G-protein (G_q-alpha subunit)	- H_1 (histamine) - α_1 (Epinephrine, norepinephrine) - V_1 (ADH) - M_1 (acetylcholine) - M_3 (acetylcholine) - GnRH, TRH, Oxytocin, Angiotensin II, Gastrin	↑ IP_3 ↑ DAG
G-protein (G_s-alpha subunit)	- D_1 (dopamine) - H_2 (histamine) - V_2 (ADH) - β_1 (Epinephrine, norepinephrine, Dobutamine, isoproterenol) - β_2 (Epinephrine, Albuterol, isoproterenol) - LH, FSH, CRH, ADH, ACTH, PTH. hCG. MSH, GHRH, Glucagon, Calcitonin	↑ cAMP
G-protein (G_i-alpha subunit)	- M_2 (acetylcholine) - α_2 (Epinephrine, norepinephrine) - D_2 (dopamine)	↓ cAMP

Table 9.2.2 - G-Protein Pathway Overview

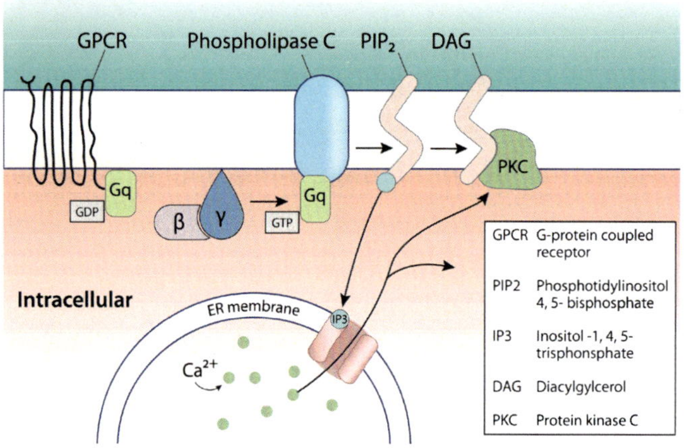

Figure 9.2.2 - G-Protein Coupled Receptor Mechanism

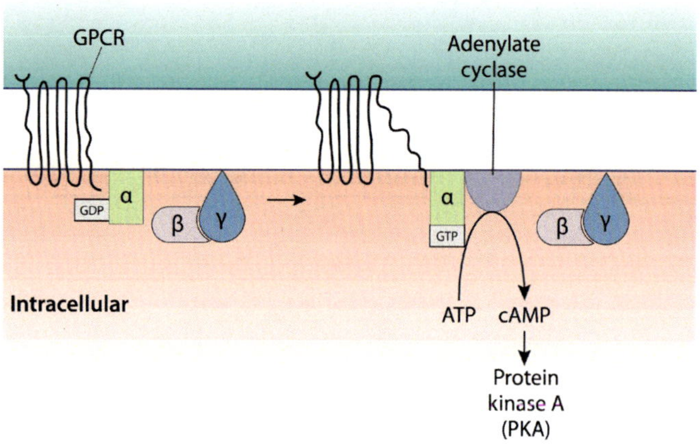

Figure 9.2.3 - Gi-Protein Coupled Receptor Mechanism

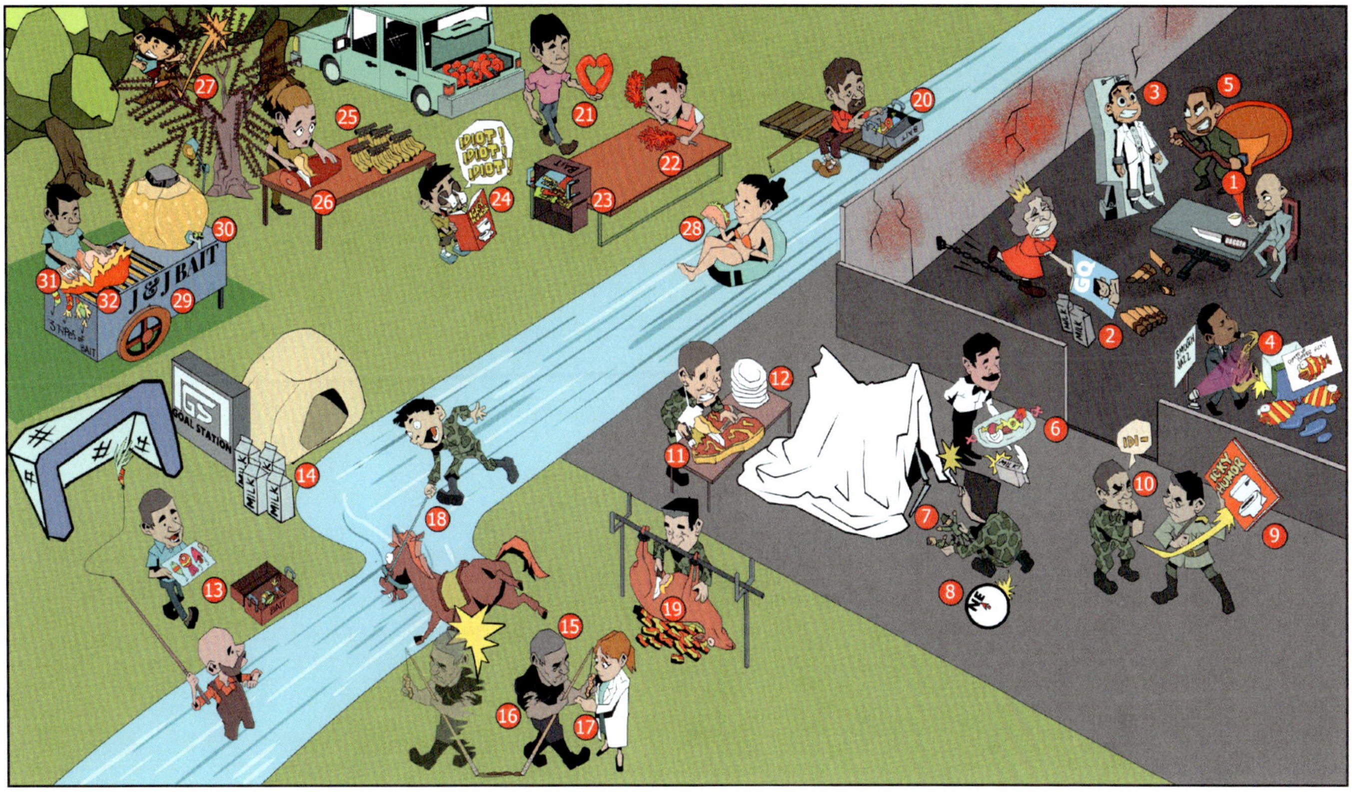

1. Evil villain drinking from teacup with single alpha-shaped handle: α_1 receptors

2. Queen of England reading GQ magazine after villain cut two of her pipes into three pieces with dagger and left them next to milk cartons: Gq protein class → phospholipase C activation → PIP_2 to Ip_3 + DAG → PKC → increased Ca^{2+}

3. Captured James Bond with wide eyes and large pupils while strapped to board: α_1 stimulation causes pupillary dilator muscle contraction → mydriasis (dilated pupils)

4. Smooth jazz musician next to deflated, constricted pufferfish with red stripes: α_1 stimulation causes vascular smooth muscle contraction → vasoconstriction

5. Villain's henchman squeezing shut hose leading from bladder-shaped tank, about to waterboard Bond: α_1 stimulation causes internal urethral sphincter muscle contraction

6. Butler holding tray with two alpha-shaped handles: α-1 receptors

7. Henchman dressed up as GI Joe taking down tent while butler knocks over carton of milk: Gi protein class → adenylate cyclase inhibition → decreased CAMP → decreased PKA → decreased Ca^{2+}

8. Broken compass pointing to northeast: α_1 stimulation decreases NE release (negative feedback)

9. Supervisor confiscating Icky Humor magazine from henchman: α_1 stimulation decreases aqueous humor production (decreased IOP)

10. Henchman inhibiting himself from saying an insult: α_1 stimulation decreases insulin release

11. Chef breaking his knife while trimming fat from meat: α_1 stimulation decreases lipolysis

12. Several plates stacked on top of each other: α_1 stimulation increases platelet aggregation

13. Man fishing with one piece of bait on fishing rod and bait box with two handles while other man offers him three varieties of extra bail: β_1, β_2, and β_3 receptors

14. Fisherman setting up tent and goal station box near milk cartons: Gs protein class → adenylate cyclase stimulation → increase CAMP → increased PKA → increased Ca^{2+}

15. Henchman fishing in relaxation area with one piece of bait on pole: β_1

16. Henchman contracting his bicep while trying to put one piece of bait on hook: β_1 stimulation increases contractility (positive inotropic)

17. Medical personnel checking pulse of pacing henchman with fishing rod: β_1 stimulation increases heart rate (positive chronotropic)

18. Horse bucking henchman off and upwards with reins in the air: β_1 stimulation increases renin

19. Henchman trimming fat off roasting deer: β_1 stimulation increases lipolysis

20. Fisherman with bait tackle box with two handles: β_2

21. Buff civilian doing balloon art and making red heart-shaped balloon: β_2 stimulation increases vasodilation in skeletal muscles and coronary arteries

22. Relaxed, sleeping cheerleader with lung-shaped pom poms: β_2 stimulation increases bronchodilation/ bronchial relaxation

23. Beta 2 tackle box containing Icky Humor magazine: β-2 stimulation increase aqueous humor production (increased IOP)

24. Kid saying "Idiot!" several times in a row: β_2 stimulation increases insulin release

25. Bunches of bananas: β_2 stimulation increases cellular K^+ uptake

26. Mom trimming fat off meat: β_2 stimulation increases lipolysis

27. Kid falling out of tree with glycogen-like branches β_2 activation stimulates glycogenolysis

28. Pregnant woman on tube eating taco: β_2 stimulation decreases uterine tone

29. "J&J Bait" booth: β_3

30. Distended bladder-shaped tank with yellow water on J&J Bait booth: β_3 stimulation causes relaxation of detrusor smooth muscle → increased bladder capacity

31. Bait salesman trimming fat off fish: β_3 stimulation increases lipolysis

32. Fish with exposed muscle catching fire while cooking: β_3 stimulation increases thermogenesis in skeletal muscle

See Figure 9.2.1 - Autonomic Nervous System Overview (Autonomic Pharmacology, Section 1, Page 28)

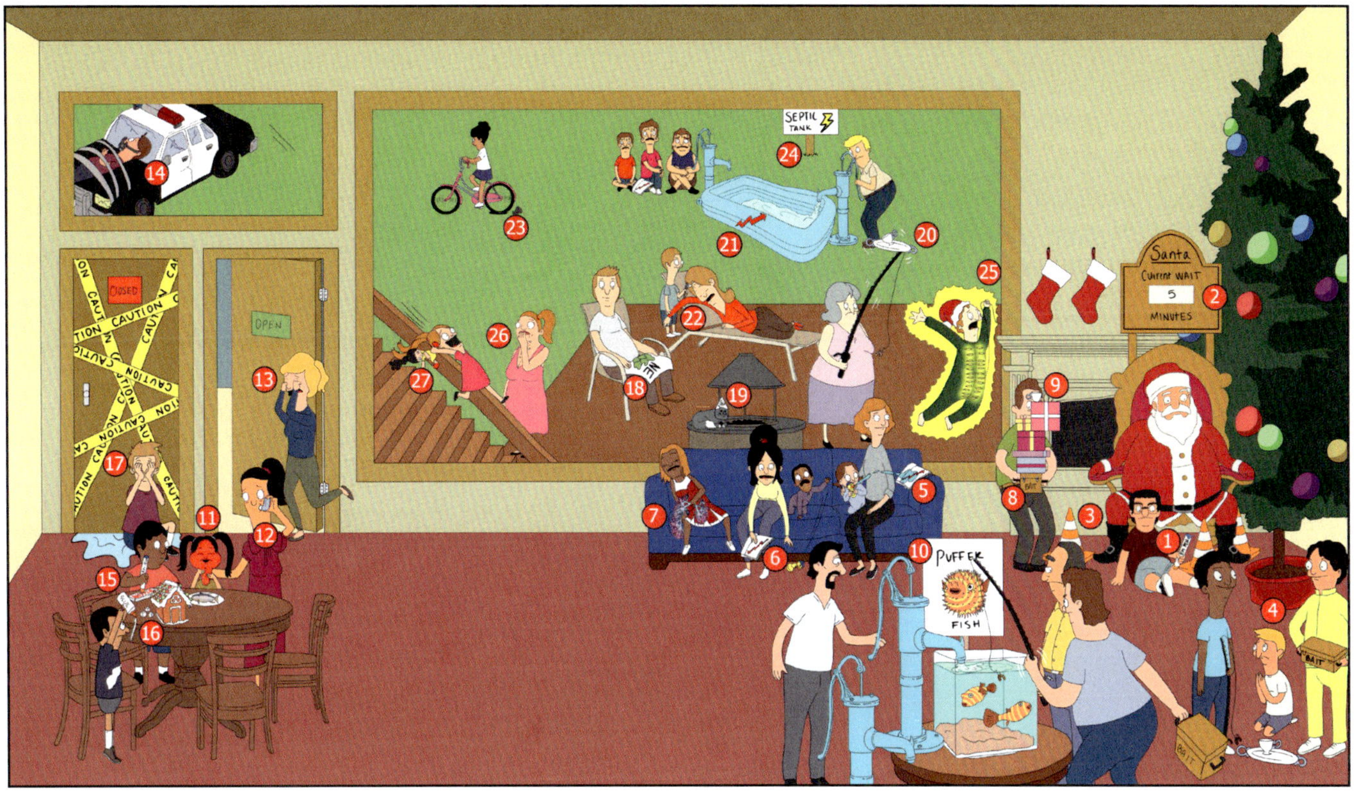

1. Kid with EpiPen in line to see Santa: Epinephrine

2. "Current wait 5 minutes: sign: Epinephrine has the shortest half-life of the catecholamines

3. Orange construction cones around Santa's chair: Produced by the adrenal medulla

4. Two boys with baited fishing pole and two-handled tackle box standing higher than boy with alpha-handle teacup and tray: Epinephrine's relative stimulation of adrenergic receptors at normal doses: β-1 = $\beta_2 > \alpha$

5. Baby actively squeezing water pump toy into magazine with increasing stock market graph: Epinephrine increases systolic blood pressure

6. Second baby refusing to use water pump toy next to magazine with decreasing stock market graph: Epinephrine decreases diastolic blood pressure

7. Sleeping cheerleader with bronchial-shaped pom poms: Epinephrine causes bronchodilation (bronchial relaxation)

8. Two-handled bait box at bottom of present stack: At low doses, β_2 effects predominate

9. Alpha-shaped teacup teetering at top of present stack: At high doses, α_1 effects predominate

10. Rude guest trying to catch constricted pufferfish from fish tank while other guests confiscate bait box and pole and refill tank from one of two water pumps: Epinephrine given with β blockers causes α_1 vasoconstriction to dominate diastole and systole → high systolic blood pressure and high diastolic pressure

11. Little girl at table struggling to breath with red, swollen neck: Use epinephrine for anaphylaxis

12. Little girl's mom panicking and using asthma inhaler: Use epinephrine for asthma

13. Woman squeezing eyes in pain from chili peppers while running towards open bathroom door: Use epinephrine for open-angle glaucoma

14. Rowdy guest being arrested and tied to hood of police car: Use for cardiac arrest

15. Kid trying to open Nestle chocolate bar wrapper with EpiPen: Epinephrine can enhance the anesthetic effect when injected alongside a local anesthetic

16. Kid with liver-shaped glue stain on shirt unable to reach sugar and glue placed high on table: Epinephrine can cause an elevation of plasma glucose due to an increased in hepatic glucose output

17. Kid squeezing eyes in pain while running towards closed bathroom door with caution tape: Epinephrine is contraindicated in closed-angle glaucoma

18. Compass pointing towards northeast: Norepinephrine (NE)

19. Mean cat playing with coal in triangular fire pit: Norepinephrine is a catecholamine and neurotransmitter produced in the adrenal medulla (and noradrenergic neurons)

20. Grandma balancing alpha-handle teacup on tray on top of baited fishing pole: $\alpha_1 > \alpha_2 > \beta_1$

21. Guests using one of two hand pumps to pump water into pool with upward stock market graph: Norepinephrine increases systolic and diastolic blood pressure

22. Kid checking sleeping mom's pulse and reflexes: Norepinephrine can cause reflex bradycardia

23. Deflated tire on new bike in backyard: Use norepinephrine for hypotension

24. "Septic tank" sign with lighting bolt: Use for septic shock (first line vasopressor in septic shock)

25. Guy in Christmas onesie with nerve-like pattern getting zapped: Use for neurogenic shock

26. Anxious mom biting nails while supervising daughter: Norepinephrine can cause anxiety

27. Daughter sliding down stair railing while holding doll with fluttering eyes: Norepinephrine can decreased REM sleep

Receptor	Actions
α_1	Mydriasis Vasoconstriction (↑ BP, ↑ VR to heart) Internal urethral sphincter contraction
α_2	↓ NE release (negative feedback) ↓ Aqueous humor production (↓ IOP) ↓ Lipolysis ↓ Insulin release ↑ Platelet aggregation
β_1	↑ Heart rate and contractility ↑ Renin release (RAAS) (↑ BP) ↑ Lipolysis
β_2	Vasodilation (skeletal muscles) Bronchodilation ↑ Aqueous humor production (↑ IOP) ↑ Insulin **release** ↑ Lipolysis
β_3	↑ Bladder capacity ↑ Thermogenesis ↑ Lipolysis

Table 9.2.1 - Adrenergic Receptors and Actions

See Figure 9.2.1 - Autonomic Nervous System Overview (Autonomic Pharmacology, Section 1, Page 28)

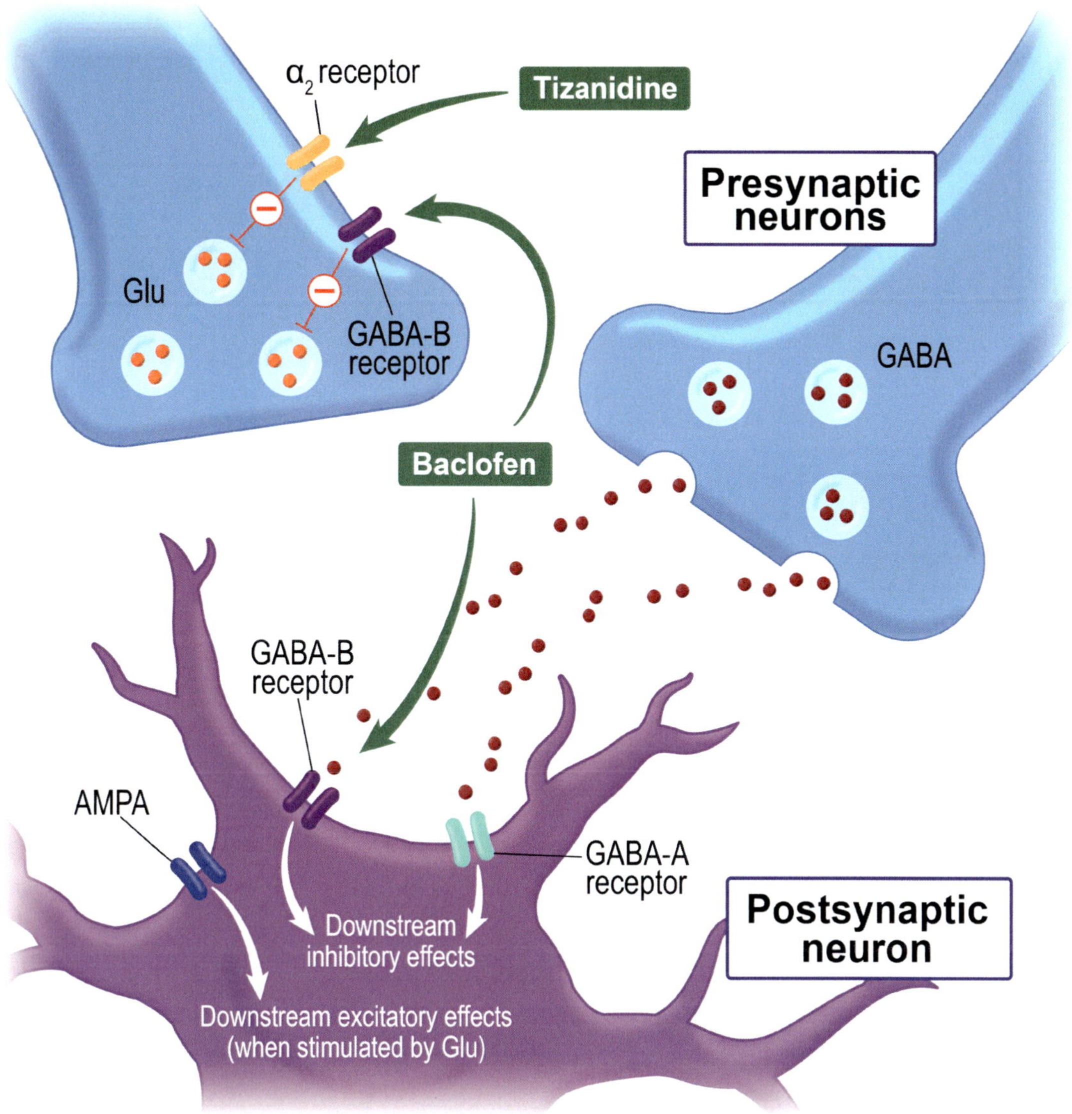

Figure 9.2.4 - Tizanidine and Baclofen Mechanism

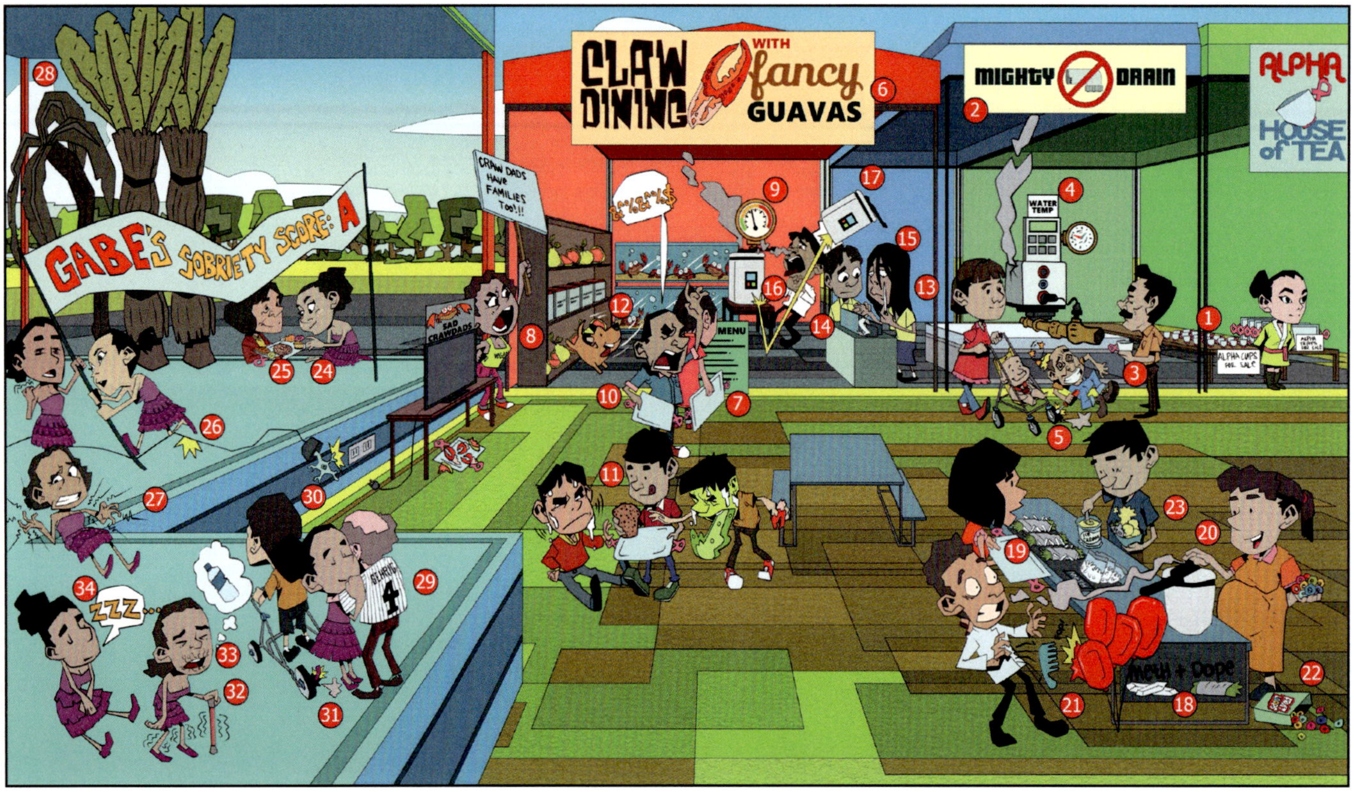

1. Teacups with single alpha-shaped handle: Alpha agonists

2. "Mighty Drain" plumbing booth: Midodrine

3. Alpha one teacup in front of Mighty Drain booth: α_1 agonist

4. Automatic Mighty Drain machine leaking and unable to control water flow: Use midodrine for autonomic insufficiency

5. Man getting dizzy after standing up and accidentally deflating stroller wheel: Use midodrine for postural hypotension

6. "Claw dining with fancy guavas" booth: Clonidine and guanfacine

7. Woman holding alpha two tray next to "claw dining with fancy guavas" booth: Clonidine and guanfacine are α_2 agonists

8. Vegan protester trying and failing to gain sympathy for her message: Clonidine and guanfacine are sympatholytic (inhibits sympathetic nervous system)

9. Pressure cooker with gauge in yellow zone, but not in red zone yet: Use clonidine and guanfacine for hypertensive urgency (not first line)

10. Teenager with twitching head and neck who is shouting profanities: Use clonidine and guanfacine for Tourette syndrome

11. Sweating, vomiting, and irritable kids after booth runs out of poppyseed muffins: Use clonidine and guanfacine for symptom control in opioid withdrawal

12. Overactive pup with short attention span running around booth: Use clonidine and guanfacine for attention-deficit hyperactivity disorder (ADHD)

13. Bored cashier falling asleep with head on table: Clonidine and guanfacine can cause CNS depression

14. Coworker taking pulse of sleeping cashier: Clonidine and guanfacine can cause bradycardia

15. Pin lying on table close to cashier's eye: Clonidine and guanfacine can cause miosis

16. Chef choking on claw with guava: Clonidine and guanfacine can cause respiratory depression

17. Pressure cooker bouncing upwards after being dropped on ground: Abrupt cessation of clonidine and guanfacine can cause rebound hypertension

18. "Meth + Dope" booth: α-methyldopa

Customer holding alpha two tray near drug booth: α_2 agonist

19. Pregnant woman making meth and dope in pressure cooker: Use α-methyldopa for hypertension in pregnancy

20. Patron accidentally popping RBC-like balloons with comb: α-methyldopa is a direct Coombs test positive (specifically a warm autoimmune hemolytic anemia)

21. Pregnant woman knocking over and spilling Froot Loops: α-methyldopa can cause drug-induced lupus

22. Spilled ice cream on man's chest: α-methyldopa can cause hyperprolactinemia

23. Dancers with tinsel outfits: Tizanidine

24. Piece of brain on alpha two tray with snacks: Tizanidine is an α_2 agonist that acts centrally

25. Dancer tripping over neuron-shaped unplugged cord while holding banner that reads "Gabe's sobriety score: A": Presynaptic α_2 stimulation → decreased excitatory neurotransmitter release (e.g. glutamate) → overall increase in GABA-A activity (overall inhibitory effect)

26. Dancer with muscle spasms in hands: Use tizanidine for relief of spasticity

27. Dying, unwrapped palm tree prop: Use tizanidine for multiple sclerosis

28. Lou Gehrig baseball uniform: Use tizanidine for ALS

29. Kid with cerebral palsy watching his sister dance: Use tizanidine for cerebral palsy

30. Deflated tire on kid's wheelchair: Tizanidine can cause hypotension

31. Weak dancer using cane to walk after tiring routine: Tizanidine can cause weakness

32. Thirsty dancer with dry mouth after tiring routine: Tizanidine can cause xerostomia

33. Dancer falling asleep after tiring routine: Tizanidine can cause sedation

See Figure 9.2.1 - Autonomic Nervous System Overview (Autonomic Pharmacology, Section 1, Page 28)

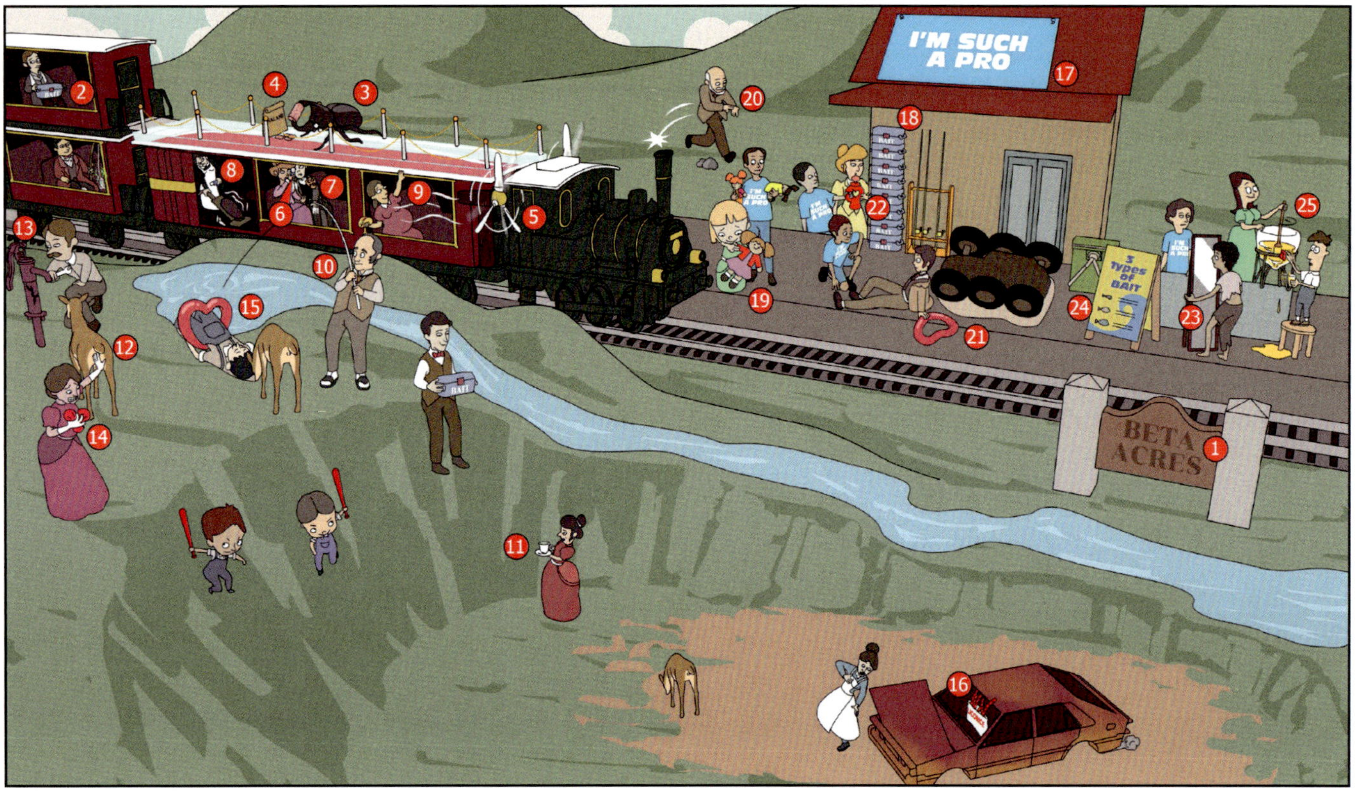

1. "Beta Acres" sign at train station: Beta agonists

2. Double-decker train car with guy in top compartment holding two-handled bait box and guy in bottom compartment holding fishing pole with bait already on it: $\beta_2 > \beta_1$ activity

3. Giant beetle on top of train: Albuterol

4. Beetle holding salami: Salmeterol

5. Wind turbine system powering train: Terbutaline

6. Lady using inhaler in shock after seeing giant beetle: Use albuterol, salmeterol and terbutaline for asthma

7. Lady's husband with Colorado Police Department (COPD) badge: Use albuterol, salmeterol and terbutaline for COPD

8. Vacuum with shaking airway tube: Use albuterol, salmeterol and terbutaline for bronchospasm

9. Pregnant woman holding taco: Use terbutaline as tocolysis (mainly used to delay preterm labor for up to 48 hrs)

10. Fisherman with rod at top of slope, son holding tackle box with two hands in middle of slope, and wife with alpha teacup at bottom of slope: $\beta_1 > \beta_2 > \alpha_1$ activity

11. Fisherman with rod at top of slope, son holding tackle box with two hands in middle of slope, and wife with alpha teacup at bottom of slope: $\beta_1 > \beta_2 > \alpha_1$ activity with dobutamine

12. Doe with butt facing towards fisherman's family: Dobutamine

13. Doe standing near pond with broken pump: Use dobutamine for heart failure

14. Mom squeezing heart-shaped stress ball and holding onto doe's butt while watching two toddlers playing with long red bats: Use dobutamine for cardiac stress testing

15. Doe rescuing unconscious, drowning camper with heart-shaped tube tied around his waist: Use dobutamine for cardiogenic shock

16. Lady startled by doe's butt grabbing her chest and leaning on car with clogged muffler and red licorice on dashboard: In patients with preexisting coronary artery disease, dobutamine can precipitate infarction or angina

17. "I'm such a pro" sign installed by station staff on roof of train station: Isoproterenol

18. Tackle bait boxes for rent stacked on platform up to height of fishing poles: $\beta_1 = \beta_2$ activity with isoproterenol

19. Girl checking doll's pulse with employee in "I'm such a pro" shirt helping her: Use isoproterenol for bradycardia

20. Old man skipping steps and running to catch train while checking his pulse: Use isoproterenol to evaluate tachyarrhythmias

21. Employee wearing “I’m such a pro” shirt helping man who crashed ATV: Use isoproterenol for heart block

22. Employee warning “I’m such a pro” shirt trying to help woman drink smoothie with clogged straw, buth accidentally making situation worse: Isoproterenol can worsen ischemia in coronary artery disease

23. Beggar trying to trade mirror for train ticket: Mirabegron

24. “3 types of bait” sign at kiosk: Selective β_3 receptor agonist

25. Kids spilling lemonade on ground and churning lemonade container too fast: Use mirabegron for urinary urge incontinence (overactive bladder)

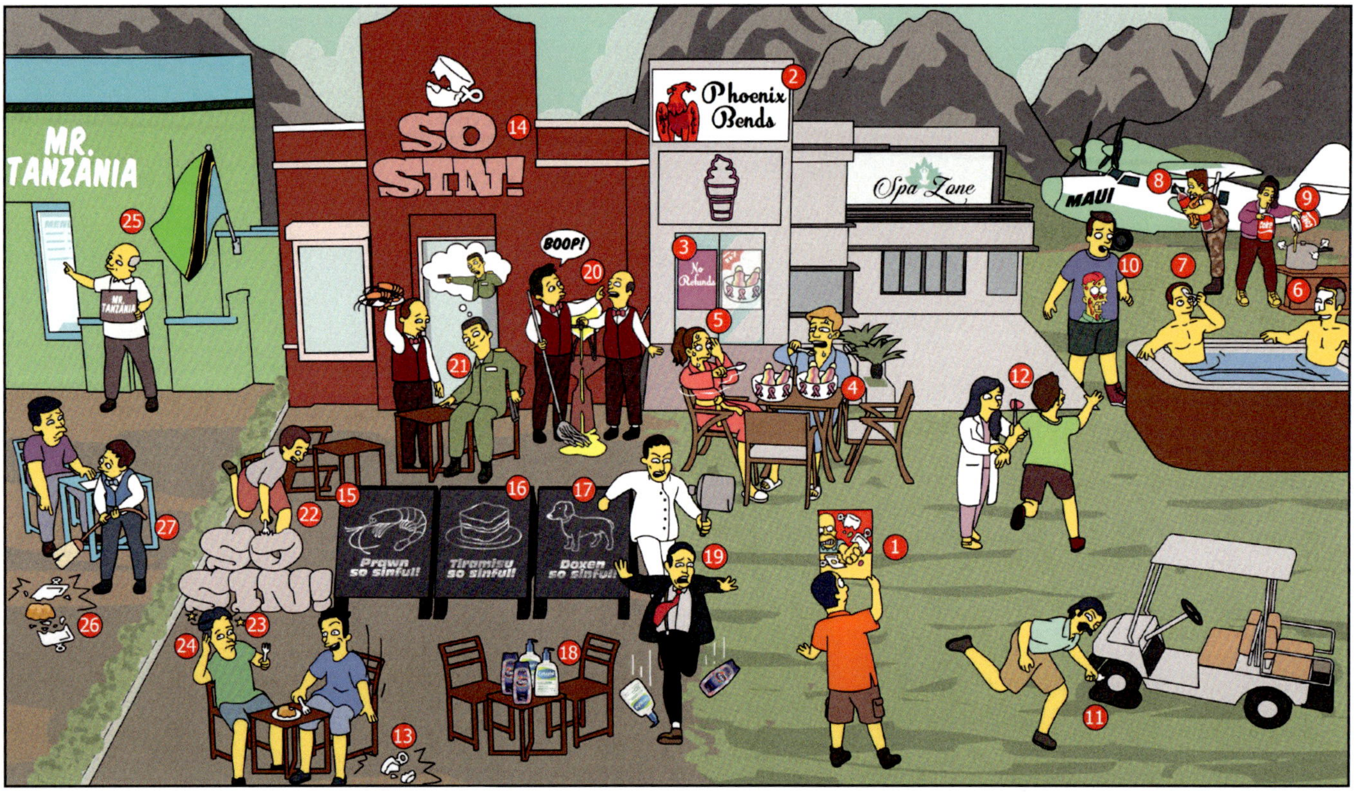

1. Man with weight loss brochure showing overweight man crushing teacup with one alpha-shaped handle and tray with two alpha-shaped handles: Nonselective alpha (α) blockers

2. "Phoenix Bends" health spa: Phenoxybenzamine

3. "No refunds" sign in Phoenix Bends window: Phenoxybenzamine is an irreversible competitive alpha blocker (nonselective)

4. Ice cream shaped like kidney and adrenal gland being served in cancer ribbon bowl: Use phenoxybenzamine preoperatively for pheochromocytoma surgery

5. Sweating, shaking lady with headache after eating ice cream: Phenoxybenzamine is used to prevent catecholamine crisis

6. Spa guest wearing half-face mud mask similar to mask in Phantom of Opera: Phentolamine

7. Other spa guest removing half-faced mud mask: Phentolamine is a reversible competitive alpha blocker (nonselective)

8. Tired marine loading wine and cheese onto MAUI charter plane with pressure cooker blasting steam in background: Use phentolamine for hypertensive crisis in patients on MAO inhibitors (MAUI) who ingest tyramine-containing food

9. Coke being poured onto pressure cooker and making pressure worse right next to spa with phantom-masked guests: Use phentolamine for severe cocaine-induced hypertension

10. Man with zombie shirt looking in direction of guests peeling off phantom masks: Use phentolamine to prevent tissue necrosis following NE extravasation

11. Dizzy guest after standing up too fast accidentally punctures golf cart tire: Phenoxybenzamine and phentolamine can cause orthostatic hypotension

12. Guy running away from physical therapist who is trying to check his pulse and reflexes with reflex hammer: Phenoxybenzamine and phentolamine can cause reflex tachycardia

13. Smashed teacup with single alpha-shaped handle on ground: α_1 selective blockers

14. "So Sin!" restaurant logo with broken alpha teacup: α1 blockers have an "osin" suffix

15. "Prawn so sinful!" poster outside restaurant: Prazosin

16. "Tiramisu so sinful!" poster outside restaurant" Terazosin

17. "Doxen so sinful!" poster outside restaurant: Doxazosin

18. Tums and lotion being sold outside restaurant: Tamsulosin

19. Vendor dropping Tums and lotion after being chased by pressure cooker chef: Use α_1 blockers for hypertension (except tamsulosin)

20. Waiter booping other waiter on nose while mopping up spilled lemonade: Use α_1 blockers to decrease urinary symptoms associated with BPH

21. Veteran being pulled out of flashback after being served prawn: Use prazosin for PTSD

22. Inflatable "So Sin!" logo being deflated by spa worker: α_1 blockers can cause orthostatic hypotension

23. Guest with spinning stars above head after hitting head on chair: α_1 blockers can cause dizziness

24. Dizzy guest holding head in pain: α1 blockers can cause headache

25. "Mr. Tanzania" restaurant: Mirtazapine

26. Angry customer shoving tray with two alpha-shaped handles off table and breaking it: Mirtazapine is a α_2 selective

27. Waiter using funny-looking, atypical broom to clean up tray and consoling depressed customer: Mirtazapine can be used as an atypical antidepressant

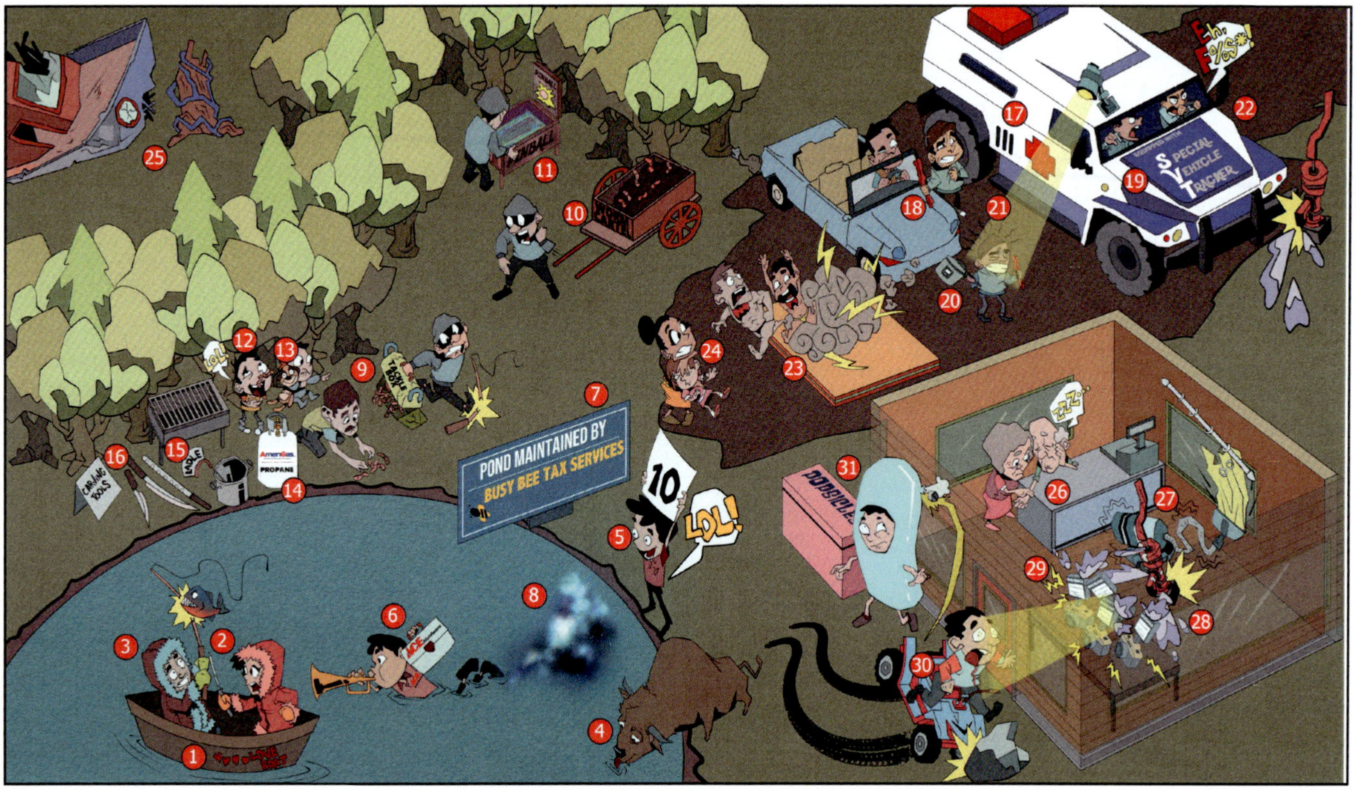

1. Hearts on fisherman's boat with fisherman holding rod with one piece of bait: β_1 selective blockers (cardioselective beta blockers)

2. Girlfriend in boat holding metal probe: Metoprolol is a beta1 selective blocker

3. Both fishers wearing Eskimo parkas: Esmolol is a beta1 selective blocker

4. Bison drinking water at edge of lake: Bisoprolol is a β_1 selective blocker

5. Tween holding up sign marked "10" and yelling "LOL" at sight of fisherman struggling: Atenolol is a β_1 selective blocker

6. ACE Hardware worker playing budgie: Acebutolol is a β_1 selective blocker

7. "Busy BEE TAX services" sign next to lake: Betaxolol is a β_1 selective blocker

8. ACE worker stirring up nebula of water: Nebivolol is a β_1 selective blocker

9. Robber stealing open two handled bait box while breaking fishing rod: Nonselective beta blockers (blocks β_1 and β_2 receptors)

10. Bait cartel transporting worms in cart: Carteolol is a nonselective beta blocker

11. Cartel member playing on pinball machine: Pindolol is a nonselective beta blocker

12. Kid laughing and yelling "LOL" while putting worms into nasal cavity: Nadolol is a nonselective beta blocker

13. Kid playing with Lion King Timon plush toy: Timolol is a nonselective beta blocker

14. Propane tank for cooking stove: Propranolol is a nonselective beta blocker

15. Ladle for stew: Labetalol is a nonselective beta blocker

16. Carving tools for meat: Carvedilol is a nonselective beta blocker

17. Heavily armored police car sent to catch cartel: Beta blockers can be used for hypertrophic cardiomyopathy

18. Peddler grabbing chest in fright while offering licorice to person in driver's seat of car with clogged tailpipe: Use beta blockers for acute coronary syndrome (unstable angina, NSTEMI, STEMI)

19. Kid scribbling over no parking sign with a ib ECG reading pattern in front of red car: Non-dihydropyridine CCBs can be used in atrial fibrillation and atrial flutter

20. Scared licorice peddler holding pressure cooker: Use beta blockers for hypertension in select situations

21. Licorice peddler holding head in pain from spotlight: Use beta blockers for migraine prophylaxis

22. Driver of armored vehicle saying "Eh F%S*!" after hitting water pump while passenger gives thumbs down in disapproval: Beta blockers reduce mortality in HFrEF (but never use in acute decompensated heart failure)

23. Male strippers wearing big red bow ties running away and kicking up a dirt storm: Use beta blockers for hyperthyroid storm

24. Mother covering girl's eyes at sight of strippers: Use beta blockers for glaucoma

25. Abandoned ship with broken porthole next to tree trunk with thick blue vines: Use nonselective beta blockers as prophylaxis for variceal bleeding in patients with portal hypertension

26. Grandma checking pulse of sleeping grandpa inside store: Beta blockers can cause bradycardia

27. Spasming vacuum in store: Beta blockers can cause bronchospasm

28. Vacuum breaking water pump and causing leak: Beta blockers can exacerbate heart failure

29. Broken Insignia-brand camera flashing spontaneously: Beta blockers can cause insomnia

30. Driver crashes ATV after being blinded by flash: Beta blockers can cause AV heart block

31. Guy wearing leaky, deflated popsicle costume: Beta blockers can cause erectile dysfunction

See Figure 9.2.1 - Autonomic Nervous System Overview (Autonomic Pharmacology, Section 1, Page 28)

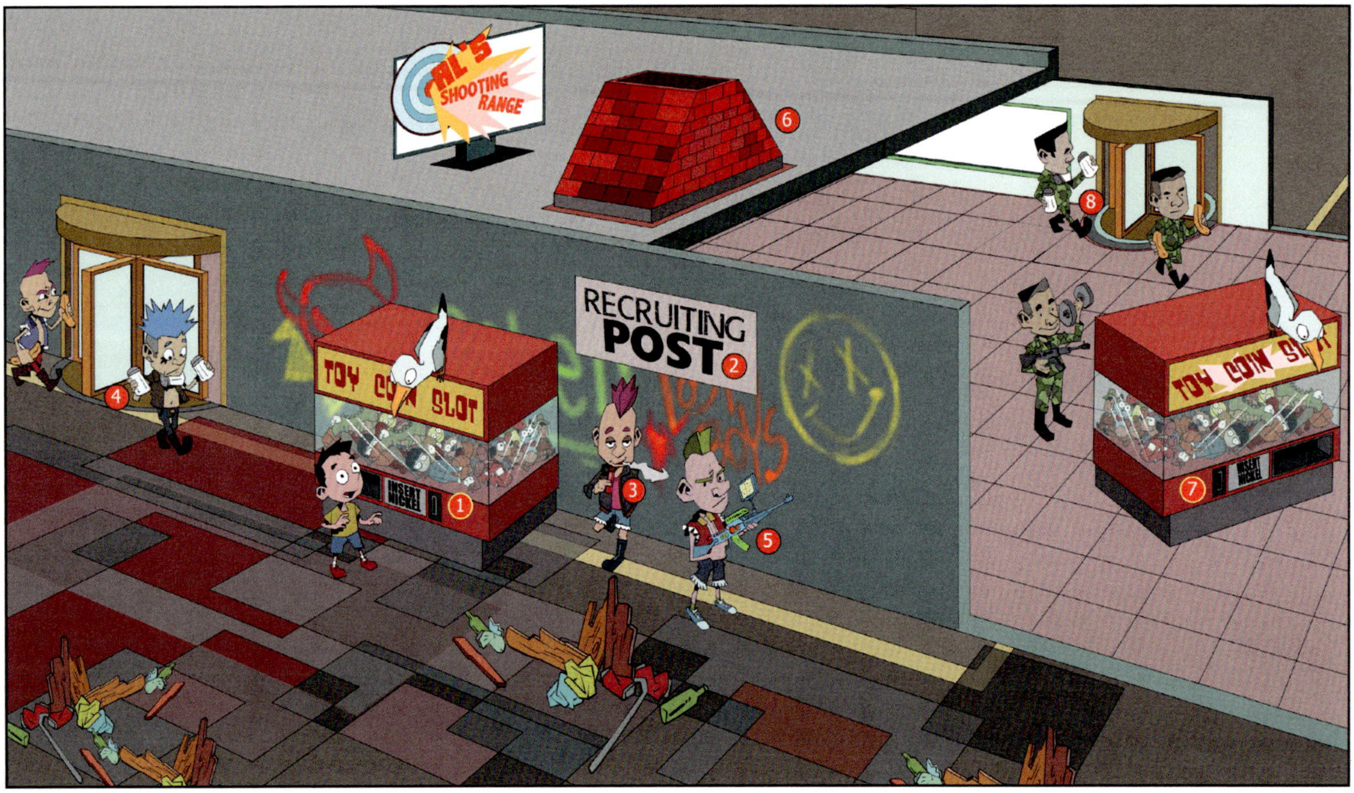

1. Seagull on top of claw machine with "insert nickel" sign: Autonomic nicotinic (Nn) ACh receptors

2. "Recruiting Post" sign next to claw machine: Nn receptors are on the postganglionic neurons

3. Teenager vaping near "Recruiting Post" sign: Activated by nicotine

4. Gang member going in through revolving door with 2 bananas and other gang member coming out through revolving door with 3 salt shakers: Autonomic nicotinic receptors are ligand-gated Na^+/K^+ channels (3 sodium exit in exchange for 2 potassium)

5. Gang member with automatic rifle standing near "Recruiting Post" sign: Found in autonomic ganglia (Nn)

6. Triangle-shaped chimney on top of building: Found in adrenal medulla (Nn)

7. Seagull on top of claw machine with "insert nickel" sign inside building while ROTC representative flexes muscles nearby: Nicotinic ACh receptors at the neuromuscular junction (Nm) of skeletal muscle

8. Second revolving door with existing soldier carrying 3 salt shakers and entering soldier holding 2 bananas: Nicotinic receptors at the neuromuscular junction of skeletal muscles and ligand-gated Na^+/K^+ channels (3 sodium exit in exchange for 2 potassium)

See Figure 9.2.1 - Autonomic Nervous System Overview (Autonomic Pharmacology, Section 1, Page 28)

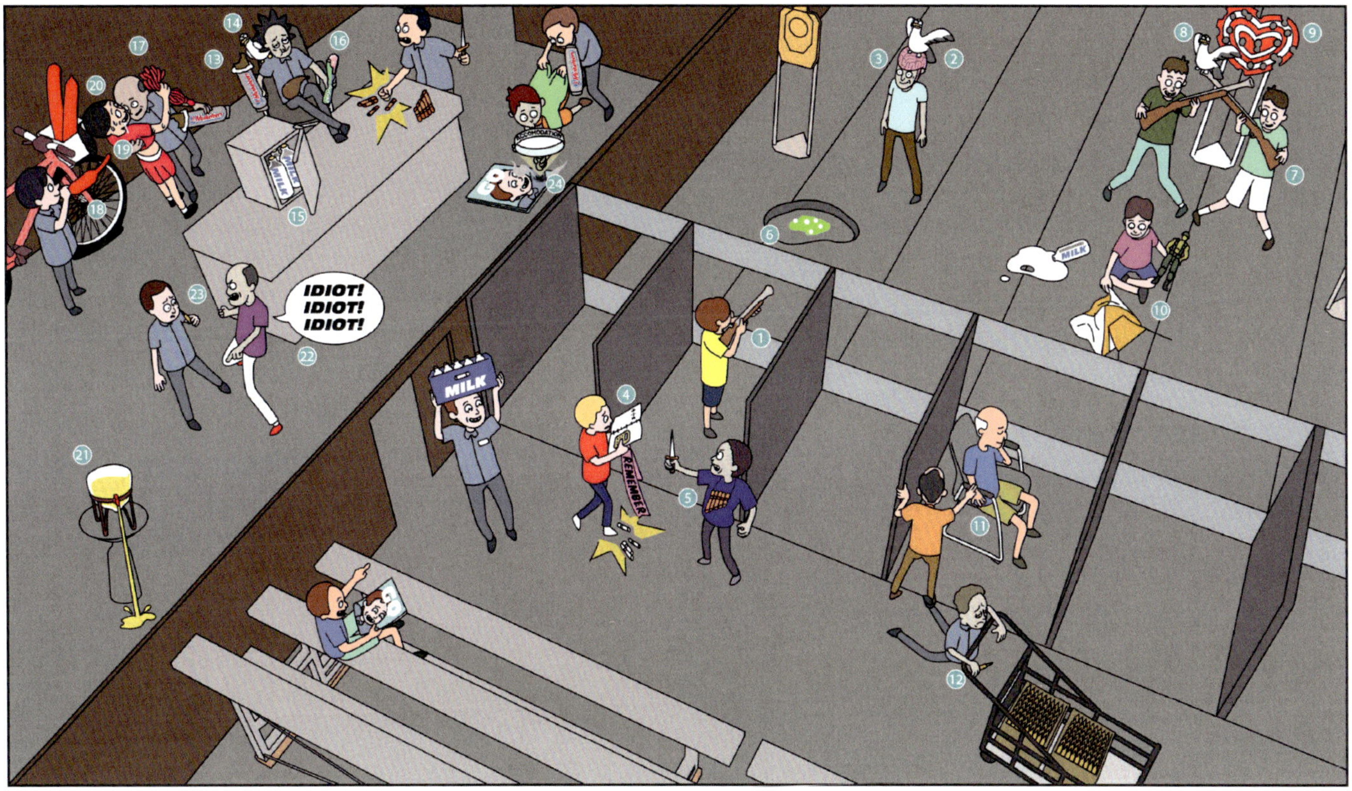

1. Kid shooting one musket at target: M_1 (muscarinic-1) receptor

2. Kid with musket shooting seagull on top of friend's head: Muscarinic receptors are stimulated by ACh

3. Kid's friend wearing helmet with brain pattern: M_1 receptors are in the brain

4. Score-keeper employee with "remember" sash, pad of paper and calculator: M_1 receptors mediate higher cognitive functions and memory formation

5. Observer with GQ magazine watching as score-keeper bumps into pipe player and breaks his pipes into three pieces, causing pipe player to take out dagger as refreshment worker arrives with milk: M_1 stimulation → Gq protein coupled → PIP_2 to IP_3+DAG → increased Ca^{2+}

6. Stomach-shaped pit in floor full of acid: M_1 stimulation increases gastric acid secretion

7. Two brother holding two muskets crossed in an X shape: M_2 (muscarinic 2) receptor

8. Seagull perched on two crossed muskets: M_2 receptors are also stimulate by ACh

9. Shot up, destroyed heart-shaped target behind two crossed muskets: M_2 receptors are on the heart

10. Son packing up campsite and tent for GI Joe figure next to spilled milk: M_2 stimulation → Gi protein coupled → decreased cAMP → decreased Ca^{2+}

11. Club member checking pulse of sleeping man: M_2 stimulation causes decreased heart rate

12. Exhausted employee slumped over bullet cart: M_2 stimulation causes decreased contractility

13. 3 Musketeers candy bar at reception desk: M_3 (muscarinic-3) receptor

14. Seagull trying to snatch 3 Musketeers bar: M_3 receptors are stimulated by ACh

15. Milk cartons and discarded GQ magazine near angry customer smashing his pipes into 3 pieces and pulling out a dagger: M_3 stimulation → Gq protein coupled → PIP_2 to IP_3+DAG → increased Ca^{2+}

16. Employee at reception desk squeezing Go-Gurt tube: M_3 stimulation causes gut peristalsis

17. Cheerleader squeezing lung-shaped pom poms: M_3 stimulation causes bronchoconstriction

18. Cheerleader's bike with deflated tire and long, red balloons in basket: M_3 stimulation causes vasodilation and hypotension

19. Salivating cheerleader looking at 3 Musketeers bar: M_3 stimulation causes salivary secretions

20. Cheerleader sweating while looking at 3 Musketeers bar: M_3 stimulation causes increased sweat production (sympathetic nervous system)

21. Lemonade spilling from bladder-shaped dispenser: M_3 stimulation causes urine voiding (detrusor muscle contraction

22. Customer yelling "Idiot!" at range employee: M_3 stimulation causes insulin release

23. Employee gesturing towards his eye with pin in his hand: M_3 stimulation causes contraction of pupillary sphincter muscle (miosis)

24. Kid with magnifying glass burning GQ magazine while employee with 3 Musketeers bar tries to stop him: M_3 stimulation causes accommodation (near focus via ciliary muscle contraction)

Receptor	Actions
M_1	CNS (higher cognitive functions) ↑ Gastric acid
M_2	↓ HR ↓ Contractility
M_3	Miosis Lens accommodation Bronchoconstriction Vasodilation (decreased BP) Salivation and lacrimation Peristalsis Bladder contraction Sweating (sympathetic) Insulin release

Table 9.2.3 - Muscarinic Receptors and Actions

See Figure 9.2.1 - Autonomic Nervous System Overview (Autonomic Pharmacology, Section 1, Page 28)

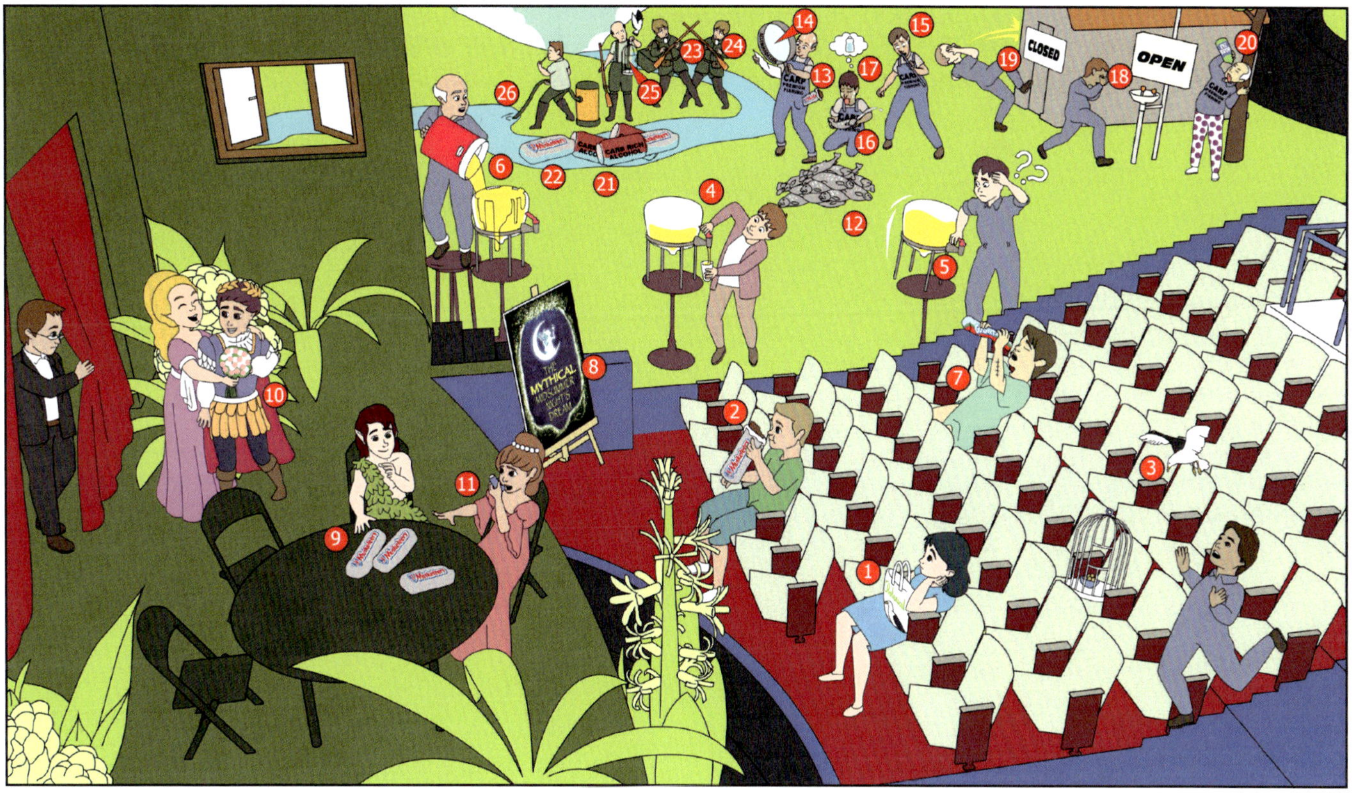

1. Lady with seagull purse watching play in botanical setting: Bethanechol

2. Audience member eating 3 Musketeers candy bar: Direct M_3 agonist

3. Theatre worker unable to trap bothersome seagull in cage: Bethanechol is resistant to AChE

4. Audience member getting lemonade out of bladder-shaped dispenser: Bethanechol causes detrusor muscle contraction

5. Broken lemonade dispenser with no visible obstruction in it: Use bethanechol for non-obstructive urinary retention

6. Overflowing lemonade dispenser: Use bethanechol for overflow incontinence

7. Patient fresh out of surgery squeezing Go-Gurt tube with nothing coming out even though there's no obstruction: Use bethanechol for postoperative and neurogenic ileus (i.e. non-obstructive ileus)

8. Mythical play: Methacholine

9. 3 Musketeers bars on stage: Methacholine stimulates M_3 receptors

10. Character with pom-pom bouquet of flowers squeezing actor very tightly: Causes bronchoconstriction via M_3 receptor stimulation

11. Critic judging nervous actress who is using inhaler: Use methacholine to diagnose asthma ("methacholine challenge")

12. Pile of carp next to river by theatre: Pilocarpine

13. Fisherman eating 3 Musketeers bar: Pilocarpine is a direct M_3 agonist

14. Fisherman using magnifying lens to read list of carp orders: Pilocarpine contracts the ciliary muscle (lens accommodation)

15. Fisherman holding pin up to eye: Pilocarpine contracts the pupillary sphincter muscle → miosis ("pinpoint pupil")

16. Crying, sweating fisherman near carp pile while water dribbles out of carp's mouth: Pilocarpine stimulates production of tears, sweat and saliva

17. Dehydrated fisherman with cracked, dry tongue dreaming of water: Use pilocarpine for xerostomia

18. Groundskeeper pressing fingers into eyes and running towards eyewash station with "open" sign: Use pilocarpine for open-angle glaucoma

19. Groundskeeper squeezing eyes after running into shed with "closed" sign: Use pilocarpine for closed-angle glaucoma

20. Fisherman with eye drops, dry mouth, and purple polka dot pants: Use pilocarpine for Sjögren's syndrome

21. "Carb rich alcohol" beer cans floating down river: Carbachol

22. 3 Musketeers bar wrappers floating down river: Carbachol binds to M_3 receptors

23. One hunter holding single musket next to two other hunters who are crossing muskets in "X" shape: Carbachol also stimulates M_1 and M_2 receptors

24. Hunters with crossed muskets vaping: Carbachol also stimulates nicotinic receptors (NN and NM)

25. Seagull inside cage while beer cans remain in river next to twin hunters: Carbachol is a "carbon copy" of acetylcholine but is resistant to AChE, unlike ACh

26. Worker using vacuum cleaner to relive pressure from trash in river and holding pin to eye: Use carbachol to constrict pupil (miosis) → relieves intraocular pressure in open-angle glaucoma

See Figure 9.2.1 - Autonomic Nervous System Overview (Autonomic Pharmacology, Section 1, Page 28)

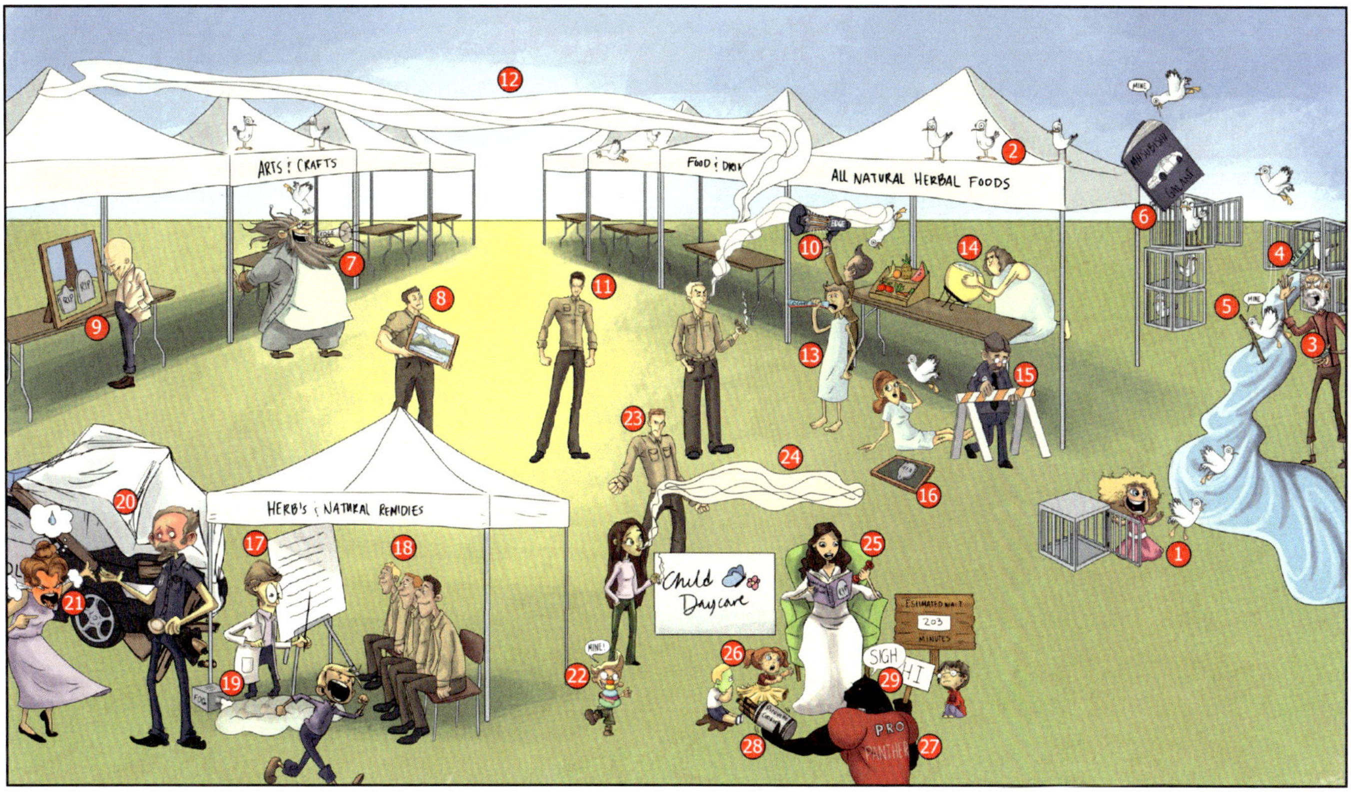

1. Girl opening seagull cage to release seagulls: Acetylcholinesterase inhibitors

2. Seagulls overrunning farmer's market: All cause an increase in acetylcholine (ACh)

3. Grumpy, confused old man yelling at Pez candy: Use as first line treatment for Alzheimer's disease

4. Old man done with Pez dispenser: Donepezil

5. Seagull carrying stick across river while squawking "mine" and freezing second seagull from cage: Rivastigmine

6. Seagull carrying Mitsubishi magazine with Galant car on cover and dropping magazine while squawking "mine": Galantamine

7. Megaphone with "EDGE" written on it: Edrophonium

8. Four charged-up US marines standing in center of market: Edrophonium is a quaternary amine (charged and hydrophilic)

9. Vendor with magnifying glass inspecting his gravestone paints: Use edrophonium to diagnose myasthenia gravis

10. "EDGE" megaphone with neon light: Neostigmine

11. Four charged-up US marines standing in center of market: Quaternary amine (i.e. charged and hydrophilic)

12. Marine puffing cloud of smoke far above everyone's heads: No CNS penetration with neostigmine or edrophonium

13. Hospital patient fresh out of surger unable to squeeze out Go-Gurt even though tube is not obstructed: Use for postoperative and neurogenic ileus

14. Broken lemonade dispenser with no visible obstruction in it: Use for postoperative urinary retention

15. Policeman removing blockade around unconscious lady in hospital gown: Use for postoperative reversal of neuromuscular junction blockade

16. Gravestone painting lying next to unconscious lady in hospital gown: Use for myasthenia gravis

17. Vendor dressed like physician selling natural remedies and holding stick: Physostigmine

18. Three US marines listening to "physician": tertiary amine (neutral)

19. "Physician" penetrating cloud from fog machine: Freely crosses blood brain barrier to penetrate CNS

20. State trooper crashing into booth near herbal vendor's booth: Use an antidote for atropine overdose

21. Vendor at destroyed booth is hot as a hare, red as a beet, dry as a bone, and mad as a hatter: Use to reverse anticholinergic toxicity

22. Toddler playing with pyramid toys while saying "mine": Pyridostigmine

23. Four charged-up US marines standing in center of market: Quatemary amine (i.e. charged and hydrophilic)

24. Parent in daycare area blowing cloud of smoke upward: No CNS penetration with pyridostigmine

25. Teacher lifting weights while reading "The Graveyard Book" to little kids: Use pyridostigmine for myasthenia gravis to increase muscle strength

26. Sick kids disgusted by storybook experiencing rash, abdominal pain, nausea, and sweating: Pyridostigmine can cause itchy rash, sweating nausea, diarrhea, and abdominal pain

27. "Pro Panther" mascot visiting daycare: Use propantheline to control pyridostigmine side effects

28. Pro panther handing out pirouette cookies to kids: Use glycopyrrolate to control pyridostigmine side effects

29. Panther sighing in exhaustion while holding "Hi" sign" Use hyoscyamine to control pyridostigmine side effects

See Table 9.2.3 - Muscarinic Receptors and Actions (Autonomic Pharmacology, Section 8, Page 45)
See Figure 9.2.1 - Autonomic Nervous System Overview (Autonomic Pharmacology, Section 1, Page 28)

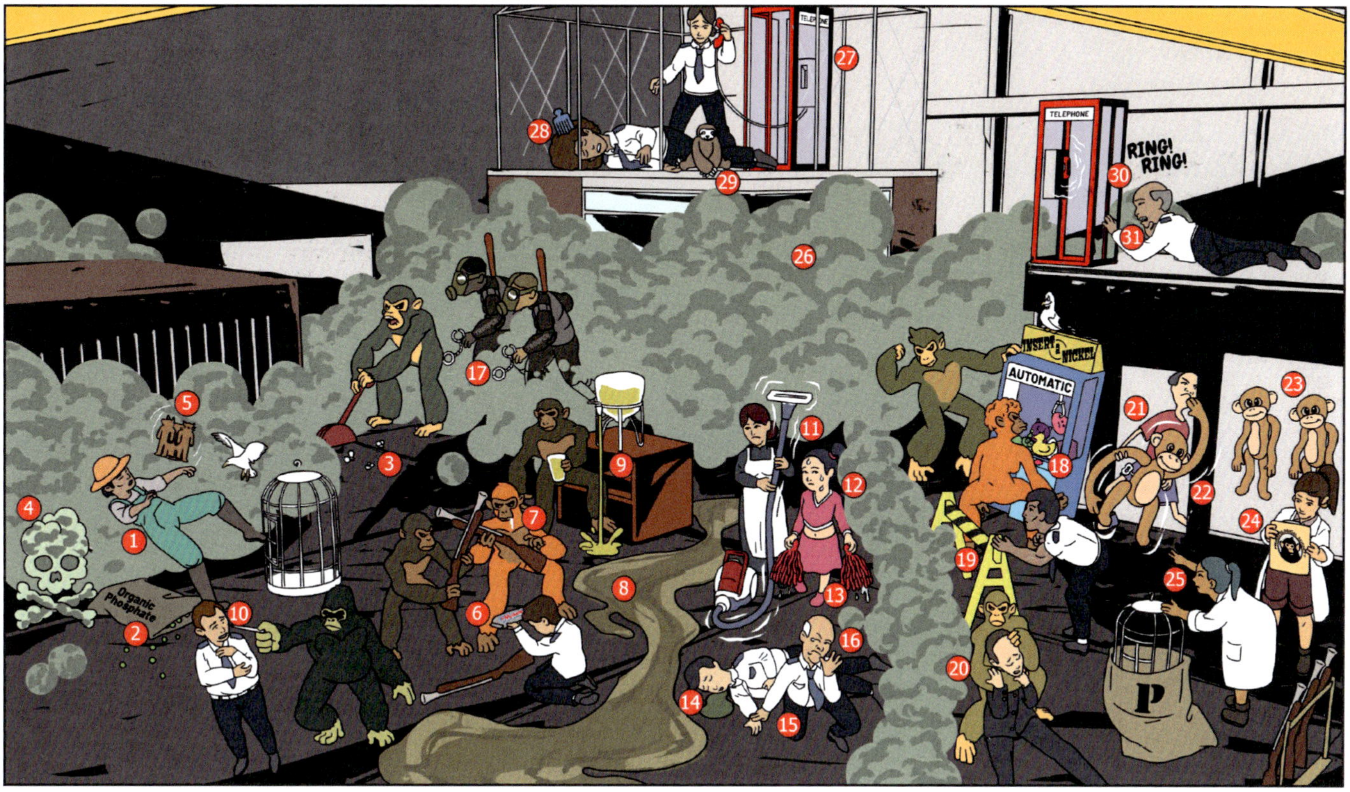

1. Ape pushing lever to release seagull from cage while guard is knocked out by gas: Anticholinesterase poisoning (i.e. AChE inhibitor poisoning) leads to increased ACh activity

2. Guard tripping over "Organic Phosphate" bag after inhaling gas: Organophosphates

3. Dead bugs killed by gas: Organophosphates are commonly used as insecticides

4. Toxic gas cloud next to farmer: Organophosphate poisoning is usually seen in farmers

5. Wooden "mate" carving of two people holding hands: Organophosphates are carbamate agents

6. Two apes holding two muskets crossed with man offering them his single musket and his 3 Musketeers bar: Anticholinesterase poisoning → higher ACh activity → increased muscarinic receptor stimulation

7. Ape salivating at sight of 3 Musketeers bar: Can cause salivation

8. Muddy brown river leaking from sewer: Can cause diarrhea

9. Leaking lemonade dispenser shaped like bladder: Can cause urination

10. Gorilla holding pin he used to escape from cage up to guard's eye: Can cause miosis

11. Cleaning lady's vacuum sucking in air: Can cause bronchospasm

12. Cleaning lady's scared daughter sweating in fear: Can cause sweating

13. Daughter holding pom poms that are getting sweaty and wet: Can cause bronchorrhea

14. Guard who threw up and fated lying on floor: Can cause emesis

15. Second guard checking pulse of fainted guard: Can cause bradycardia

16. Guard with watering eyes due to smell of vomit: Can cause lacrimation

17. State troopers cleaning up mess caused by apes: Reverse muscarinic effects with atropine which blocks muscarinic receptors

18. Seagull perched on claw machine with "insert nickel" sign: Anticholinesterase poisoning can cause nicotinic effects at autonomic ganglia (Nn) and the NMJ in skeletal muscle (Nm)

19. Officer setting up blockade to trap apes: Causes neuromuscular blockade (Similar to succinylcholine)

20. Ape choking lobby attendant until he passes out: Can cause respiratory arrest

21. Man struggling to pick up blow-up ape doll: Can cause muscle weaknessvv

22. Weak man visibly shaking: Can cause fasciculations

23. Limp, deflated blow-up ape dolls: Can cause flaccid paralysis

24. Primatologist taking notes: Reverse nicotinic effects with pralidoxime

25. Primatologist bribing apes with nickels for claw machine while locking seagull in cage: If given early, pralidoxime regenerates AChE → lower ACh → decreased muscarinic and nicotinic stimulation

26. Gas cloud that primatologists can't cross being released by ape pulling lever: Pralidoxime is a quaternary amine → does not readily cross BBB

27. Guard booth high up above gas cloud: Anticholinesterase poisoning can cause CNS effects

28. Guard passed out due to gas with comb in hair: Can cause coma

29. Stuffed toy sloth next unconscious guard: Can cause lethargy

30. Ringing phone next to incapacitated guard: Can cause seizures

31. Guard coughing and choking while trying to answer phone: Can cause central respiratory depression

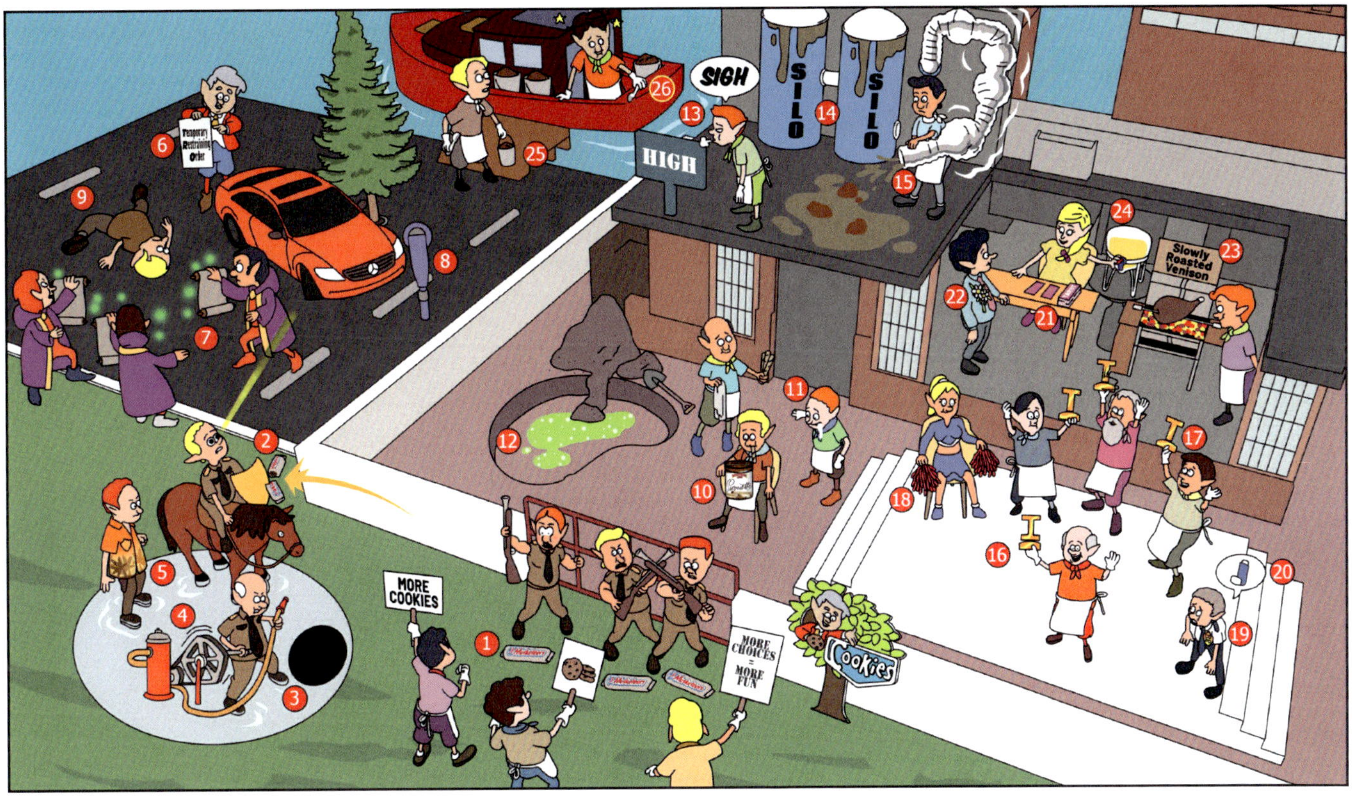

1. Elves protesting factory with one single musket plus a pair of crossed muskets while 3 Musketeers bars lie on ground: Muscarinic agents

2. Trooper staring into sky after blocking 3 Musketeers bar with shield: Blocking M_3 prevents accommodation (cycloplegia → patients can focus on distant objects but not near objects)

3. Trooper standing in eyeball-shaped puddle: Atropine (ophthalmic solutions)

4. Trooper charging wheel-powered water hose in cyclic motion: Cyclopentolate (ophthalmic solutions)

5. State trooper dressed in Hawaiian shirt: Tropicamide (ophthalmic solution)

6. Factory owner with "Temporary Restraining Order" (TRO) against protestors parking Benz next to pine tree; Benztropine

7. Three wizards practicing hex spells: Trihexphenidyl

8. Parking meter in front of owner's car: Use benztropine and trihexyphenidyl for Parkinson's disease

9. Protestor contoured by wizards' hex: Use benztropine and trihexyphenidyl for acute dystonia

10. Factory worker eating pirouette cookies: Glycopyrrolate

11. Drooling elf staring longingly at pirouette cookies: Use glycopyrrolate to reduce airway secretions and salivation

12. Stomach-shaped acid hole in factory floor: Use glycopyrrolate for peptic ulcers by decreasing gastric secretions

13. Sighing elf on roof next to "High" sign: Hyoscyamine

14. Two silos storing chocolate on roof: Dicyclomine

15. Guy shaking spazzing colon-like tube that is spewing chocolate chunks at irregular intervals: Use hyoscyamine and dicyclomine as antispasmodics for irritable bowel syndrome

16. "I trophy" shaped like I for employee receiving award: Ipratropium

17. Two "T trophies" shaped like T for employees receiving awards: Tiotropium

18. Relaxing cheerleader with lung-shaped pom poms: Ipratropium and tiotropium cause bronchorelaxation/dilation

19. Colorado Police Department (COPD) called to regulate protest: Use ipratropium and tiotropium for COPD

20. COPD officer in need of inhaler: Use ipratropium and tiotropium for asthma

Abnormally tall tarot cards: Tolterodine

21. Elf getting tarot cards read while wearing oxeye boutonniere: Oxybutynin

22. Slow-roasted venison in cafeteria: Solifenacin

23. Guy closing spigot of bladder-shaped lemonade container: Use tolterodine, oxybutynin, and solifenacin for overactive bladder

24. Factory worker putting ice cream scoops onto delivery boat: Scopolamine

25. Motion sick boat worker smelling ice cream to feel better: Use scopolamine for motion sickness

See Figure 9.2.1 - Autonomic Nervous System Overview (Autonomic Pharmacology, Section 1, Page 28)

Receptor	Actions
M_1	CNS (higher cognitive functions) ↑ Gastric acid
M_2	↓ HR ↓ Contractility
M_3	Miosis Lens accommodation Bronchoconstriction Vasodilation (decreased BP) Salivation and lacrimation Peristalsis Bladder contraction Sweating (sympathetic) Insulin release

Table 9.2.4 - Muscarinic Receptors and Actions

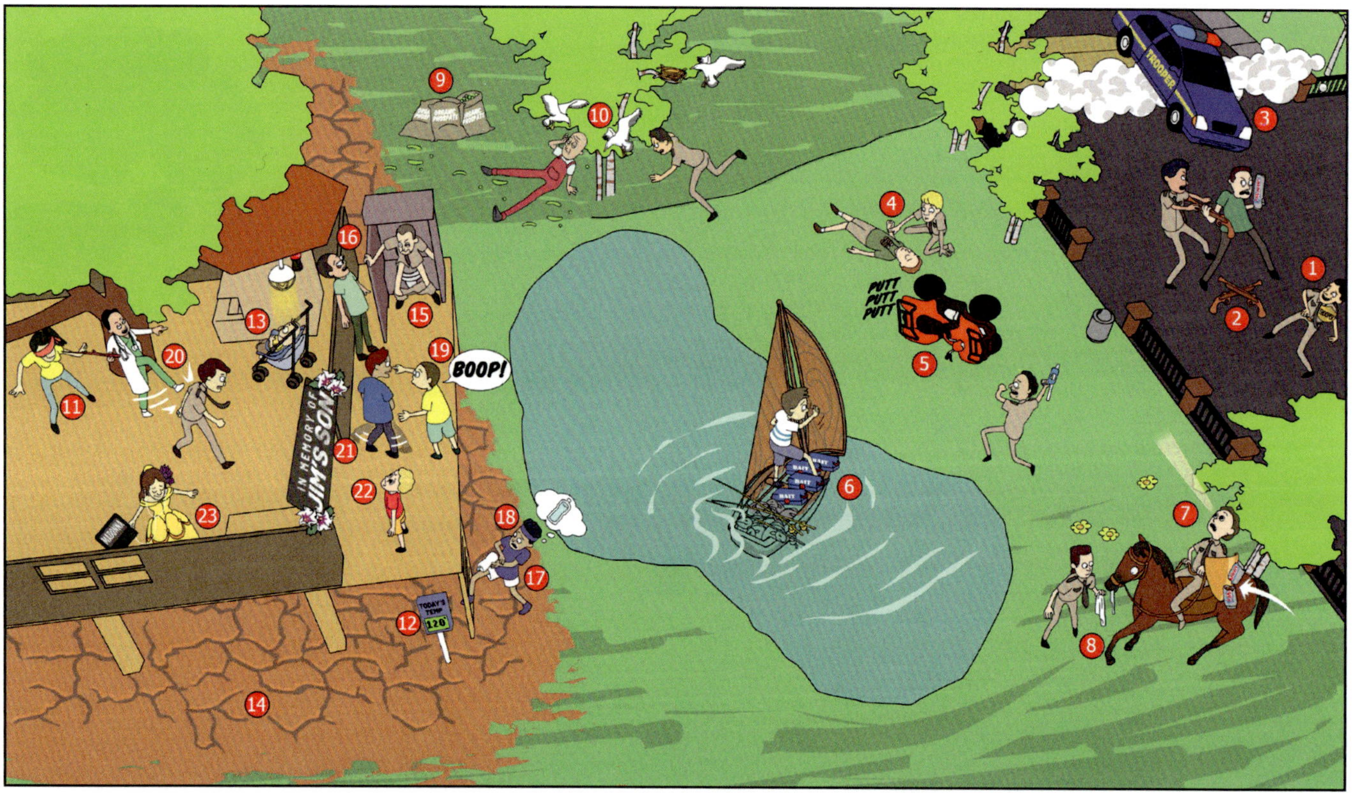

1. State trooper in statek park: Atropine

2. Hooligan holding single musket and 3 Musketeers bar with two crossed musketeers on ground nearby: Atropine is a muscarinic antagonist (M_1-M_3)

3. Trooper vehicle crossing through the cloud layer: Atropine can cross the blood-brain barrier (BBB)

4. Trooper checking pulse of sleeping bird watcher: Use atropine for bradycardia

5. ATV breaking down: Use atropine for AV block

6. Trooper trying to rescue sinking boat containing fishing poles, bait boxes, and sailing man by using glue gun: Use atropine to reverse β blocker overdose (along with saline and glucagon)

7. Dazed trooper on horseback blocking 3 Musketeers bar with shield: Atropine blocks M_3 receptors on the ciliary muscle → lens flattens to view distant objects

8. Other trooper wiping up horse drool: Use atropine to decrease salivation (e.g. during surgery)

9. "Organic Phosphate" pea bags on ground near disoriented groundskeepers: Use atropine to reverse organophosphate (anticholinesterase) poisoning (i.e. poisoning from high ACh activity)

10. Trooper shooing seagulls away from groundskeeper: Use atropine to reverse effects of AChE inhibitors

11. Blindfolded woman walking around treehouse in no particular direction: Atropine can cause disorientation

12. Thermometer next to treehouse with "high temperature" sign: Atropine can cause increased body temperature (due to decreased sweating)

13. Baby left under heat lamp: Atropine can cause hyperthermia in infants

14. Dry, cracked ground below treehouse: Atropine can cause dry, scaly, and flushed skin

15. Constipated trooper occupying restroom: Atropine can cause constipation

16. Shocked tourist with large, bulging eyes after walking in on trooper in restroom: Atropine can cause mydriasis → increased IOP (increased risk of closed-angle glaucoma)

17. Fitness nut checking pulse while running: Atropine can increase heart rate

18. Fitness nut with dry, cracked mouth thinking of water bottle: Atropine can cause dry mouth

19. Man holding in urge to urinate while being booped on nose by kid: Atropine can cause urinary retention (esp. in men with benign prostatic hyperplasia)

20. Physician chasing trooper with stick to make trooper undo mistakes in state park management: Reverse atropine overdose by inhibiting AChE (i.e. increased ACh activity) using physostigmine

21. "In memory of Jim's Son" banner: Jimsonweed (Datura Stramonium) produces effects similar to atropine

22. Kid with dilated pupils staring at banner: Jimsonweed is often called "Gardener's pupil" because it causes mydriasis

23. Girl dressed as Belle listening to Madonna with flower in hair: Belladonna flower (Atropa belladonna; deadly nightshade) produces effects similar to atropine

Receptor	Actions
D_1	- Dilates renal vascular smooth muscle → maintains renal perfusion - Activates the direct pathway of the striatum
D_2	- Inhibits the indirect pathway of the striatum (i.e. indirectly activates striatum) - Located in the chemoreceptor trigger zone (CTZ) of the area postrema → induces vomiting
H_1	- ↑ nasal mucus production - ↑ bronchial mucus production - ↑ vascular permeability → hypotension and edema - Bronchoconstriction - Activates peripheral nocireceptors → pain
H_2	- Stimulates gastric acid production
V_1	- ↑ contraction of vascular smooth muscle
V_2	- ↑ H_2O reabsorption by increasing aquaporin-2 channels in the collecting tubules - ↑ vWF release

Table 9.2.5 - Dopamine, Histamine, and Vasopressin Receptors and Actions

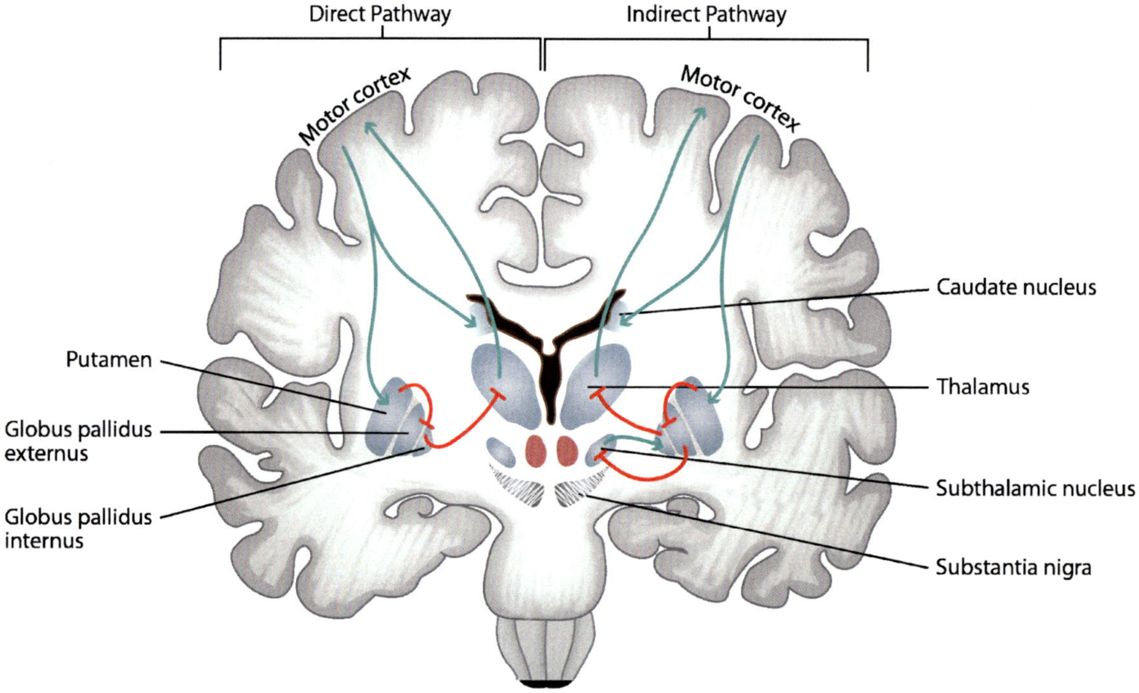

Figure 9.2.5 - Basal Ganglia and Striatum

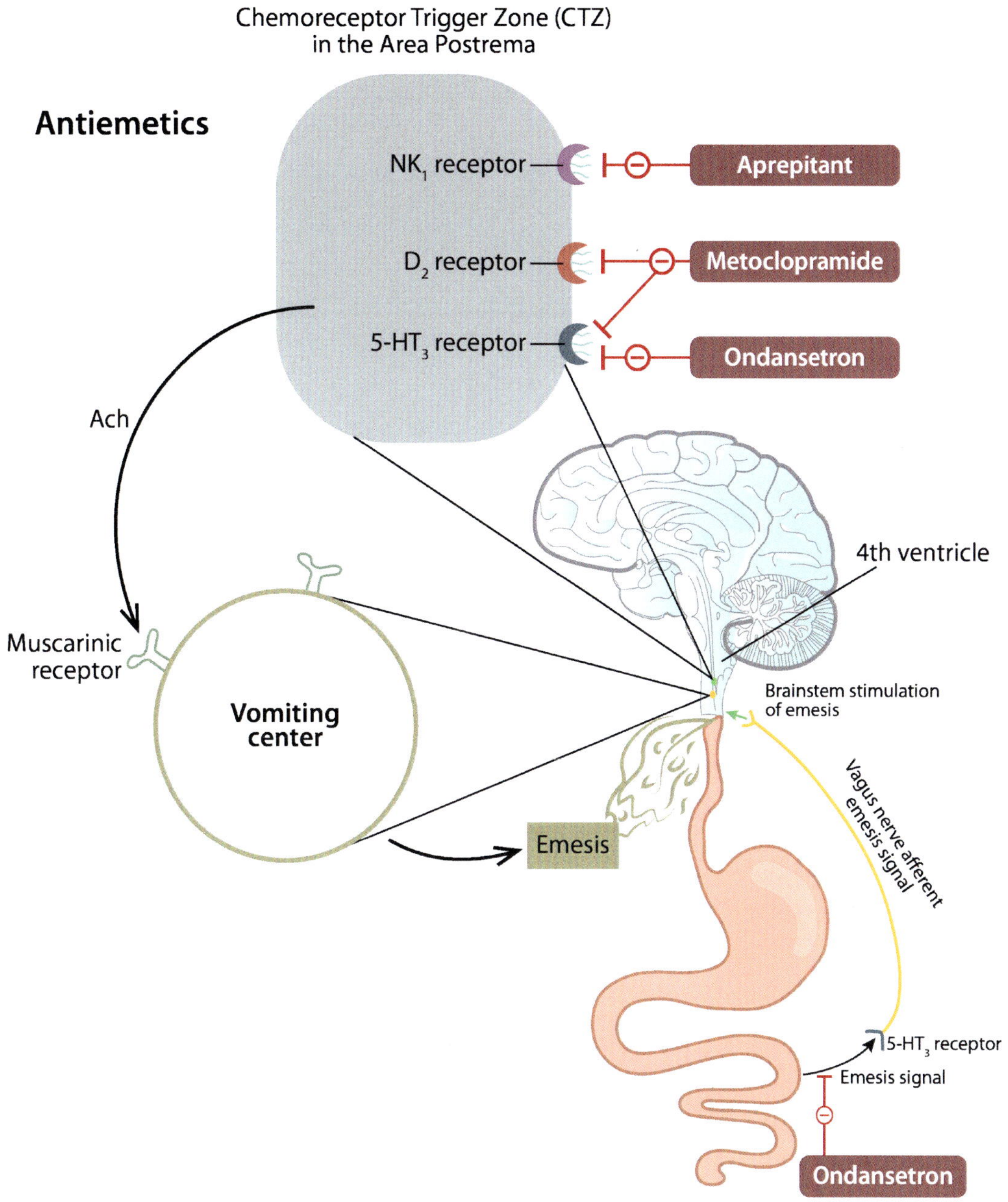

Figure 9.2.6 - Antiemetic Drug Mechanisms

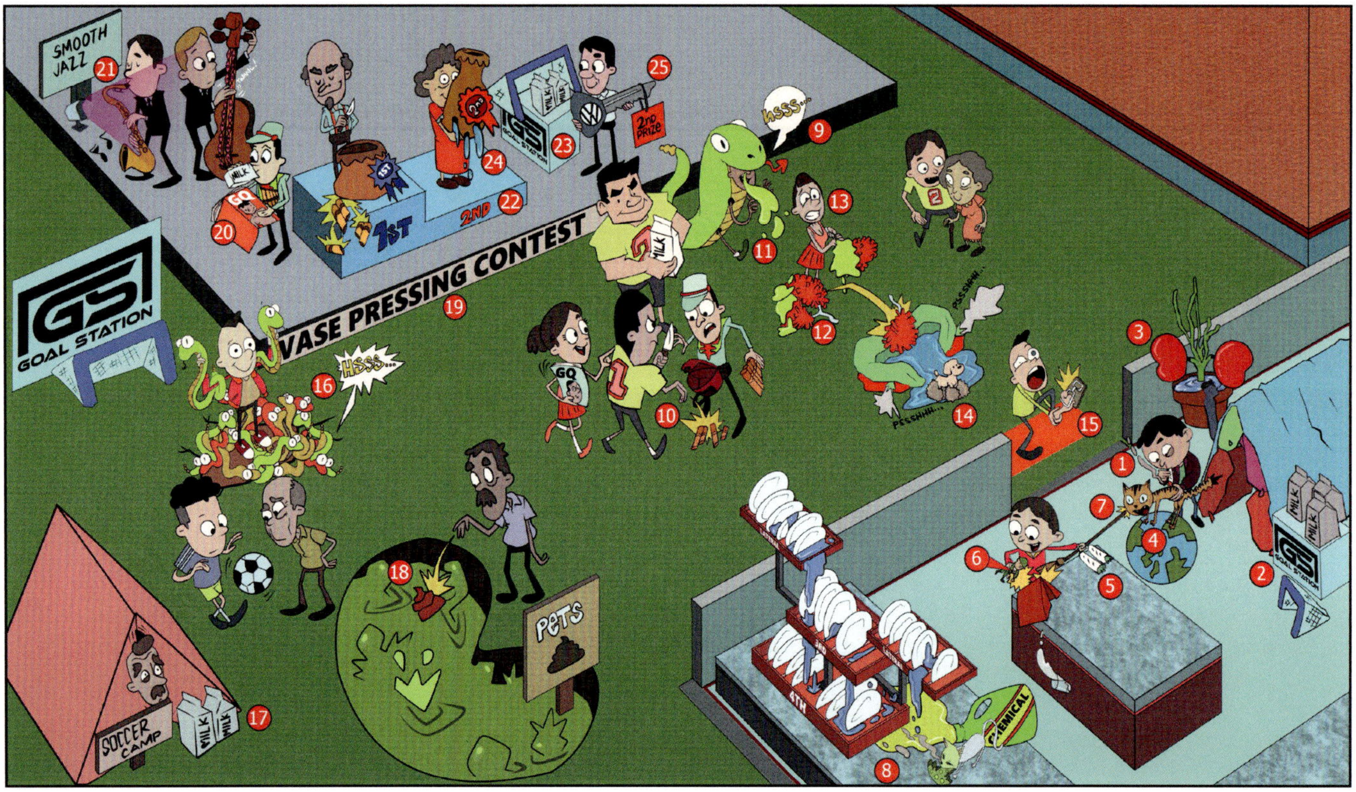

1. Teenager holding single piece of rolled dope: Dopamine-1 (D_1) receptor

2. Teenager setting up SG brand goal station box and camping tent next to milk cartons: D_1 stimulation → Gs protein class → adenylate cyclase activation → increased cAMP → PKA → increased Ca^{2+}

3. Swollen kidney bean plant next to tent: D_1 stimulation relaxes (dilates) renal vascular smooth muscle → maintains renal perfusion

4. Teenager holding agitated striped cat directly on top of globe: D_1 → activates the direct pathway of the striatum → increased motor activity

5. Two pieces of rolled dope sitting on counter: Dopamine-2 (D_2) receptor

6. Teen using GI Joe toy to knock model tent and milk off counter: D_2 stimulation → Gi protein class → adenylate cyclase inhibition → decreased cAMP → decreased PKA → Decreased Ca^{2+}

7. Teen using broom handle to hit agitated striped cat indirectly: D_2 activation → inhibits the indirect (inhibitory) pathway of the striatum → increased motor activity

8. Four-tiered drying rack on counter near spilled chemical cleaner that causes cat to vomit: Chemoreceptor trigger zone (CTZ) located in the area postrema in the 4th ventricle and adjacent vomiting center nuclei receive input and can cause vomiting

9. Single hissing snake mascot outside: Histamine-1 (H_1) receptor

10. heerleader with GQ magazine behind athlete with knife who breaks band kid's two pipes into three pieces while other athlete holds up carton of milk: H_1 stimulation → Gq protein class → phospholipase C activation → PIP_2 to IP_3 + DAG → protein kinase C → increased CA^{2+}

11. Snake mascot sneezing on cheerleader's pom poms: H1 stimulation increases nasal mucus production

12. Cheerleader's lung-shaped pom poms covered in mucus: H1 stimulation increases bronchial mucus production

13. Cheerleader squeezing pom poms to get them clean: H1 stimulation causes bronchoconstriction

14. Toy poodle absorbing water from deflating pool: H1 stimulation increases vascular permeability → hypotension and edema

15. Teen stepping on mouse trap and screaming in pain: H1 stimulation increases activation of peripheral nociceptive receptors leading to increased pain

16. Reptile club president holding two hissing snakes: Histamine-2 (H_2) receptor

17. Kids setting up GS brand goal station, tent and milk cartons for soccer camp: H_2 stimulation → Gs protein class → adenylate cyclase activation → increased cAMP → PKA protein powder → increased CA^{2+}

18. Stomach-shaped pit with bubbling acid: H_2 stimulation increases gastric acid secretion

19. "Vase pressing contest" sign near man with 1st place ribbon: Vasopressin-1 (V_1) receptor

20. First place vase winner cutting pipes into three pieces next to band kid holding GQ magazine and drinking milk: V_1 stimulation → Gq protein class → phospholipase C activation → PIP_2 to IP_3 + DAG → PKC → increased Ca^{2+}

21. "Smooth jazz" sign next to bass player tightening strings: V_1 stimulation increases vascular smooth muscle contraction

22. Old lady with 2nd place ribbon from vase pressing contest: Vasopressin-2 (V_2) receptor

23. GS brand goal station given to 2nd place winner as prize: V_2 stimulation → Gs protein class → adenylate cyclase activation → increased cAMP → PKC → increased Ca^{2+}

24. 2nd place vase contains holes that are leaking water: V_2 increases H_2O permeability and reabsorption

IMMUNOLOGY PHARMACOLOGY

Section I - Cyclosporine

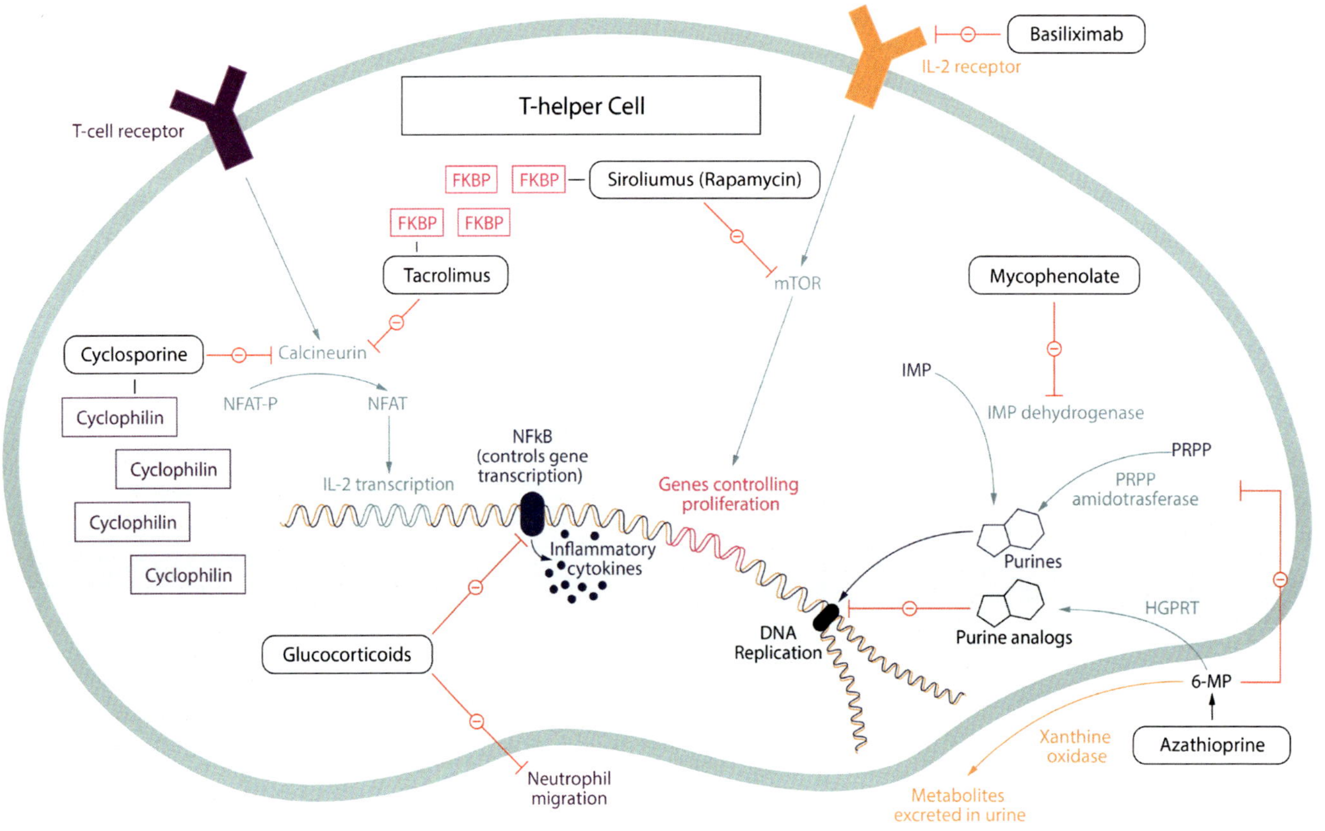

Figure 9.3.1 - Immunosuppressive Drug Targets

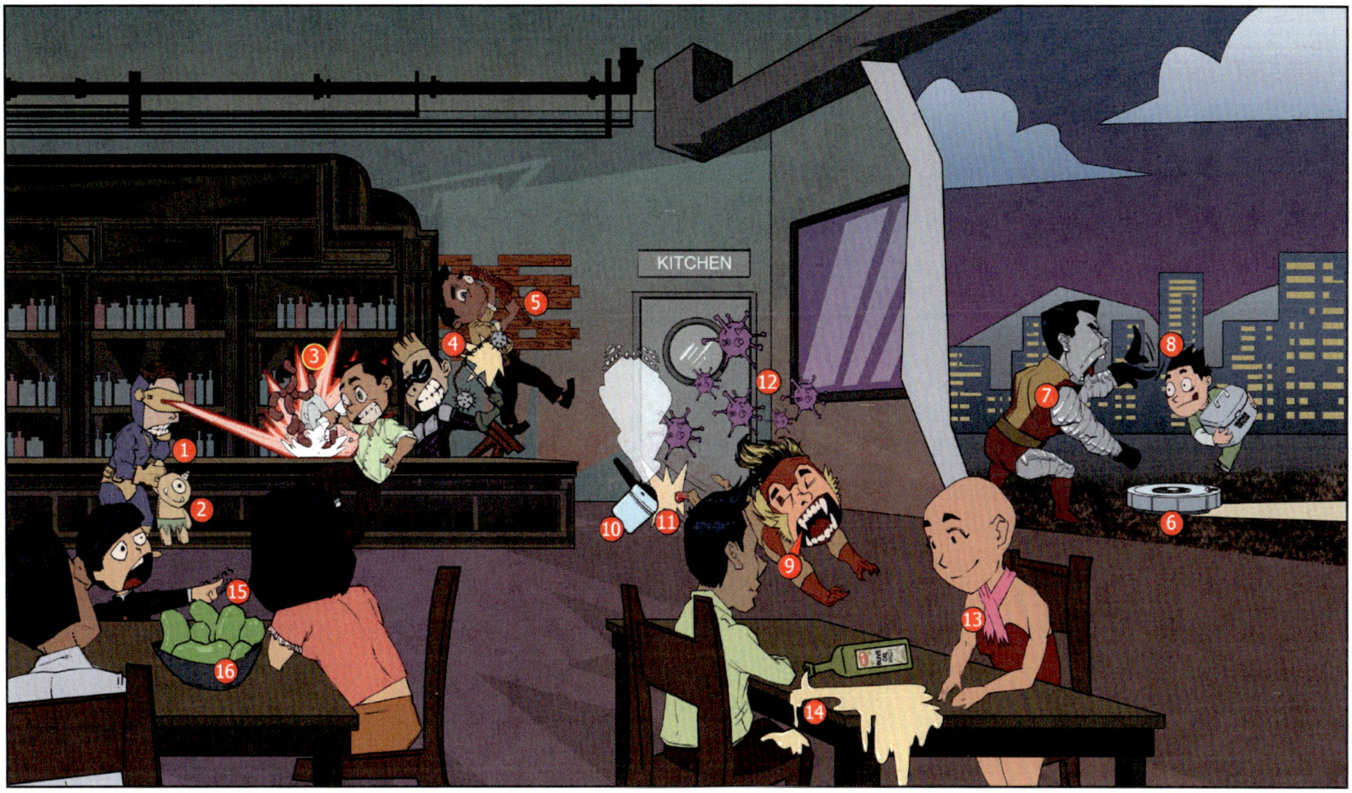

1. Cyclops: Cyclosporine

2. Stuffed cyclops bear: Binds to cyclophilin

3. Milk and sausage links getting blasted: Inhibits calcineurin

4. T-shaped flail: Blocks T-cell activation

5. Two interlocking wooden tiles: Blocks IL-2 gene transcription

6. Roomba: Used to treat rheumatoid arthritis

7. Colso-guy: Used to treat psoriasis

8. Rejecting organ harvester: Used to reduce acute transplant rejection

9. Exposed gums: May cause gingival hyperplasia

10. Pressure cooker: May cause hypertension

11. Burned toe: May cause gout

12. Purple dust: Increases the risk of infection

13. Cancer hope ribbon: Increases the risk of malignancy

14. Dripping oil: May cause hyperlipidemia

15. Trembling: May result in neurotoxicity (e.g. tremor)

16. Kidney beans: May result in nephrotoxicity and renal tubular acidosis

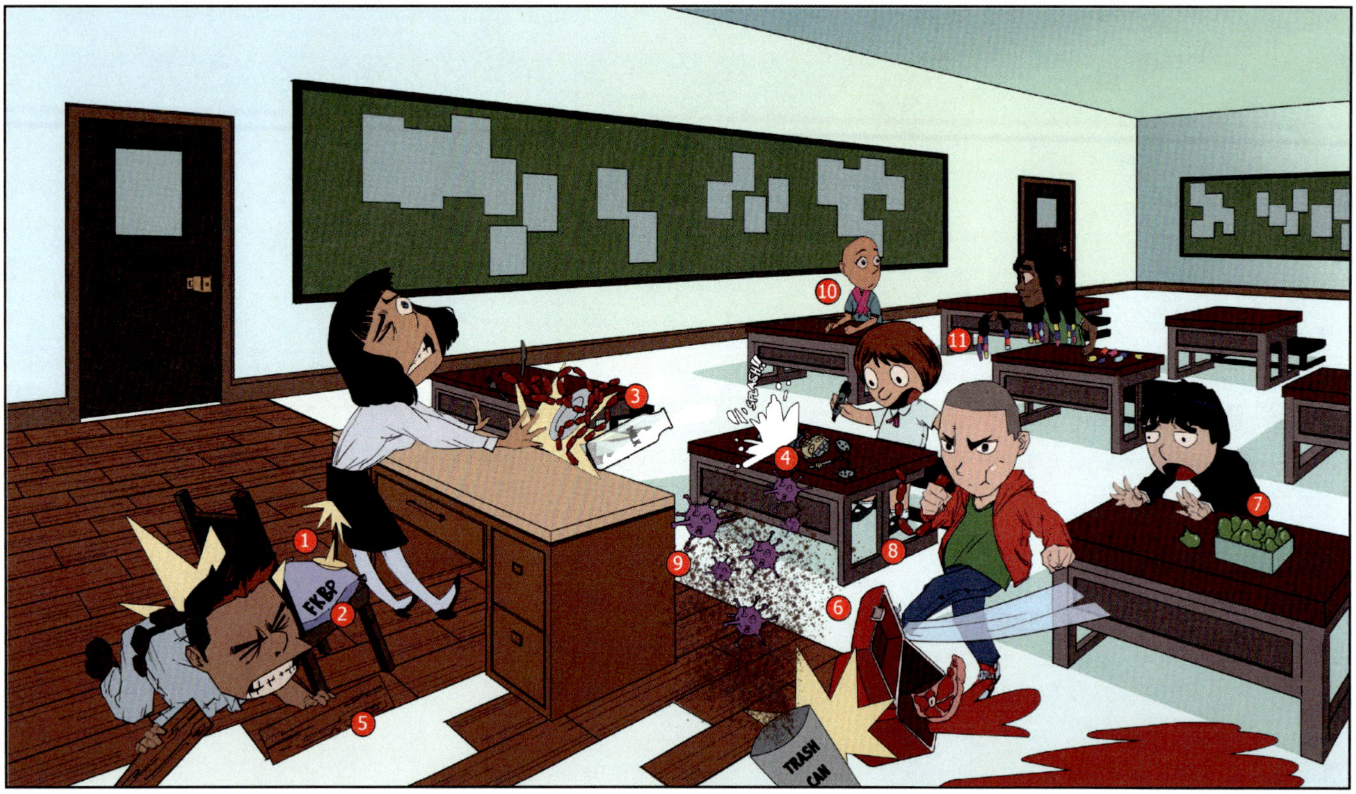

1. Thumbtack: Tacrolimus

2. Fluffy, kumfy, butt pad: Binds *FK506* binding protein (FKBP)

3. Milk and sausage links: Inhibits calcineurin

4. T-shaped flail splattered in milk: Blocks T-cell activation

5. Guy laying down two interlocking panels is hit by chair: Prevents IL-2 transcription

6. Bully kicking lunchbox resembling transplant cooler with raw meat: Used for acute transplant rejection

7. Kidney beans: Nephrotoxic

8. Sausage link: Neurotoxic

9. Dust and infectious particles; Increases the risk of infection

10. Cancer hope ribbon: Increases the risk of malignancy

11. Dyed beads: Increases the risk of diabetes

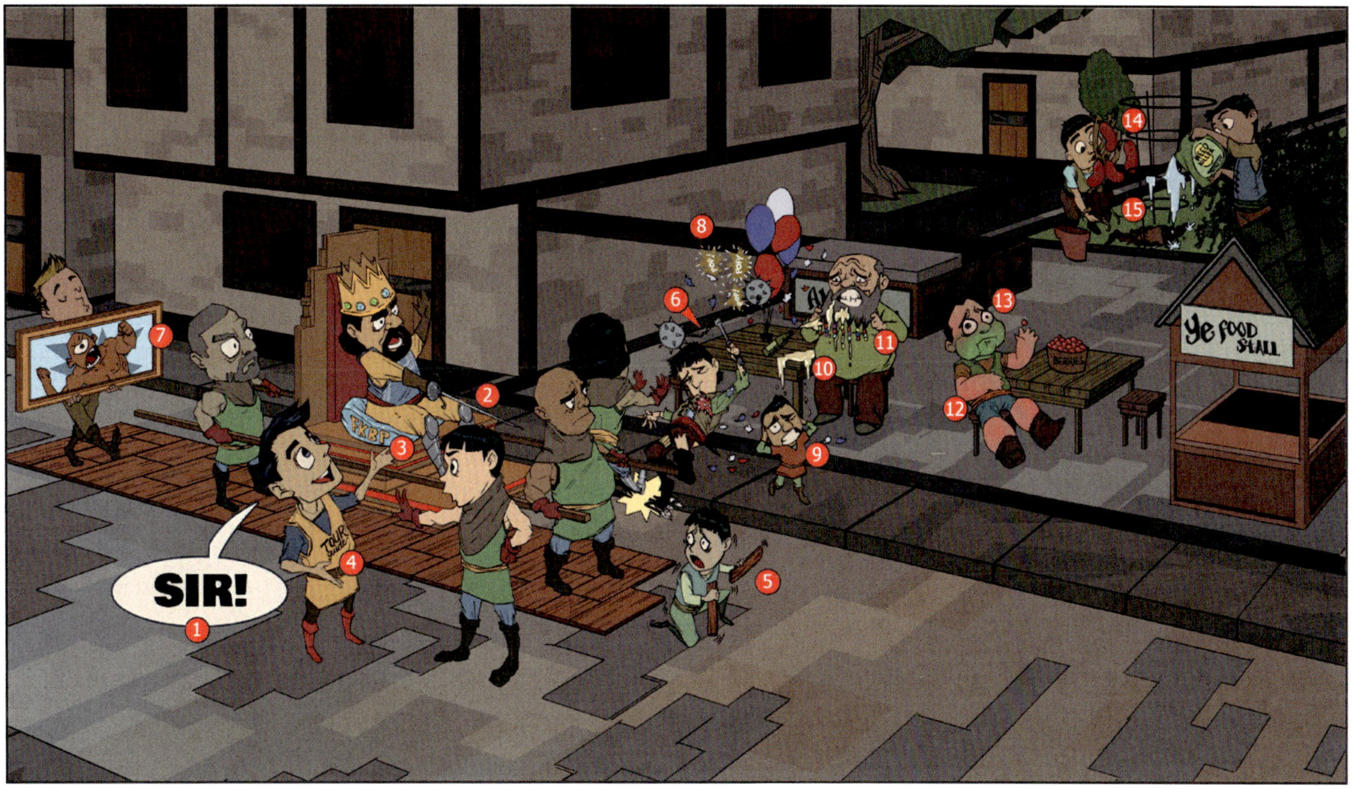

1. Sir: Sirolimus

2. Rapier: Rapamycin

3. Fluffy, kumfy butt pad: Binds to FKBP

4. Shirt with the word "TOUR": Inhibitors mTor pathway

5. Two interlocking tiles: Blocks IL-2 response

6. Falling man with the T-shaped flail and broken arrows: Blocks T and B cell activation

7. Cyclops painting: Sirolimus (rapamycin) acts synergistically with cyclosporine

8. Popped balloons: Can cause pancytopenia

9. Kid holding his head: Can cause headaches

10. Dripping oil: Can cause hyperlipidemia

11. Dyed beads: Can cause diabetes

12. Allergic reaction to berries: Can cause peripheral edema

13. Belly ache and nausea: Can cause GI distress

14. Transplanting the kidney plant: Used for kidney transplants

15. Plant cage drenched in weed-killer: Used in drug-eluting stents

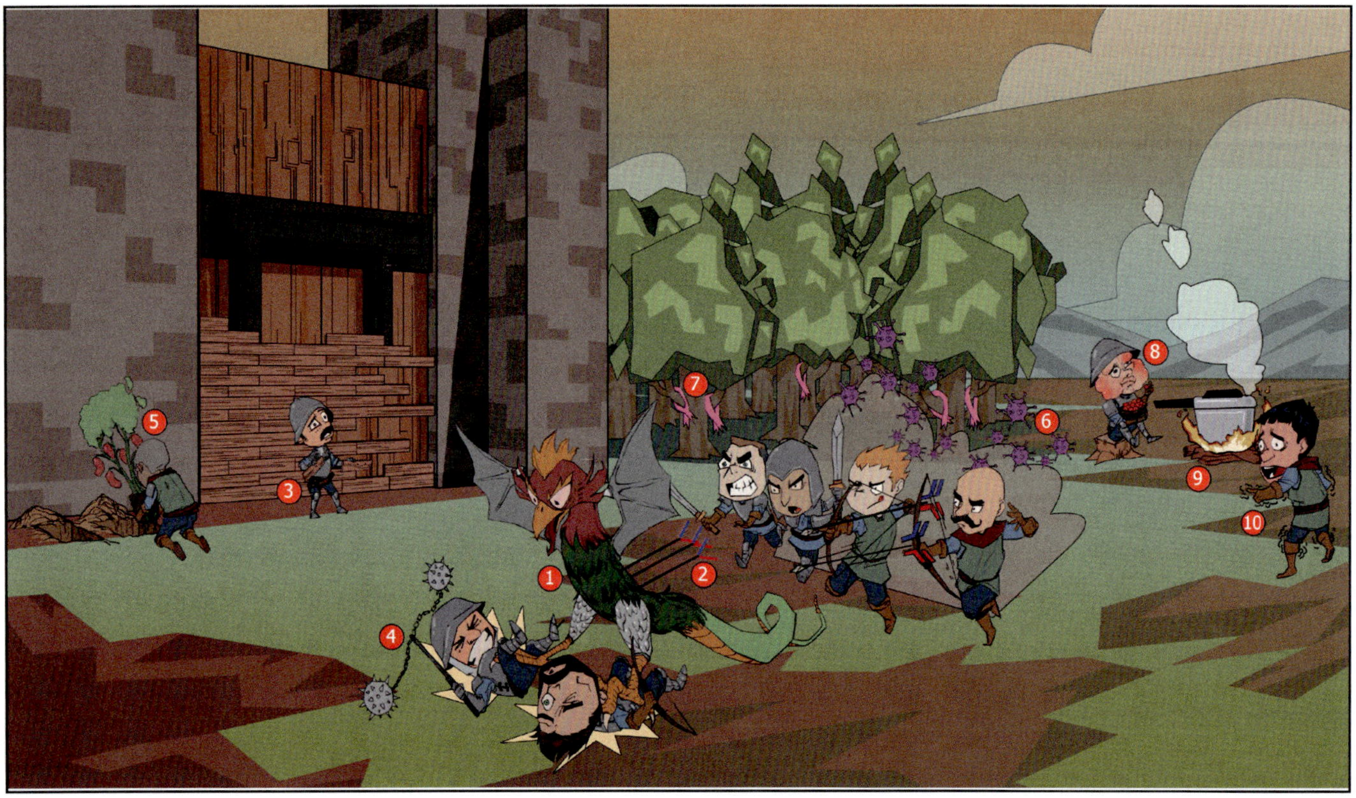

1. **1.** Basilisk: Basiliximab
2. **2.** Arrows: Monoclonal antibody
3. **3.** Two interlocking floor panels: Blocks the IL-2 receptor
4. **4.** Destroyed archer and T-shaped flail: Blocks B-cell and T-cell (lymphocyte) proliferation/activation
5. **5.** Transplanting kidney beans: Use for acute kidney transplant rejection
6. **6.** Dust and infectious particles: Increase the risk of infection
7. **7.** Cancer hope ribbons: Increases the risk of malignancy
8. **8.** Swollen face: May cause edema
9. **9.** Pressure cooker: May cause hypertension
10. **10.** Frightened soldier trembling: May cause tremors

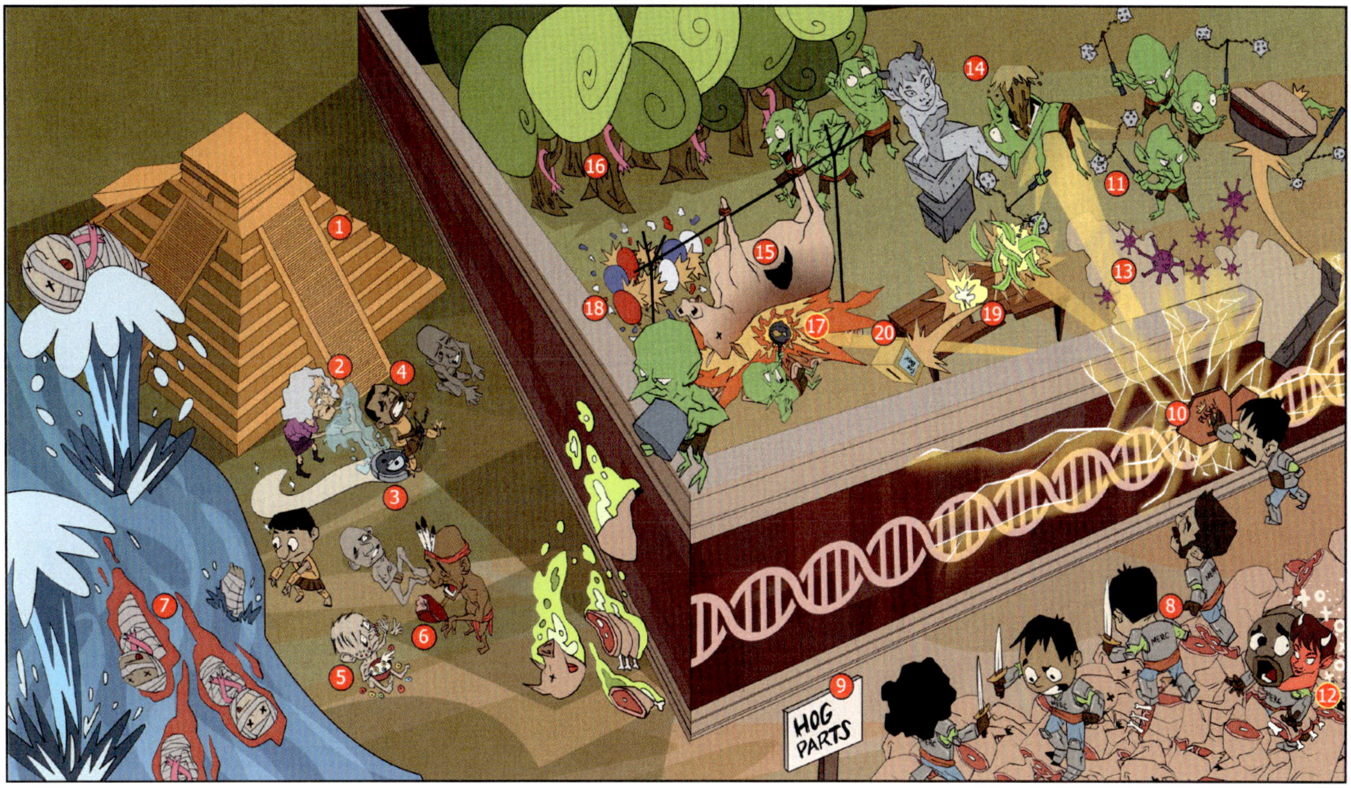

1. Aztec: Azathioprine

2. Old crohn: Used to treat Crohn disease

3. Roomba: Used to treat rheumatoid arthritis

4. Roomba causing warrior to fire an arrow into his foot: Used to treat many autoimmune conditions

5. Spilled fruit loops and crumbs on cheeks: Used to treat systemic lupus erythematosus (SLE)

6. Shaman with cow heart and sick man rejecting it: Used to prevent organ transplant rejection

7. Bloody water, cancer ribbons and blasting geysers: Used to treat acute lymphoblastic leukemia (ALL)

8. 6 mercenary captains: Azathioprine is converted to 6-mercaptopurine (6-MP)

9. Hog parts: HGPRT acts on 6-MP

10. Purine shaped boulder destroying DNA wall: HGPRT converts 6-MP into a purine analog (purine antagonist) which disrupts DNA synthesis and cell proliferation

11. Death of the globins wielding the T-shaped flails: Azathioprine and 6-MP preferentially inhibit T-cell proliferation

12. Succubus kissing and hugging the captain: Xanthine oxidase (XO) deactivates 6-MP

13. Infection particles: Can increase risk of infection

14. Vomiting: Can cause GI distress

15. Cow with liver-shaped spot: Can cause hepatitis

16. Cancer ribbon: Can increase risk of malignancy

17. Flame engulfing pan: Can cause pancreatitis

18. Balloons popping: Can cause pancytopenia

19. Exploding table with aloe vera: Co-administration with allopurinol can increase toxicities due to xanthine oxidase inhibition

20. Fee box: Co-administration with febuxostat can increase toxicities due to xanthine oxidase inhibition

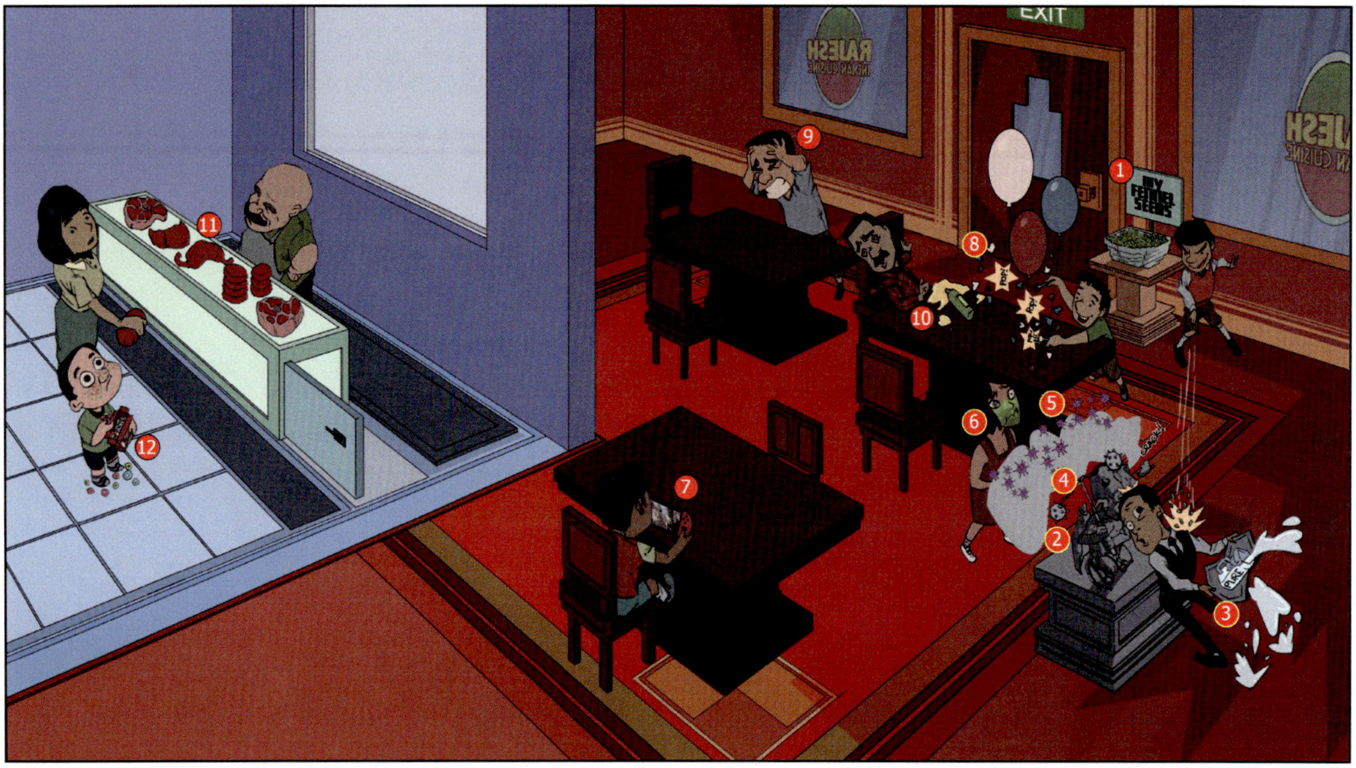

1. "My Fennel Seeds" sign: Mycophenolate

2. Broken imp statue: Inhibits IMP dehydrogenase

3. Purine shaped tray with pure water: Inhibits purine synthesis

4. Broken imp statue holding a T-shaped flail and a quiver of arrows on its back: Inhibits proliferation of B and T-cells

5. Infectious particles; Can predispose patients to infection

6. Green face: Can cause GI distress

7. Video game showing battle with Megatronix (CMV image mnemonic): Can cause invasive CMV infection

8. Popped balloons of various colors: Can cause pancytopenia

9. Grabbing head: Can cause headaches

10. Dripping oil: can cause hyperlipidemia

11. Organs: Use for organ transplant

12. Fruit loops and raw kidney: Use for lupus nephritis

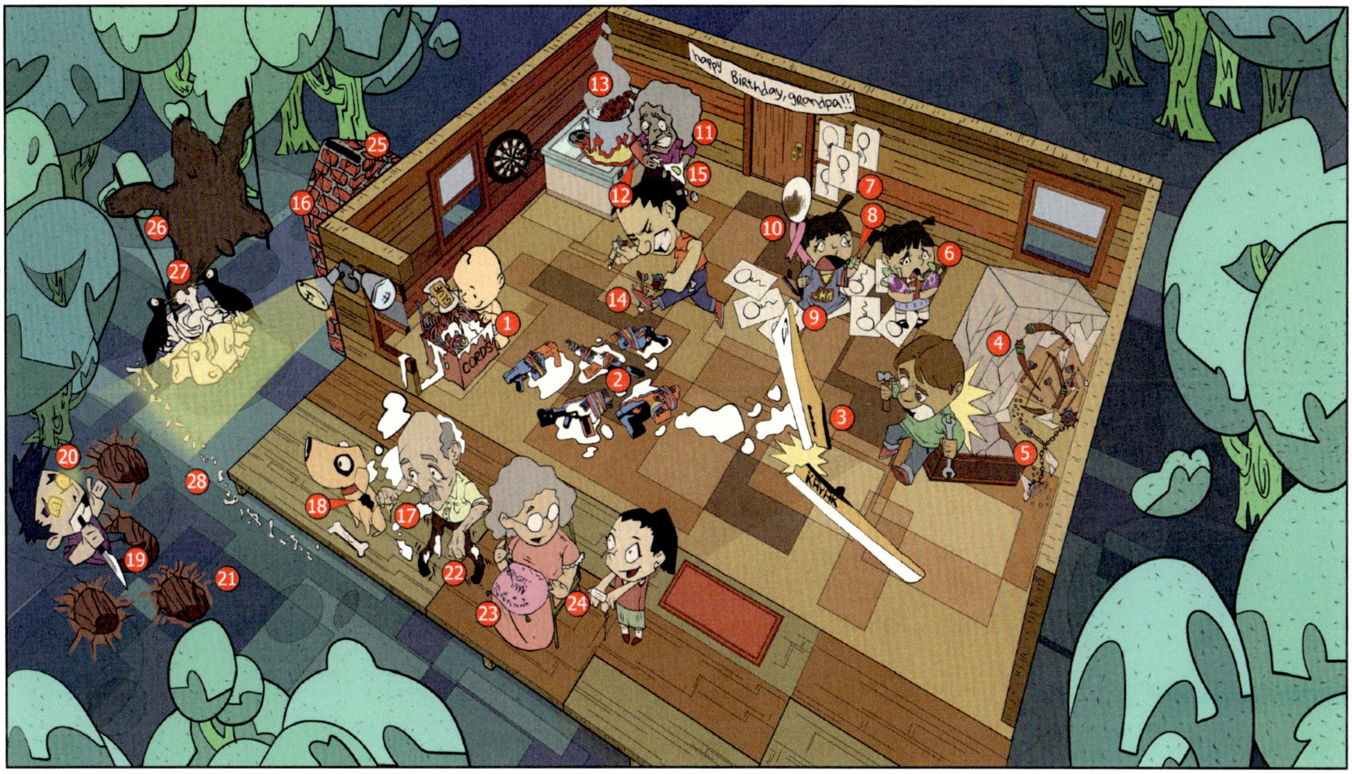

1. Glue and cords: Glucocorticoids

2. Nerf guns wrapped in cords and covered in glue: Glucocorticoids inhibit NF-kappaB

3. Broken kayak on its side: By inhibiting NF-kappaB, glucocorticoids prevent cytokine release

4. Broken glass case containing T-shaped flail and bows and arrows: Glucocorticoids suppress T-cells, B-cells and antibodies

5. Disintegration of the T-shaped flail: Glucocorticoids induce T-cell apoptosis

6. Turtles with shells resembling neutrophils trying to get free: Glucocorticoids inhibit neutrophil chemotaxis

7. Pretend balloons drawn on white paper: Glucocorticoids cause artificial leukocytosis by causing demargination of neutrophils

8. Inhaler: Glucocorticoids can be used to treat asthma

9. NHL jersey: Glucocorticoids can be used to treat non-Hodgkin lymphoma (NHL)

10. Smudged white balloon with pink cancer ribbon: Glucocorticoids can be used to treat chronic lymphocytic leukemia (CLL)

11. Old crone: Glucocorticoids can be used to treat Crohn disease

12. Arm burned by flame: Glucocorticoids can be used to treat many inflammatory conditions

13. Intestines on stove with ulcers in them: Glucocorticoids can be used to treat ulcerative colitis

14. Arrow dart impaling foot: Glucocorticoids can be used to treat many autoimmune conditions

15. Egg on skin: Glucocorticoids can be used to treat eczema

16. Breaking triangular chimney top: Glucocorticoids can be used to treat adrenal insufficiency

17. Old man covered in glue: Glucocorticoids can cause hyperglycemia

18. Dog with liver-shaped spot: Glucocorticoids upregulate gluconeogenesis in the liver

19. Psycho: Glucocorticoids can cause psychosis

20. Light reflecting off eyes: Glucocorticoids can cause cataracts

21. Holes in the ground: Glucocorticoids can cause gastric ulcers

22. Old man trying to stand up and being weak and wobbly: Glucocorticoids can cause myopathy (weakness)

23. Embroidered seat cushion: Glucocorticoids can cause Cushing syndrome

24. Grandma refusing tampon: Glucocorticoids can cause amenorrhea

25. Chimney on the edge of the house: Glucocorticoids can cause adrenal atrophy

26. Thinning bear skin hanging with striae: Glucocorticoids can cause skin thinning and striae

27. Crows eating with flesh on the femoral head: Glucocorticoids can cause osteonecrosis of the femoral head

28. Broken bones and bone fragments; Glucocorticoids can cause osteoporosis

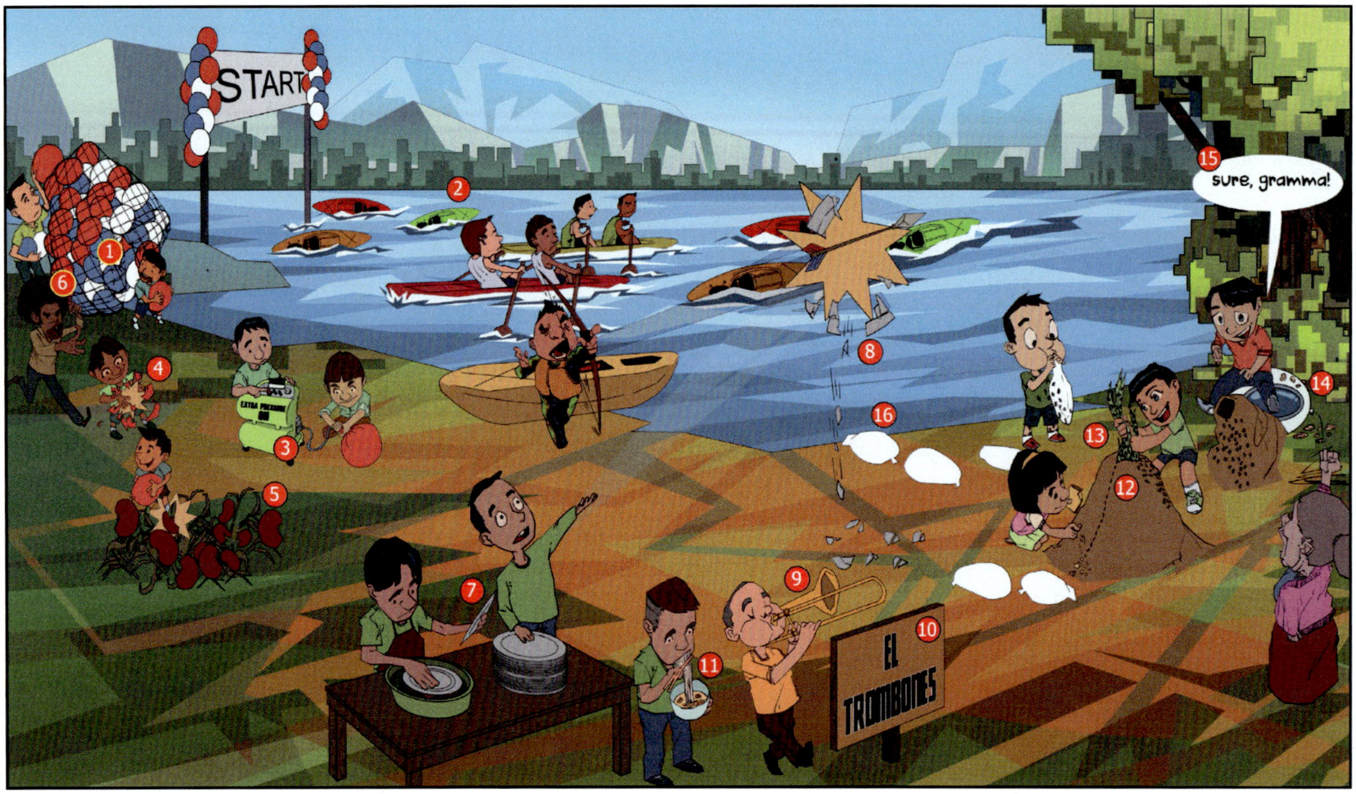

1. Balloons getting shoved into a big container: Bone marrow stimulation

2. Kayaks tipped over on their sides: Recombinant cytokines can stimulate bone marrow production

3. "Extra pressure on": Erythropoietin (EPO) stimulates RBC development

4. Popped red balloons: Use recombinant EPO in cases of anemia

5. Destroyed kidney beans: Anemia that results from kidney failure warrants recombinant EPO administration

6. Afro: Epoetin alpha is a recombinant EPO

7. Plates: Platelets

8. Arrow shattering plates: Recombinant cytokines should be used in cases of autoimmune thrombocytopenia

9. Trombone: Thrombopoietin (TPO) stimulates platelet development

10. El Trombones: Eltrombopag is a TPO receptor agonist

11. Ramen noodles: Romiplostim is a TPO analog

12. Colony of ants exiting the anthill: Granulocyte colony-stimulating factor (G-CSF) stimulates granulocyte production

13. Filling the hole with grass: Filgrastim is a recombinant G-CSF

14. Grains of bread and unique ball: Granulocyte-monocyte stimulating factor (GM-CSF) increases granulocyte and monocyte levels

15. "Sure, gramma!": Sargramostim is a recombinant GM-CSF

16. White, deflated balloons covered in ants: Consider Sargramostim or Filgrastim in cases of leukopenia

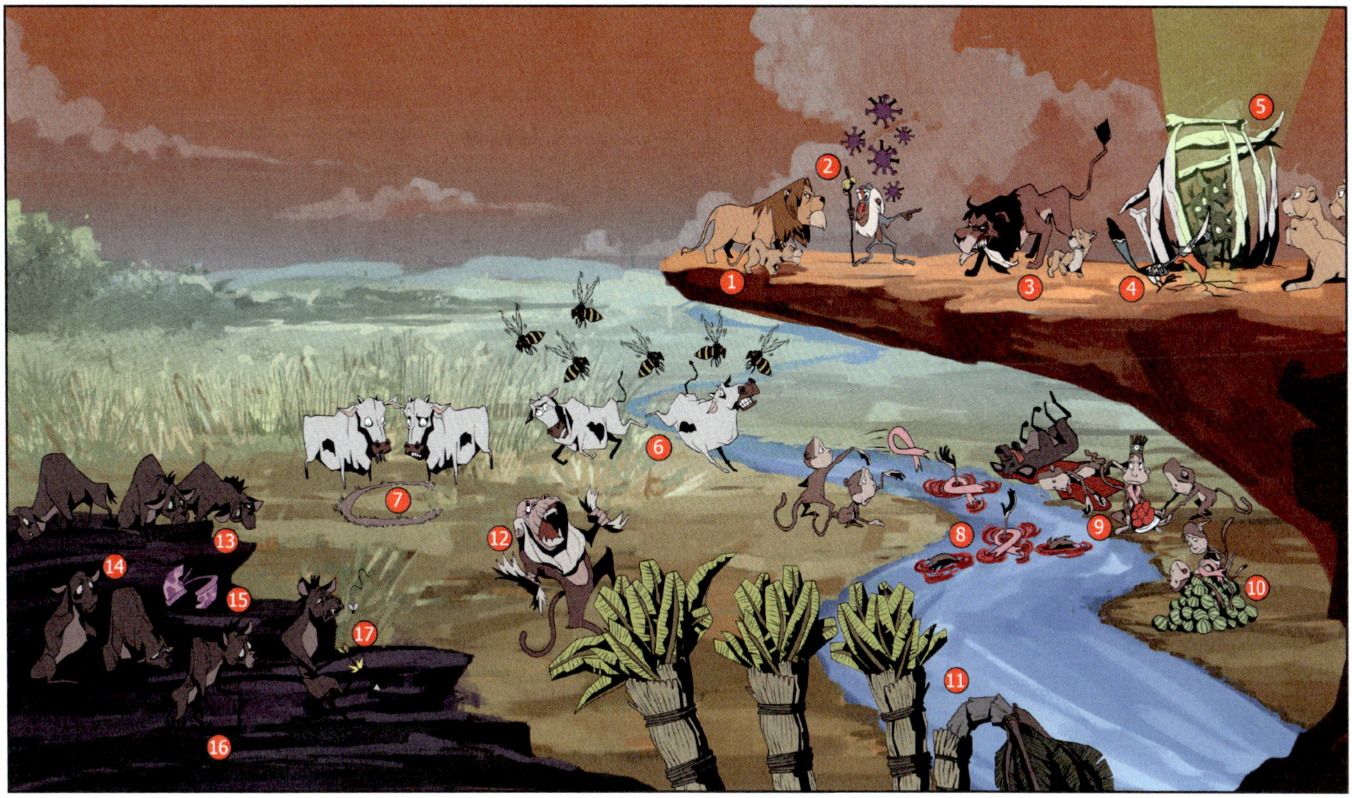

1. Alpha lion and smaller beta cub: Interferon alpha and beta

2. Virally sick baboon interacting with two lions: Infected cells release interferon alpha and beta

3. Murderous lion trying to kill lion cub: Interferon alpha and beta activate natural killer cells

4. Bird with "TH1" feathers smashing beak on ground, emitting green rays: Th1 cells release interferon gamma

5. Green rays beaming on bone cage: Interferon gamma activates macrophages to increase phagocytosis

6. Liver-spotted cows tormented by killer bees: Interferons can be used pharmacologically to treat hepatitis B infections

7. Liver-spotted cows with C-shaped crop circle: Interferons can be used pharmacologically to treat hepatitis C infections

8. Monkeys throwing pink cancer ribbons in bloody water with tufts of fur: Interferons can be used pharmacologically to fight hairy cell leukemia

9. Monkey with pink ribbon being served kidney beans: Interferons can be used pharmacologically to treat renal cell carcinoma

10. Monkey placing pink ribbon over dead monkey that is resting on a pile of melons: Interferons can be used pharmacologically to fight melanoma

11. Palm tree that's dying because it doesn't have enough insulative wrapping: Interferons can be used pharmacologically to treat multiple sclerosis

12. Grandpa monkey ripping chest hair: Interferons can be used pharmacologically to fight chronic granulomatous disease

13. Depressed hyenas: Interferons can cause depression

14. Tired hyena with headache: Interferons can cause malaise and flu-like symptoms

15. Empty neutrophil-looking turtle shell: Interferons can cause low neutrophil counts

16. Weak hyena: Interferons can cause muscle weakness

17. Hyena stabbing himself in foot with arrow: Interferons can cause autoimmunity

ANTIBIOTICS

Antibiotics | Section 1 - Penicillin

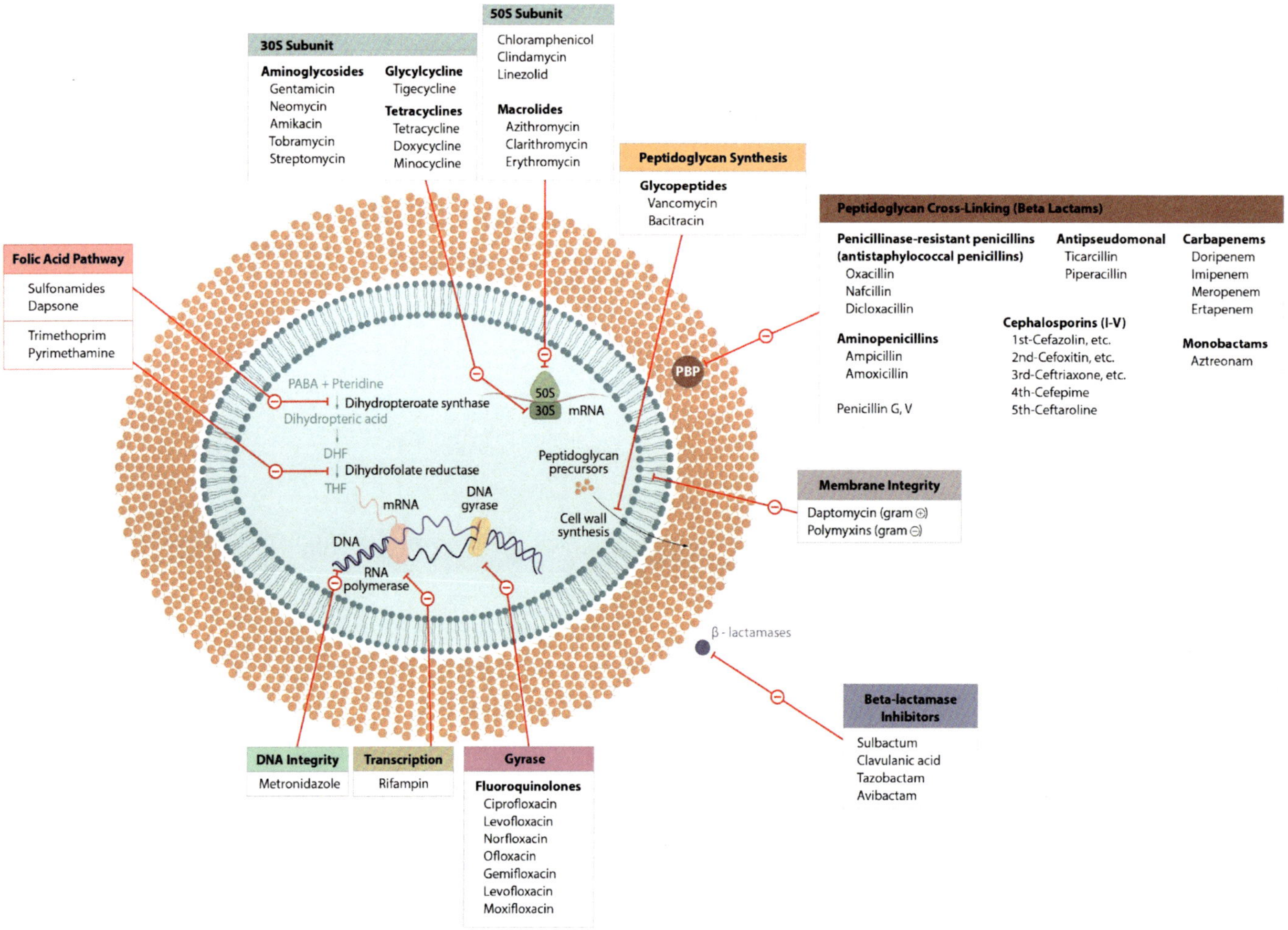

Figure 9.4.1 - Antibiotic Mechanisms

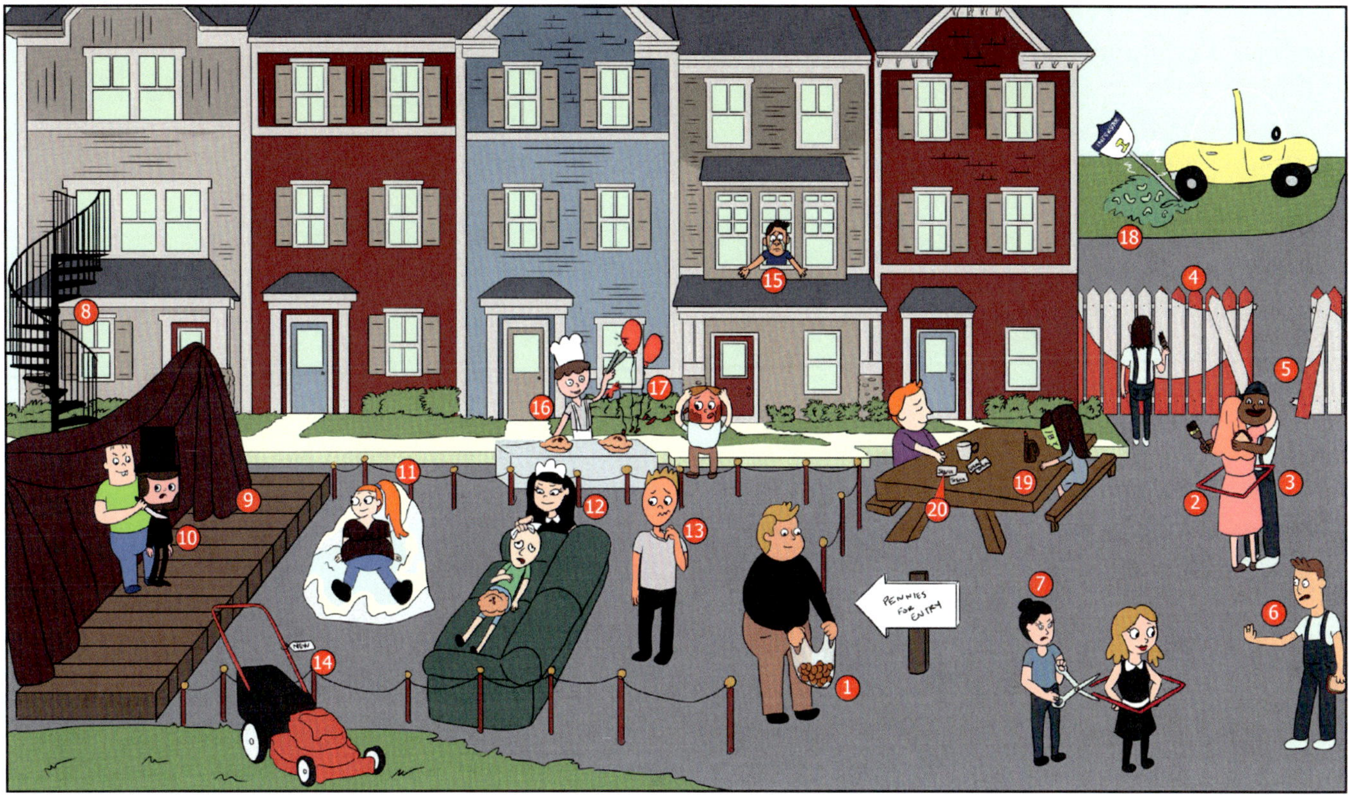

1. Bag of pennies: Penicillin

2. Square hula hoop on lady with pink dress: Beta lactam rings

3. Hula hoop girl hugging PB&J holding boyfriend: Penicillins (and all beta lactams) bind to PBP (penicillin binding protein) on bacterial cell walls

4. Incomplete wall: Penicillin prevents cell wall cross-linking

5. Peppermint color fence next to painters and girl hugging boyfriend; When bound to penicillin, PBP cannot cross link peptidoglycan in the bacterial walls

6. Man holding a PB&J sandwich and resisting the hula girl: Bacteria can develop resistance by mutating the PBP on their cell wall, preventing beta lactams from binding

7. Girl cutting square hula hoop on rejected girl: Bacteria can also develop resistance through using beta lactamases, which break down beta lactams

8. Spiral staircase: Penicillin can treat Syphilis

9. Acting stage: Penicillin can treat Actinomyces

10. Mugger holding knife to Abe Lincoln's throat: Penicillin can treat Neisseria meningitidis

11. Pregnant women sitting on glacier: Pregnant patients with *S. agalactiae* infections should be given penicillin during the intrapartum period

12. Maid bringing pie to sick groundskeeper on couch: Penicillin can treat rheumatic fever caused by *Strep pyogenes* M protein

13. Co-worker pulling at collar next to couch: Penicillin treats *S. pharyngitis*

14. New red mower: Penicillin can treat *S. pneumoniae*

15. Sensitive, crying man in window: Penicillin can cause hypersensitivity reactions

16. Popping red balloons: Penicillin can cause direct autoimmune hemolytic anemia (AIHA)

17. Boy having allergic reaction from pies next to popping red balloons: Penicillin can cause some people to have severe allergic reactions

18. Destroyed kidney beans and interstate sign: Can cause acute interstitial nephritis

19. Syrup induced sickness: Penicillin can cause serum sickness

20. Stevia packets on table: Penicillin can cause Stevens-Johnson syndrome

See Figure 9.4.1 - Antibiotics Mechanisms (Antibiotics, Section 1, Page 69)

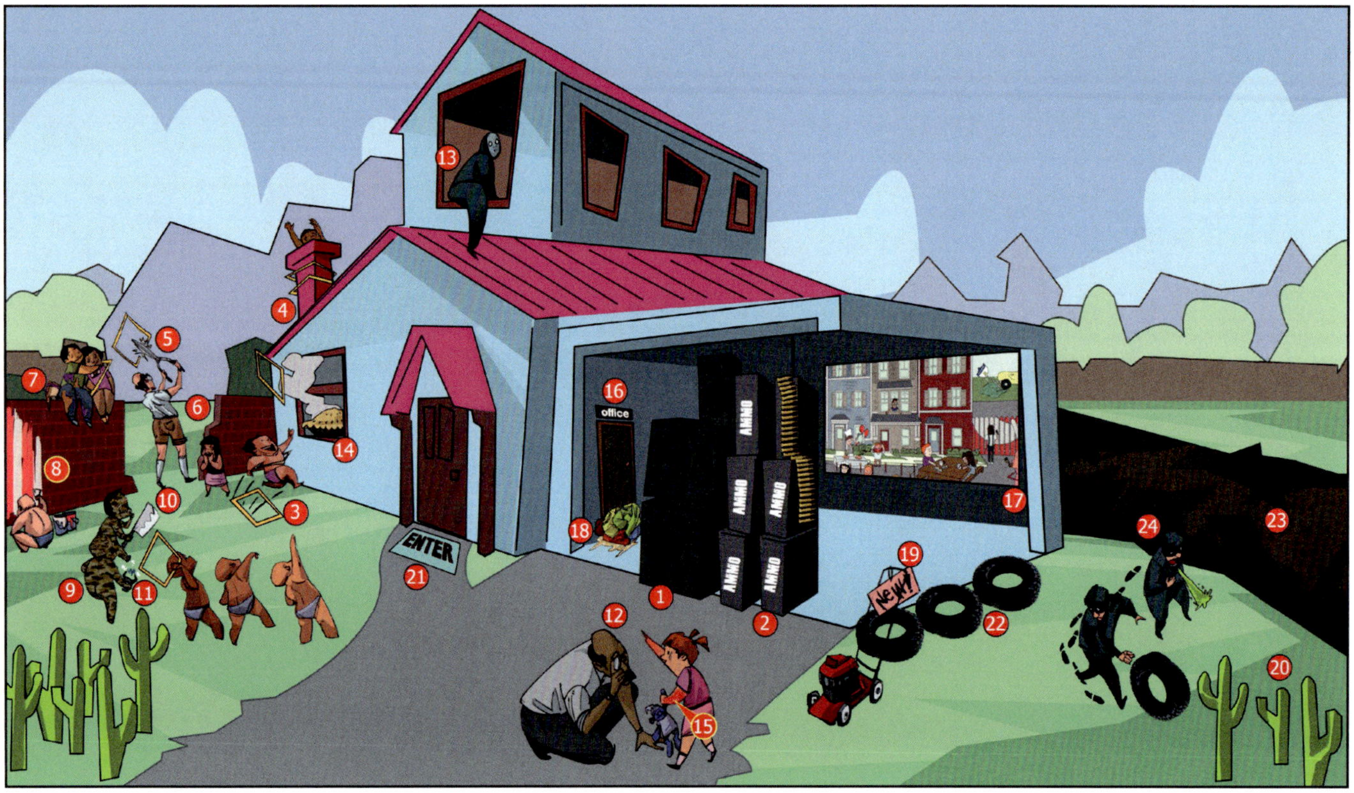

1. Amps stacked from floor to ceiling: Ampicillin

2. Ammo: Amoxicillin

3. Square hula hoops: Beta lactam

4. Kid sliding through pink chimney: Increased uptake into gram negative bacteria through porins

5. Scissors: Aminopenicillins are beta lactams that are penicillinase-sensitive

6. Brick wall with huge gap in it: Penicillins lead to cell wall lysis

7. Boy covered in PB&J hugging his girlfriend who is wearing one of the square hula hoops: Beta lactams bind to penicillin-binding protein (PBP) on cell wall

8. Peppermint pattern: Amoxicillin and ampicillin work by disrupting peptidoglycan on the cell wall

9. Kids dressed like soldiers: Combine with sulbactam to protect against penicillinase

10. Cleavert: Combine with clavulanic acid to protect against penicillinase

11. Taser: Combine with tazobactam to protect against penicillinase

12. Monocle: Used to treat listeria monocytogenes

13. Burglar: Used to treat Borrelia burgdorferi

14. Pie: used for Strep pyogenes

15. Rash from dirty Elve's Blue Village (EBV) toy: Amoxicillin can cause a maculopapular rash in patients infected with EBV (mononucleosis)

16. "Office" sign: Can treat Haemophilus influenzae

17. Painting of the hypersensitive man from the penicillin story: Causes hypersensitivity reactions

18. Pile of dirty clothes: Can treat *H. pylori*

19. New mower: Can treat *S. pneumoniae*

20. Cacti: Can treat Moraxella catarrhalis

21. "Enter" mat: Can treat Enterococcus

22. Thief rolling away a tire: Can cause pseudomembranous colitis

23. Muddy river: Can cause diarrhea

24. Thief throwing up: Can cause vomiting

See Figure 9.4.1 - Antibiotics Mechanisms (Antibiotics, Section 1, Page 69)

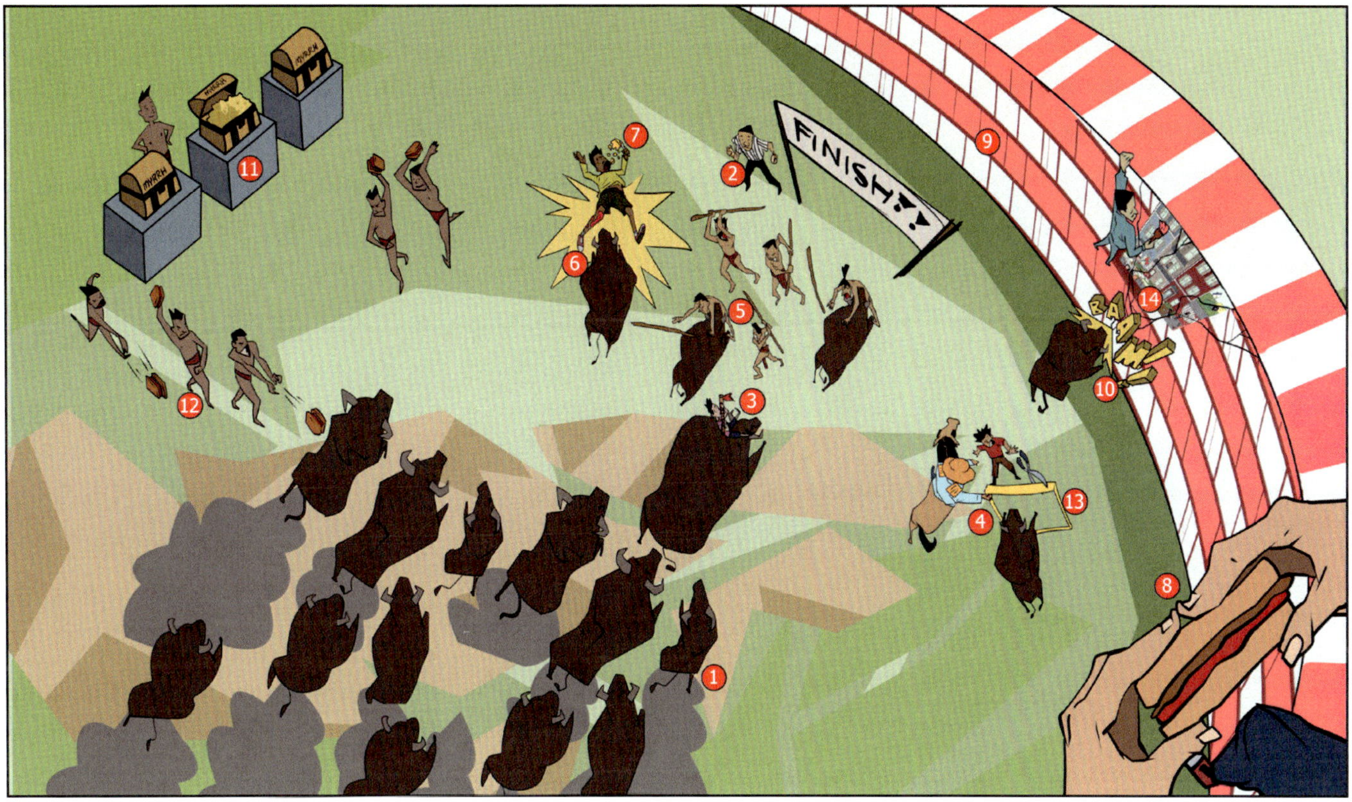

1. Oxen: Ocacilin

2. 2 clocks/stopwatches held by official: Dicloxacillin

3. Native American flute (NAF) played by man on lead oxen: Nafcillin

4. Oxen jumping through square hula hoop: Beta lactam

5. Staffs used by protesters: These anti-staph penicillins treat Staph aureus effectively

6. Raised sore on spectator's leg attacked by oxen: Can treat cellulitis (often caused by *S. aureus*)

7. Honey surrounded around mouth of spectator: Can treat impetigo (often caused by *S. aureus*)

8. PB&J sandwich on top of peppermint wall: Bind to PBP (penicillin binding protein)

9. Peppermint paint: Peptidoglycan

10. Oxen hits peppermint wall causing crack: By blocking peptidoglycan cross-linking, these drugs cause lysis of the cell wall

11. Chests of myrrh not near oxen: Cannot treat MRSA

12. People guarding myrrh throwing PB&J sandwiches at oxen: MRSA is resistant to anti-Staph penicillins

13. Spectator trying to cut square hula hoops with scissors, but the hoop is too thick: Anti-staph penicillins are beta lactamase resistant due to the drug's bulky R group

14. Hypersensitivity mural on peppermint wall: Can cause some hypersensitivity reactions

See Figure 9.4.1 - Antibiotics Mechanisms (Antibiotics, Section 1, Page 69)

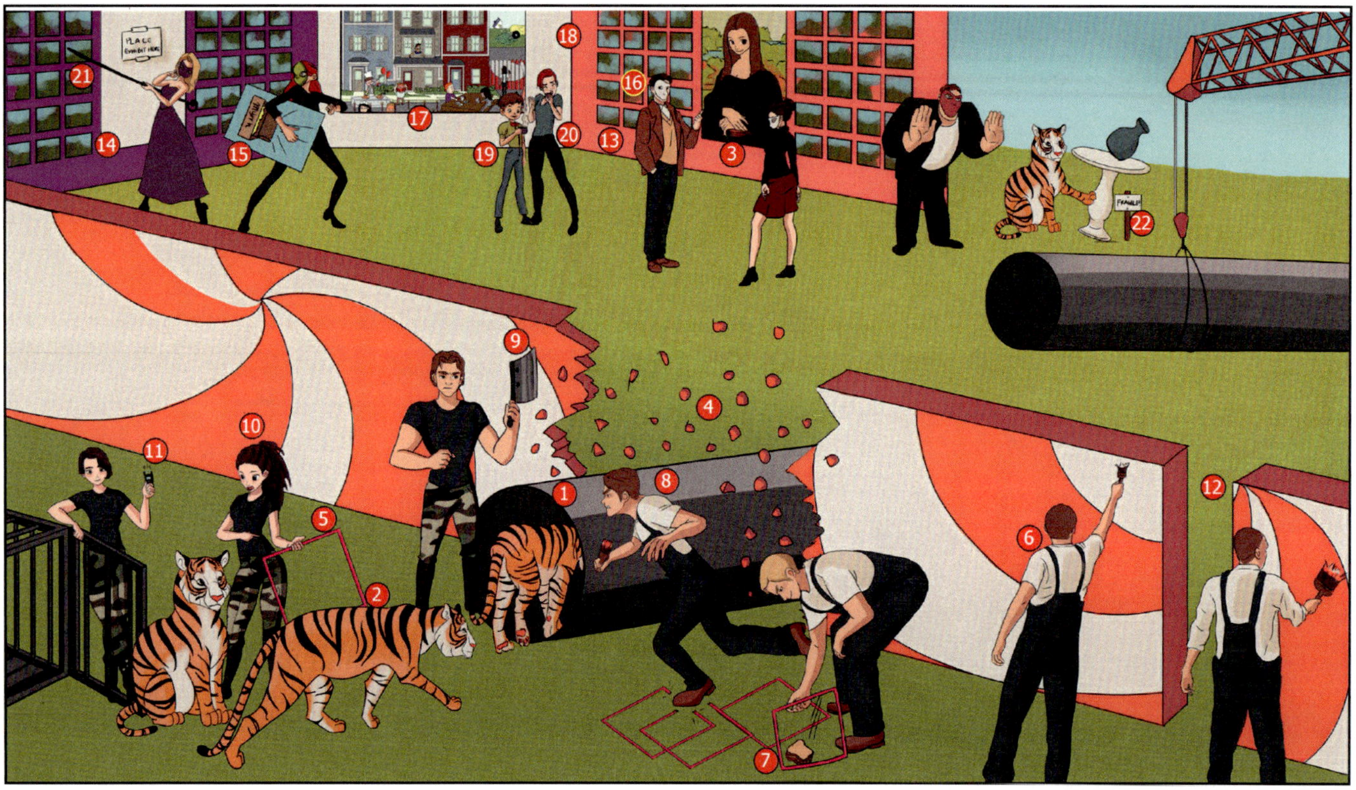

1. Pipe swinging from construction line through peppermint wall: Piperacillin

2. Tigers: Ticarcillin

3. Tigers entering damaged pipe to the Mona Lisa: Piperacillin and ticarcillin are penicillins designed to attach Pseudomonas

4. Pipe crashes into wall, creating red debri enveloping pipe: Piperacillin and ticarcillin can enter porins in gram negative bacteria

5. Soldiers tries to convince tiger to jump into pipe through square hula hoop: Piperacillin and ticarcillin are beta lactams

6. Two painters painting red and white peppermint: Peptidoglycan

7. City worker trying to pick up square hula hoop, but dropped his PB&J: PBP binds the beta lactams

8. City man running towards tiger and breaks square hula hoops on ground: Beta lactamase can destroy beta lactams

9. Soldier with big cleaver next to damaged pipe: Antipseudomonal penicillins can be combined with clavulanic acid (beta lactamase inhibitor)

10. Soldiers wearing camouflage pants: Sulbactam is a beta lactamase inhibitor

11. Soldier releasing tigers with taser: Tazobactam is a beta lactamase inhibitor

12. The painters allow a rift in the wall: Beta lactams kill the bacteria by causing lysis of the cell wall

13. Mona Lisa pinkish wall covered by smaller paintings: Antipseudomonal penicillins cover most gram negative bacteria, including Pseudomonas

14. Purple wall with small paintings: Piperacillin and ticarcillin can cover most gram positive organisms

15. Painting of box of myrrh being stolen off of purple wall: Antipseudomonal penicillins cannot cover MRSA

16. People in gallery are wearing masks: Antipseudomonal penicillins cover anaerobic bacteria

17. White wall with image of hypersensitivity reactions: Antipseudomonal penicillins can cause hypersensitivity reactions

18. Pink and purple walls: Antipseudomonal penicillins are broad-spectrum

19. Young guest sipping on hot chocolate in front of white wall: Can be used for sepsis

20. Taller guest next to hot chocolate coughing from steam: Can be used for pneumonia

21. Guest pointing her staff to purple wall: Piperacillin and ticarcillin treat typical strains Staph. Aureus

22. Tiger knocking over fragile vase next to pink wall: Antipseudomonal penicillins can treat Bacteroides fragilis

See Figure 9.4.1 - Antibiotics Mechanisms (Antibiotics, Section 1, Page 69)

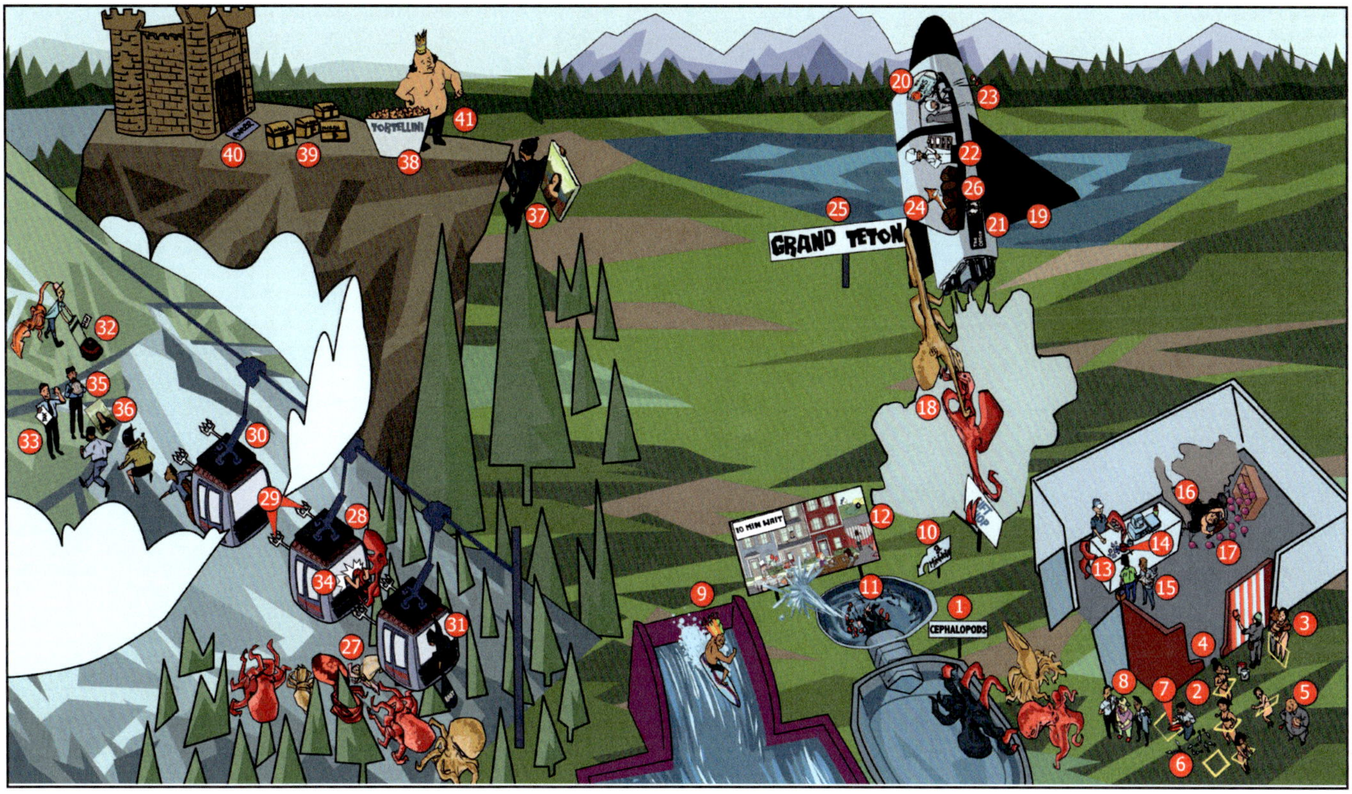

1. Cephalopods escaping tank: Cephalosporins

2. Girls dancing in square hula hoops: Cephalosporins are beta lactams

3. Two painters with PB&J painting peppermint wall and hanging girlfriend: Beta lactams bind to PBP

4. Unfinished brick wall next to hula hoop girls: Binding to PBP prevents peptidoglycan cross-linking, causing cell lysis

5. Overweight painter eating PB&J next to repulsed hula hoop girl: Bacteria can resist beta lactams via altered PBP

6. Owner cutting square hula hoop surrounded by scissor pieces: Cephalosporins are usually resistant to lactamases

7. Owner's big red scissors: most organisms, even gram negative bacteria, do not produce extended spectrum beta lactamases

8. Krusty the clown is handcuffed: Cephalosporins can cause a vitamin K deficiency

9. Dyed hair surfer: Cephalosporins can cause a disulfiram reaction

10. "A minnow" sign next to pond: Aminoglycosides

11. Kidney beans smashed by invasive cephalopod in minnow pond: Cephalosporins cause increased nephrotoxicity with aminoglycosides

12. Splashed water from cephalopod onto hypersensitivity mural with wait time of "10 min": Cephalosporins can cause hypersensitivity reactions in 10% of patients who would develop hypersensitivity reactions when exposed to penicillins

13. Cephalopods in gift shop interfering with sapphire exchange: Cephalexin is a 1st generation cephalosporin

14. Cephalopod steals man's fez hat: Cefazolin is a 1st generation cephalosporin

15. Man in line with small stature of Greek God Proteus: Can treat proteus mirabilis

16. Man in hole covered in coal mine dust with big club: Can treat *E. coli* and klebsiella

17. Coal covered man bumps purple balls: Can treat gram positive cocci, such as Streptococcus and Staphylococcus species

18. Two Cephalopods clinging onto shuttle: 2nd generation cephalosporins

19. Top cephalopods hold onto pterodactyl size wing of shuttle while bottom cephalopod holds onto gift shop sign: 2nd generation cephalosporins cover enterobacter, in addition to organisms covered by 1st generation cephalosporins

20. MARS on screen inside shuttle: Can treat serratia marcescens

21. "The Office" sticker on shuttle: Can treat haemophilus influenzae

22. Chef with knives inside the shuttle: Can treat neisseria infections

23. Apple core thrown out of shuttle: Cefaclor is a 2nd generation cephalosporin

24. Pet fox on shuttle: Cefoxitin is a 2nd generation cephalosporin

25. "Grand Teton" sign: Cefoteton is a 2nd generation cephalosporin

26. Four rocks inside of shuttle: Cefuroxime is a 2nd generation cephalosporin

27. Three gondolas leveled with gift shop: 3rd generation cephalosporins

28. "Gondolas": Can treat Neisseria Gonorrhoeae

29. Two tridents on roofs of gondolas: Ceftriaxone is a 3rd generation cephalosporin

30. Gondolas emerge through clouds: 3rd generation cephalosporins can cross the blood brain barrier

31. Burglar entering in first gondola: Can treat Borrelia burgdorferi (Lyme disease)

32. Cephalopod removing hat off of man with new mower near highest gondola: Can treat strep: pneumoniae, and meningitis

33. Tax Collector greeting people off gondola: Cefotaxime is a 3rd generation cephalosporin

34. Feet being grabbed by cephalopod on gondola: Cefpodoxime is a 3rd generation cephalosporin

35. Man tasting dime: Ceftazadime is a 3rd generation cephalosporin

36. Dime taster holding Mona Lisa painting: Ceftazadime can treat pseudomonas infections

37. Bandit with Mona Lisa painting on pine tree: Cefepime is a 4th generation cephalosporin used primarily for pseudomonas

38. Fat man with crown eating huge bowl of tortellini: Ceftaroline is a 5th generation cephalosporin

39. Chests of myrrh next to fat man with tortellini: Ceftaroline can treat MRSA

40. "Enter" mat in front of castle: Ceftraoline can treat Enterococcus

41. Fat man with tortellini rejecting bandit: Ceftaroline does not cover pseudomonas infections

See Figure 9.4.1 - Antibiotics Mechanisms (Antibiotics, Section 1, Page 69)

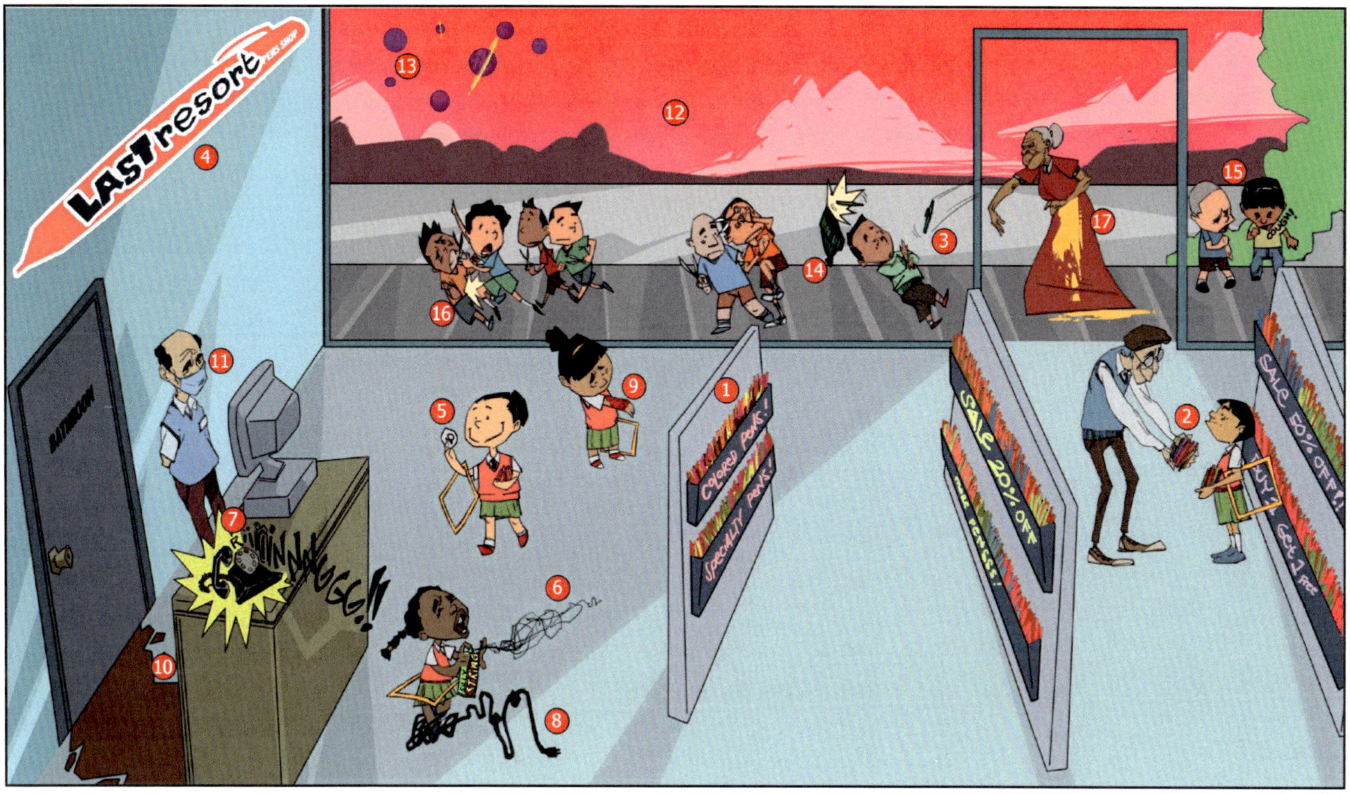

1. Pens: Carbapenems

2. Square hula hoop: carbapenems are beta beta lactams

3. Old woman resisting the hooligans by throwing pens: Resistant to beta lactamases

4. "Last Resort" pen shop: Use carbapenems as a last resort

5. DIME: Doripenem, Imipenem, Meropemen and Ertapenem

6. Silly string: Take with cilastatin

7. Shaking phone: Can cause seizures

8. Cords shaped like a nephron: Dehydropeptidase I in the nephron can deactivate carbapenems (prevent this with cilastatin)

9. Rash: Carbapenems can cause a rash

10. Diarrhea: Can cause GI distress

11. Hospital face mask: Covers anaerobes

12. Red and pink sky: Covers gram negative rods

13. Purple planets: Covers gram positive cocci

14. Pen knocking beanie off of head: Can be used for meningitis

15. Smoke causing kids to cough: Can be used for pneumonia

16. Painful blow to the gut: Can be used for intra-abdominal infections

17. Urine on crotch: Can be used for UTIs

See Figure 9.4.1 - Antibiotics Mechanisms (Antibiotics, Section 1, Page 69)

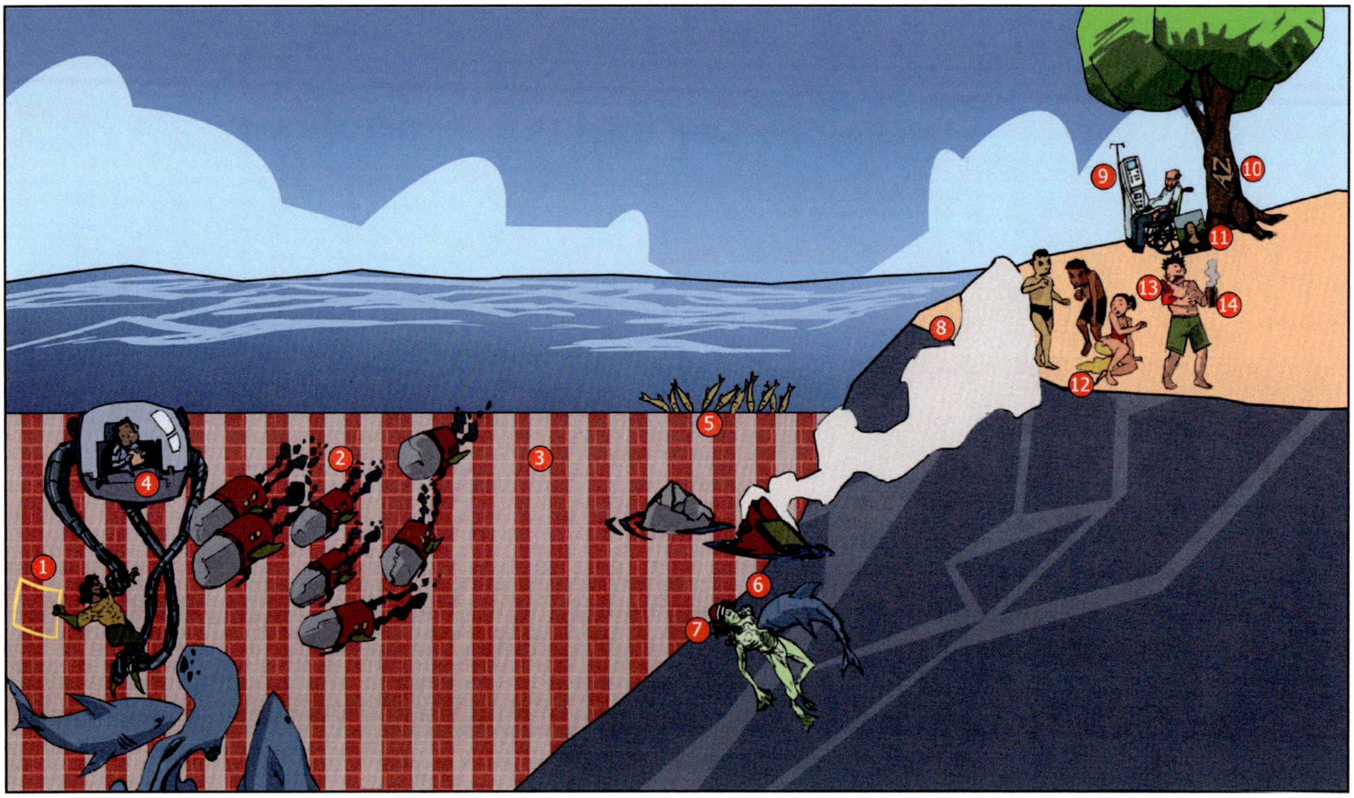

1. Aquatic man carrying one square hula hoop: Monobactams

2. Red underwater ships fight off aquatic man: Monobactams work against gram negative bacteria

3. Aquatic man attempting to breach peppermint wall: monobactams target the peptidoglycan within the cell wall

4. PB&J eating pilot in pod with 3 tentacles in front of peppermint wall: monobactams target penicillin-binding 3 (PBP-3) to prevent peptidoglycan cross-linking

5. Minnows trying to break the wall: monobactams work synergistically with aminoglycosides

6. Shark tearing up insides of pilot: Can be used for intra-abdominal infections

7. Dead pilot's helmet: Can be used to treat meningitis

8. Smoke causing breach goers to cough: Can be used to treat pneumonia

9. Old man with dialysis machine: Can be used in patients with renal insufficiency

10. "AZ" letters on love tree: Azteronam is the primary monobactam used clinically

11. Mona Lisa painting next to old man: Can be used to treat pseudomonas aeruginosa

12. Girl urinating herself next to coughing beach goers: Can be used to treat urinary tract infections

13. Red shrapnel metal burns man's arm: Can be used to treat gram negative skin infections

14. Burned man sipping hot drink: Can be used for gram negative sepsis

See Figure 9.4.1 - Antibiotics Mechanisms (Antibiotics, Section 1, Page 69)

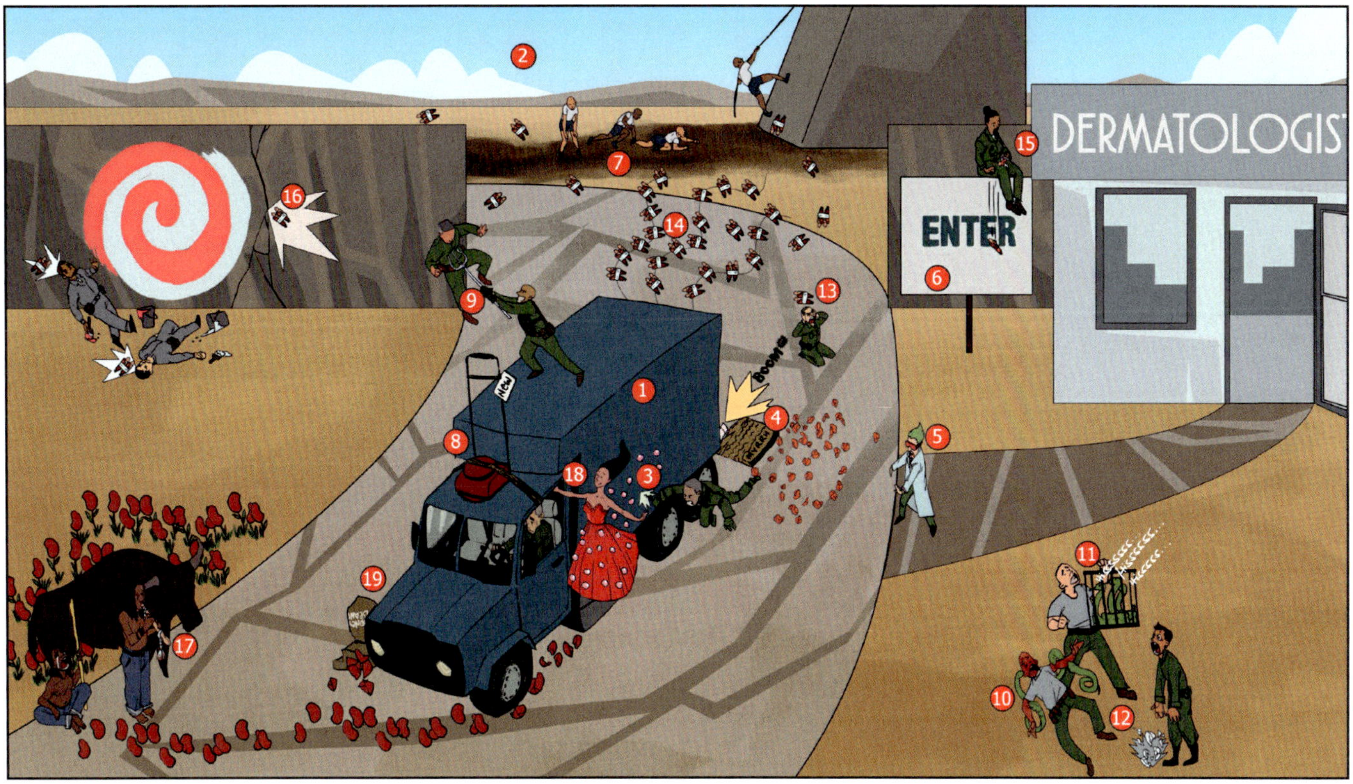

1. Van: Vancomycin

2. Purple van and sky: Vancomycin covers gram positive organisms

3. Van destroys scissors: Vancomycin is resistant to beta lactamases

4. Chest of myrrh crushed by van: Vancomycin treats MRSA

5. Animal dermatologist: Vancomycin treats Staph. Epidermidis

6. Enter sign: Vancomycin treats Enterococcus spp.

7. Difficult training camp: Vancomycin treats C. difficile

8. New lawnmower: Vancomycin treats S. pneumoniae

9. Trident fending off officer with hat: Vancomycin is given with ceftriaxone empirically for bacterial meningitis

10. Hissing snakes biting man causing him to turn red: Histamine can cause mast cell degranulation, which can cause red man syndrome (flushing)

11. Locked up hissing snakes: Flushing can be prevented with antihistamines

12. Shattered plates: Vancomycin can cause thrombocytopenia

13. Military officer holding ears in agony following the loud burst: Vancomycin can cause ototoxicity

14. Dalai Lama statues in pairs trailing the van: Vancomycin works by binding to D-Ala-D-Ala

15. Single Dalai Lama resting on top of girl on enter sign: Enterococcus can develop vancomycin resistance by substituting D-Ala-D-Lac

16. Peppermint style mural on cracked wall: Vancomycin works by inhibiting cell wall peptidoglycan formation

17. An ox, a man playing a flute, and a man holding a staff: Vancomycin should be downgraded to nafcillin or oxacillin in patients infected with a sensitive strain of Staph aureus (MSSA)

18. Dress with pink eosinophile sequins: Vancomycin can cause DRESS syndrome which is marked by eosinophilia

19. Scattered and damaged kidney beans: Vancomycin is nephrotoxic

See Figure 9.4.1 - Antibiotics Mechanisms (Antibiotics, Section 1, Page 69)

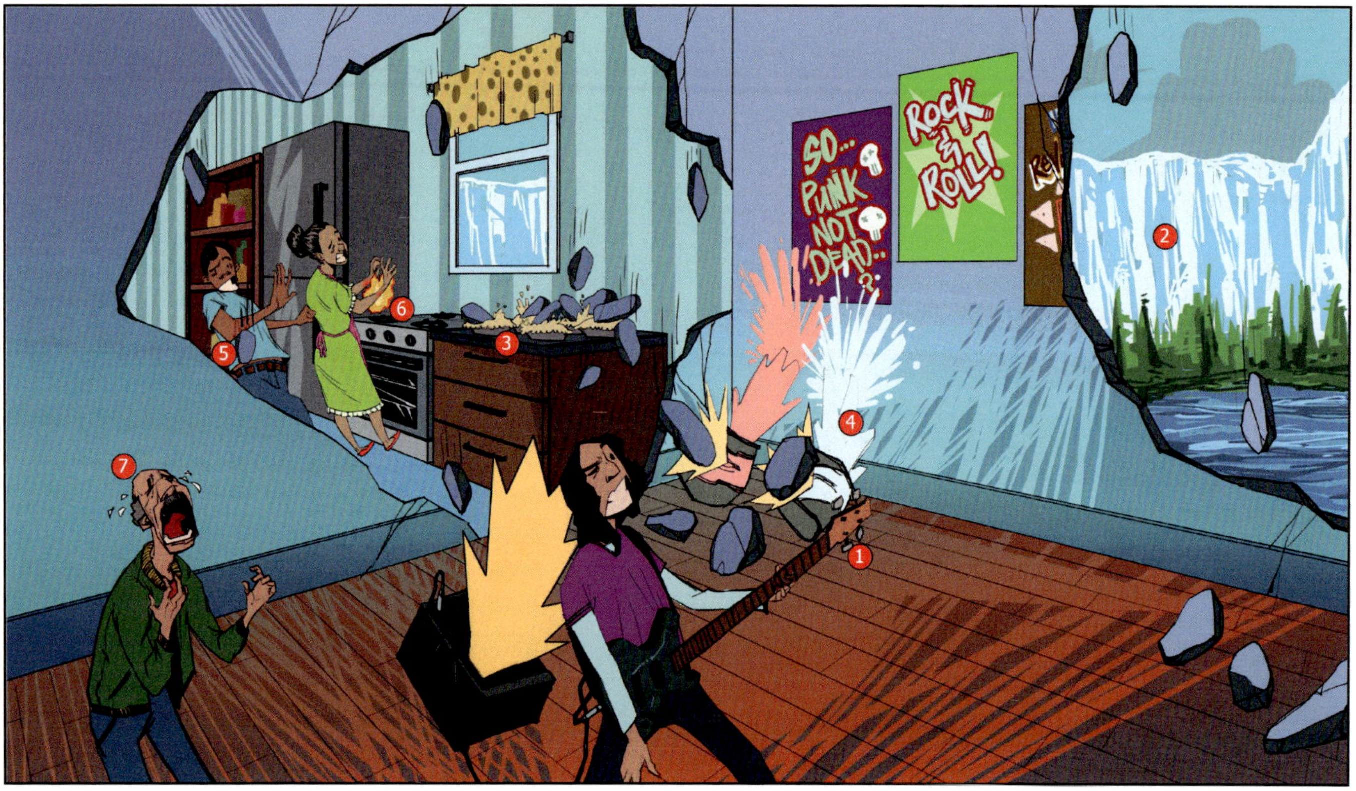

1. Bass guitar: Bacitracin

2. Glacier outside of house: Streptococcus agalactiae is bacitracin-resistant

3. Pie getting destroyed: Streptococcus pyogenes is bacitracin-resistant

4. White and pink paint near broken wall: Prevents peptidoglycan synthesis which disrupts the bacterial cell wall

5. Scrape on arm: Use for minor cuts and scrapes

6. Burned by stove top: Use for minor burns

7. Dad crying: May cause hypersensitivity reactions

See Figure 9.4.1 - Antibiotics Mechanisms (Antibiotics, Section 1, Page 69)

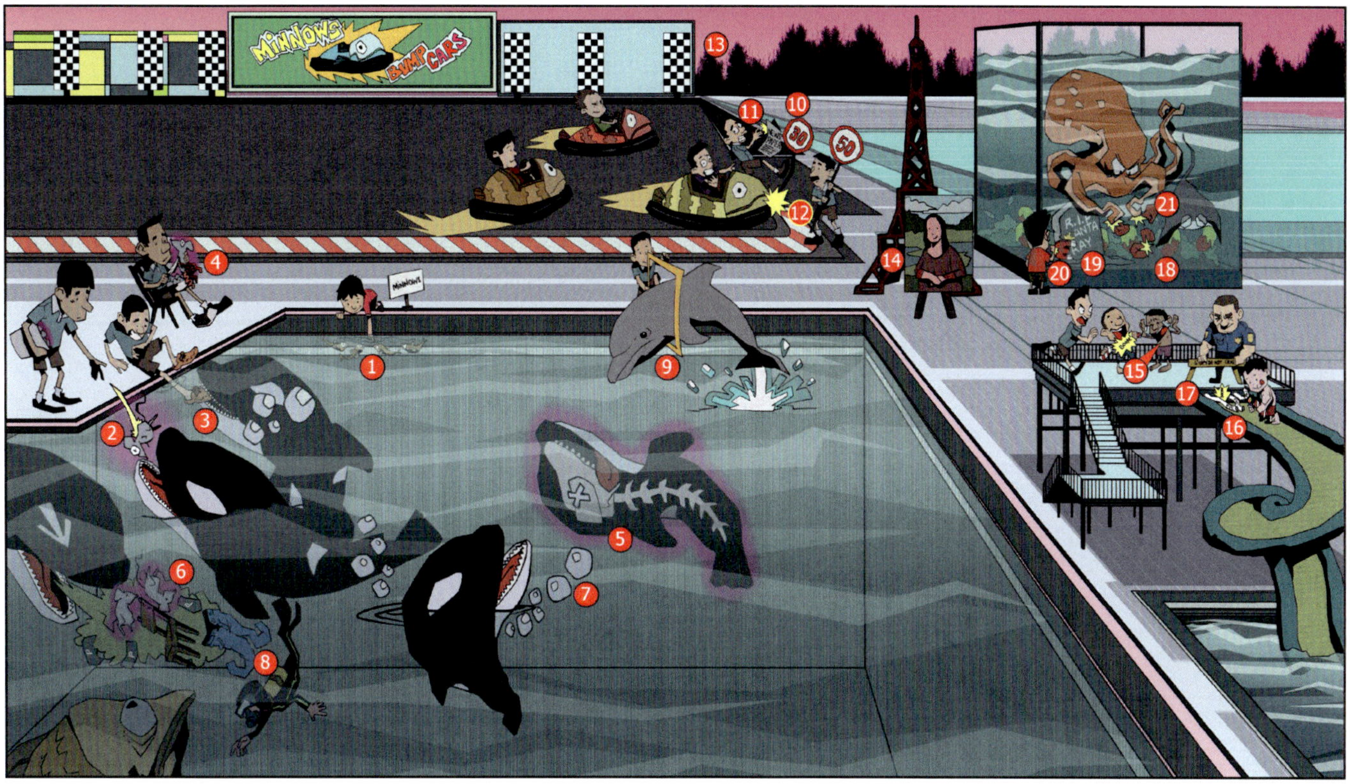

1. Minnows: Aminoglycosides

2. Toxic purple mice being fed to whale: Most aminoglycoside drug names end with the suffix "-mycin"

3. Moccasins being eaten by whale: Aminkacin

4. Knife cut, spilling toxic mouse guts on chair man's knees: Neomycin can be used for bowel surgery

5. Dead poisoned whale with purple aura: Aminoglycosides are bactericidal

6. Whale self-induced vomiting and vomits purple mice, chair, tickets with the letter "P", and denim jeans: Bacteria develop resistance to aminoglycosides via phosphorylation, acetylation, or adenylation of the drug

7. Oxygen bubbles: Aminoglycosides require O_2 for uptake

8. Fish and scuba diver with mask at bottom can't get mice: Are ineffective against anaerobes

9. Dolphins jump out of water through square hula hoops: Are synergistic with beta-lactam antibiotics

10. Bumper cars decorated in minnow fish with one bumper car hitting 30 MPH sign: Inhibit the 30S ribosomal subunit

11. Employee reading by sign disrupted from his newspaper: Directly disrupts the ability of the organism to read mRNA

12. Company man tries to change 30MPH sign for 50 MPH, but kid won't move and sticks out all 5 fingers: Inhibit formation of the initiation complex

13. Pink sky in background: Can be used for severe gram negative rod infections

14. Mona Lisa near the mini Eiffel tower: Can be used to treat pseudomonas and francisella

15. Kid covering his ears from exploding firework on loopy water slide: Risk of aminoglycoside-induced ototoxicity is increased when combined with loop diuretics

16. Firecracker explosion causes PVC pipe to break apart at start of loopy water slide: Are nephrotoxic and most commonly damage the proximal convoluted tubule

17. Buff policeman sets up blockade in front of water slide: May cause neuromuscular blockade

18. Kidney bean plants covered in green goop in fish tank: Nephrotoxic

19. Gravestone in tank: Contraindicated among patients who have myasthenia gravis

20. Falling "M" magnet on grave because kid pounds on tank: Can cause hypomagnesemia

21. Octopus destroys kidney bean plants in tank: Increased nephrotoxicity when used with cephalosporins

See Figure 9.4.1 - Antibiotics mechanisms (Antibiotics, Section 1, Page 69)

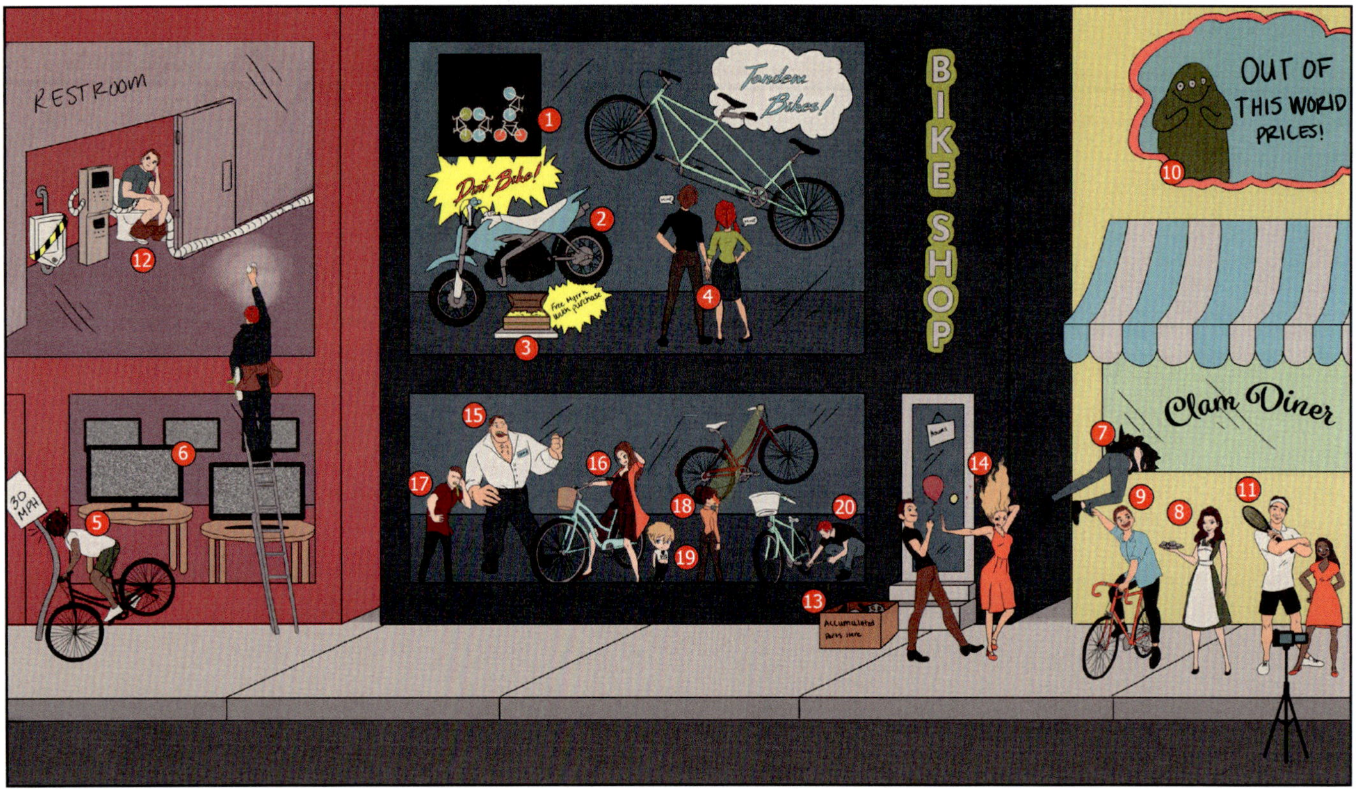

1. Tetris bicycle picture: Tetracycline

2. Dirt bike: Doxycycline

3. Open chest of myrrh under dirt bike: Doxycycline can be used for MRSA infections

4. "The bicycle is mine": Minocycle

5. Boy on bike crashing into 30 MPH speed limit sign: Tetracyclines bind to 30S ribosome and prevents attachment of aminoacyl-tRNA

6. Static televisions: Tetracyclines are bacteriostatic

7. Burglar being grabbed by man on bike: Tetracyclines are used to treat lyme disease, or *Borrelia burgdorferi*

8. Clams being held by woman: Tetracyclines are used for Chlamydia

9. Acne on burglar-catching man: Tetracyclines are used to treat acne

10. Green, plasma-filled alien on sign: Tetracyclines are used to treat Mycoplasma

11. Tennis racquet held by tennis player next to clams: Tetracyclines are used to treat *Rickettsia* species

12. Man with dialysis machine using toilet next to closed off urinal: Tetracyclines are eliminated through stool, not urine (i.e. safe in renal failure)

13. Accumulated bicycle parts inside box in front of bike shop: Accumulates inside cells, making these drugs effective at dealing with intracellular pathogens

14. Girl avoiding boyfriend with "plus sign" shape, sparkles falling out of static hair: Avoid cations within 2 hours of taking these medications

15. Salesman on bottom floor with discolored teeth: Tetracyclines can cause teeth discoloration

16. Pregnant woman told to get off of bike: Tetracyclines should be avoided in pregnancy

17. Vomiting man by salesman: Tetracyclines can cause vomiting and GI distress

18. Light shining off bike, causing skin to burn: Tetracyclines can cause photosensitivity

19. Kid wearing shrunk skull and crossbones shirt: Tetracyclines can inhibit bone growth in kids

20. Air coming out of bike tire on bottom floor: Bacteria can resist tetracyclines through efflux or influx pumps

See Figure 9.4.1 - Antibiotics Mechanisms (Antibiotics, Section 1, Page 69)

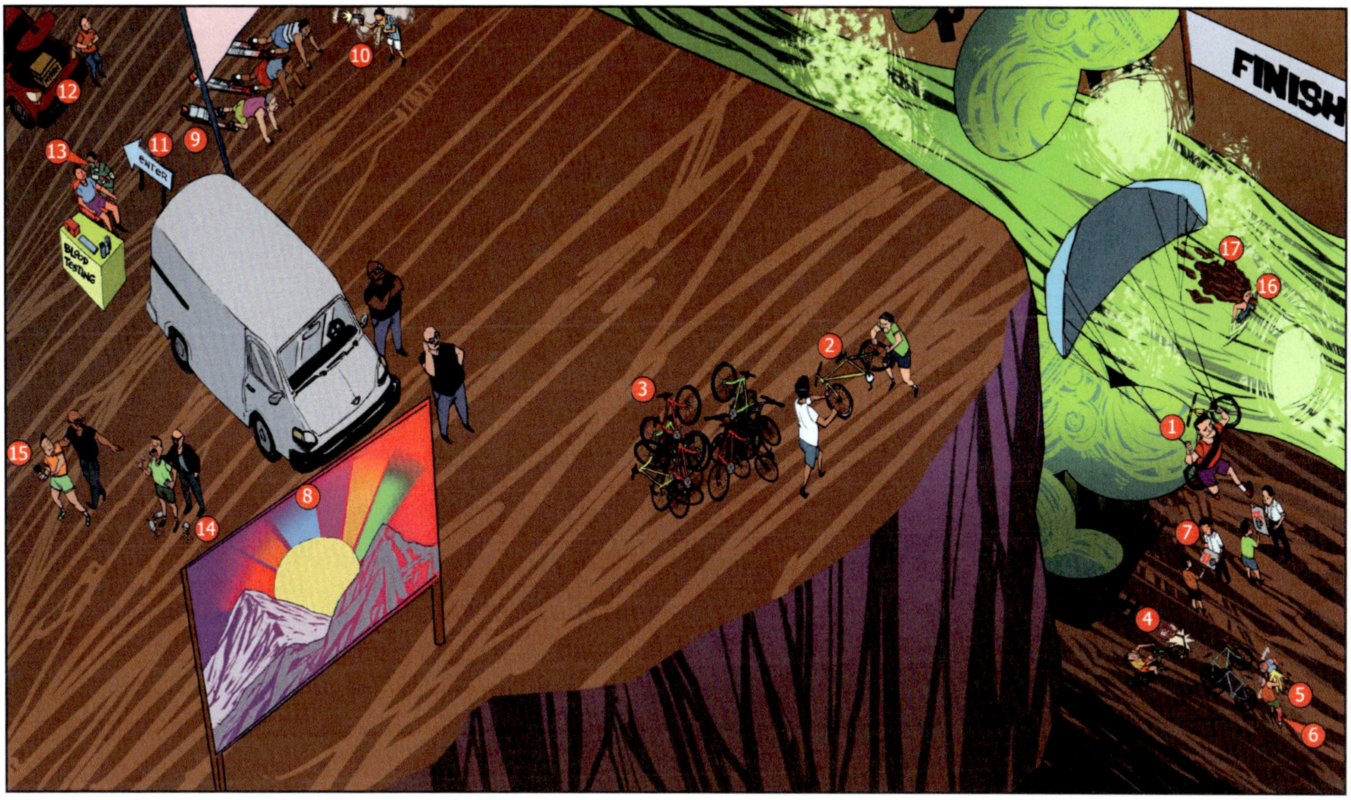

1. Gliding with a cycle: Glycylcyclines

2. Tugging the cycle: Tigecycline

3. Bikes stacked like the tetris game: A tetracycline derivative

4. Knocked over "30" speed limit sign: Binds to the 30S ribosomal subunit

5. Punching in the abdomen: Use for intra-abdominal infections

6. Scraped leg: Use for complicated skin infections requiring deep penetration

7. Death waivers with skulls: U.S. boxed warning on tigecycline (increase mortality)

8. Sunset with a mix of red and purple colors: Broad spectrum coverage included gram-negative and gram-positive organisms

9. Contestants holding completely still: Bacteriostatic

10. Cough: Used to treat pneumonia

11. Security guards by van and enter sign: Used to treat vancomycin-resistant Enterococcus

12. Myrrh chest: Used to treat MRSA infections

13. Mask: Anaerobic coverage

14. Bottles of pills: Use for multidrug-resistant organisms

15. Guy with protein bar being rejected: Inhibit protein synthesis

16. Vomit: May cause nausea and vomiting

17. Brown watery river: May cause diarrhea

See Figure 9.4.1 - Antibiotics Mechanisms (Antibiotics, Section 1, Page 69)

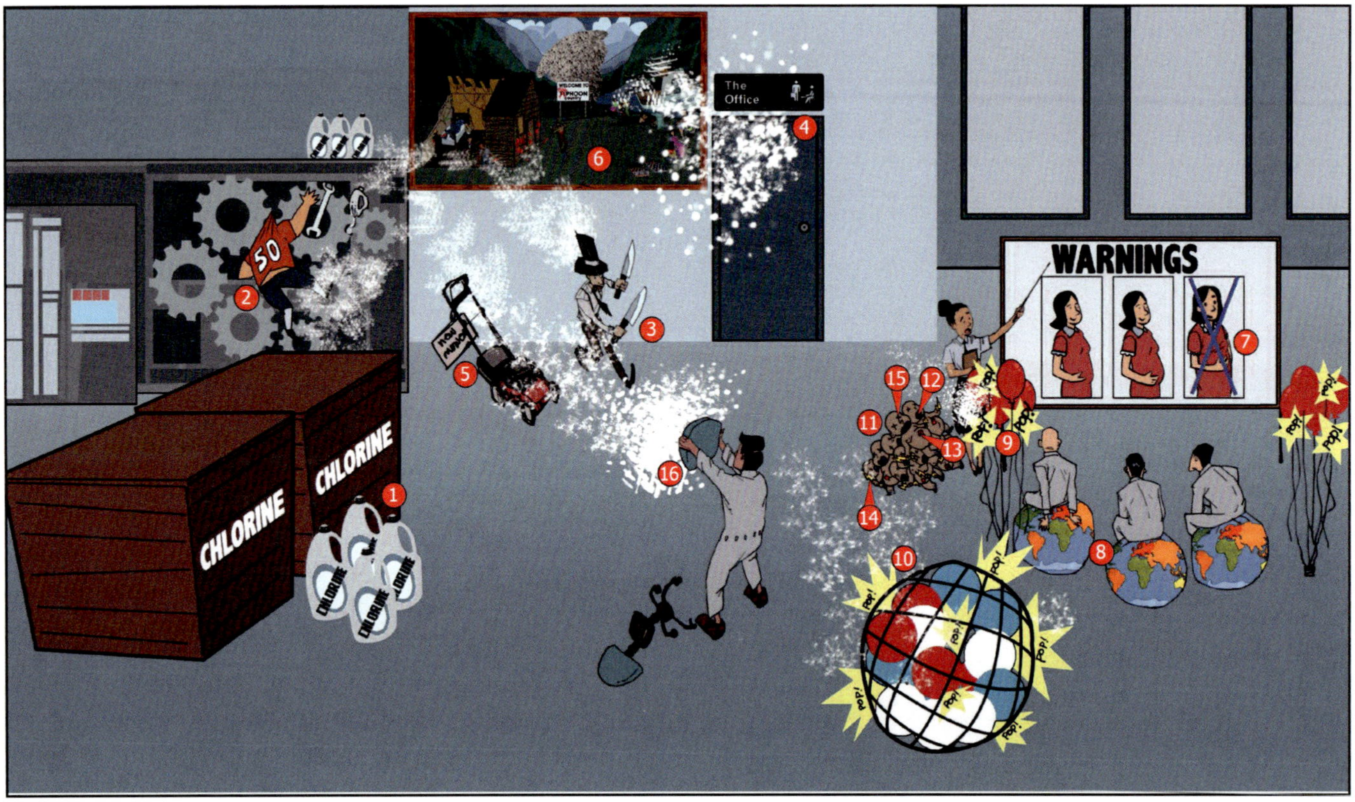

1. Chlorine: Chloramphenicol

2. Mauled player wearing the number 50 jersey: Blocks the 50S ribosomal subunit

3. Knives and hat: Used to treat neisseria meningitidis

4. Office sign: Can treat *Haemophilus influenzae*

5. New mower: Treats *S. pneumoniae*

6. Rocky Mountain painting: Treats Rickettsial diseases

7. Third column of sign: Do not use in 3rd trimester of pregnancy

8. Blow-up globes: Used predominantly in developing countries

9. Popping red balloons: Anemia is a side effect of chloramphenicol

10. Net containing balloons: Can cause aplastic anemia

11. Gray, stuffed babies: Can cause gray baby syndrome

12. Dark blue lips: Cyanosis can occur in infants exposed to chloramphenicol in utero

13. Belly rubies: Bilirubin metabolism is immature in infants due to decreased activity of UDP-glucuronosyltransferase

14. Lightning bolts: Gray baby syndrome can present with shock

15. Xs over eyes: Gray baby syndrome can cause death

16. Seat transferred from the chair to shield against the chlorine: Resistance via plasmid-encoded acetyltransferase inactivates the drug

See Figure 9.4.1 - Antibiotics Mechanisms (Antibiotics, Section 1, Page 69)

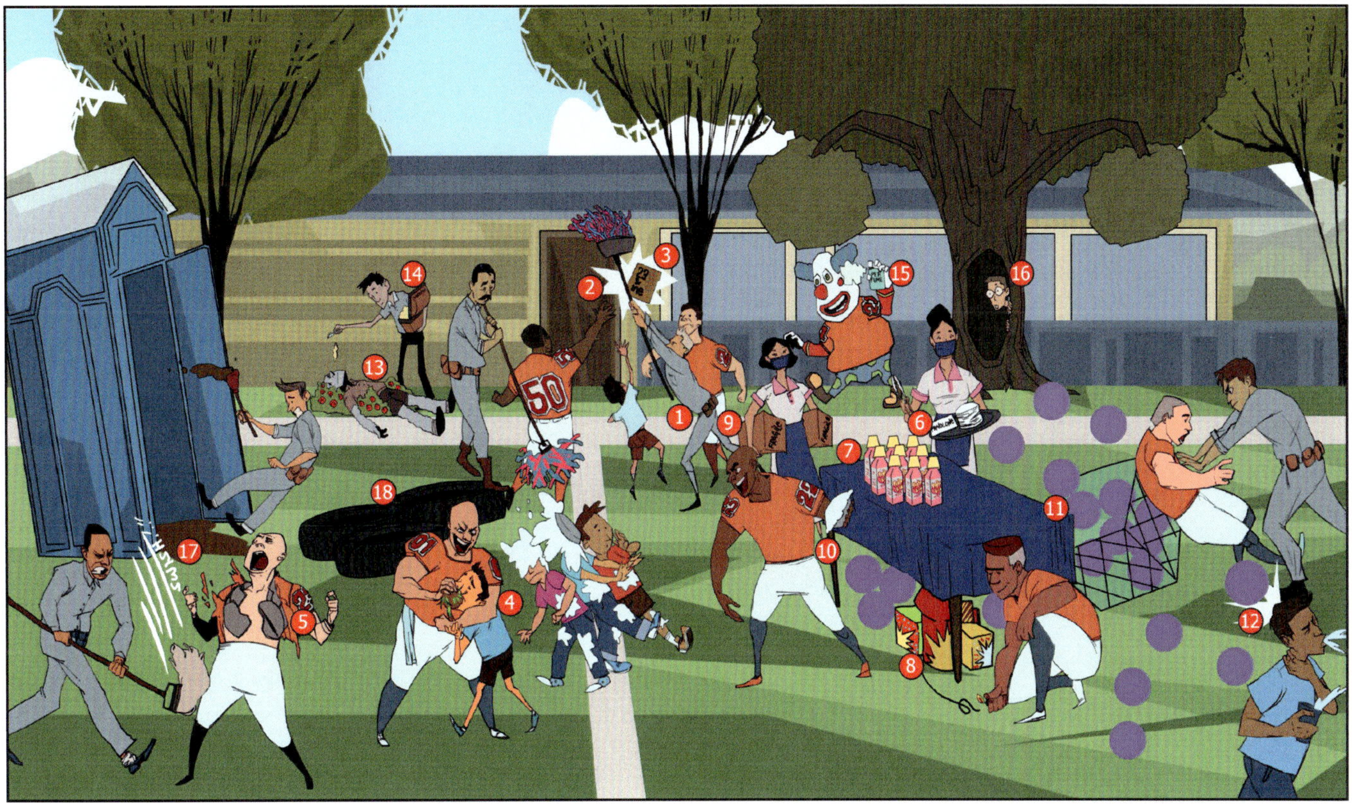

1. Cleaner: Clindamycin

2. Cleaning man blocking throw from the player with the "50" on his jersey: Clindamycin blocks translocation at the larger ribosome (50S ribosome)

3. Blocking the "23 & Me" notebook: Clindamycin binds to 23S rRNA of 50S ribosome

4. Grass and dirt in mouth: Used for anaerobic oral infections

5. Football pads shaped like lungs: Can be used for lung abscesses

6. School cafeteria worker serving provolone cheese: Clindamycin can treat *Prevotella species*

7. Pepto Bismol: Can treat *Peptostreptococcus species*

8. Lighting the fuse: Can treat *Fusobacterium species*

9. Boxes labeled "Fragile": Can treat *Bacteroides fragilis*

10. Pie splattering all over kids: Can be used for invasive *Strep pyogenes*

11. Dodgeball spilling: Used for gram positive cocci

12. Kid hit in the head right as he was drinking: Can be used to treat aspiration pneumonia

13. Garden with decomposing stippling body similar to clue cell: Can treat *gardnerella vaginalis*

14. Cleaning man sprinkles decomposing body with myrrh: Can treat MRSA

15. Clown spraying perfume: Can treat *clostridium perfringens*

16. Guy hiding in hollow tree trunk with two large tree branches: Can be used for endometritis

17. Diarrhea spraying all over from portable restroom: Can cause diarrhea

18. Cleaning man falling into tires: Can cause pseudomembranous colitis

See Figure 9.4.1 - Antibiotics Mechanisms (Antibiotics, Section 1, Page 69)

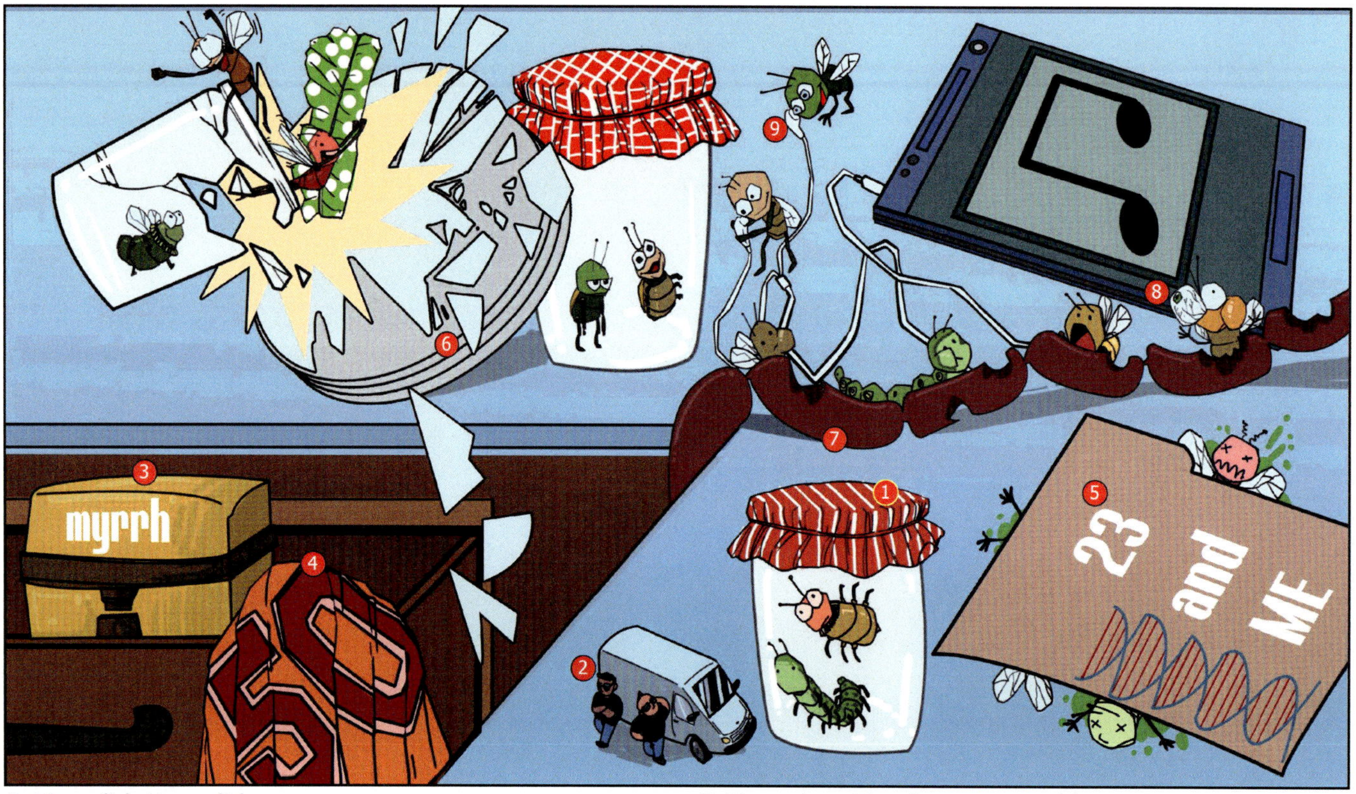

1. Linen lid: Linezolid

2. Toy van with two toy bodyguards: Used to treat vancomycin-resistant organisms

3. Chest of myrrh in drawer: Used to treat MRSA

4. Dirty football jersey with the number "50" on it: Works by blocking the activity of the 50S ribosomal subunit of bacteria

5. Folder that reads "23 and Me" that has squished some of the bugs: Bacteria can develop resistance to linezolid through point mutations on the 23S rRNA gene which prevents binding to the 50S ribosome

6. Plates breaking from escaped bugs: Can cause thrombocytopenia

7. Neuron-like sausage links being eaten by bugs: Can cause peripheral neuropathy

8. Bulging eyes of bug eating sausage link: Can cause optic neuropathy

9. Two bugs sharing a tune: Can cause serotonin syndrome

See Figure 9.4.1 - Antibiotics Mechanisms (Antibiotics, Section 1, Page 69)

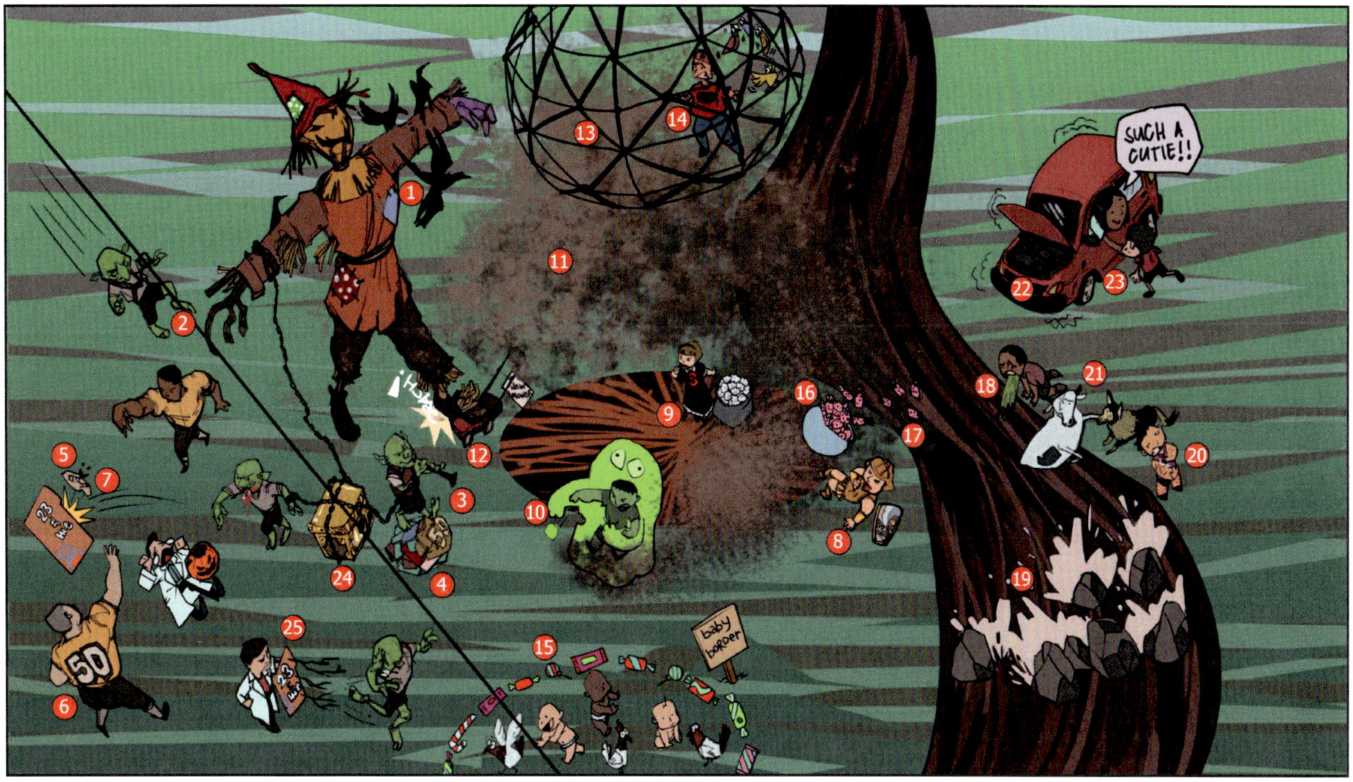

1. Crows and scarecrow: Macrolides

2. Zip line with goblin: azithromycin

3. Clarinet being played by goblin: Clarithormycin is a macrolide

4. Clarinet playing goblin on top of pile of dirty jerseys: Clarithrobycin can treat H. pylori

5. "Ear throw" by goblin next to clarinet: Erythromycin

6. #50 footballer throwing "23 and Me" binder, and ear knocking binder off course: Macrolides bind to the 23S rRNA on the 50S ribosomal subunit

7. Binder set off course by colliding ear: By blocking translocation, macrolides halt protein production

8. Kid in the pit dressed like solider from Roman legion: Macrolides can treat legionella

9. Little girl with "S" on her shirt standing next to bag of clams in the pit: Macrolides can treat STI chlamydia

10. Plasma looking alien: Macrolides can treat mycoplasma

11. Three costumed children coughing from giant dirt cloud: Macrolides can treat atypical pneumonia

12. New mower near scarecrow: Macrolides treat Strep pneumoniae

13. aviary near scarecrow containing man and birds: Macrolides can treat Mycobacterium avium-intracellulare (MAC)

14. Man with band-aid on his head in aviary wearing 50 United States shirt: Prophylactically administer macrolides to AIDS patients if $CD4^{+}$ counts are < 50

15. Babies and hens surrounded by border of candy: Macrolides can treat Babesia. bordetella pertussis, and bartonella henselae

16. Little round pink candies spilled by Roman solider: Macrolides can cause eosinophilia

17. Muddy river: Macrolides can cause diarrhea

18. Vomiting kid near river: Macrolides can cause nausea

19. Waves in river violently crashing against rocks: Macrolides can cause motility issues

20. Scraped arms and red wounds of kid near vomit: Macrolides can cause a maculopapular rash

21. Collie saving the liver-spotted cow from drowning: Cholestatic hepatitis

22. Shaking car owned by woman saying, "Such a cutie!!": Macrolides can cause cardiac arrhythmia

23. Kid getting face stretched by woman calling him a cutie: Causes QT prolongation

24. Pandora's box between clarinet playing and ear-throwing goblins: Clarithromybin and erythromycin inhibit cytochrome P-450

25. Sticks in the other "23 and Me" binder chasing away goblin: Methylation of 23S rRNA makes bacteria resistant to macrolides

See Figure 9.4.1 - Antibiotics Mechanisms (Antibiotics, Section 1, Page 69)

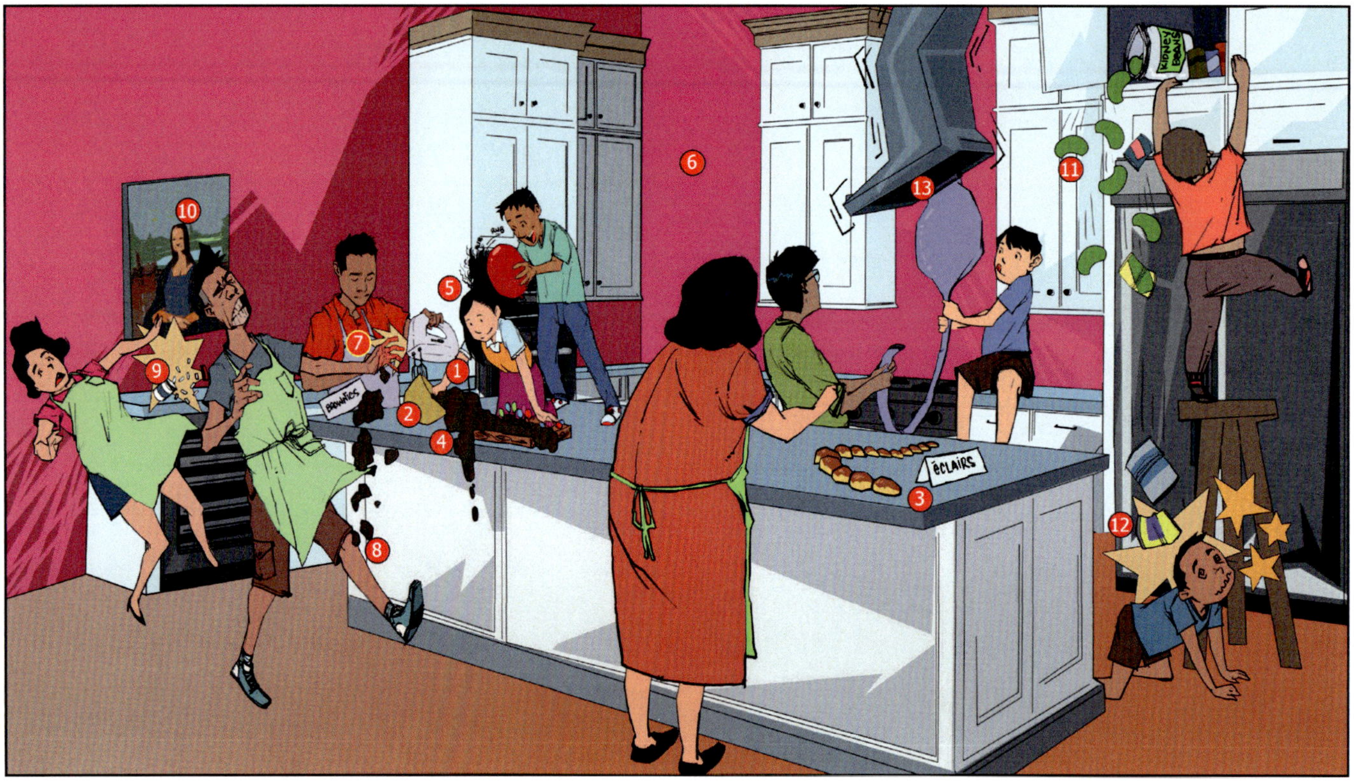

1. Mixer: Polymyxins

2. Mixing brownies: Polymyxin B

3. Eclairs: Colistin (polymyxin E)

4. Dum dums that resemble phospholipids and brownie batter leaking: Binds to phospholipids on the cell membrane → disruption of cell membrane → leakage of cellular contents → cell death

5. Boy rubbing balloon on sister's hair: Polymyxins are cation polypeptides

6. Pink walls: Use for gram-negative bacteria

7. Guy getting hand caught in mixer: Use for superficial skin infections

8. Brownie batter landing on knee: Polymyxin B is a component of triple antibiotic ointment (e.g. Neosporin)

9. Girl slipping and knocking over pills: Use for gram-negative multidrug-resistant bacteria

10. Mona Lisa: Use to treat Pseudomonas

11. Jar of kidney beans: May cause nephrotoxicity

12. Cans fallon on head: May cause neurotoxicity (e.g. slurred speech, weakness)

13. Hose sucking up air and shaking: May cause bronchospasm

See Figure 9.4.1 - Antibiotics Mechanisms (Antibiotics, Section 1, Page 69)

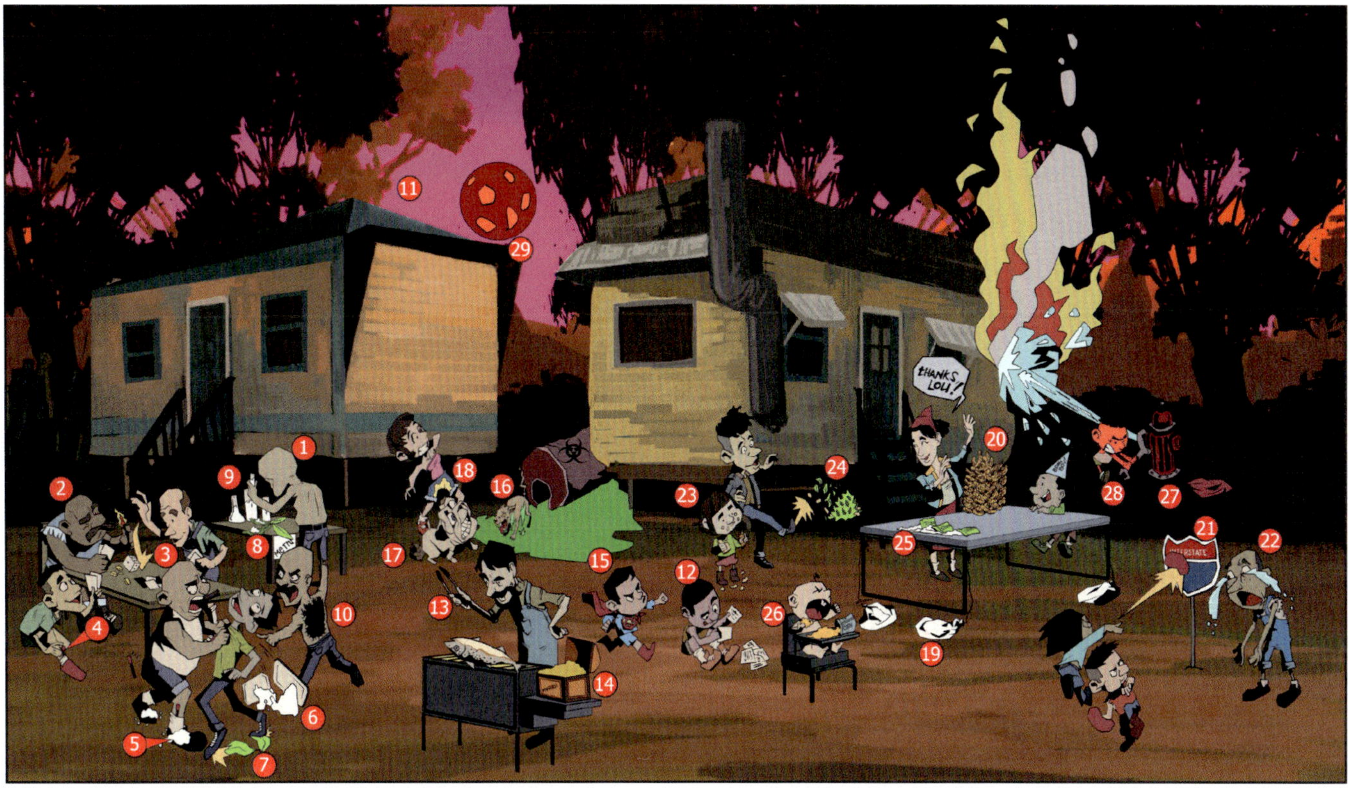

1. Table labeled "Meth": Trimethoprim (TMP)

2. Sulfur match mustache man is using: Sulfonamide

3. Dice rolled near sulfur match: Sulfadiazine

4. Sulfur match in man's socks: Sulfisoxazole

5. Meth spilled on sock because of dropped sulfur match: Sulfamethoxazole

6. Man grabs high meth user causing him to drop 2 trays of meth: Sulfonamides inhibit dihydropteroate synthase

7. High meth user steps on two leaves of foliage: Sulfonamides prevent the formation of dihydrofolic acid (DHF)

8. Two of four pieces of foliage on "Meth" table have meth on them: Trimethoprim inhibits dihydrofolate reductase

9. Foliage's congruent pattern of 4 is ruined on "Meth table": Trimethoprim prevents the formation of tetrahydrofolate (THF)

10. Man who needs a back-trim pointing at "Meth" table and meth sock: Bactrim is the name for TMP and SMX combined

11. Sky shade of purple at the top and pink towards the horizon: Use for gram positive and gram negative bacteria

12. Note cards being used by kid: Use for Nocardia

13. Salmon being grilled: Use for salmonella

14. Chest of myrrh next to grilled salmon: Use for MRSA

15. Kid dressed up as superman/hero: Use for pneumocystis jiroveci (PCP)

16. Toxic green ooze covering feral cat: Use for toxoplasmosis prophylaxis

17. Dog shit near green ooze: Use for shigella

18. Urine on meth cook wive's pants: Use for UTIs

19. Deflated white balloons tied to party table: Can cause leukopenia

20. Pile of free birthday bananas on party table: Can cause hyperkalemia

21. Kidney bean destruction on interstate sign: Can cause interstitial nephritis

22. Crying man next to interstate sign: Can cause hypersensitivity reactions

23. Grains falling from sister's mouth next to party table: Can cause low granulocytes (granulocytopenia)

24. Lou covers scatters grains under foliage: Leucovorin (form of folic acid) prevents granulocytopenia

25. Stevia on party table: Can cause Steven-Johnson syndrome

26. Angry baby's neck covered in corn: Kemicterus

27. Deflated red balloon tied to hydrant can cause hemolysis in patients with G6PD deficiency

28. Super red and sunburnt kid near hydrant: Causes photosensitivity

29. Blood moon: Can cause megaloblastic anemia

See Figure 9.4.1 - Antibiotics Mechanisms (Antibiotics, Section 1, Page 69)

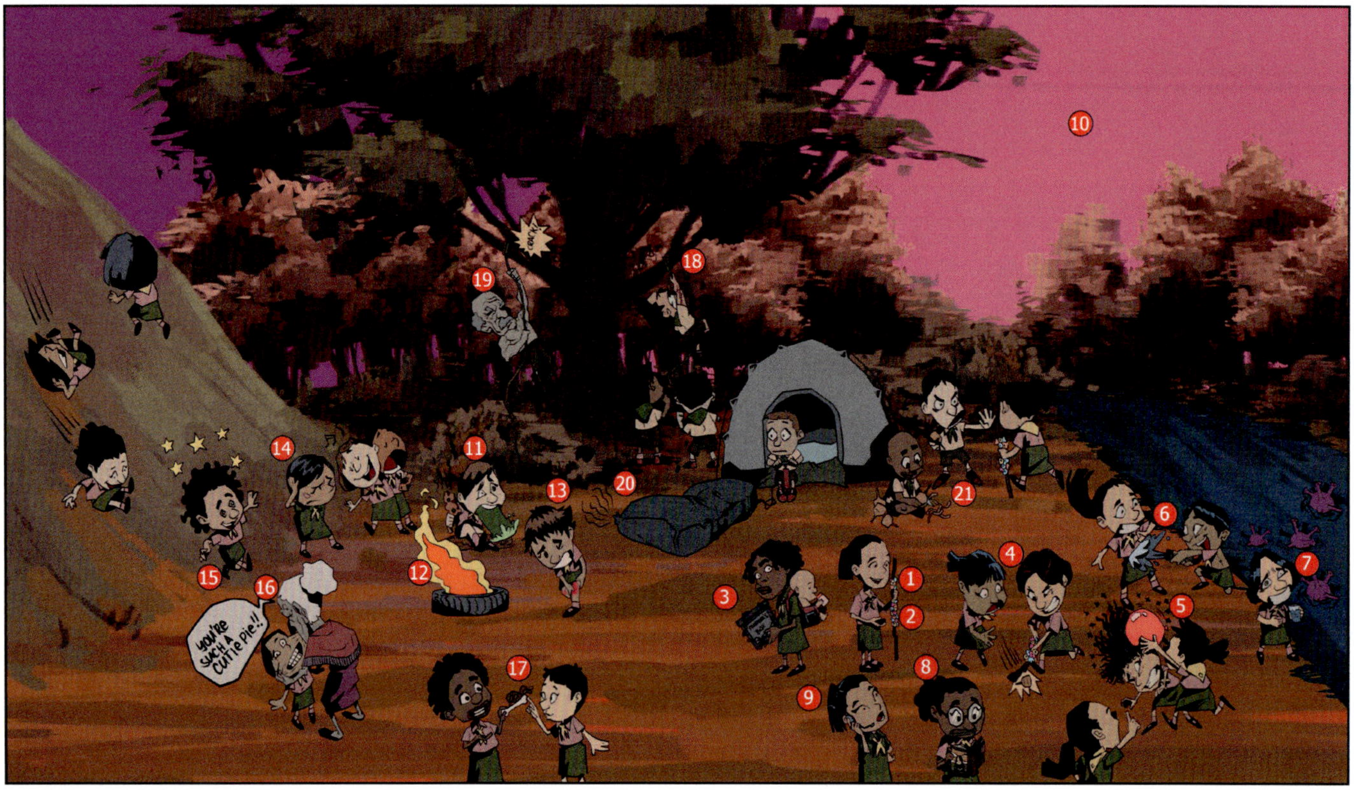

1. Flower staff: Fluoroquinolones

2. Flower: Most fluoroquinolones drug names end with the suffix "floxacillin" (e.g. ciprofloxacin, norfloxacin, ofloxacin, gemifloxacin, levofloxacin, moxifloxacin)

3. Girl scout carrying Pandora's Box covered in chains with toddler drinking juice from a sippy on her back: Ciprofloxacin is a CYP-450 inhibitor

4. Spinning top: Ciprofloxacin is a CYP-450 inhibitor

5. Positively charged hair: Fluoroquinolones should not be taken with cations such as antacids (e.g. calcium carbonate) because they chelate and inactivate the drug

6. Water getting sprayed on crotch: Fluoroquinolones are used to treat UTIs

7. Girl scout drinking from river with infectious particles: Fluoroquinolones are used to treat GI infections

8. Mona Lisa: Fluoroquinolones are used to treat Pseudomonas

9. Headset: Fluoroquinolones are used to treat otitis extema

10. Pink and purple sky: fluoroquinolones are a relatively broad group of antibiotics that can be used to treat both gram negative rods (e.g. *Pseudomonas, E. coli*) as well as some gram positive organisms (e.g. *Streptococcus pneumoniae, Bacillus anthracis*)

11. Vomiting: Fluoruinolones can cause vomiting and/or GI upset

12. Tire: Prolonged use of fluoroquinolones may cause superinfections (e.g. pseudomembranous colitis)

13. Redness on leg: Fluoroquinolones may cause skin rashes and myalgias

14. Holding head in distress: Fluoroquinolones may cause headaches

15. Dizzy girl scout: Fluoroquinolones may cause dizziness

16. Elderly woman saying, "You're such a cutie pie": Fluoroquinolones may cause QT prolongation

17. Tarantula crawling on bone: Fluoroquinolones are teratogenic and should be avoided in pregnancy, nursing mothers, and children due to the possibility of cartilage damage

18. Boy scout with bulging veins and tendons while climbing tree: Fluoroquinolones may cause tendonitis or tendon rupture

19. Old man on steroids with bulging veins and tendons causing tree branch to crack: Fluoroquinolones are more likely to cause tendonitis or tendon rupture in those over 60-years-old and those who are taking steroids

20. Air coming out of mattress: Resistance to fluoroquinolones may occur via efflux pumps

21. Top and boy rejecting girl scout: Resistance to fluoroquinolones via alterations in DNA gyrase

See Figure 9.4.1 - Antibiotics Mechanisms (Antibiotics, Section 1, Page 69)

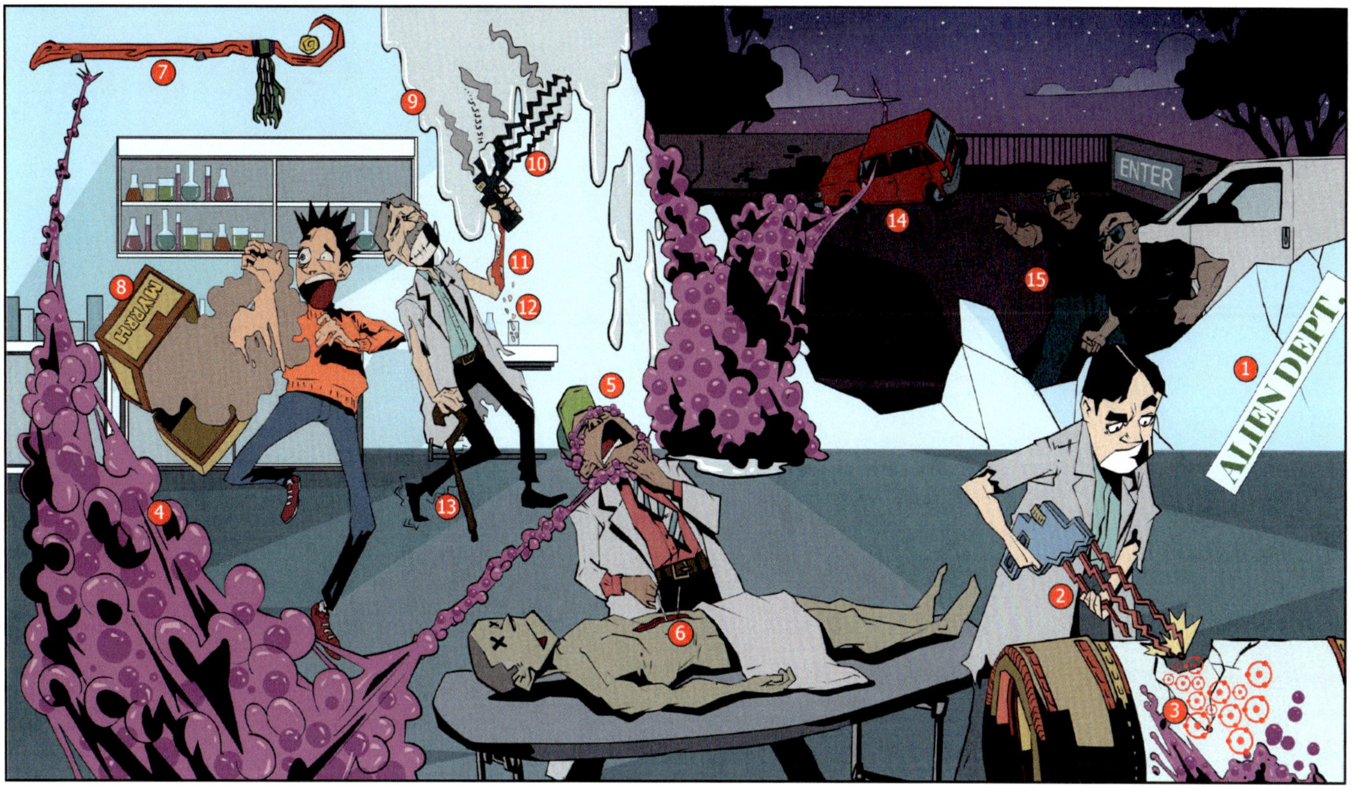

1. "ALIEN DEPT.": Daptomycin

2. Weapon that looks like lipopeptide: Daptomycin is a lipopeptide

3. Hole in container where ions are spewing out: Transmembrane channel causes an ion disturbance which kills DNA, RNA and protein synthesis

4. Alien symbiote that's made of purple spheres: Daptomycin attacks gram positive cocci

5. Scientist wearing a hat and getting choked by alien: Treats meningitis

6. Abdominal dissection: Intra-abdominal infection

7. Ancient alien staff: Use for Staph infections

8. Chest of myrrh spilling onto skin: Use for severe MRSA skin infections

9. Fluid coating wall surface: Surfactant

10. Lipopeptide weapon malfunctioning after touching the fluid on the wall: Daptomycin is deactivated by surfactant

11. Muscles in the arm of the scientist bursting through the skin: Daptomycin can cause rhabdomyolysis

12. Pieces of muscle dropping into a lab vial: Monitor CPK to assess muscle breakdown

13. Body going limp from weakness: Can cause myopathy

14. Symbiote lifting up car: Daptomycin can treat gram positive organisms responsible for endocarditis

15. Security guards outside of van: Can be used for vancomycin resistant Enterococcus (VRE)

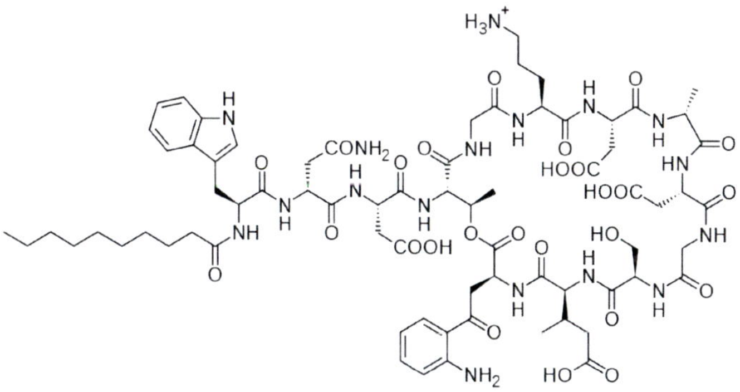

Photo Credit: Public domain via Wikimedia

Figure 9.4.2 - Example of a Lipopeptide

See Figure 9.4.1 - Antibiotics Mechanisms (Antibiotics, Section 1, Page 69)

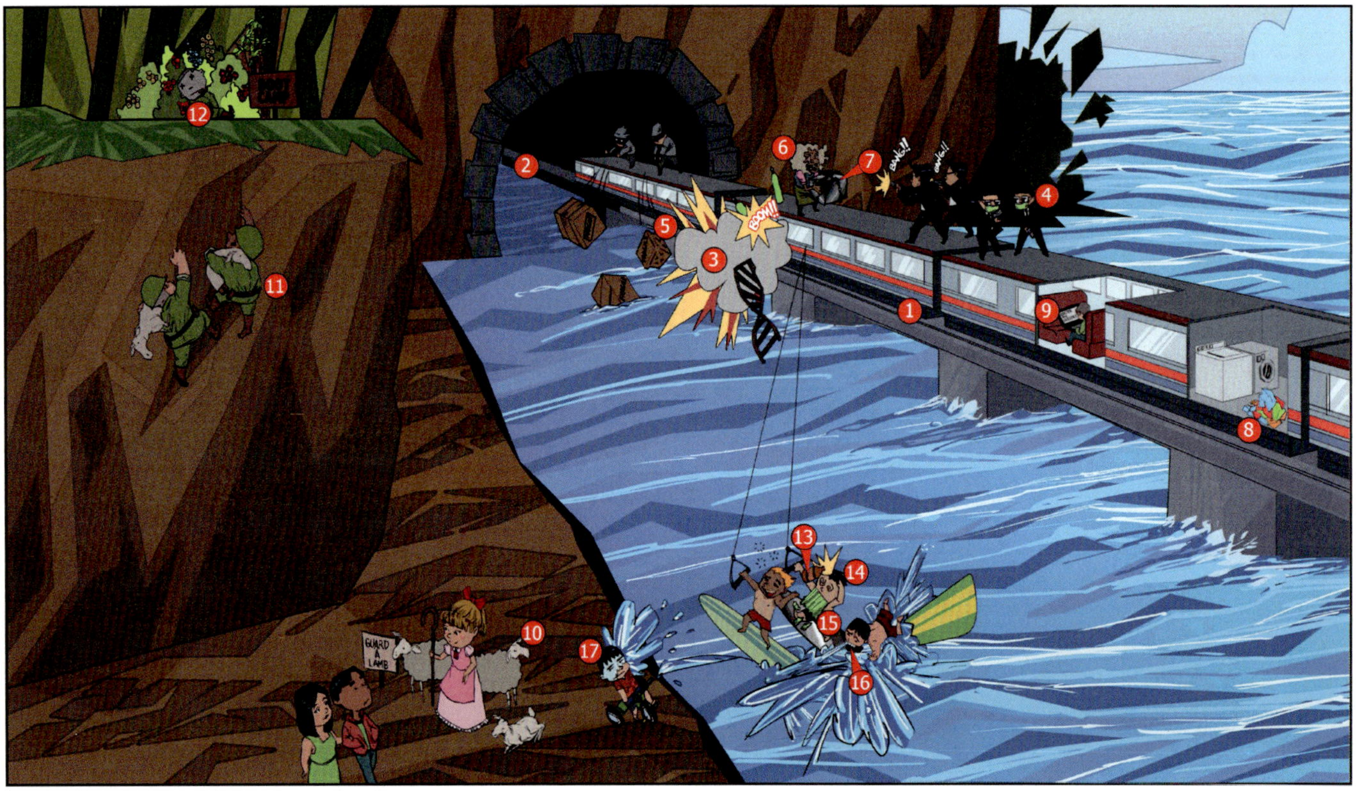

1. Metro: Metronidazole

2. Metro traveling underneath tunnel that resembles the diaphragm: Used to treat infections below the diaphragm

3. Reactive oxygen tank damaging train track that resembles DNA: Forms free radical metabolites that damage bacterial DNA (bactericidal)

4. Agents with masks: Used to treat anaerobes

5. Fragile box: used to treat *bacteroides fragilis*

6. Old crone: Used to treat Crohn disease

7. Chrome-ornate box locked with chains: Cytochrome P-450 inhibitor

8. Pile of clothes on ground: Used to treat *Helicobacter pylori*

9. Man working on "Enter my History" site: Used to treat Entamoeba histolytica

10. "Guard a Lamb" sign: Used to treat *Giardia lamblia*

11. Soldiers at difficult boot camp that are climbing cliff: Used to treat *Clostridium difficile*

12. Dead soldier: Used to treat *Gardnerella vaginalis*

13. Surfer discarding alcohol: Disulfiram-like reaction (tachycardia, hypotension, and flushing) with alcohol

14. Bottle hitting head: May cause headaches

15. Vomit: May cause vomiting

16. Teeth colliding with metallic-colored surfboard: My cause metallic taste

17. Boy with tricycle and moaning: Used to treat *Trichomonas vaginalis*

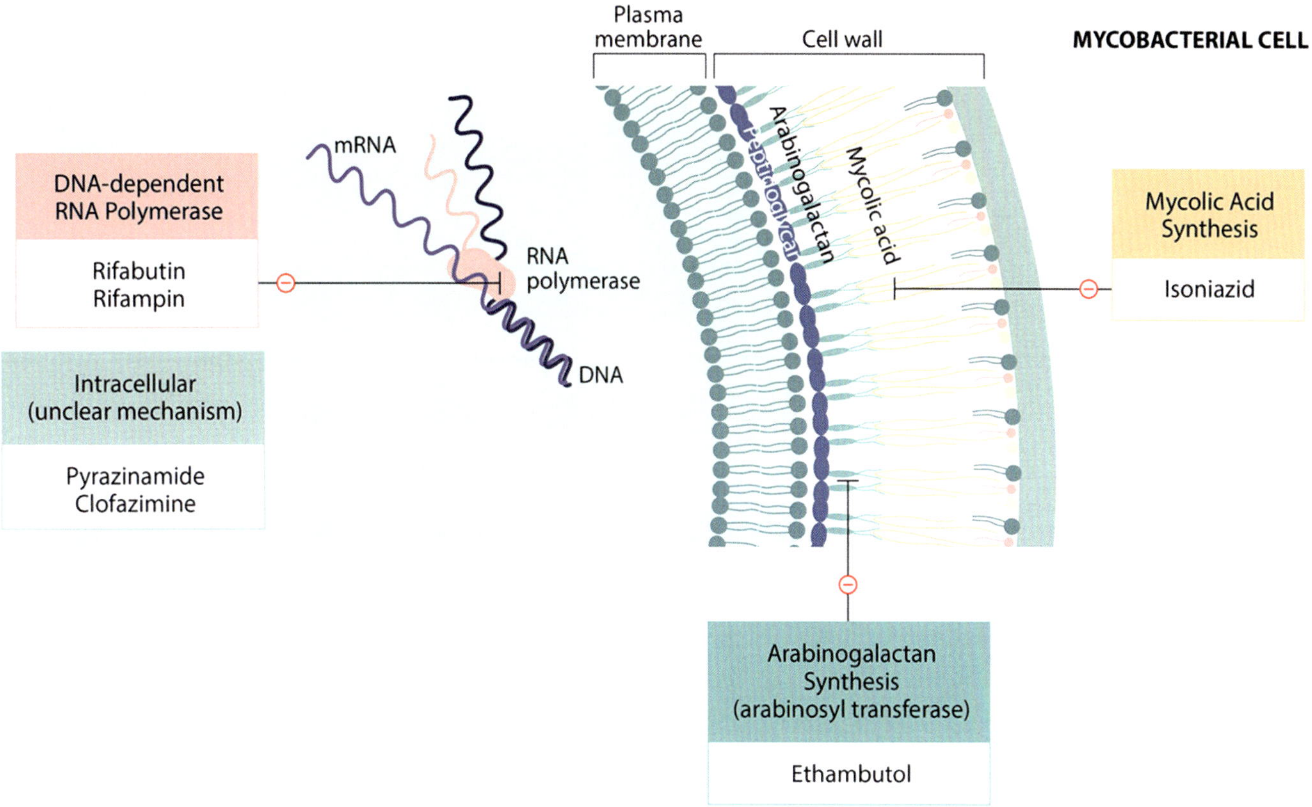

Figure 9.4.3 - Overview of Antimycobacterials

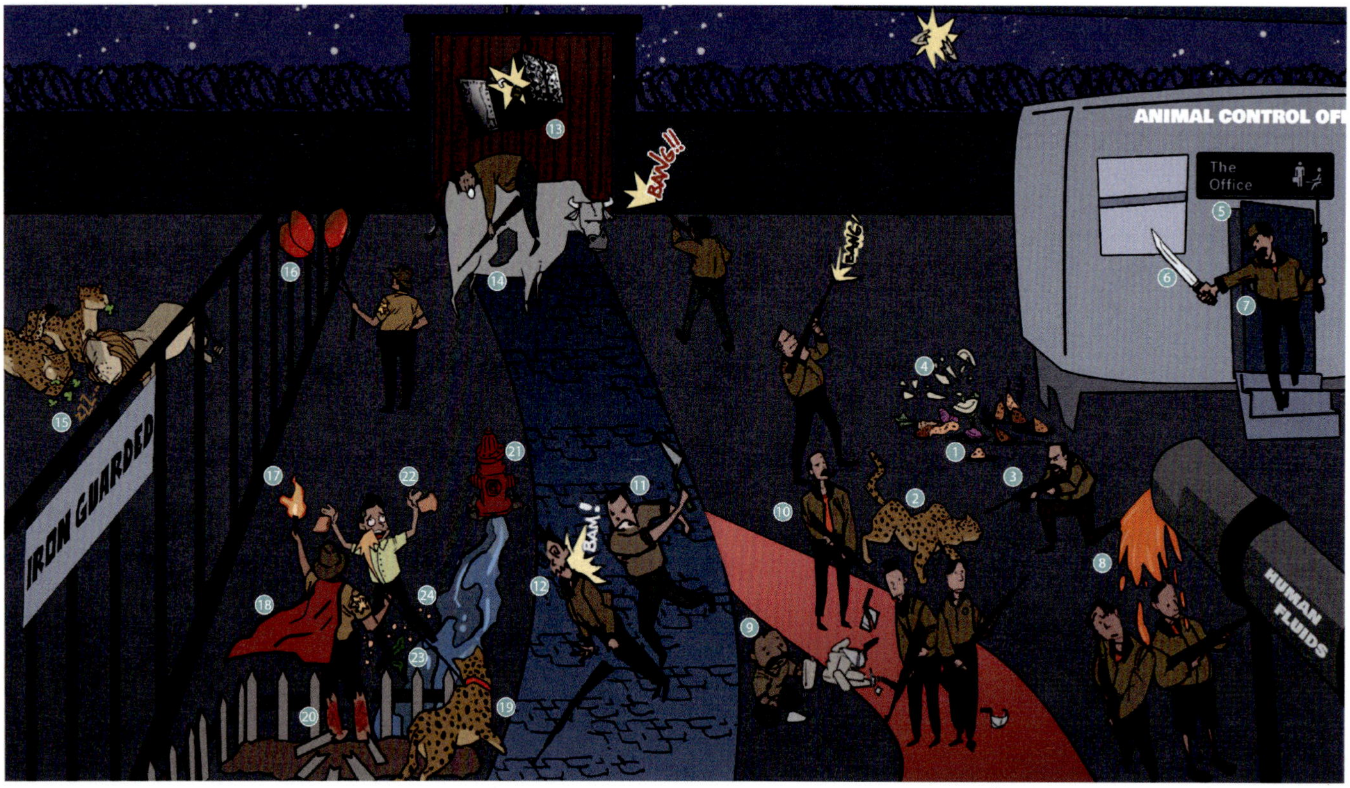

1. Tubers on ground: *Mycobacterium tuberculosis*

2. Leopard: *Mycobacterium leprae* (Leprosy)

3. Rifle held by animal keeper: Rifampin can be used to treat tuberculosis and leprosy

4. Broken plates near tubers: Can cause thrombocytopenia

5. "The Office" sign above head animal keeper: Can be used to treat *Haemophilus influenzae*

6. Hat and knife of head animal keeper: Can be used to treat *Neisseria meningitidis*

7. Head animal keeper, Rasputin look-alike: Rifabutin is another rifamycin

8. Orange fluid from "Human Fluids" pipe: Can cause orange body fluids

9. Bricks from blue walkway to build red walkway: Bacterial DNA dependent RNA polymerase

10. Rifleman blocking brick layer: Rifampin blocks bacterial DNA-dependent RNA polymerase

11. Brick layer hitting isolated rifleman: Bacteria can develop resistance against rifampin via mutations of DNA dependent RNA polymerase

12. Rifleman standing alone: Bacterial resistance is rapid when rifampin is used as monotherapy

13. Chrome box being blasted open: is a cytochrome P-450 inducer

14. Drunk man on pregnant, liver-spotted cow: Rifampin can cause hepatitis in alcoholics and pregnant woman

15. Leopards chewing on clovers next to sleepy lion: Clofazimine is added to the regimen in cases of lepromatous leprosy

16. Deputy holding 3 red balloons turning brown by touching iron bars: Dapsone can oxidize Fe^{2+} in hemoglobin to Fe^{3+}, making the blood appear brownish (methemoglobinemia)

17. Deputy holding up sulfur match: Dapsone is a sulfonamide

18. Hero deputy: Dapsone can be used to treat *pneumocystis jiroveci pneumonia* (PCP)

19. Leopard held by deputy: Dapsone can treat leprosy

20. Rash on deputy's leg from destroying "villi-like" fence slats: Dapsone can treat *dermatitis herpetiformis* in celiac disease

21. Fire hydrant watering garden: Dapsone can cause hemolysis in G6PD deficiency

22. High man dropping 2 slices of bread: Inhibits dihydropteroate synthase

23. Two pieces of foliage destroyed by high man: Prevents formation of dihydrofolate (DHF)

24. Falling bread grains from high man: Can cause granulocytopenia

See Figure 9.4.3 - Overview of Antimycobacterials (Antibiotics, Section 22, Page 92)

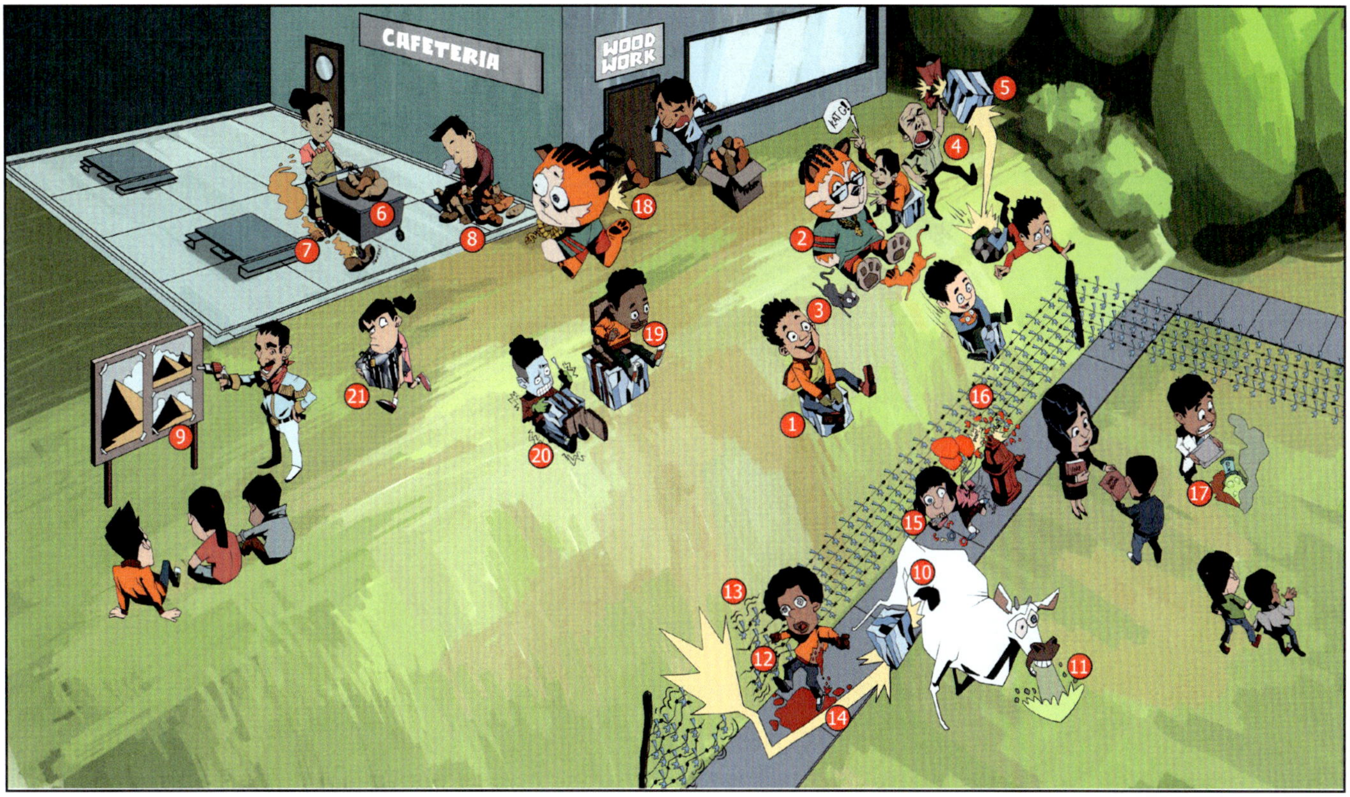

1. Kid sitting on ice block: Isoniazid

2. Cat mascot looks like a “gansta” called Kat G: *KatG* is a mycobacterial gene

3. Small cats surrounding Kat G sliding down hill: *KatG* produces catalase which activates isoniazid

4. Microphone hld by faculty member: Mycolic acid gives strength to the mycobacterial cell wall

5. Flung ice from falling kid hitting microphone: Isoniazid decreases synthesis of mycolic acid in fungal cell wall

6. Lunch lady wheeling big tray of tubers: Isoniazid is used to treat tuberculosis

7. Ripe tubers smashed by wheels of cart, leaving trail of fruit joists: Isoniazid is used in conjunction with RIPE therapy

8. Asleep tuber delivery man on a pile of tubers: Isoniazid can be used as monotherapy in latent TB

9. Teacher pointing with six shooter to pictures of pyramids: Isoniazid is always given with pyridoxine (vitamin B6)

10. Ice block from out of control kid slamming into cow that has a big liver-shaped spot: Isoniazid can cause hepatotoxicity

11. Ice block collision inside gate causing cow to vomit: Isoniazid can cause GI symptoms

12. Dazed kid wearing gloves grabbing barb wire fence without pain: Isoniazid can cause peripheral neuropathy

13. Shaking barb wire fence: Isoniazid can cause seizures

14. Blasted looking road rash on dazed kid inside gated area: Isoniazid can cause sideroblastic anemia

15. Fruit loops spilling from little girls mouth inside gated are: Isoniazid can cause drug-induced SLE (lupus)

16. Little girl tripping over fire hydrant and popping red balloons: isoniazid causes hemolysis in patients with G6PD

17. Kid inside gate dropping beaker with acid, causing gap in yearbook line: Isoniazid can cause anion gap metabolic acidosis

18. Spare Kat G costume on top of hill having tubers thrown at it: Tuberculosis can develop resistance by under expressing their *KatG* gene

19. Kid on hill securing wooden seat on top of his ice block: Isoniazid is metabolized and excreted via liver acetylation

20. Kid on hill shivering as he slowly adds chair to his ice block: Some patients acetylate slower which gives them greater side effects

21. Suspicious girl on hill holding padlocked chrome box, evading wood shop: Isoniazid inhibits cytochrome P-450

See Figure 9.4.3 - Overview of Antimycobacterials (Antibiotics, Section 22, Page 92)

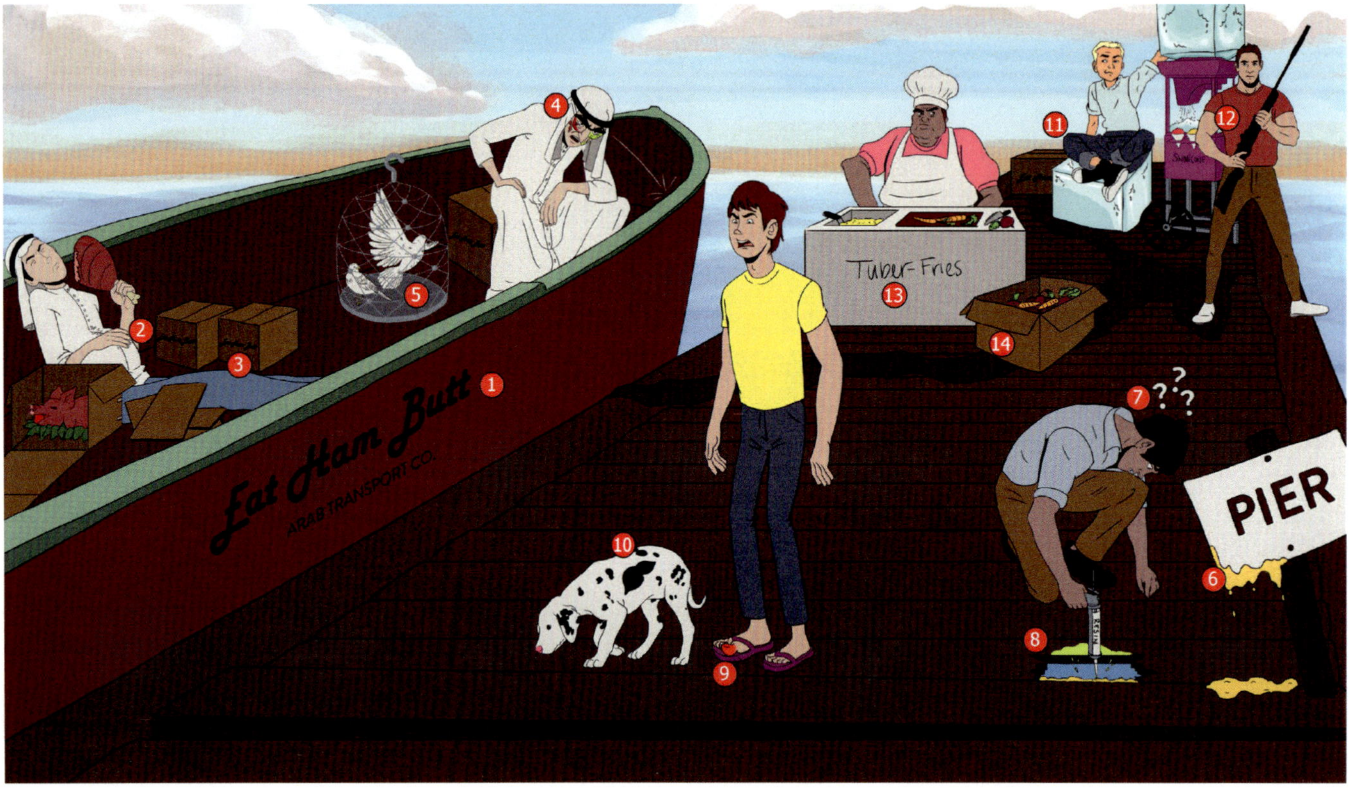

1. "Eat ham butt" boat: Ethambutol

2. Muslim ham stuffed man in the Arab Transport Co. boat: Ethambutol blocks arabinosyltransferase

3. Unfinished cardboard boxes containing ham: By blocking arabinosyltransferase, ethambutol prevents carbohydrate polymerization in the fungal cell wall

4. Blood in one eye and green snot in the other of the broken glasses man: Ethambutol can cause red and green color-blindness, as well as decreased visual acuity (optic neuropathy)

5. Little aviary: Ethambutol can be used against mycobacterium avium-intracellulare (MAC)

6. Pier and yellow rezin: Pyrazinamide

7. Confused doc worker on pier: Pyrazinamide has an unknown mechanism

8. Resin repairing pier ruined by acidic water: Pyrazinamide works best in acidic pH

9. Tourist stubbing big red toe on pier: Pyranizamide can cause gout

10. Liver-spotted dalmatian: Pyrazinamide can cause hepatotoxicity

11. Man sitting on block of ice: Isoniazid

12. Rifle held by man next to ice: Rifampicin

13. "Tuber-fries" stand: Ethambutol and pyrazinamide are used for tuberculosis

14. Ripe food next to food stand: RIPE stands for rifampin, isoniazid, pyrazinamide, and ethambutol

ANTIFUNGALS

Section 1 - Amphotericin B and Flucytosine and Nystatin

Antifugal therapy

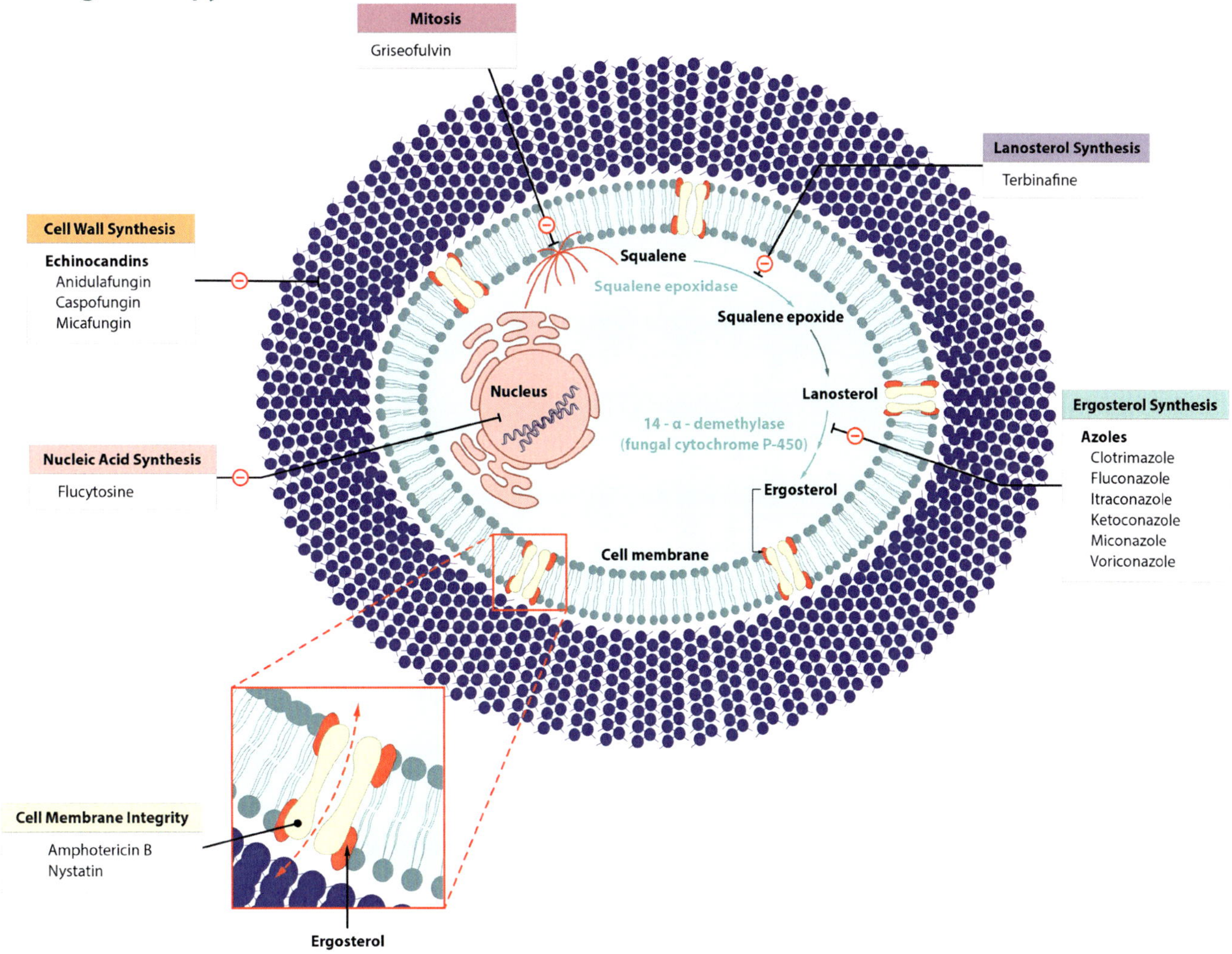

Figure 9.5.1 - Mechanisms of Antifungal Medications

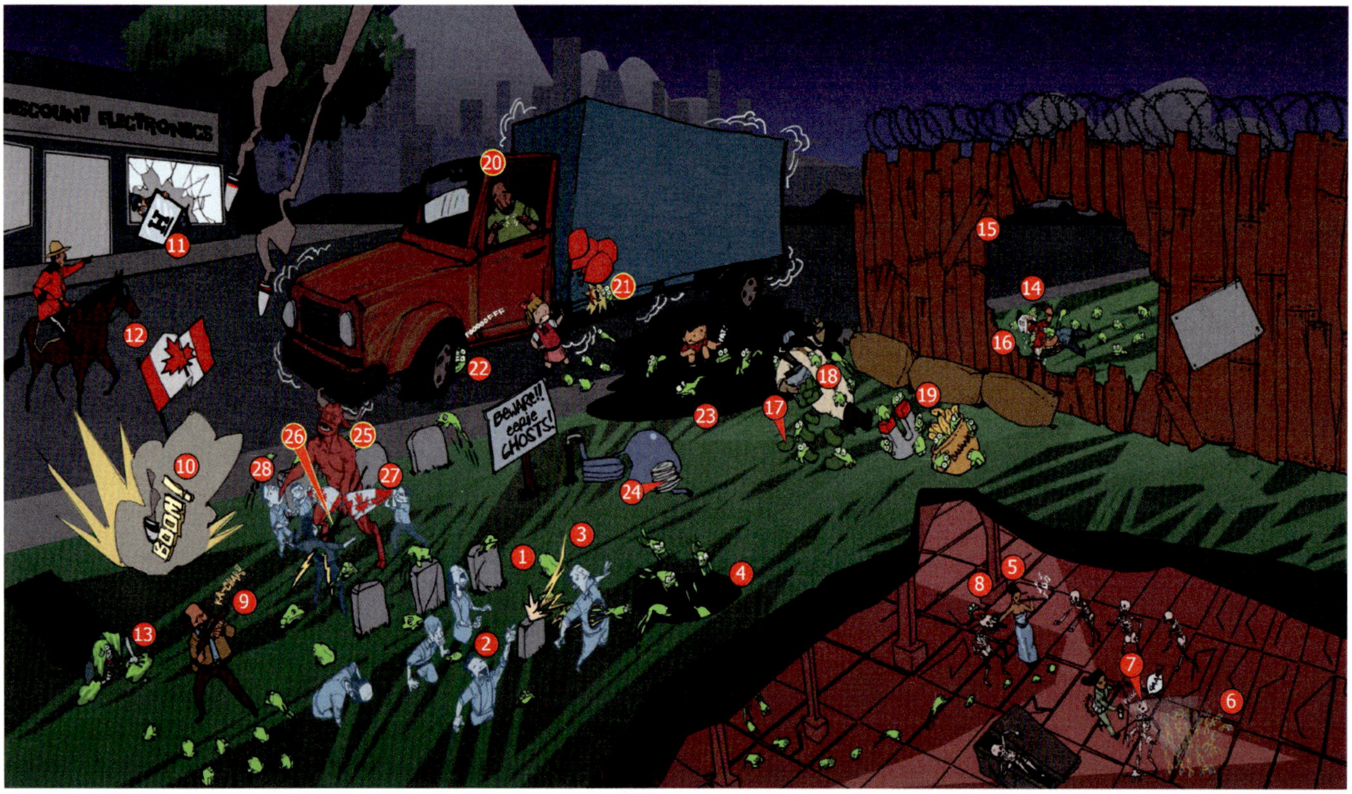

1. Amphibians: Amphotericin B

2. Amphibians jumping on eerie ghost headstones: Amphotericin B binds to ergosterol on cell membrane

3. Lightning strike causing amphibian to jump through a ghost, creating a hole: Forms pores in the cell membrane and causes electrolyte leakage

4. Crypt: Used to treat cryptococcus

5. Flute player wielding a sai: Use flucytosine with Amphotericin B to treat Cryptococcus

6. Dental hygienist spraying plants with fluoride: Flucytosine is converted to 5-Fluorouracil which then blocks DNA and RNA synthesis

7. Skeleton melting from fluoride: Flucytosine can cause bone marrow suppression

8. Flute-sai woman and amphibian attacking the brain: Use flucytosine and Amphotericin B intrathecally for meningitis

9. Shotgun being cocked: Amphotericin B is used to treat Coccidioidomycosis

10. Blasting bomb: Amphotericin B can treat Blastomycosis

11. History channel on plasma TV: Amphotericin B can treat Histoplasmosis

12. Canadian mountie: Amphotericin Be can treat Candida

13. Zombie covered in mucous: Amphotericin B can treat Mucor

14. Amphibians attacking the human eating a cholesterol-rich burger: Symptoms caused by binding to human cholesterol

15. Amphibians creating a hole in the wall: Amphotericin B binds to human cholesterol and causes pores

16. Guard looking sick: Can cause fever and chills

17. Dropped kidney beans: Can cause kidney damage

18. Kidney beans in water: Stay hydrated to decrease nephrotoxicity

19. Magnet and sack of bananas: Regularly monitor serum magnesium and potassium levels

20. Car engine rattling: Can cause arrhythmia

21. Red balloon popping: Can cause anemia

22. Frog biting hole in tire: Can cause hypotension

23. Spilled oil causing amphibians to be harmless: Liposomal Amphotericin B is less toxic

24. Plates causing water buildup in hose: Can cause thrombophlebitis

25. Satan: Nystatin

26. Satan's trident stabbing hole in an eerie ghost and lightning bolts close by: Nystatin binds to ergosterol, creates pores and electrolyte leakage

27. Flag strapped around groin: Nystatin is used topically for vaginal and diaper Candida infections

28. Ghost stuffing Satan's hand in mouth: Use nystatin for esophageal and oral Candidiasis

See Figure 9.5.1 - Mechanisms of Antifungal Medications (Antifungals, Section 1, Page 96)

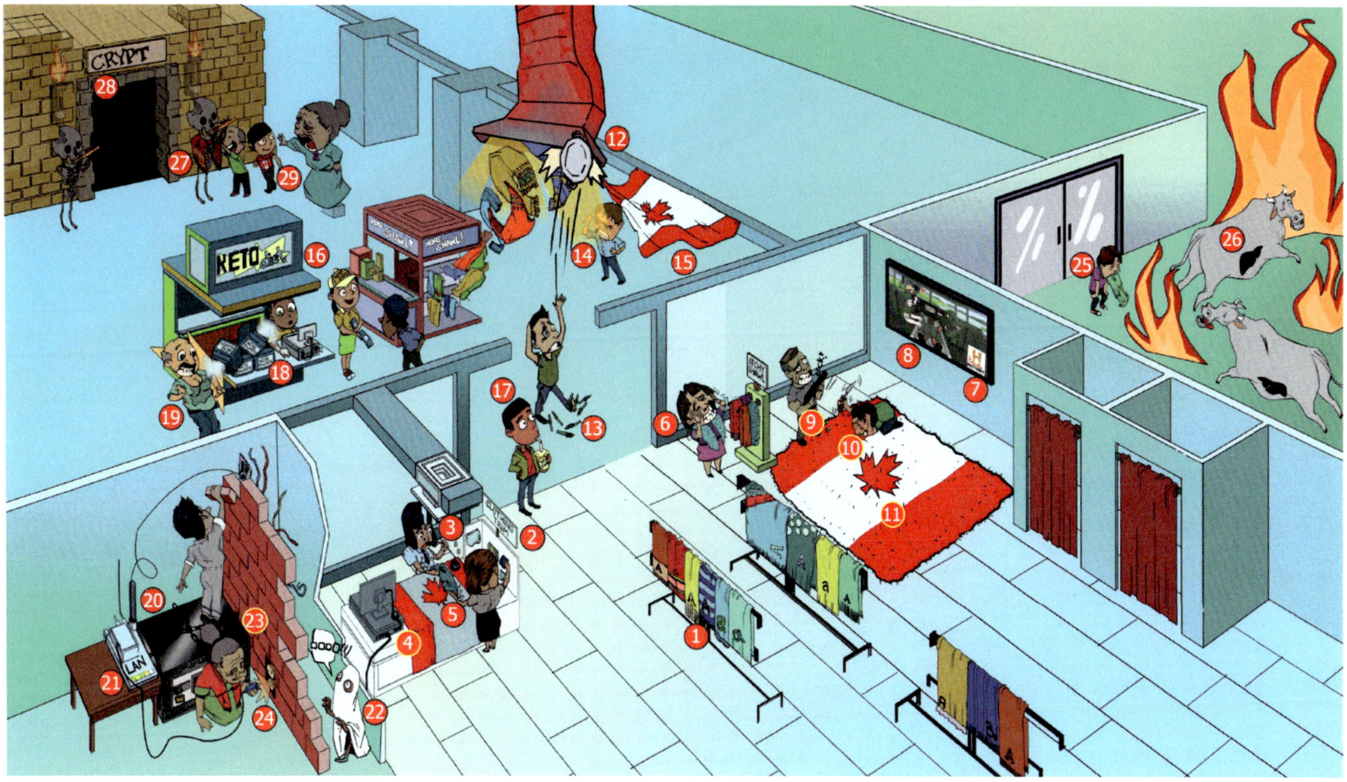

1. Different color "A" shawls: Azoles

2. "Clothing trim" sign on the checking counter: Clotrimazole

3. Microphone that store clerk is speaking into: Miconazole

4. Store clerk using the microphone and customer looking through the clothing trim both touching Canadian flag: Miconazole and clotrimazole can treat Candida infections

5. Vent leaking water onto the skin of the store clerk and the customer: Miconazole and clotrimazole can be used for topical infections

6. Itchy blue shawl on customer in front of store: Itraconazole can treat fungi

7. Plasma TV with History channel: Itraconazole can treat Histoplasma infections

8. Army blast on TV: Itraconazole can treat Blastomyces

9. Cocking of gun by customer in front of TV: Itraconazole can treat coccidioides

10. Sporadic waving of shank of customer in front of TV: Itranconazole can treat *Sporothrix schenckii*

11. Itchy shawls next to Canadian rug: Itraconazole can treat Candida infections

12. Vortex of shawls outside of clothing store: Voriconazole

13. Spilled asparagus in below vortex of shawls: Voriconazole can treat Aspergillus infections

14. Light from vent shining on man's eyes: Voriconazole causes vision changes

15. Canadian flag being sucked into the vortex: Voriconazole can treat Candida

16. Keto diet kiosk outside of clothing store: Ketoconazole

17. Onlooker sipping keto drink staring at itchy shawls: Systemic ketoconazole is used for these same diseases that itraconazole covers

18. Keto powder on kiosk counter spilling on workers hand: Topical ketoconazole treats skin infections

19. Spilled keto powder from kiosk on growing breasts: Ketoconazole can cause gynecomastia due to blocking testosterone synthesis

20. Chained chrome box: Azoles inhibit cytochrome P-450

21. LAN router next to chained chrome box: Lanosterol

22. LAN line getting hooked up to the wall space containing the eerie ghost: Fungi convert lanosterol to ergosterol

23. Man standing on chrome box: Fungal cytochrome P-450 converts lanosterol to ergosterol

24. Old woman wearing shaw unplugging LAN router from the wall space containing the eerie ghost: Azoles block cytochrome P-450 which prevents lanosterol conversion to ergosterol

25. Vomiting kid outside of mall: Azoles can cause GI distress

26. Liver-spotted cows in fire: Azoles cause liver inflammation

27. Flute playing, shawled skeleton: Fluconazole

28. Flute-shawl skeletons with damaged skulls outside the Crypt store: Fluconazole can treat Cryptococcal meningitis in AIDS patients

29. Shirt with Canadian flag next to flute-shawl skeleton: Fluconazole can treat Candida

See Figure 9.5.1 - Mechanisms of Antifungal Medications (Antifungals, Section 1, Page 96)

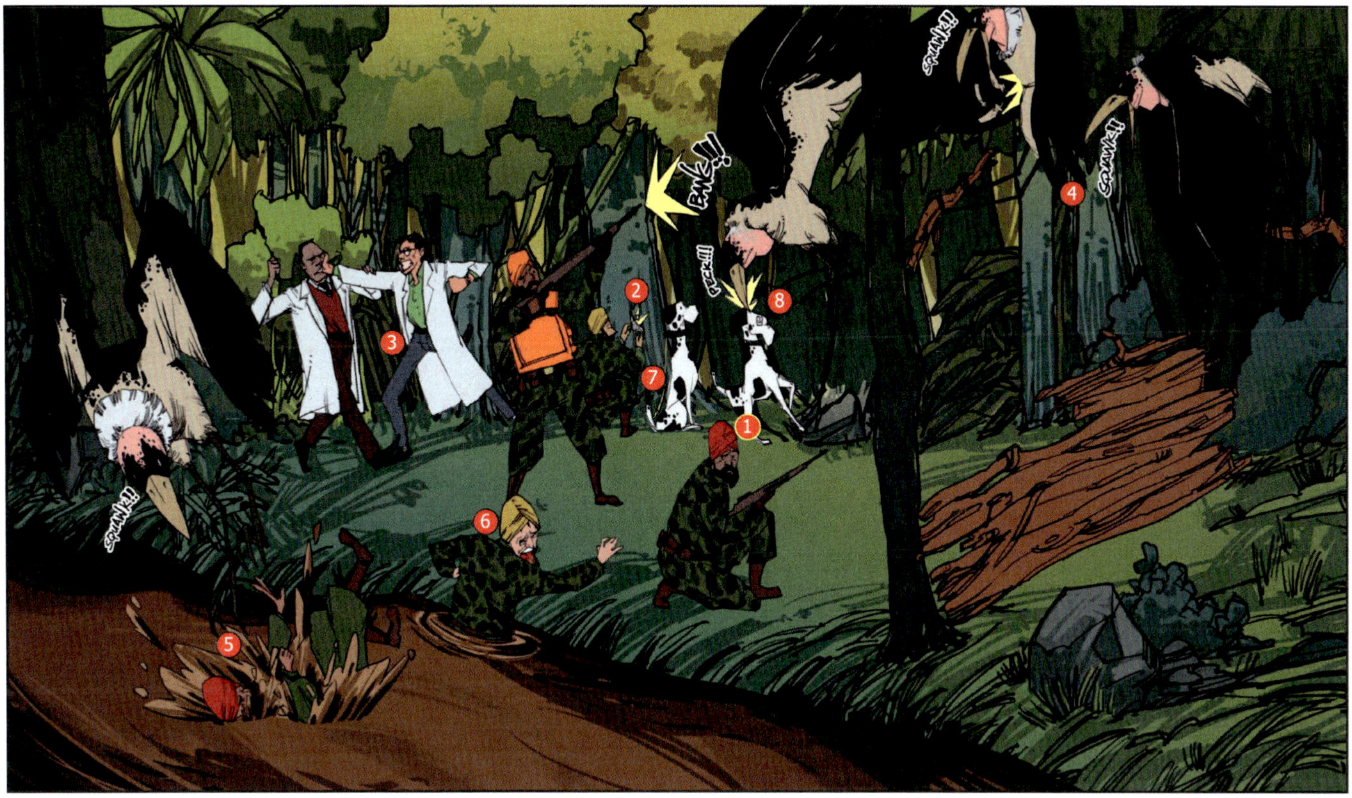

1. Turbans: Terbinafine

2. Large nail: can be used to treat onychomycosis

3. Fighting dermatologists: Can be used for all dermatophytes

4. Squawking birds flying over wall while being shot at: Terbinafine inhibits squalene epoxidase which is required to create ergosterol for the fungal cell wall

5. Muddy brown river: Terbinafine can cause diarrhea and GI upset

6. Gagging and spitting: Taste disturbance can result from terbinafine

7. Liver-shaped spot: Hepatotoxic

8. Dog being pecked on head: Causes headache

See Figure 9.5.1 - Mechanisms of Antifungal Medications (Antifungals, Section 1, Page 96)

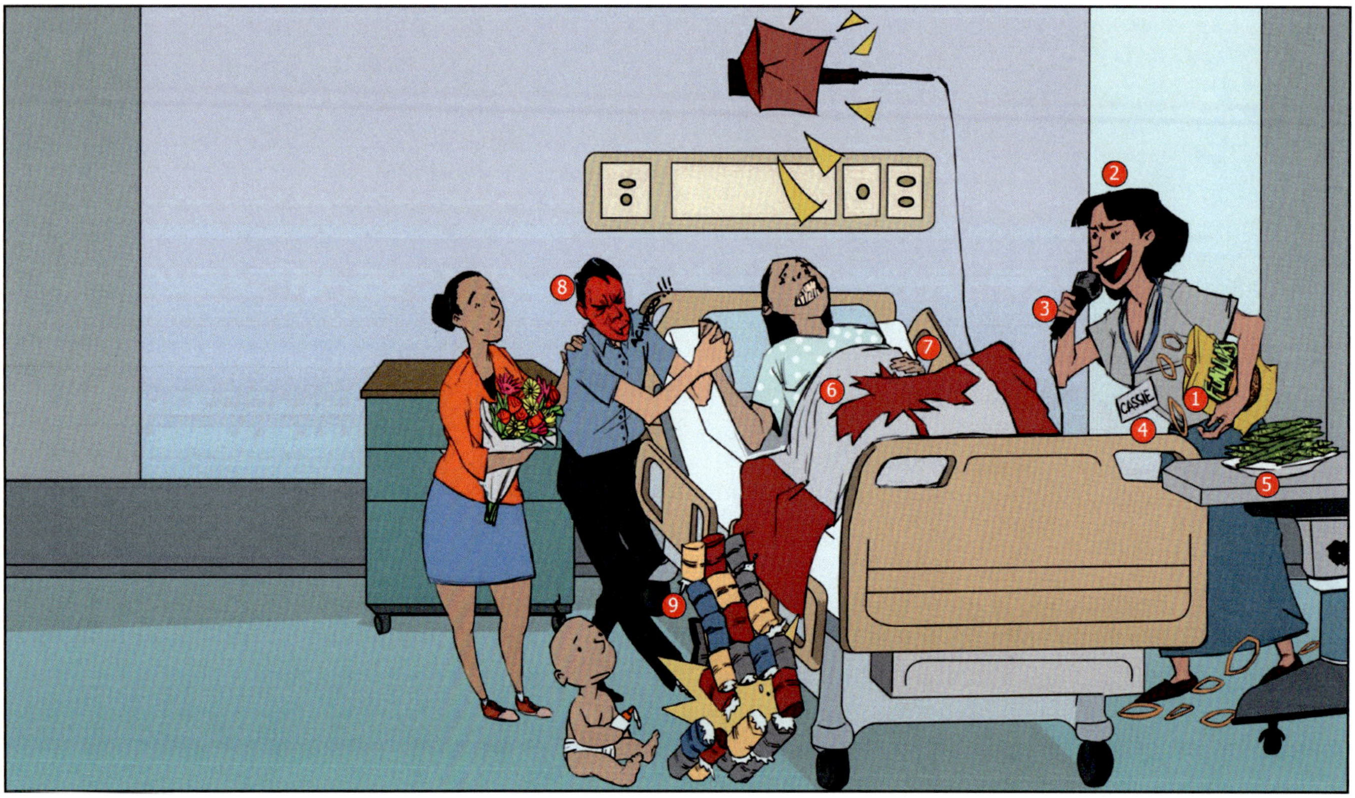

1. Funyuns: The suffix of all echinocandins if "fungin"

2. Doula: Anidulafungin

3. Microphone: Micafungin

4. Cassie: Caspofungin

5. Asparagus: Echinocandins can treat Aspergillus infections

6. Canadian themed blanket: Echinocandins can treat Candida infections

7. Stomach pain: Can cause stomach pain

8. Facial flushing: Can cause a histamine release and facial flushing

9. Glued cans: Echinocandins specifically target β-glucan with the cell wall

See Figure 9.5.1 - Mechanisms of Antifungal Medications (Antifungals, Section 1, Page 96)

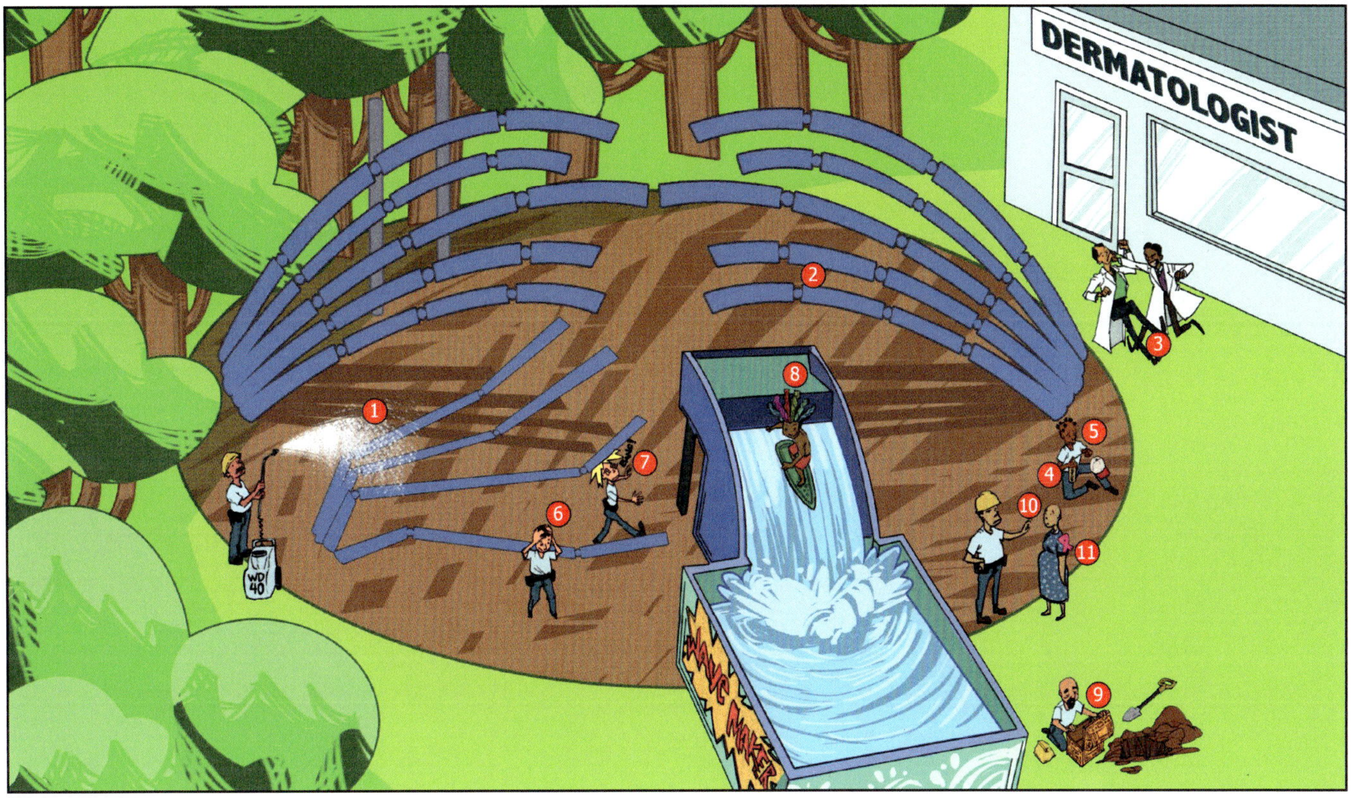

1. WD-40 grease: Griseofulvin

2. Tubes in a mitotic spindle formation: Griseofulvin targets microtubules to prevent mitosis

3. Dermatologists fighting: Griseofulvin treats dermatophyte infections

4. Sand in fingernails: Griseofulvin deposits in tissue containing keratin

5. Guy with bald spots and baseball cap: Griseofulvin is first line for tinea capitis infections

6. Man grabbing his head in pain: Griseofulvin can cause headaches

7. Confused man: Griseofulvin can cause confusion

8. Dyed hair and surfing: Griseofulvin can cause disulfiram reactions

9. Open Pandora's box: Griseofulvin induces the activity of cytochrome P-450

10. Pregnant woman getting turned away: Griseofulvin should be avoided during pregnancy

11. Pregnant cancer patient: Griseofulvin is carcinogenic

ANTIPARASITIC DRUGS

Section I - Malathion, Permethrin, and Lindane

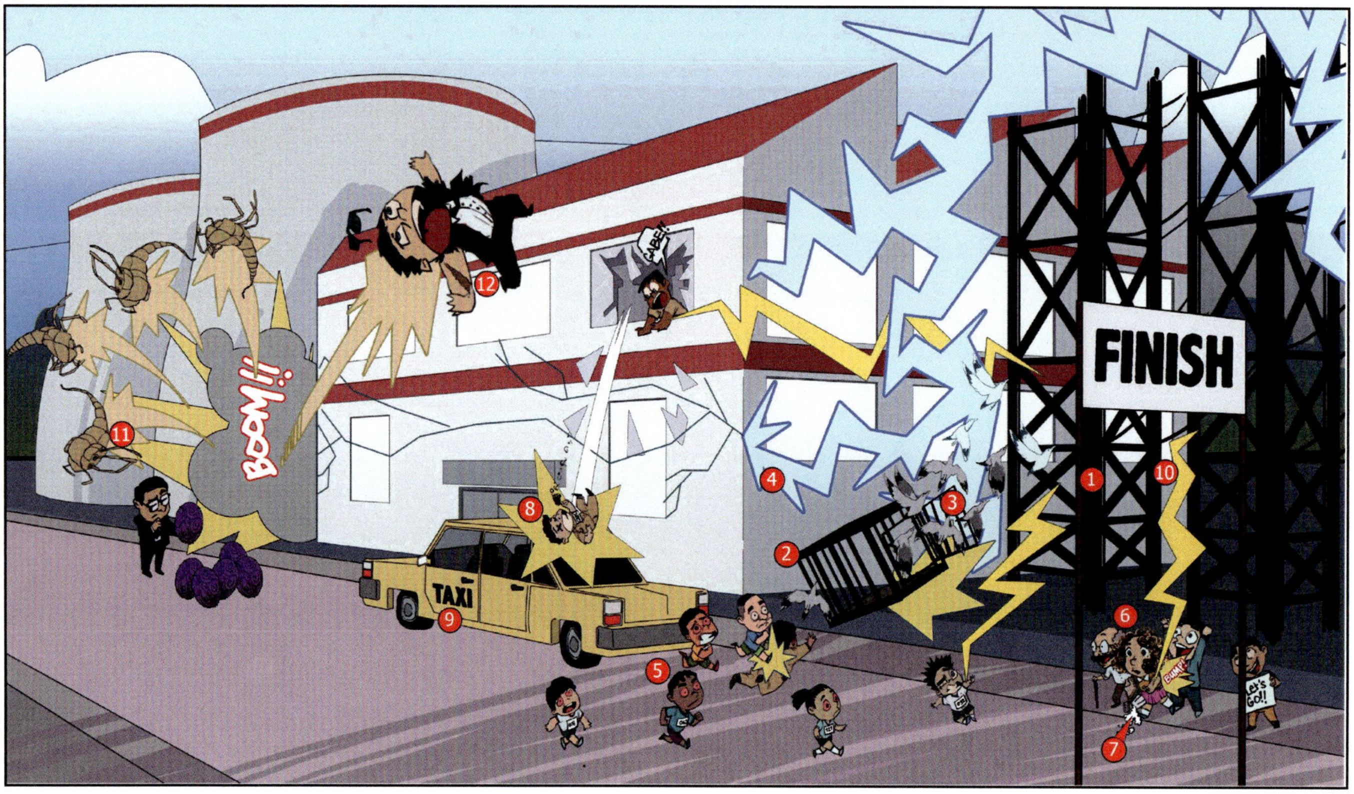

1. Electrical power plant: Neuronal synapse is the target of the drugs

2. Seagulls in a cage: Acetylcholinesterase normally decreases the synaptic levels of acetylcholine

3. Marathon runners causing cage to drop and seagulls to be released: Malathion blocks activity of acetylcholinesterase which leads to elevated acetylcholine

4. Seagull-induced electrical dysfunction: The net effect of malathion is to cause neurotoxicity through excessively high acetylcholine levels

5. Marathon runners with bloodshot eyes: Malathion can cause conjunctivitis if it contacts the eye

6. Family supporter with perm: Permethrin

7. Spilled salt with popped off lid: Permethrin causes neurotoxicity by blocking sodium channel deactivation

8. Gabe falling out of window while holding onto lint: Lindane causes neurotoxicity by blocking GABA

9. Gabe landing on top of taxi: Lindane is absorbed through the skin and cause ataxia

10. 3 Electricity bolts burning skin of plant worker, marathon runner, and girl with perm: Lindane, permethrin and malathion can cause a sensation of burning on the skin

11. FBI agents investing aliens and alien eggs during explosion: Lindane, malathion, and permethrin are used for pediculus infections (lice)

ANTIVIRALS

Section I - Oseltamivir & Zanamivir

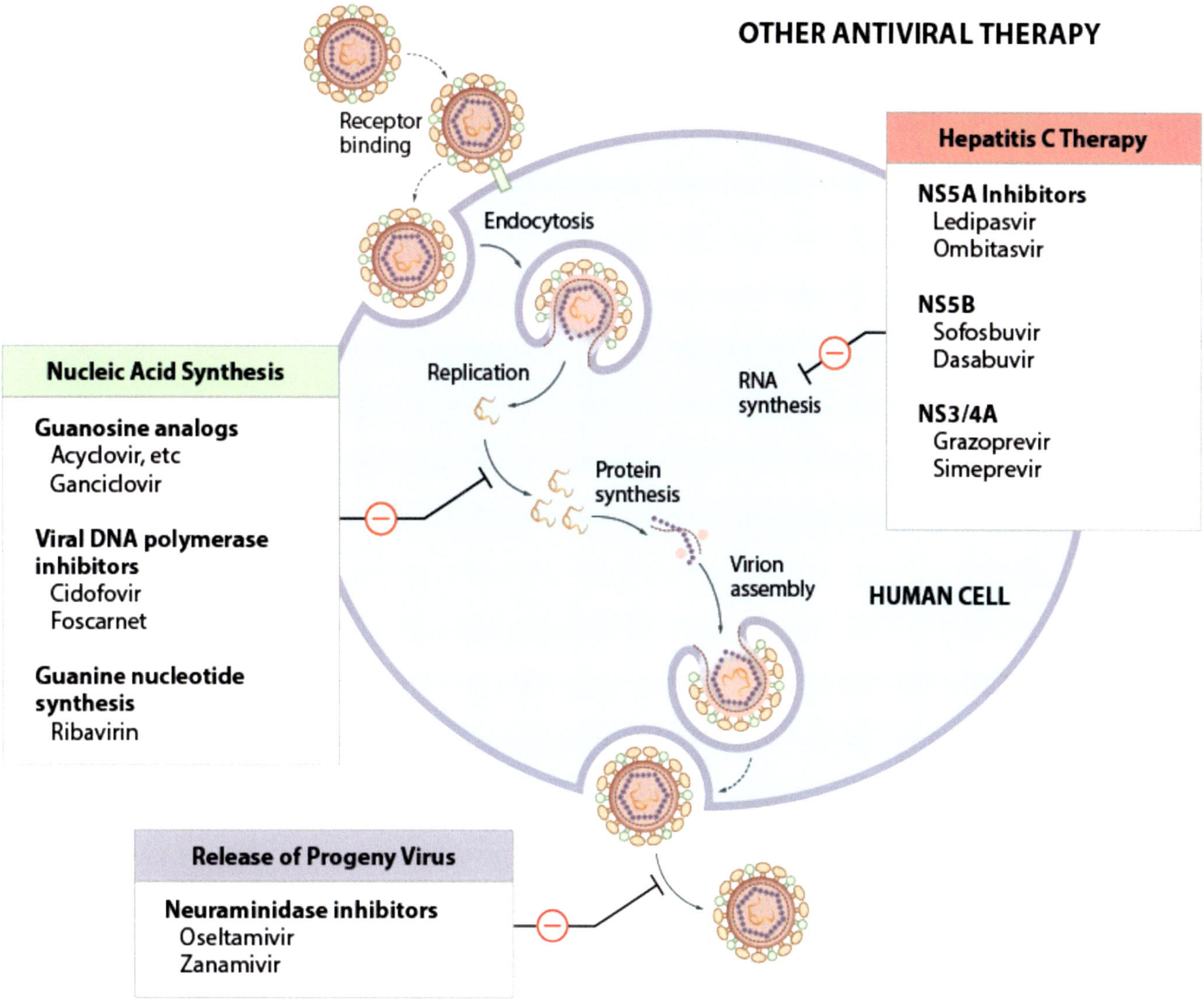

Figure 9.6.1 - Overview of Antivirals

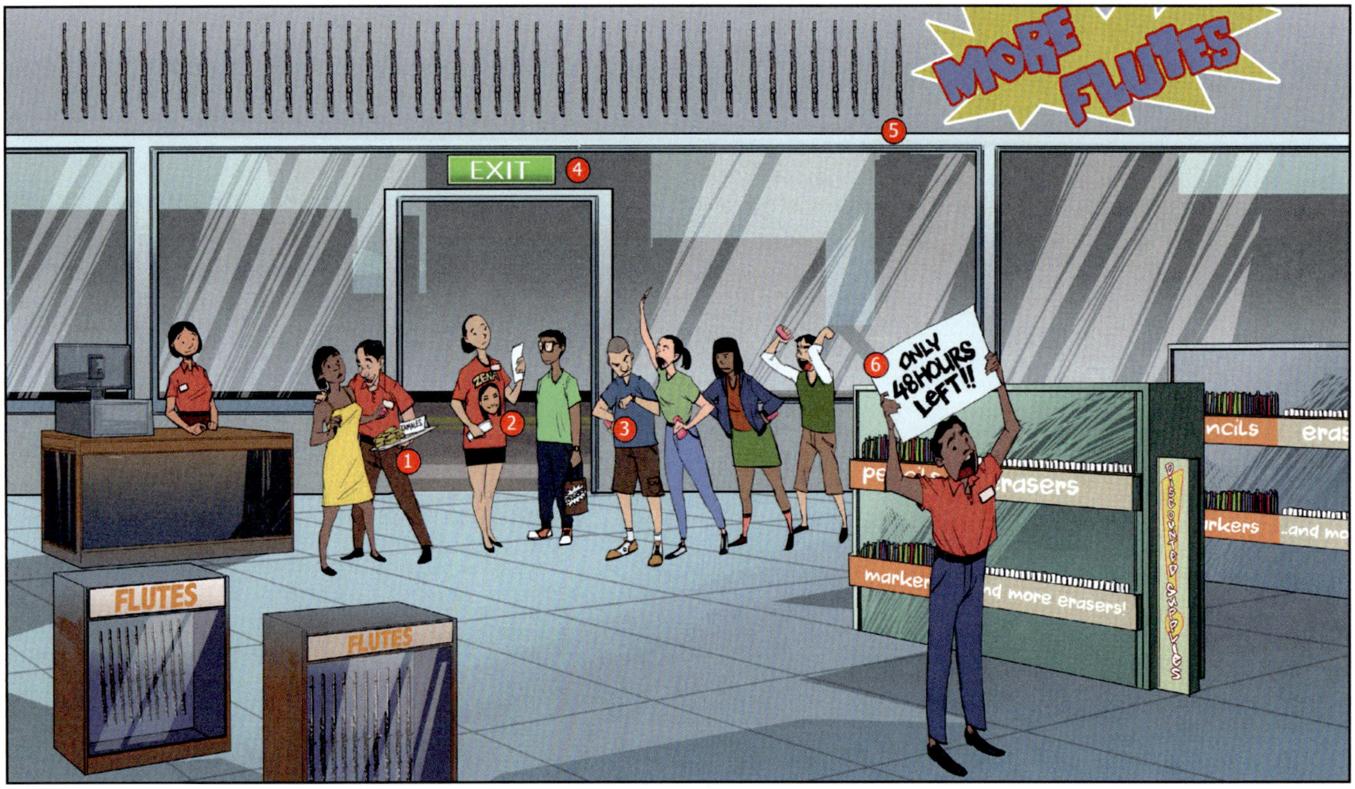

1. Tamales: Tamiflu (oseltamivir)

2. "Zena" shirt: Zanamivir

3. "New eraser": Inhibit neuraminidase

4. Unable to leave through exit door: Decreased release of viral progeny

5. Flute: Used to treat influenza A and B

6. Employee holding "only 48 hours left" sign: May shorten the duration of illness if begun within 48 hours of symptom onset

See Figure 9.6.1 - Overview of Antivirals (Antivirals, Section 1, Page 104)

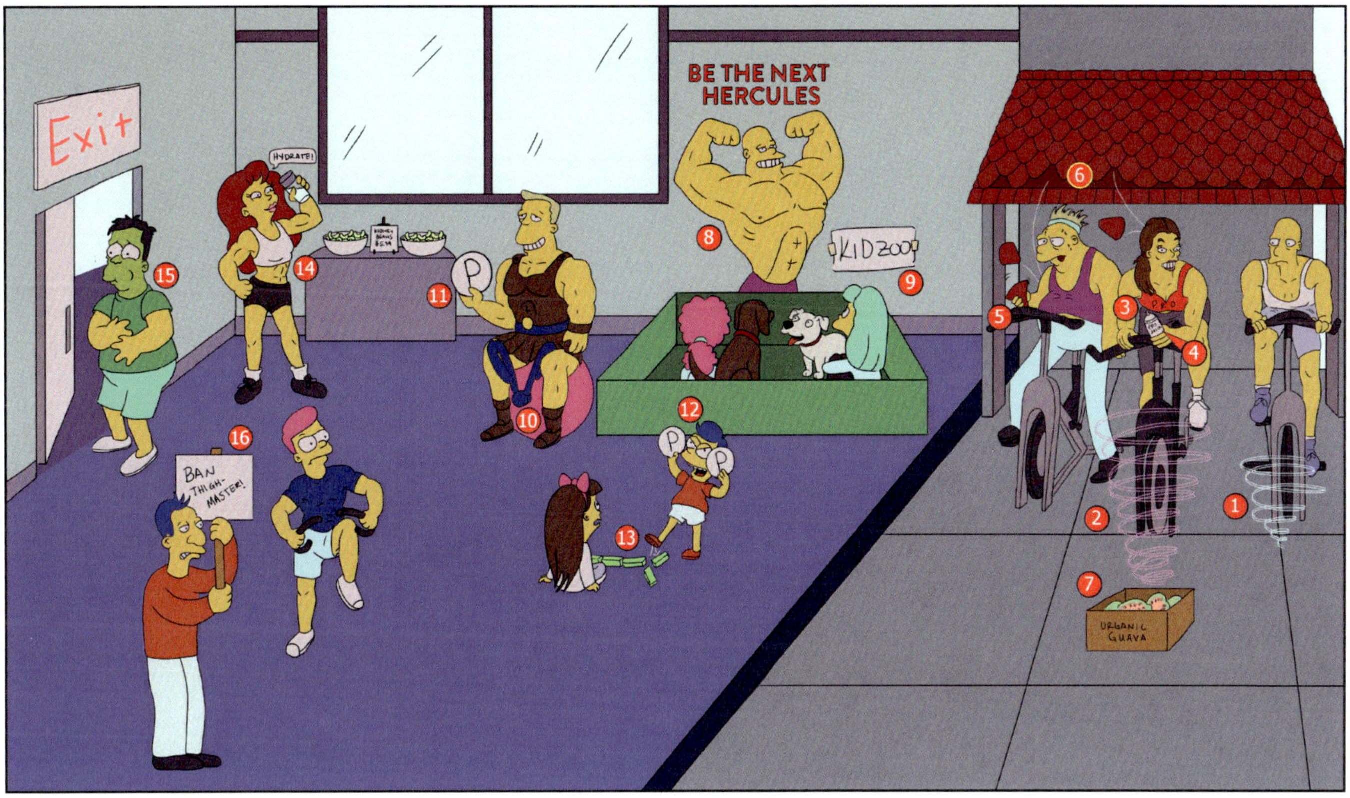

1. Stationary bike generating a cyclone: Acyclovir

2. Violet-colored bike creating a cyclone: Valacyclovir

3. Woman with red "pro" shirt and drinking a bottle labeled "pro juice": Valacyclovir is the prodrug of acyclovir

4. "Pro Juice": Valacyclovir can be taken orally because it has better bioavailability

5. Dough-boy fanning himself with red fan on currently unused cycle: Famiclovir

6. Falling red shingles on woman and Dough-boy: Famciclovir or valacyclovir are used to treat shingles (Herpes Zoster)

7. Box of guavas in front of cycles: Acyclovir, Valacyclovir, and famciclovir are guanosine analogs

8. "Be the next Hercules" poster: Used to treat herpes simplex virus (including HSV-1 and HSV-2)

9. "Kid zoo" label: Treats varicella zoster virus (VZV), or chicken pox

10. Man dressed as Hercules using thigh master right next to the kid zoo and hercules poster: Thymidine kinase is an enzyme produced only by virus infected cells

11. Guy dressed as Hercules holding one "P" pass: Thymidine kinase monophosphorylated the drug

12. Kid holding 2 "P" passes in front of kid zoo: Triphosphorylation is completed by normal cellular enzymes which fully activates the drug

13. Boy holding 2 "P" passes kicking girl's green block road that looks like DNA: Once fully activated, the drug will inhibit viral DNA polymerase by terminating the growing DNA chain

14. Trainer standing near table of kidney beans reminding everybody to stay hydrated: Hydration can prevent kidney injury while using these drugs

15. Green-faced man next to exit sign: These drugs can cause nausea and vomiting

16. Two protestors with picket and pink hair breaking black thigh master with knees: Resistance to these drugs can develop through alteration of viral thymidine kinase

See Figure 9.6.1 - Overview of Antivirals (Antivirals, Section 1, Page 104)

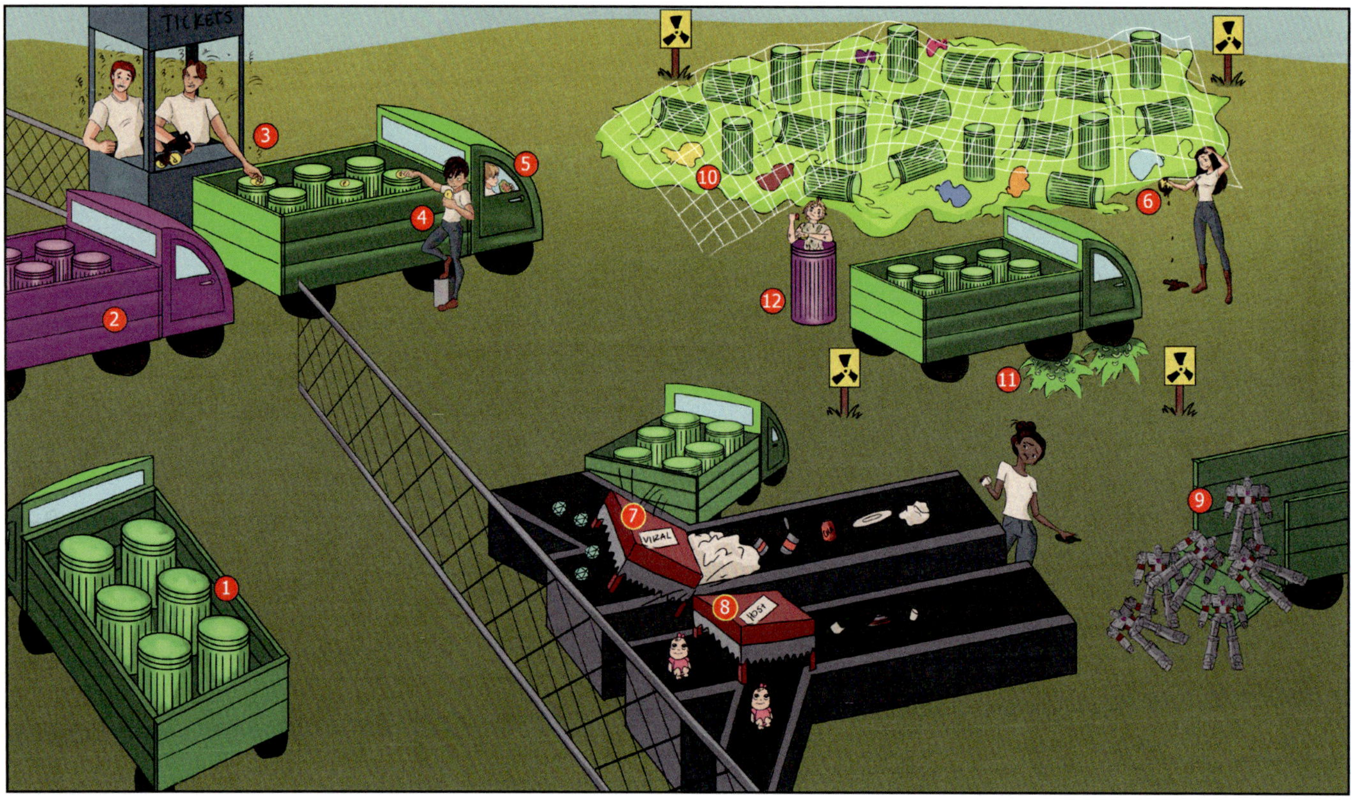

1. Garbage: Ganciclovir

2. Violet garbage truck: Valganciclovir

3. Dirty ticket booth handing out "P" passes: Ganciclovir and valganciclovir must be activated by viral kinases

4. Additional two "P" stickers: Ganciclovir and valganciclovir require 3 phosphate groups (1 added via viral kinase and 2 added via cellular kinases) in order to become fully activated

5. Guae: Guanosine analog

6. Coffee spilled on the "P" tickets: Viruses develop resistance to ganciclovir and valganciclovir via mutated viral kinases

7. Viral compactor on DNA conveyor belt: Ganciclovir and valganciclovir primarily inhibit the viral DNA polymerase

8. Violet compactor bumping host compactor: Ganciclovir and valganciclovir inhibit the host DNA polymerase to a lesser degree

9. Megatron action figures: Ganciclovir and valganciclovir can be used to treat CMV

10. Hazardous waste area and deflated balloons covered by net: Ganciclovir and valganciclovir may cause bone marrow suppression as a toxic side effect

11. Green truck running over kidney beans: Ganciclovir and valganciclovir may cause renal toxicity

12. Homeless person inside of the violet garbage: Valganciclovir has better bioavailability than ganciclovir

See Figure 9.6.1 - Overview of Antivirals (Antivirals, Section 1, Page 104)

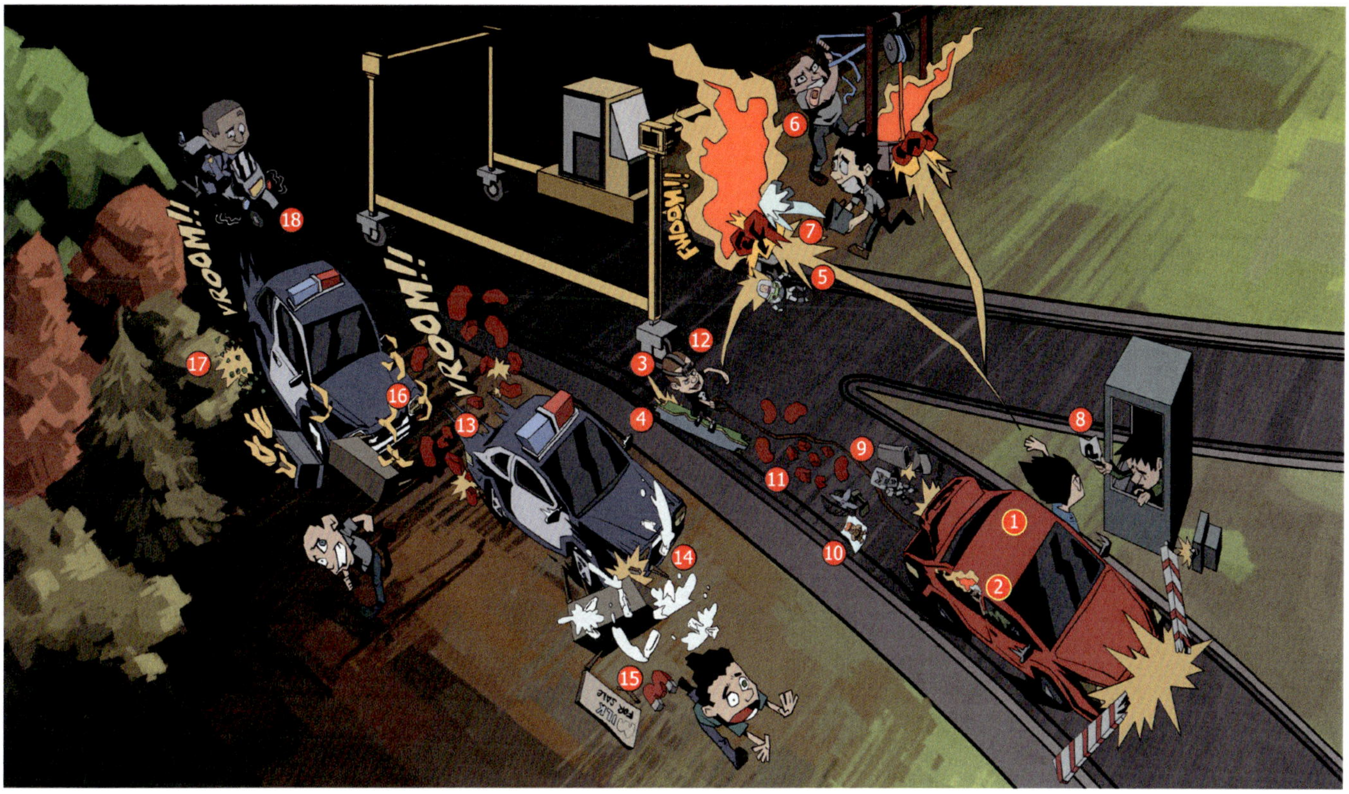

1. Fast car: Foscarnet

2. Paper burning outside fast car's pyro passenger: Foscarnet is a pyrophosphate analog

3. Sid from "Toy Story": Cidofovir

4. Long board that Sid is riding: Cidofovir has a long half-life

5. Crane at fork of road being hit by fire and toy: Foscarnet and cidofovir work by inhibiting viral DNA polymerase

6. Fire hitting red rope of well white construction worker with bandaid pulling on blue well rope: Foscarnet inhibits both viral DNA polymerase and reverse transcriptase

7. Construction worker throwing water at flame: Foscarnet and cidofovir develop resistance by mutating DNA polymerase

8. Car breaking through barricade bypassing "P" ticket: Foscarnet and cidofovir do not require intracellular activation by viral or cellular kinases

9. Megatronix and garbage can falling from fast car's trunk: Foscarnet and cidofovir can be used to treat ganciclovir-resistant CMV infections

10. Cyclone fan and Hercules drawing falling from fast car's trunk: Foscarnet and cidofovir can be used to treat acyclovir-resistant HSV infections

11. Sid destroying kidney beans: cidofovir is nephrotoxic

12. GoPro on Sid's head: Cidofovir should be administered with probenecid and IV saline to reduce nephrotoxicity

13. Fast police cars smashing into kidney beans: Foscarnet is nephrotoxic

14. Fast police car destroying milk stand: foscarnet can cause hypocalcemia

15. Magnet falling off milk stand: Foscarnet can cause hypomagnesemia

16. Fast police car destroying bananas from produce stand: Foscarnet can cause hypokalemia

17. Peas getting destroyed from produce stand: Foscarnet can cause hypophosphatemia

18. Patrol man's shaking motorcycle: Foscarnet may cause seizures

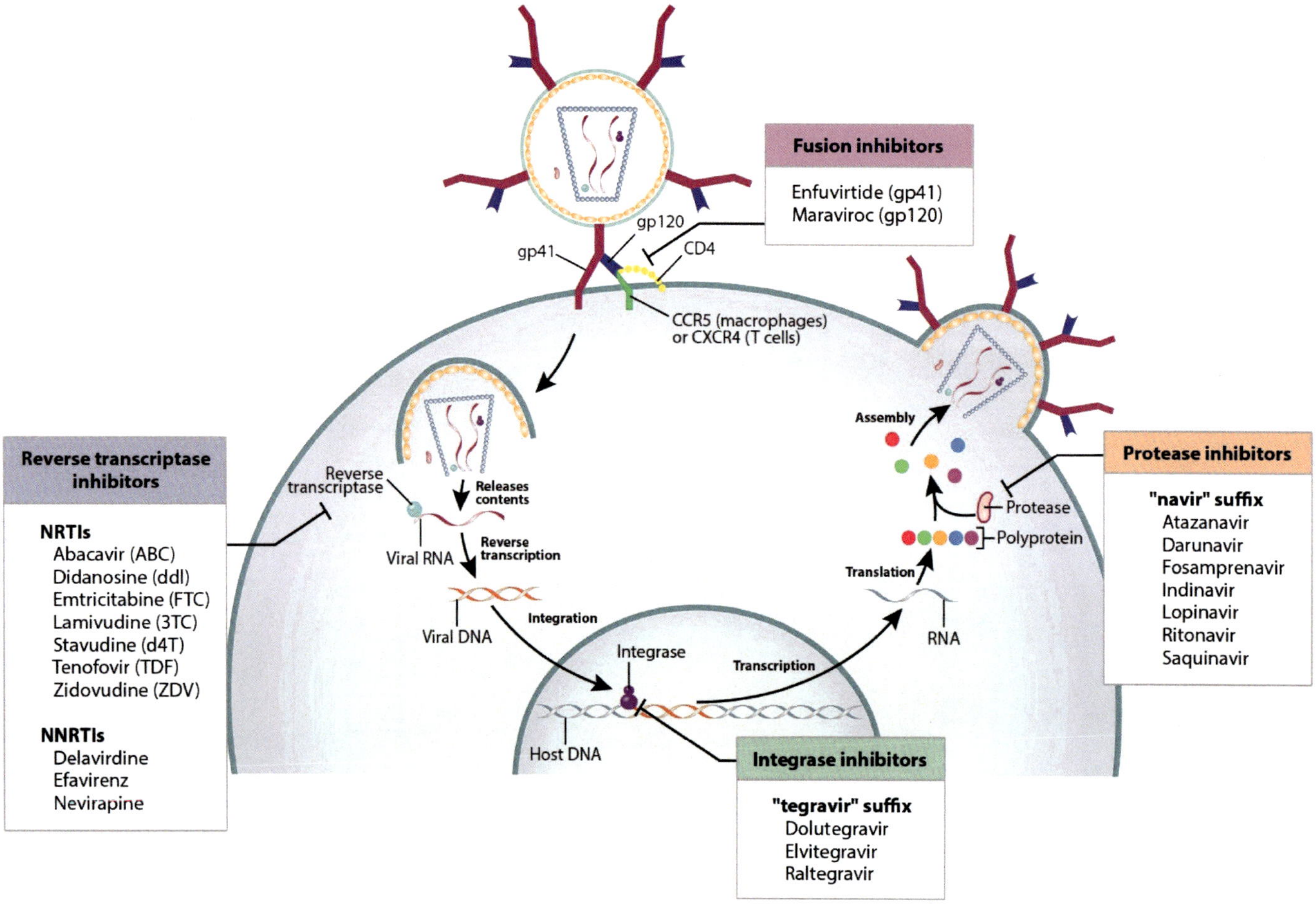

Figure 9.6.2 - HIV Therapy Mechanisms

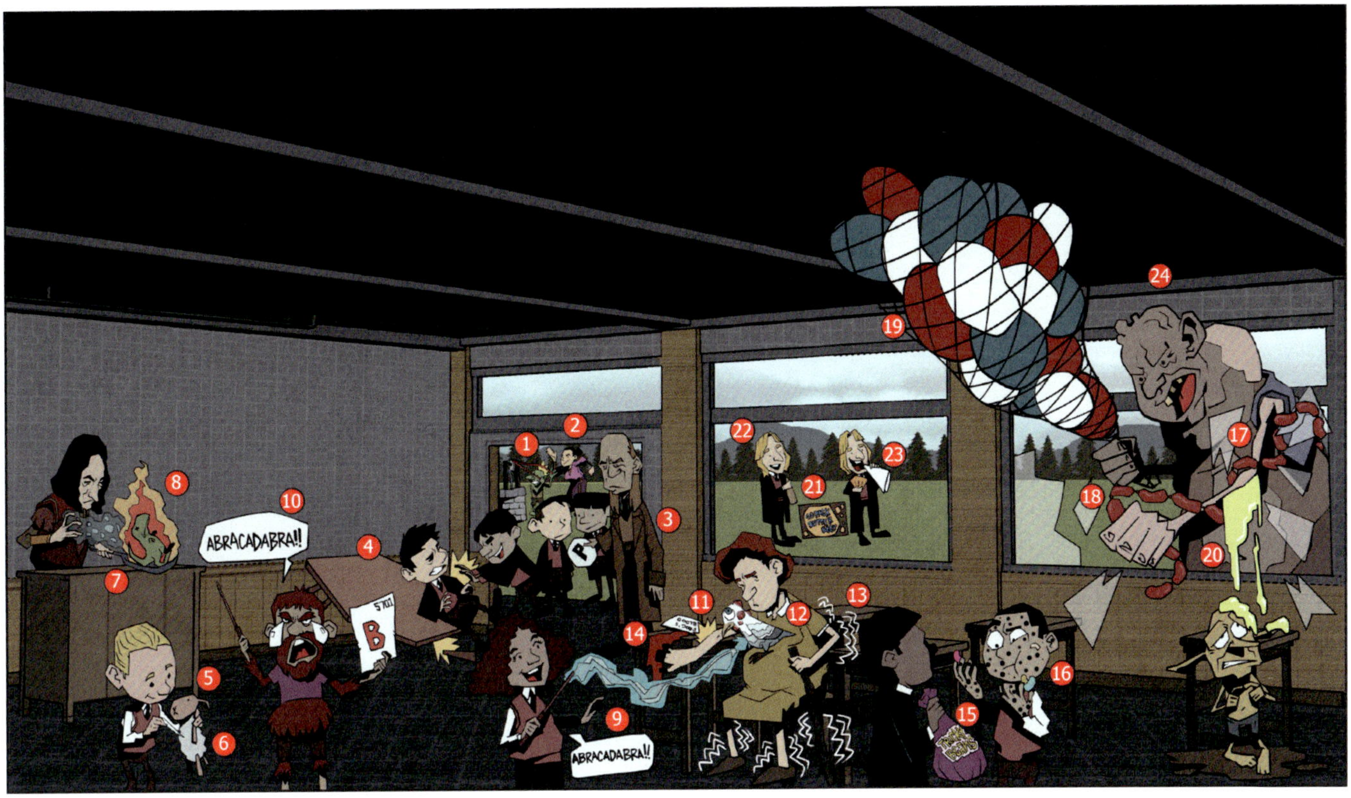

1. Well with 2 red ropes and 1 blue rope outside of school: Reverse transcriptase

2. Witch hitting house elf on the head to release ropes: Nucleoside reverse transcriptase inhibitor (NRTI)

3. School caretaker handing "P" cards to kids to enter school: Nucleosides must be phosphorylated

4. Young wizard being pushed and breaking hexagon table leg: Lacks a 3' OH group

5. Lamb voodoo doll played with blond hair wizard: Lamivudine

6. Stabbing the lamb voodoo doll: Stavudine

7. Dead dinosaur being cooked by professor: Didanosine

8. Dead dinosaur on fire in pan: Didanosine can cause pancreatitis

9. Young witch yelling, "Abracadabra": Abacavir

10. Hairy, large, and angry wizard crying and yelling, "Abracadabra" while holding paper with B grade and student ID 5701: *HLA B5701* mutation causes hypersensitivity reactions with abacavir

11. Zit covered dove being zapped by young witch: Zidovudine

12. Zit-dover sitting on pregnant witch's belly: Zidovudine is safe in pregnancy and helps reduce fetal transmission

13. Weak, pregnant witch trying to arise from chair: Zidovudine cna cause myopathy

14. Pregnant witch spilling frog's blood beside her: Zidovudine can cause anemia

15. Tricky beans inside purple bag: Emtricitabine

16. Wizard breaking out in black spots after eating tricky beans: 32 % of peds patients get hyperpigmentation with emtricitabine

17. Troll with skinny arms and fat face breaking through window: All NRTIs can cause lipodystrophy

18. Chain of sausage links around troll's skinny arms: All NRTIs can cause peripheral neuropathy

19. Net trapping balloons of different colors held by troll: All NRTIs can cause bone marrow suppression

20. Acid blood spilling from troll's arm on house elf's head, causing him to lose his faculties like a laxative: Lactic acidosis can be caused by all nucleoside NRTIs

21. "Ten of beer" shared by rambunctious twins outside of school: Tenofovir

22. Twins didn't get their "P" pass: Tenofovir is a nucleotide and does not need to be phosphorylated

23. Fan and cone by rambunctious twin: Tenofovir can cause Fanconi syndrome

24. Troll is inside and outside where kids are: Tenofovir can cause bone marrow suppression, lipodystrophy, and peripheral neuropathy

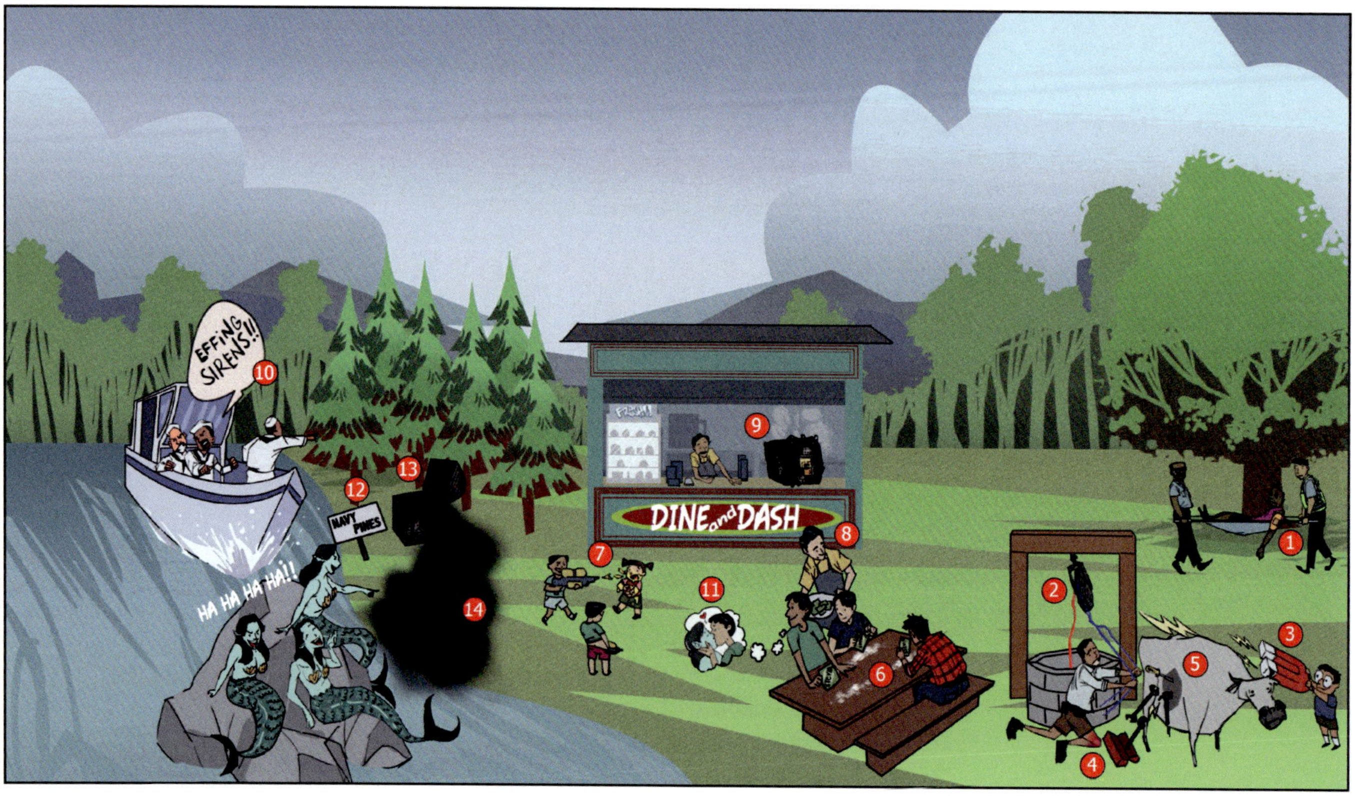

1. Bandaid on injured parkour man: NNRTIs are used for AIDS

2. Park attendant reversing damage on two blue ropes and one red rope on well: Reverse transcriptase

3. Kid with magnet aiming at well pulley: Non-nucleoside reverse transcriptase inhibitor (NNRTI)

4. Road rash on park attendant's knees: NNRTIs can cause rashes

5. Park attendant's tools impaling liver-spot on cow: NNRTIs can cause hepatotoxicity

6. Stevia spilled on picnic table: NNRTIs can cause Stevens-Johnson Syndrome

7. Little girl's body squirted with urine from squirt gun: NNRTIs can cause jaundice

8. Delivery guy next to picnic table; Delavirdine

9. Padlocked pandora's box on "Dine and Sash" countertop: Delavirdine inhibits cytochrome P-450

10. "Three effing sirens": Efavirenz

11. Daydreaming hiker on picnic table: Efavirenz can cause vivid dreams

12. "Navy pines" sign next to navy men: Nevirapine

13. Open chrome box: Nevirapine induces cytochrome P-450

14. Black could: Efavirenz induces cytochrome P-450

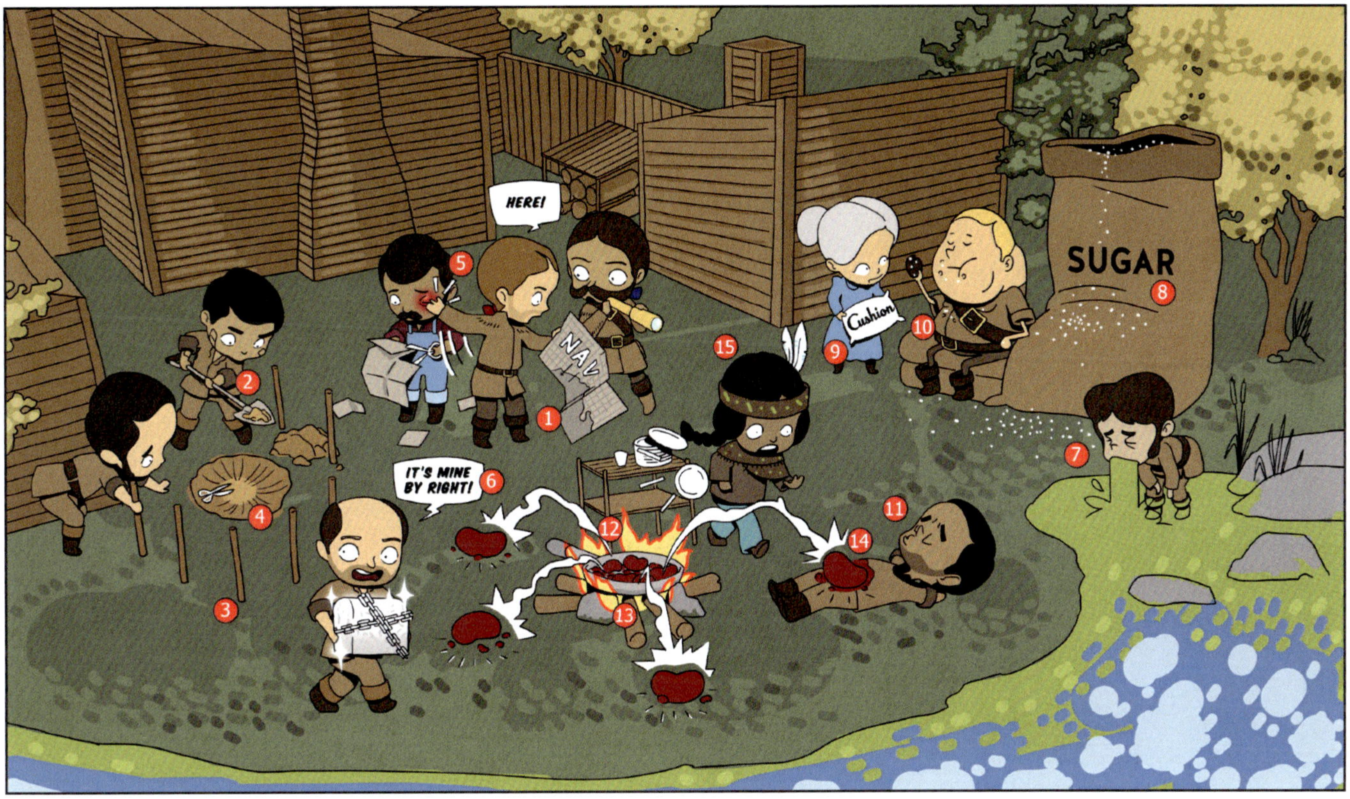

1. Leader looking at the "NAV" point on the map while saying, "Here!": All protease inhibitors have a name that ends with "navir"

2. Member digging well with band-aids on his cheeks: Protease inhibitors are used to treat HIV

3. Poles built around the well hole: HIV pol gene

4. Man stabilizing himself with his pole while reaching for the scissors in the well hole: Protease is a protein that comes from the HIV pol gene

5. Map writer with scissors getting hit in the eye by leader holding "NAV" map: Normal function of protease is to cleave HIV polyproteins into functional protein for viral progeny

6. Chrome treasure box held by a bald member saying, "It's mine by right!": Ritonavir inhibits Cytochrome P-450

7. Vomiting party member next to giant bag of sugar: Protease inhibitors can cause nausea and diarrhea

8. Bag of sugar next to fat man: Protease inhibitors can cause hyperglycemia

9. Cushion handed over by the fat man's older assistant: Protease inhibitors can cause a cushing-like syndrome

10. Buffalo hump, round face, and skinny arms of the fat man: Cna cause lipodystrophy (lipoatrophy and lipo deposition)

11. Sleeping cooking member passed out next to vomiting party member: Protease inhibitors can cause fatigue

12. Flames from campfire engulfing pan: Protease inhibitors can cause pancreatitis

13. Burning red kidney beans over campfire: Protease inhibitors can cause kidney damage

14. Red kidney popping onto crotch of sleeping cooking member: Protease inhibitors can cause hematuria

15. Indigenous person knocking over plates while running to help sleeping member: Indinavir can cause thrombocytopenia

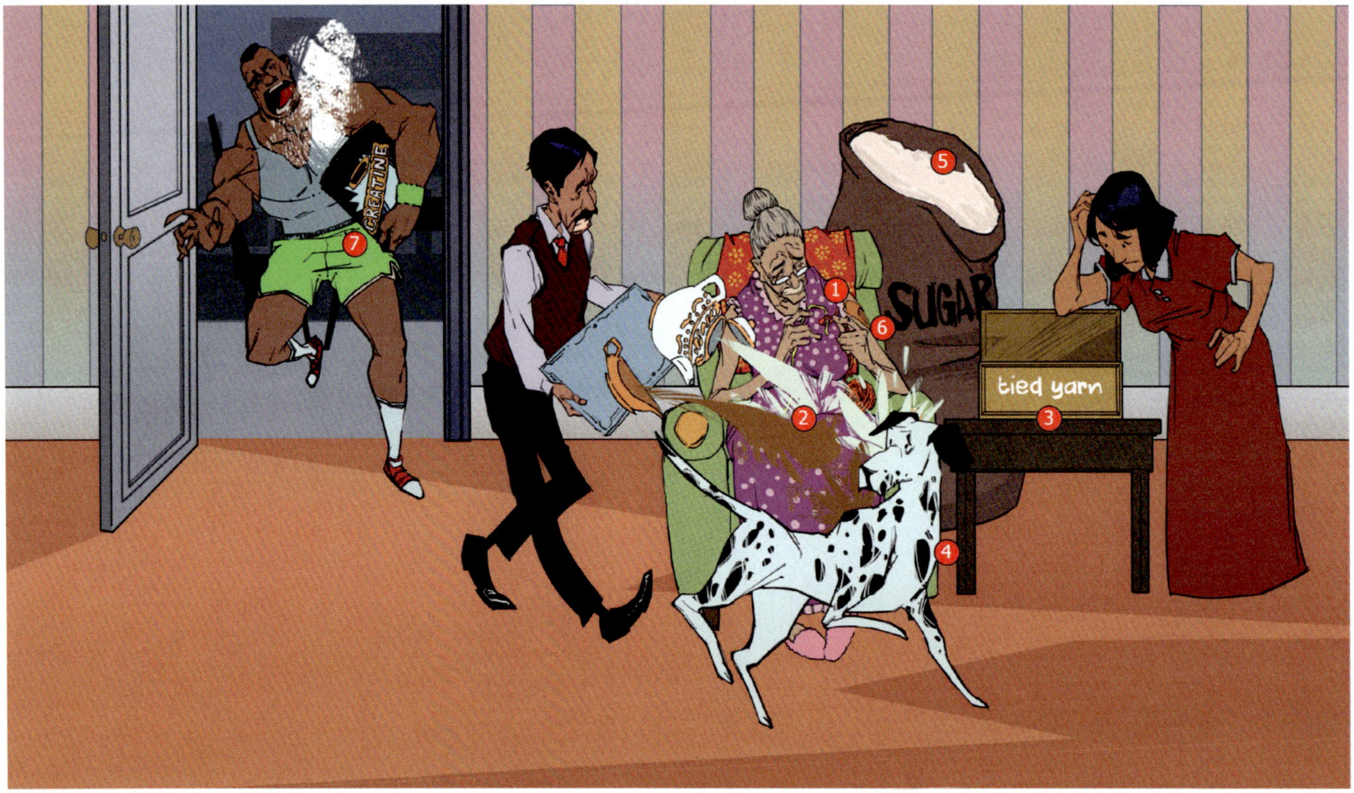

1. Elderly woman integrating yarn: Integrase

2. Tea and gravy: Name of integrase inhibitors end with "tegravir"

3. "Tied yarn" box: Prevent propagation of HIV

4. Dalmatian with liver-shaped shot: Can cause liver inflammation

5. Big bag of sugar: Can cause hyperglycemia

6. Bandaids: used to treat HIV and AIDS

7. Spilled creatine: Integrase inhibitors can increase creatine kinase (CK)

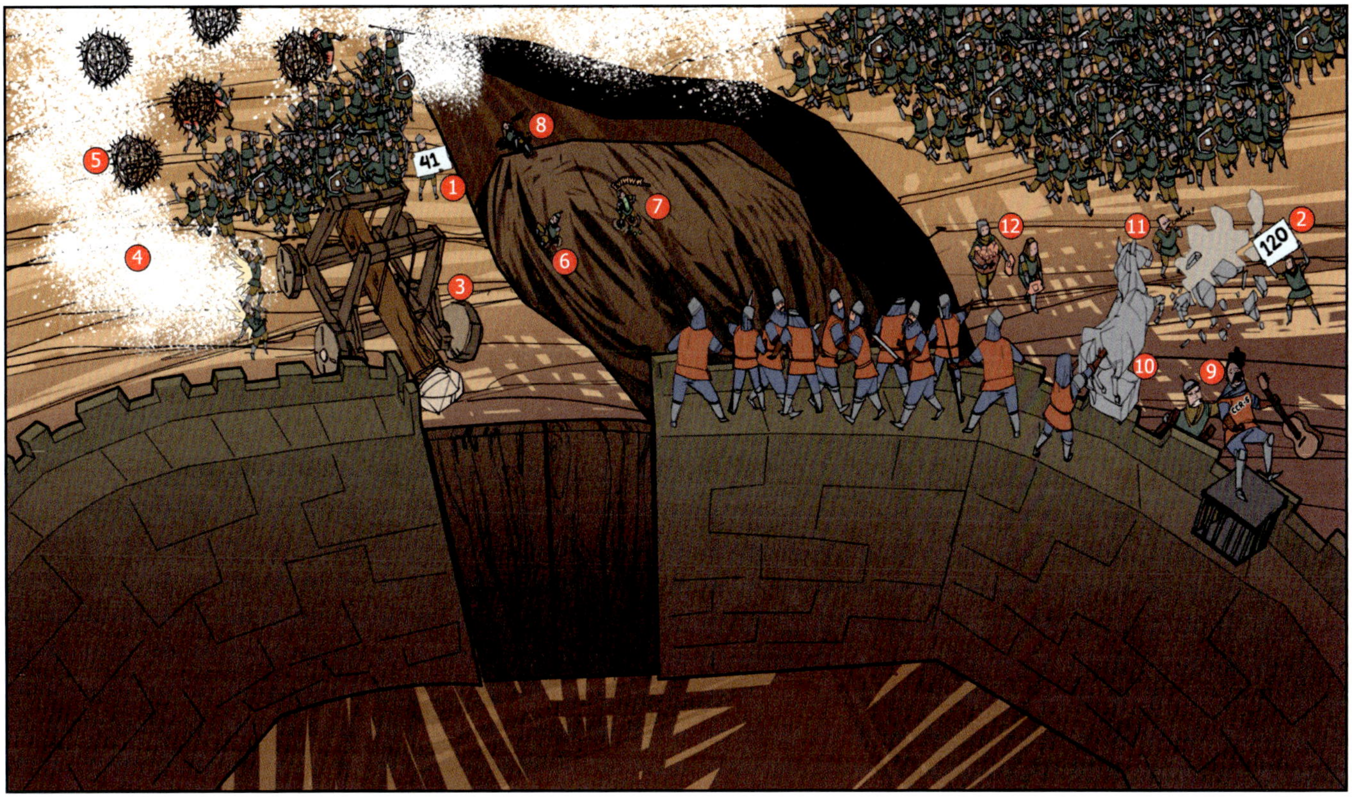

1. Army of 160 men: HIV uses two glycoproteins (*GP41* and *GP120*) to fuse to host cells

2. Two armies that add up to 160: *GP41* and *GP120* are cleaved from *GP160*

3. Battering ram: *GP41* permits HIV to enter the host cell

4. Enchanted cotton: Enfuviride

5. Thorny tumbleweeds within enchanted cotton: Skin reaction at enfuvirtide injection site

6. Moat filled with brown human waste: Enfuvirtide can cause diarrhea

7. Throwing up in disgust: Enfuvirtide can cause nausea and vomiting

8. Exhausted attacker: Enfuvirtide can cause fatigue

9. CCR singer standing on cage: *GP120* acts by binding to the CCR-5 surface protein on macrophages

10. Mare-shaped rock crushing attackers from the army of 120: Maraviroc blocks the activity of *GP120*

11. Mare rock causing dust and coughing: Maraviroc can cause upper respiratory infections

12. Bandaids: Enfuvirtide and maraviroc are used to treat HIV and AIDS

See Figure 9.6.1 - Overview of Antivirals (Antivirals, Section 1, Page 104)

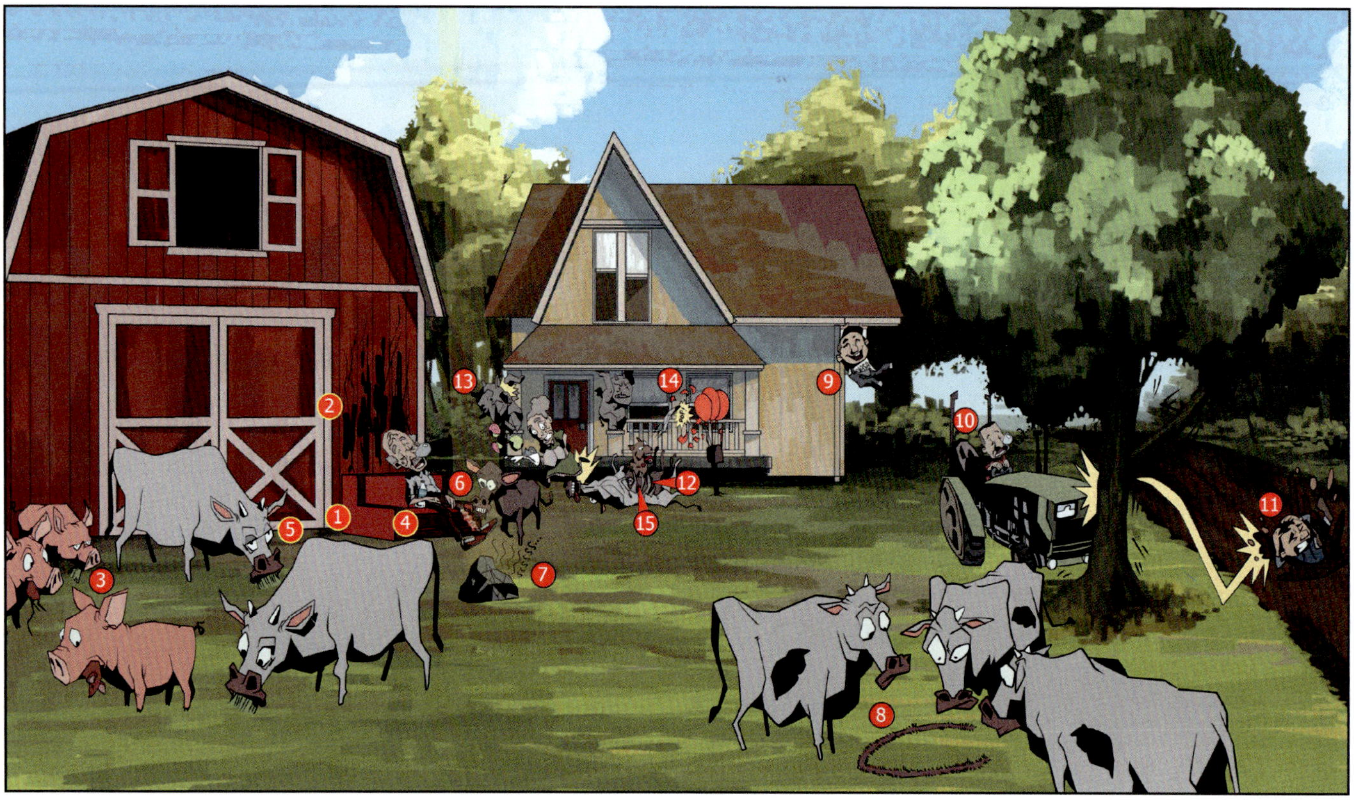

1. Sofa: Sofosbuvir

2. Lead paint peeling behind sleepy farmer: Ledipasvir

3. Omnivore pigs: Ombitasvir

4. Dasani water that sleepy farmer is holding: Dasabuvir

5. Grazing cows: Grazoprevir

6. Grazing calf causing sleepy farmer to get awful sunburn: Grazoprevir can cause photosensitivity and rash

7. Simmering rock under hot sun: Simeprevir

8. Liver spotted cows investigating the "C" crop circle: Used to treat Hepatitis C

9. Farmer's son swinging from house wearing NASA shirt being covered by overalls: These drugs inhibit replication by inhibiting one of these proteins: *NS5A*, *NS5B*, or *NS3/4A*

10. Farm-hand falling asleep while driving tractor: Can cause fatigue

11. Boy smashing head before falling into muddy river: Can cause headaches and diarrhea

12. Ribs of decaying cow: Ribavirin may also be used in conjunction with one of the other drugs

13. Ramer's wife tripping on ribs, spilling guava, ,pur water, and breaking the imp: Ribavirin inhibits IMP dehydrogenase by preventing guanine (purine) formation

14. Popped red balloon from flying rib: Ribavirin can cause hemolytic anemia

15. Unborn dead calf: Ribavirin is teratogenic

CARDIAC PHARMACOLOGY

Section I - Hypertension Treatment

HTN Type	Thiazide Diuretics	Loop Diuretics	ACE Inhibitors	ARBs	Ca 2+ Channel Blockers	Beta Blockers	Aldosterone Antagonists	Notes
Primary (Essential)	✔		✔	✔	✔			
With Heart Failure		✔	✔	✔		✔	✔	- Use β-blockers with caution in decompensated HF. - β-blockers are contraindicated in cardiogenic shock. - Combine ARBs with sacubitril (neprilysin inhibitor).
With Diabetes Mellitus	✔		✔	✔	✔	✔		- ACE inhibitors and ARBs protect against diabetic nephropathy. - β-blockers can mask symptoms of hypoglycemia.
With Asthma	✔			✔	✔	✔		- Avoid nonselective β-blockers to prevent negative side-effects such as β2-receptor-induced bronchoconstriction. - Avoid ACE inhibitors to prevent confusion as to causes of cough (drug or asthma-related).
During Pregnancy								- **<u>Memory hook</u>**: *"Moms Like Neonate Hugs"* (Methyldopa, Labetalol, Nifedipine, Hydralazine)

Table 9.7.1 - Hypertension Types and Treatments

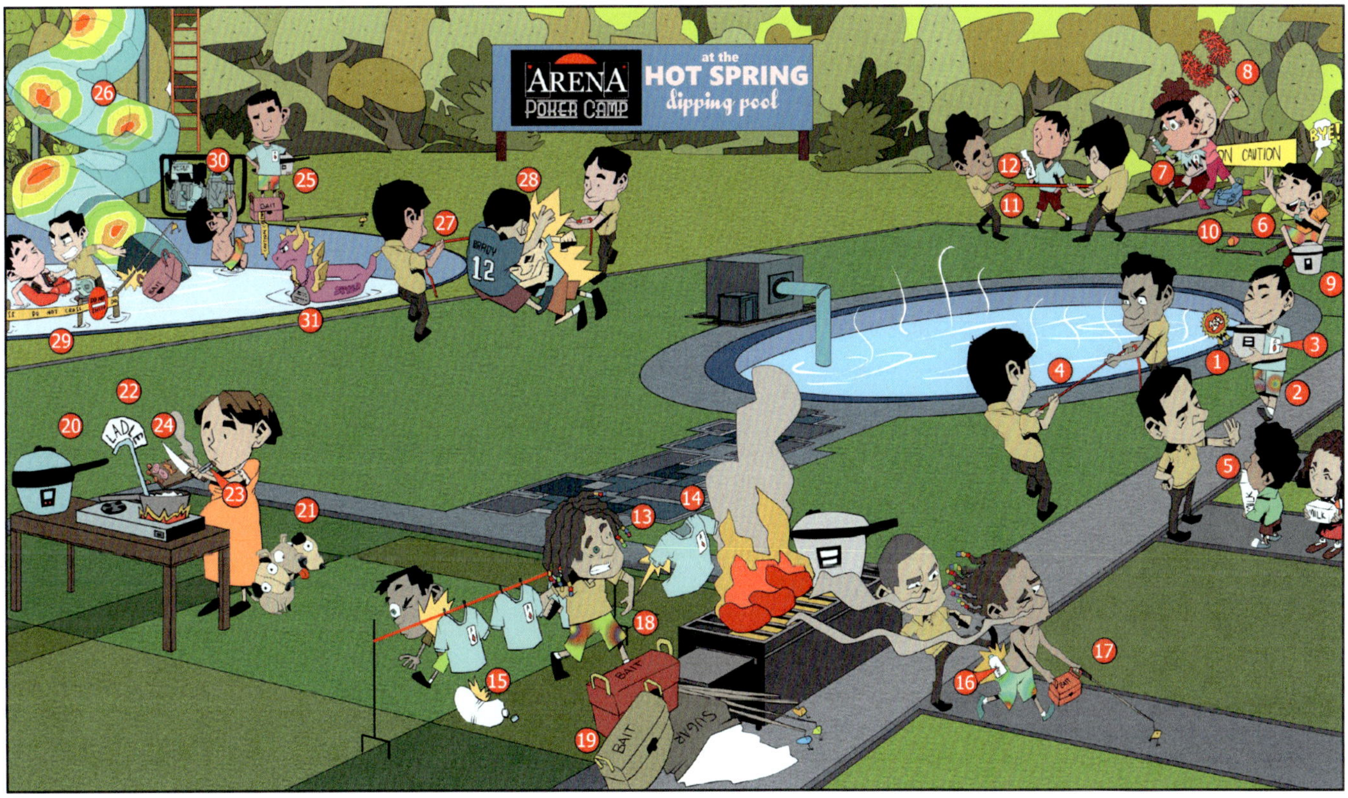

1. 1st place ribbon pn pressure cooker: Primary (essential) hypertension treatment

2. Tie-dye shorts worn by 1st place camper: Thiazide diuretics

3. Ace card camp T-shirt: Ace inhibitors

4. Counselors tightly holding red rope blocking the pool: Angiotensin II receptor blockers (ARBs)

5. Counselor blocking kids from entering with milk: Ca^2 channel blockers

6. Camper with inhaler and pressure cooker: Hypertension with asthma

7. Asthmatic camper being tightly hugged with ace shirt from crossing caution tape: Avoid ACE inhibitors to prevent confusion between drug-related cough and asthma-related cough

8. Cheerleader on top of two handled bait box with bronchiole pom poms: Avoid β_2 blockade to prevent bronchoconstriction

9. Kid with inhaler and pressure cooker wearing tie-dye pants: Use thiazide diuretics

10. Kid with inhaler sitting next to broken fishing pole with bait: Use cardioselective β-blockers (β_1 blockers)

11. Counselors tightly holding red rope blocking the pool on asthma side: Use ARBs

12. Counselors with red ropes blocking kid with milk: Use Ca^{2+} channel blockers

13. Counselor with dreadlocks and dyed beads cooking with pressure cooker: Hypertension with diabetes melitus

14. Dyed beads counselor throws ACE camp shirt to smother flaming kidney beans: Use ACE inhibitors are protective against diabetic nephropathy

15. Camper trying to sneak kidney-shaped water bottle smacked in the face by tense ace camp shirt clothesline: ARBs are protective against diabtic nephropathy

16. Counselor kicking out dye bead camper with milk in his pocket: Calcium channel blocker

17. Dyed bead camper with broken fishing rod with bail: β-blockers

18. Tie-dye shorts worm by dyed bead counselor and camper: Thiazide diuretics

19. Broken fishing poles on top of spilt sugar next to dyed bead counselor: β-blockers can mask hypoglycemia symptoms, so use cautiously

20. Pregnant counselor with pressure cooker: Hypertension in pregnancy

21. Three headed hydra-looking dog costume next to pregnant counselor: Hydralazine

22. Ladle being used by pregnant counselor: Labetalol

23. Pregnant counselor smoking metal dope: Methyldopa

24. Knife being used to cut and dip vegetables into boiling pan: Nifedipine

25. Counselor with pressure cooker staring at broken water pump: Hypertension with heart failure

26. Tie-dye color loops on water slide: Thiazide and loop diuretics

27. Camp counselors holding red rope taut near water slide: ARBs

28. Football player getting sacked while wearing a Tom Brady jersey next to a tense rope: ARBs (valsartan) can be combined with sacubitril for heart failure

29. Man tossing fishing pole and bait to save camper on heart shaped tube behind caution tape: β-blockers contraindicated in cardiogenic shock

30. Out of breath and swollen swimmer grabbing broken water pump next to fishing pole and bait with hanging caution tape: Use β-blockers cautiously in decompensation heart failure

31. Spyro with epitaph necklace tube: Aldosterone antagonists

Cardiac therapy overview

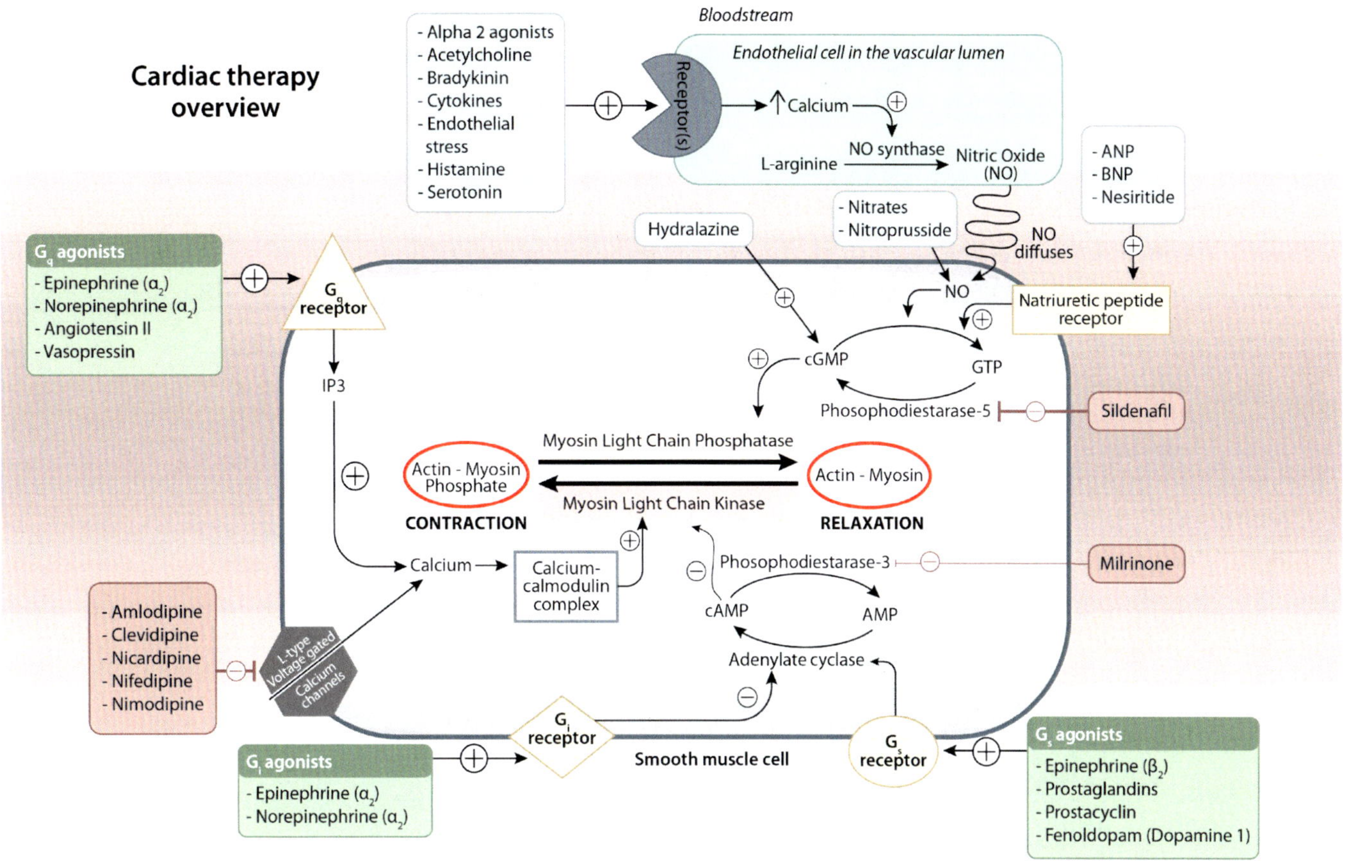

Figure 9.7.2 - Pharmacologic Effects on Smooth Muscle

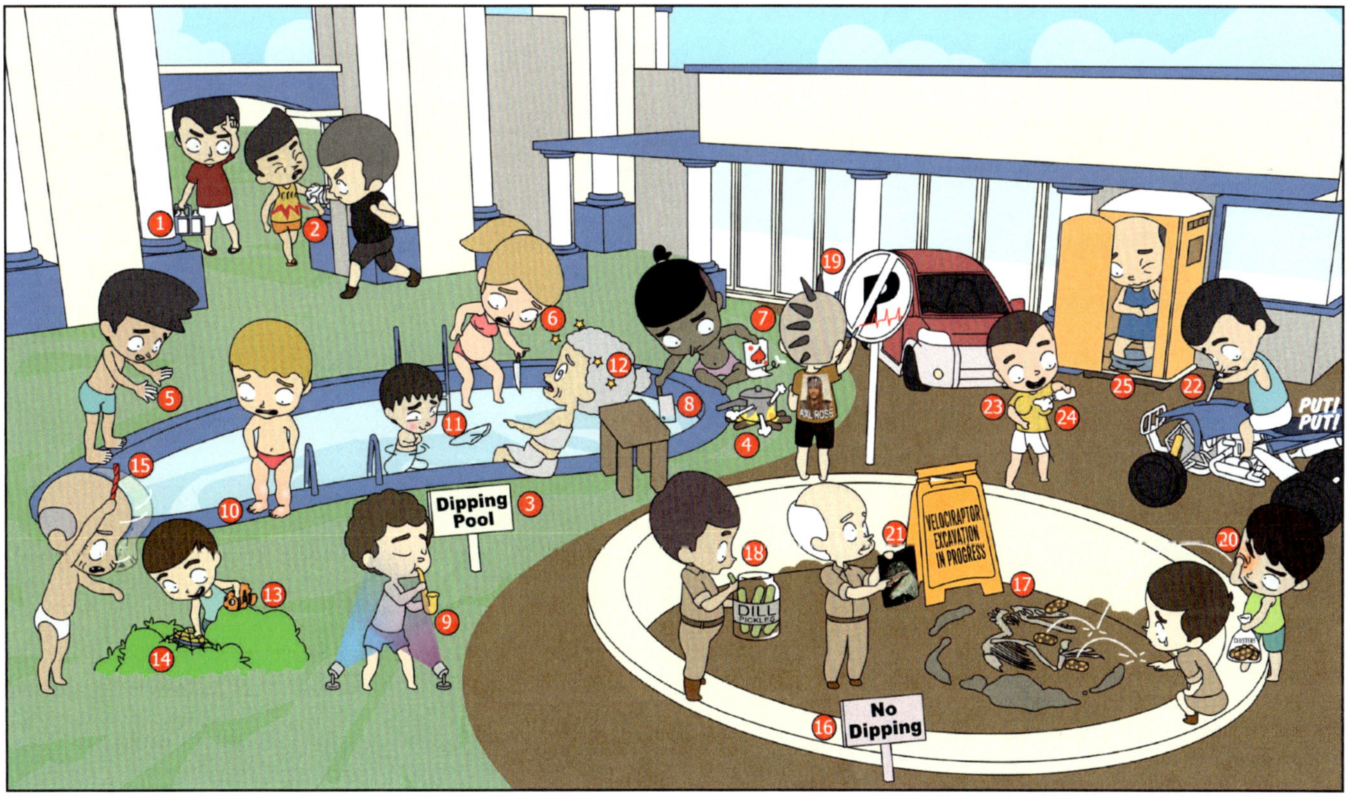

1. Teenager with milk holding "L" on his forehead because he is stopped by bouncer: All CCBs block voltage gated L-type calcium channels

2. Bouncer leaving prints from metal punch on kid's chest: CCB can be used for angina, including prinzmetal (vasospastic) angina

3. "Dipping Pool" sign: Dihydropyridine CCBs end with the suffix "-dipine"

4. Campfire with pressure cooker: Dihydropyridines CCBs can be used for hypertension

5. Kid with pale fingers and toes diving into pool: Dihydropyridine CCBs can be used for Raynaud's phenomenon (primary and secondary)

6. Pregnant lady handing knife dipping into pool: Nifedipine is a dihydropyridine CCB that can be used in pregnancy

7. Guy with hot pressure cooker got distracted by empty box of cards: Nicardipine is a dihydropyridine CCB that can be used in hypertensive emergency or urgency

8. Cleaver being washed in dipping pool near hot pressure cooker: Clevidipine is a dihydropyridine CCB that can be used in hypertensive emergency or urgency

9. Guy playing smooth jazz: Dihydropyridine CCBs act on vascular smooth muscle

10. Guy climbing out of pool who has bilateral pedal edema: Dihydropyridine CCBs can cause peripheral edema

11. Boy who blushes because he lost his swim trunks: Dihydropyridine CCBs can cause flushing

12. Dizzy old lady falling back: Dihydropyridine CCBs can cause dizziness

13. Kid playing with Nemo toy: Nimodipine is another dihydropyridine CCB

14. Kid pretending that Nemo is saving a submarine stuck in webs: Nimmodipine can treat subarachnoid hemorrhage (SAH)

15. Old guy shaking red licorice in front of disinterested kid: Nimodipine is used against SAH because it prevents cerebral vasospasm

16. "No Dipping" sign: Non-dihydropyridine CCBs

17. Velociraptor excavation: Verapamil is a non-dihydropyridine CCB

18. Archaeologist eating dill pickles: Diltiazem is a non-dihydropyridine CCB

19. Kid scribbling over no parking sign with a fib ECG reading pattern in front of red car: Non-dihydropyridine CCBs can be used in atrial fibrillation and atrial flutter

20. Archaeologist hit in face with peanut cluster and crying out of one eye: Verapamil can be used as prophylaxis in cluster headaches

21. Archaeologist focusing on teeth and prominent gums of velociraptor: Verapamil causes gingival hyperplasia

22. ATV with broken engine on dirty ground: Verapamil and diltiazem can cause cardiac depression or AV block

23. Obnoxious boy shoving balloons up shirt to look like breasts: Verapamil and diltiazem can cause gynecomastia

24. Kid pouring milk over fake breasts: Verapamil and diltiazem can cause hyperprolactinemia

25. Constipated guy on portable toilet: Verapamil and diltiazem can cause constipation

See Figure 9.7.2 - Pharmacologic Effects on Smooth Muscle (Cardiac Pharmacology, Section 2, Page 117)

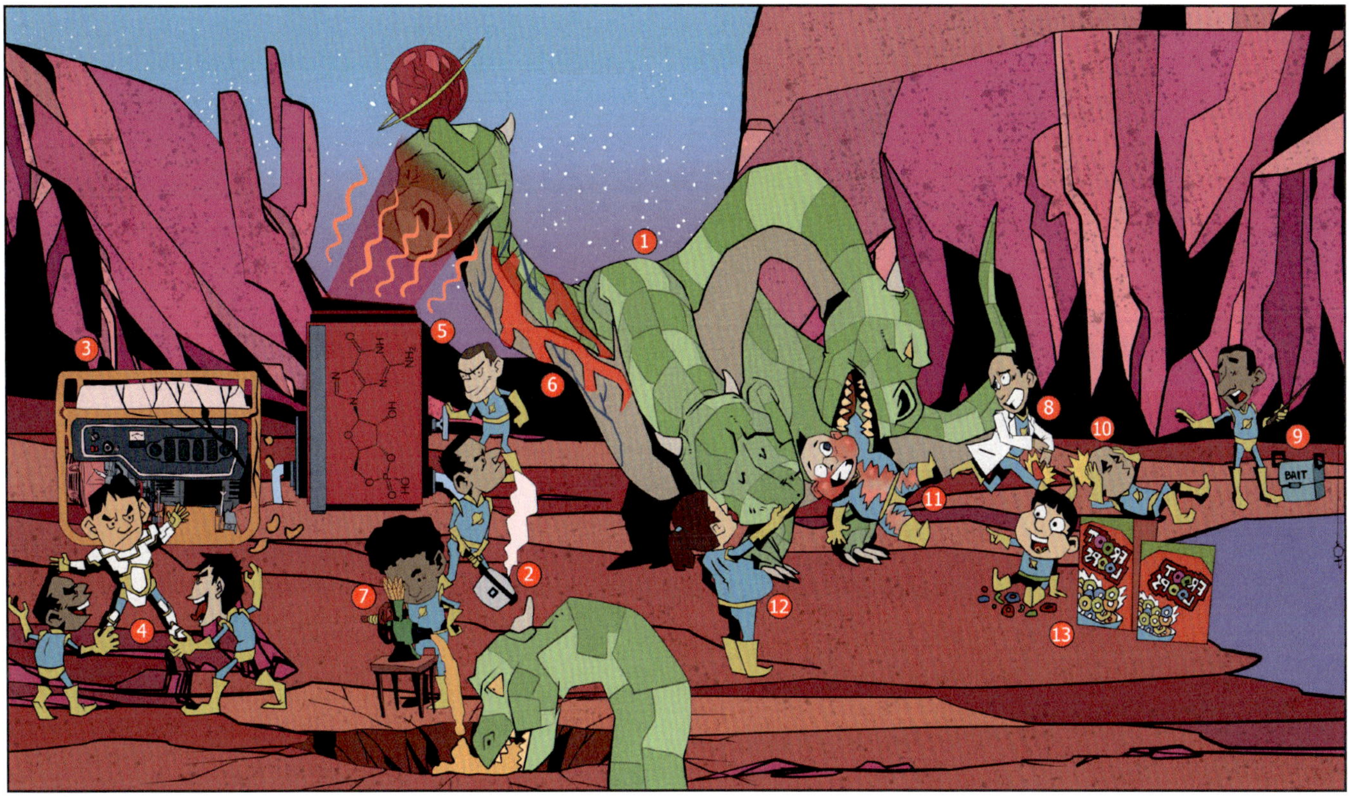

1. Three headed hydra alien: Hydralazine

2. Pressure cooker held by camp's cook: Use for severe hypertension

3. Broken pump: Use for heart failure

4. Armored isolation warrior defending broken pump against two warriors: In case of heart failure, use hydralazine alongside isosorbide dinitrate (ISDN)

5. Warrior cranking cyclic generator that is relaxing hydra: Increases cGMP which relaxes smooth muscle

6. Dilated red blood vessels on hydra are visibly larger than blue vessels: Dilation of arteries > veins

7. Assistant hand grinding wheat into crater that hydra is eating out of: Decreased afterload

8. Doctor running away from hydra with reflex hammer while checking his pulse: Can cause reflex tachycardia

9. Soldier with fishing pole and two handled bait box blocking running doctor: Prevent reflex tachycardia with beta blockers

10. Sleeping guy holding head in pain: Can cause headaches

11. Solder allergic to hydra bites with swollen leg: Can cause edema

12. Pregnant soldier petting hydra: Safe in pregnancy

13. Little boy eating froot loops: Can cause drug-induced SLE (lupus)

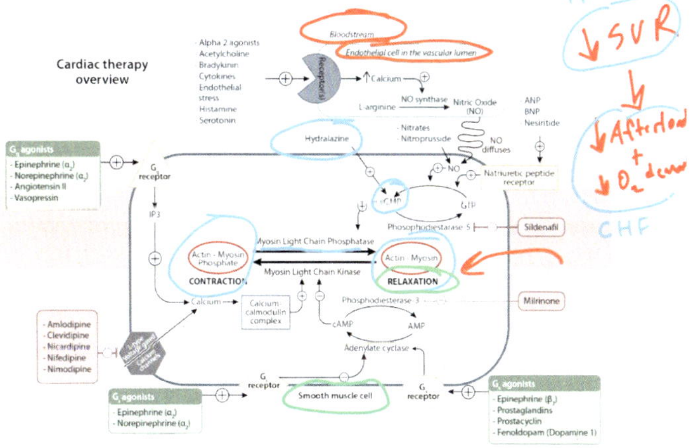

See Figure 9.7.2 - Pharmacologic Effects on Smooth Muscle (Cardiac Pharmacology, Section 2, Page 117)

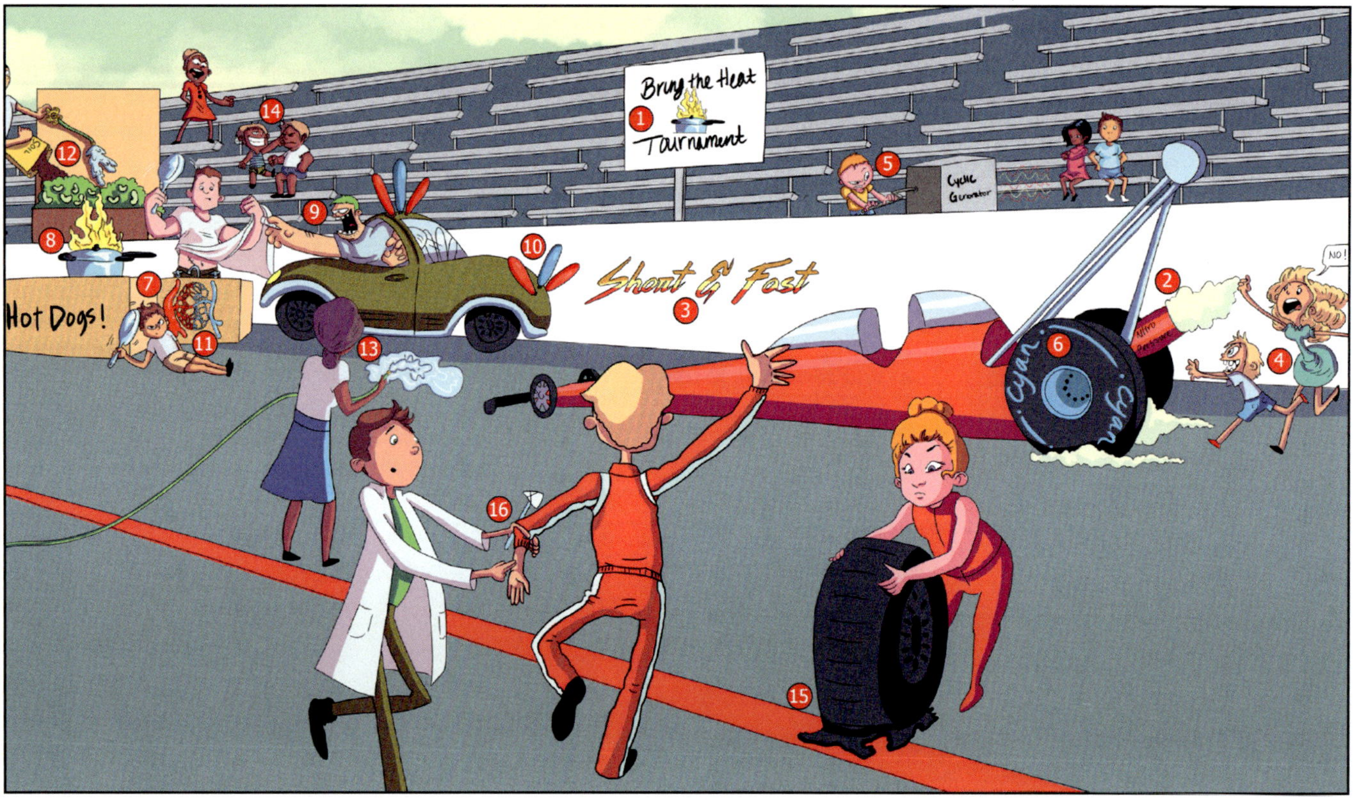

1. Flaming pressure cooker symbol on tournament sign: Hypertensive emergency

2. "Nitro Pressure" brand exhaust pipe: Nitroprusside

3. "Short & Fast" graphic near exhaust: Nitroprusside is a fast-acting and acts for a short duration

4. Mom screamed "NO!" while chasing her child: Nitroprusside directly increases release of NO (nitric oxide)

5. Worker cranking "Cyclic Generator" heater: Nitroprusside increases cGMP

6. "Cyan" tire brand: Can cause cyanide toxicity because part of it gets metabolized into cyanide

7. Hot dog worker fanning himself with pan: Fenoldopam

8. Pressure cooker next to hot dog worker who had surgery: Use fenoldopam for postoperative hypertension

9. Driver forcing dope on hotdog worker: Fenoldopam agonizes dopamine (D1) receptors

10. Long red and blue balloons tied to dope driver's dar: Fenoldopam dilates coronary vasculature

11. Kid fanning himself with pan, causing the red plumbing to swell: Fenoldopam dilates peripheral vasculature

12. Owner watering healthy kidney bean plants nearing flaming pressure cooker: Fenoldopam helps maintain renal perfusion during hypertensive emergency

13. Worker using hose to clean up spill: Fenoldopam promotes natriuresis

14. Kid sticking finger in brother's eye while mom is getting mad at them: Avoid fenoldopam in patients with glaucoma

15. Pit crew rolling flat tire: Both nitroprusside and fenoldopam can cause hypotension

16. Doctor with reflex hammer checking pulse of running driver: Both nitroprusside and fenoldopam can cause reflex tachycardia

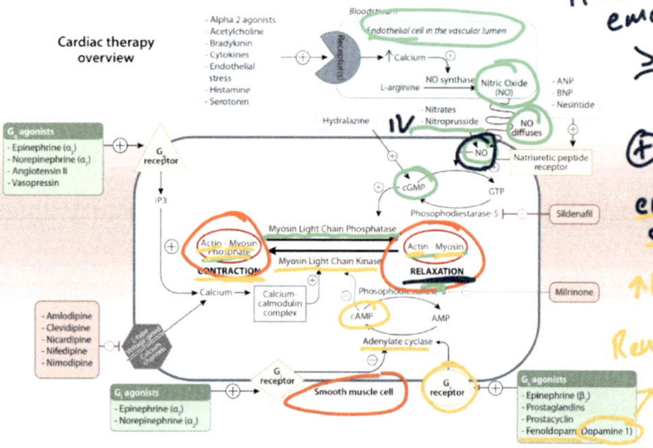

HTN emergency
≥180/120
⊕ signs of end-organ damage
↑RBF
↑
Renal vasc.

See Figure 9.7.2 - Pharmacologic Effects on Smooth Muscle (Cardiac Pharmacology, Section 2, Page 117)

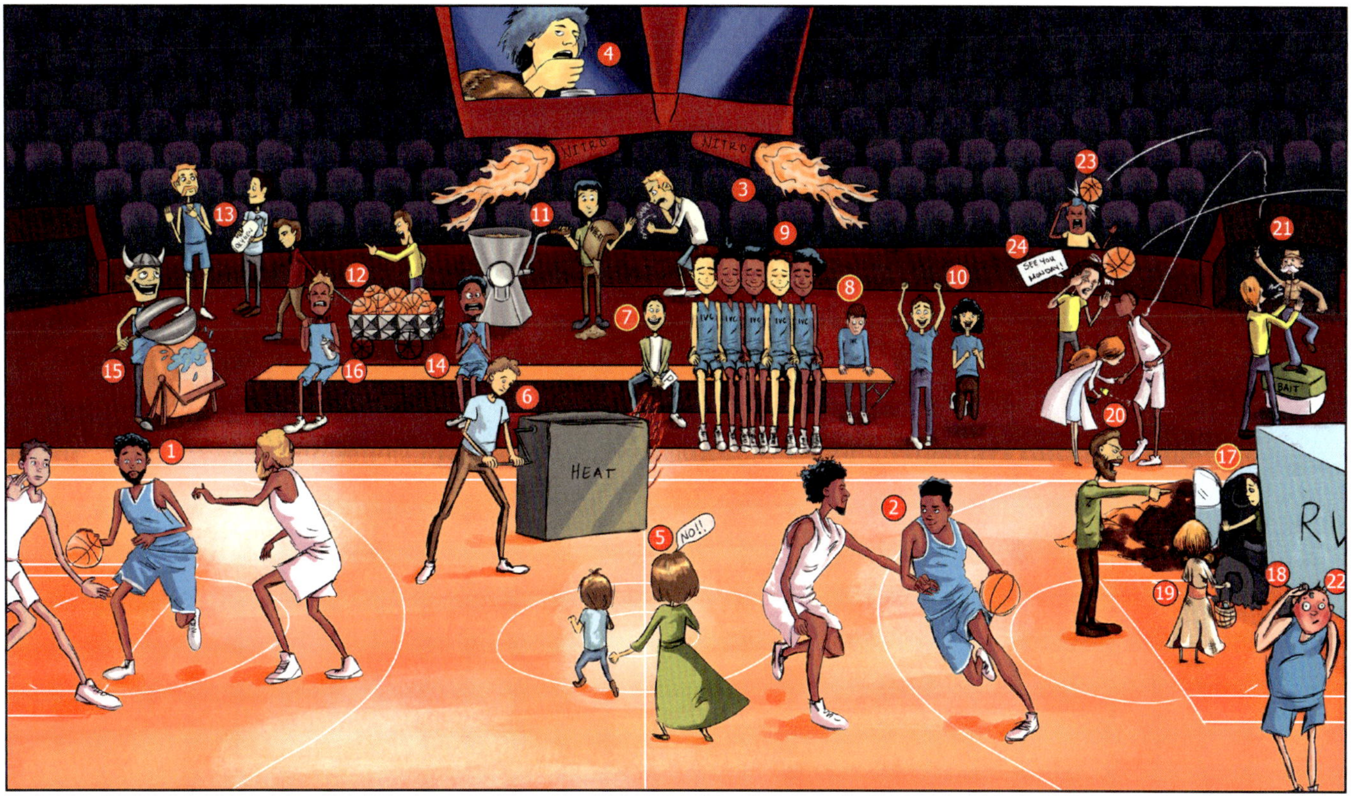

1. Isolated basketball player in blue blocked by two other players: Isosorbide dinitrate

2. Other player in blue only be being blocked by one opposing player: Isosorbide mononitrate

3. Nitro Flame throwers above court: Nitroglycerin

4. Man on jumbotron eating food: Nitroglycerin is ingested because it has better bioavailability

5. Mom chasing after her child screaming "No!!": Increases nitric oxide (NO)

6. Staff cranking cyclic heater: Increases cGMP

7. Happy and relaxed fan sitting on player's bench next to heater: Higher cGMP leads to myosin light-chain dephosphorylation → smooth muscle relaxation

8. Water boy in blue shirt with makeshift bench: Increases venous capacitance

9. Basketball players tacked tightly on bench looking relaxed with IVC jerseys: Dilated larger veins including the IVC

10. Smaller, excited team assistants. Smaller veins aren't relaxed (dilated) as much as the larger veins

11. Mad fan knocking wheat out of wheat grinder salesman's hand: Decreased preload

12. Employee being yelled at by boss while carrying basketballs in armored cart: Nitrates contraindicated in hypertrophic obstructive cardiomyopathy (HOCM)

13. Player with hand on chest turning down oxygen: Myocardial oxygen demand is also decreased → relief of pain

14. Player clutching his chest in pain: Used for angina/ ACS

15. Mascot sharpening lung-shaped ax on wet stone: Used for fluid overload/pulmonary edema

16. Player drinking water, but his throat is spasming: Used for diffuse esophageal spasm

17. Viking Coach yelling at RV driver who smashed into the court: Contraindicated in RV infarction

18. Punctured RV tire: Can cause hypotension

19. Foster kid being stopped by RV driver who doesn't want to buy her dyed eggs: Hypotension can be a life-threatening in a patient that is also taking a phosphodiesterase inhibitor

20. Doctor checking pulse and examines knee of player in white with a reflex hammer: Can cause reflex tachycardia

21. Fisherman mascot standing on bait box and pretending to hook a player while being blocked: Treat reflex tachycardia with beta blockers

22. Flushed out of shape player: Can cause cutaneous flushing

23. Concessions worker holding head in pain: Can cause headaches

24. Angry worker who quits and shouts, "See you Monday!": Can cause "Monday disease" (headache, dizziness, and tachycardia from vasodilation upon restarting the medication on Monday)

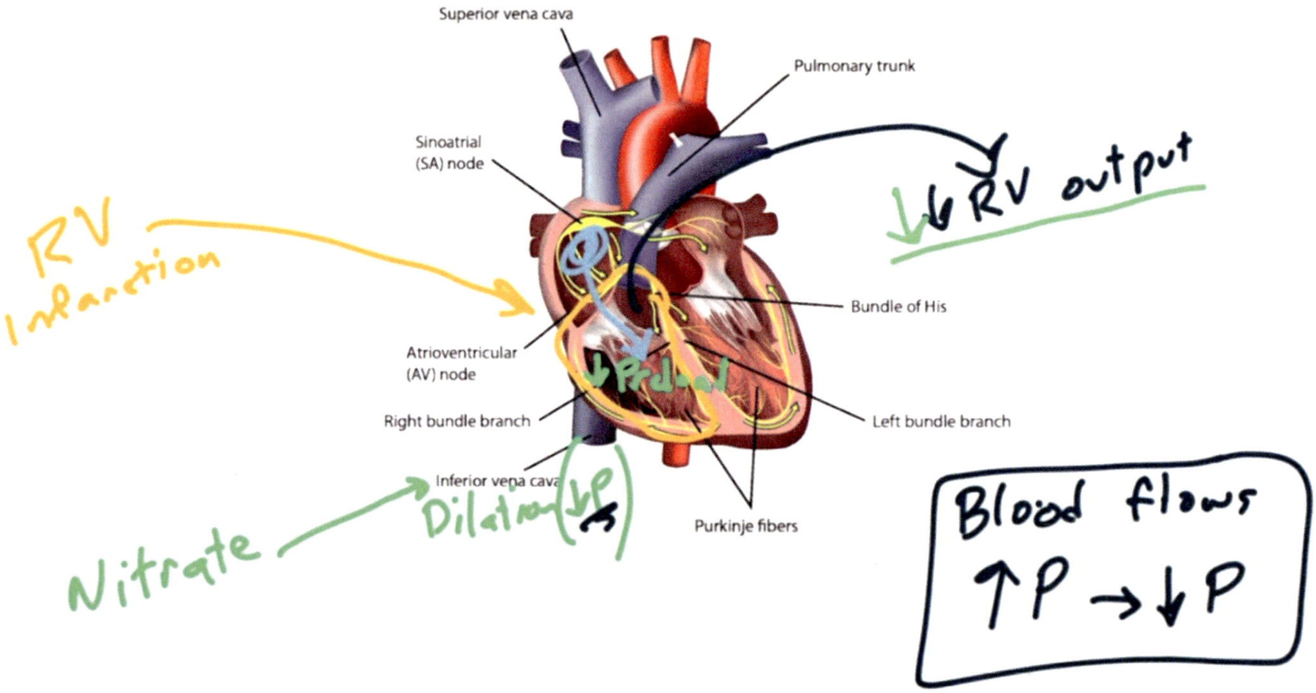

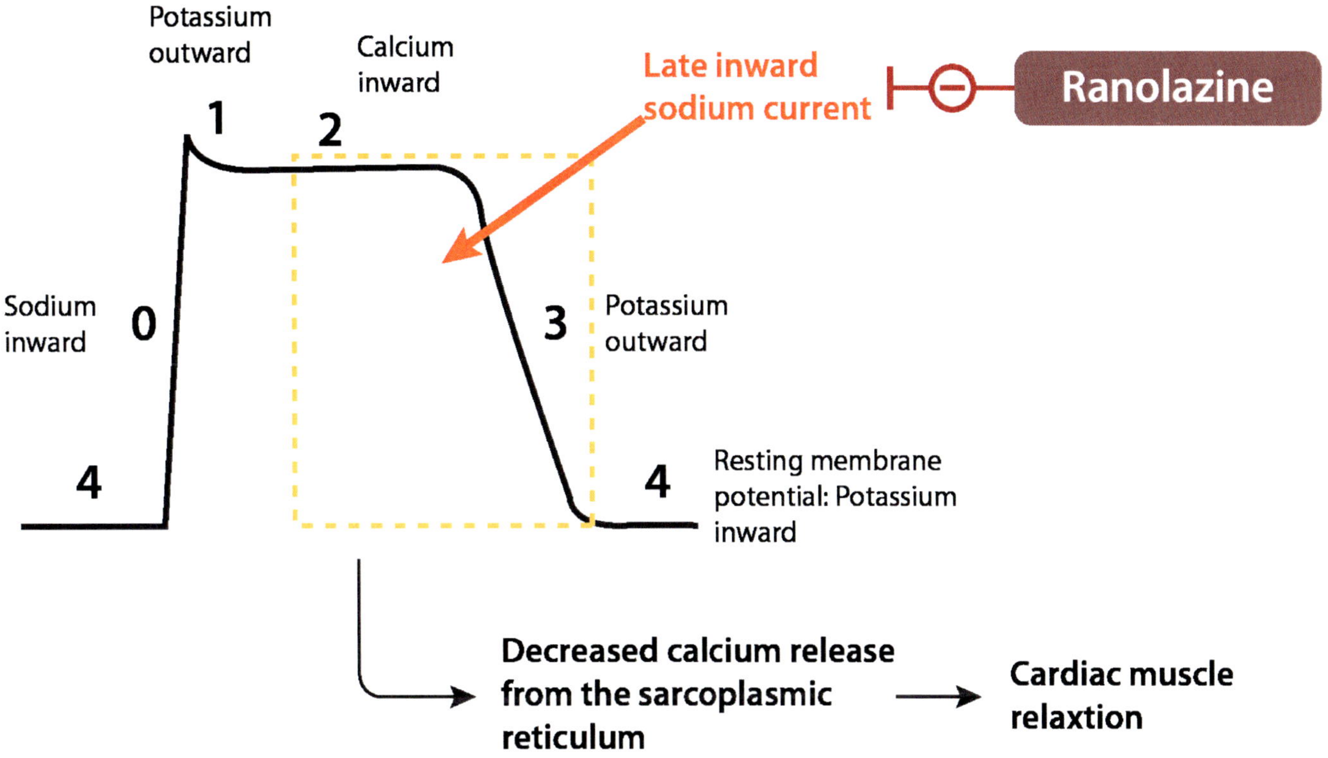

Figure 9.7.3 - Effect of Ranolazine on Ventricular Action Potentials

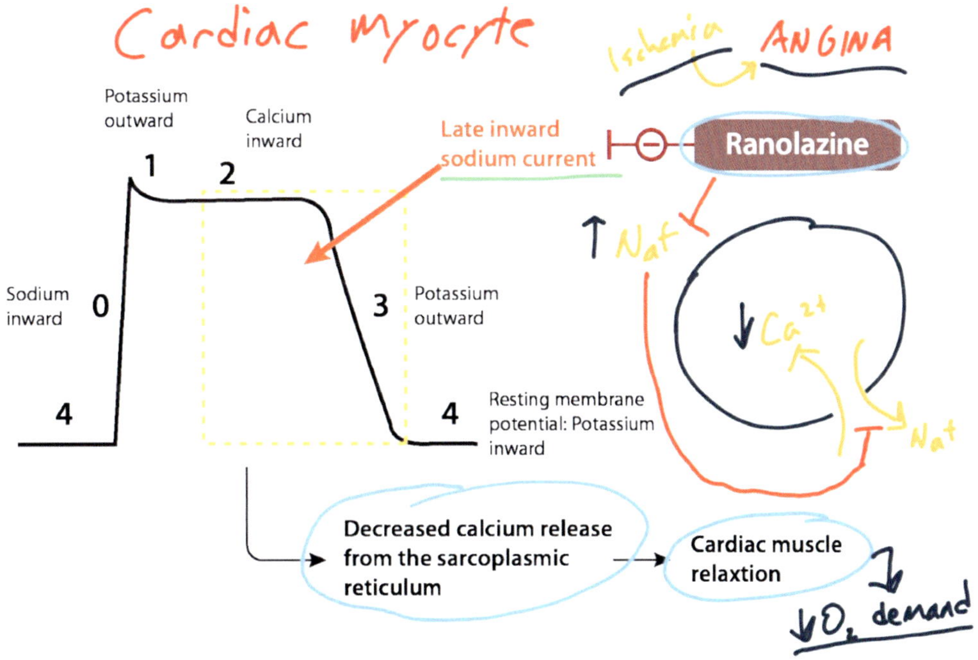

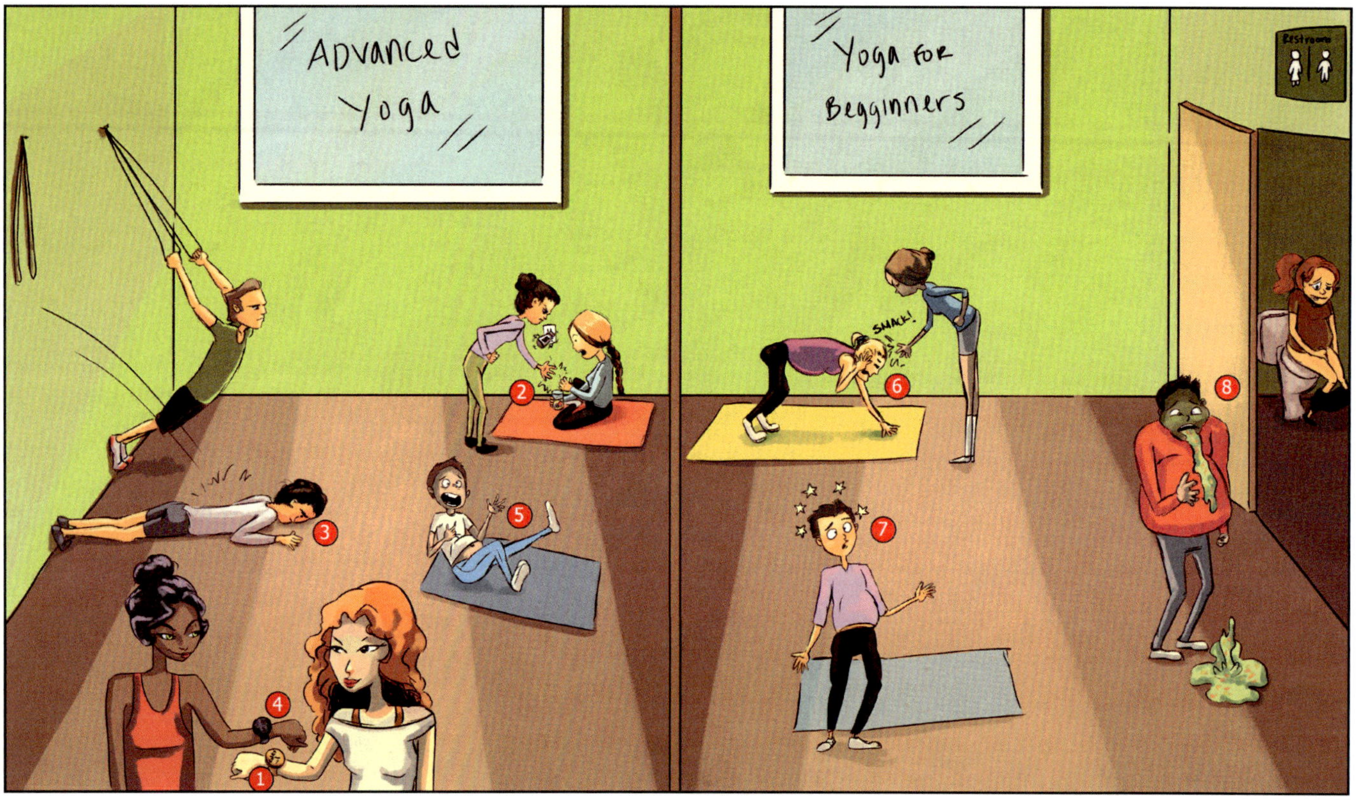

1. Gold Rolex watch: Ranolazine

2. Instructor slaps salt shaker out of student's hand: Inhibits the last phase of the inward sodium current

3. Women distracted by Rolex loses tension from band and falls over on face: Reduces diastolic wall tension and oxygen consumption

4. Women compares Apple watch, which can monitor heart rate, with Rolex watch: Does not affect heart rate or blood pressure

5. Out of shape student with distended belly grabbing his chest: Used for angina refractory to other medical therapies

6. Instructor smacking beginner student on head in beginner area: Can cause headaches

7. Dizzy beginner student: Can cause dizziness

8. Student vomiting on floor because there is a constipated student already in bathroom: Can cause constipation and vomiting

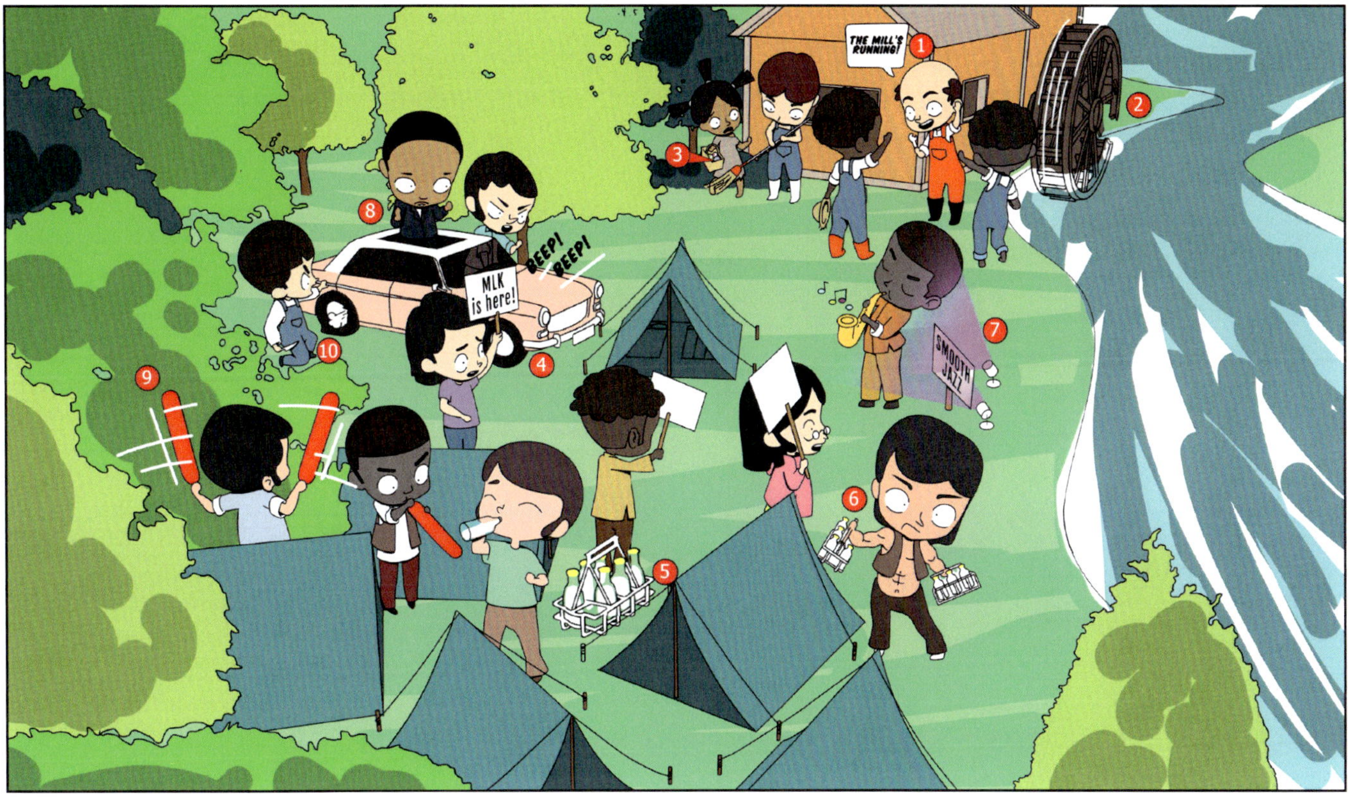

1. Man yelling "The mill's running!": Milrinone

2. Old mill missing a section: Used for acute decompensated heart failure

3. Foster kid with dyed eggs and three ponytails being blocked by worker: Selectively blocks PDE-3

4. Car by tents: Increased cAMP accumulation in cardiac myocytes

5. Camper drinking calcium rich milk: Higher cAMP leads to more calcium entering the myocyte

6. Flexing muscle man with milk: Increased inotropy or contractility

7. Man playing smooth jazz by tents and car: Increases cAMP accumulation in vascular smooth muscle

8. Group of tents blocking MLK's approach: Higher cAMP blocks MLCK activity

9. Inflated, red noise makers: Causes vasodilation

10. Man stabbing hole in tire of MLK's car: Avoid in severely hypotensive patients

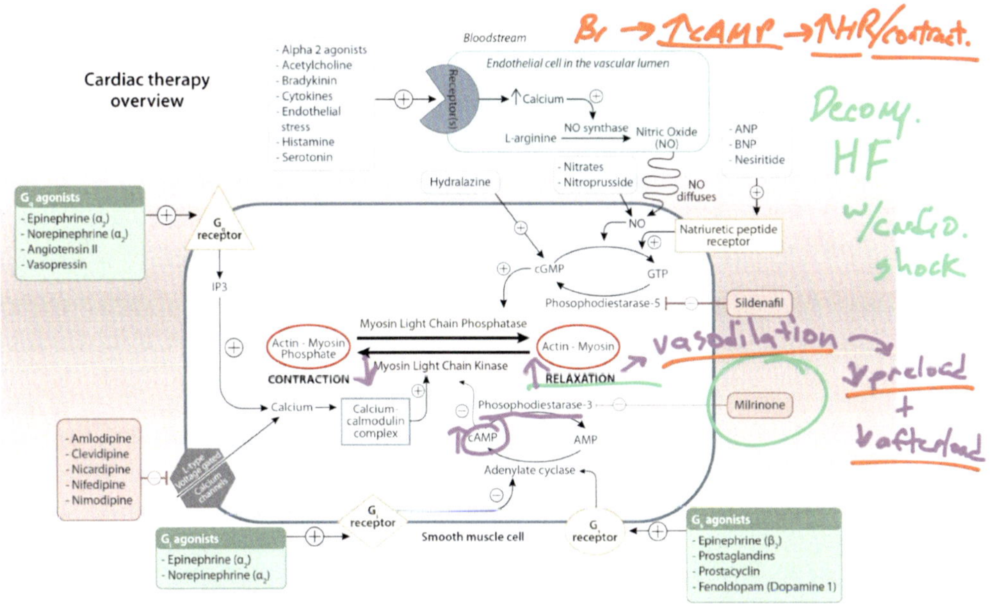

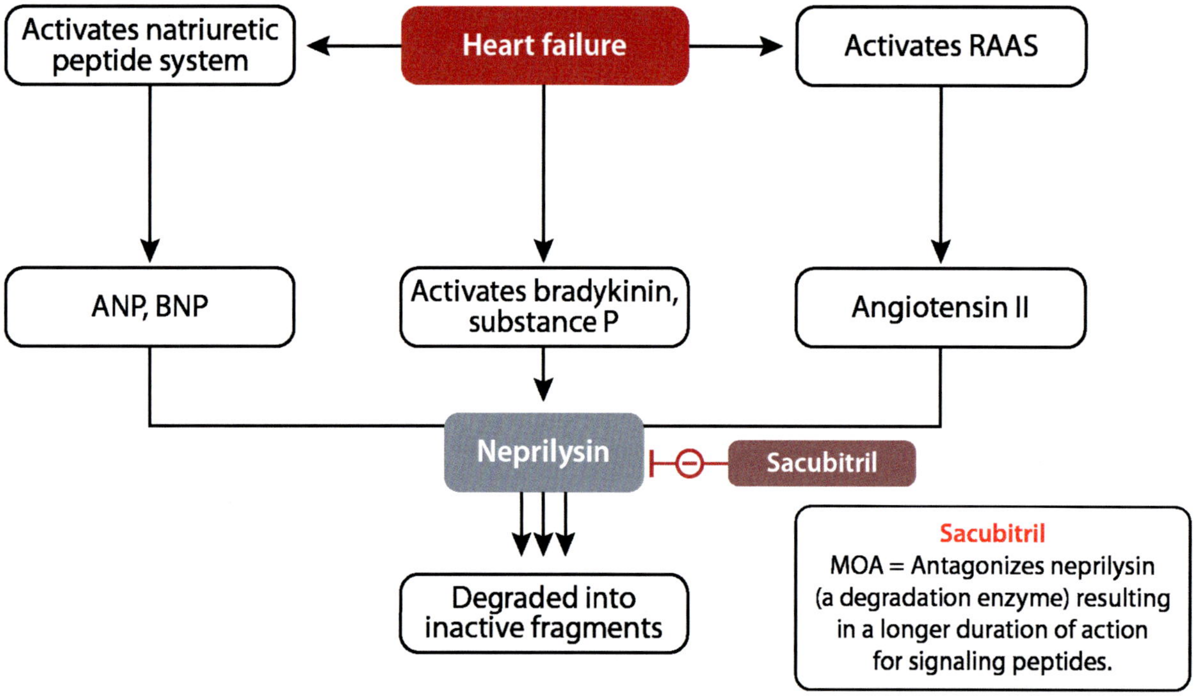

Figure 9.7.4 - Effects of Sacubitril in Heart Failure

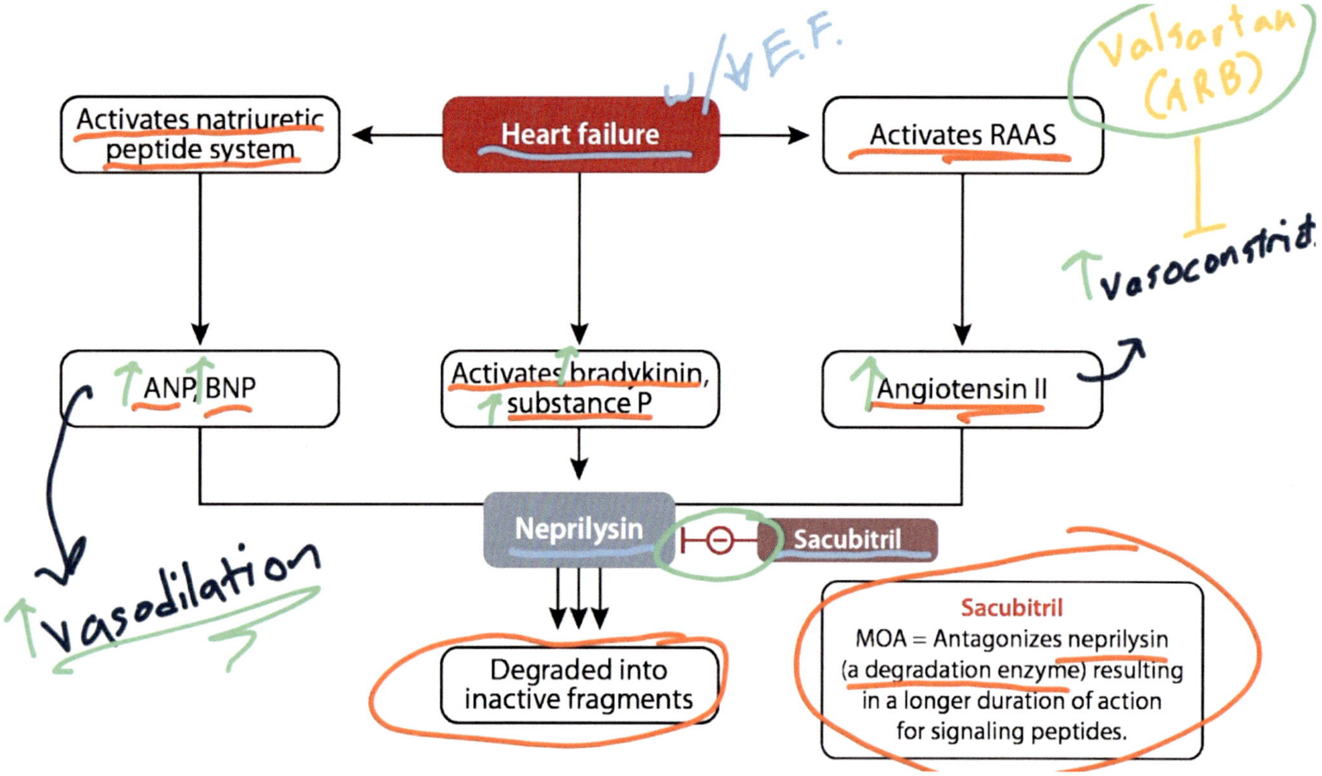

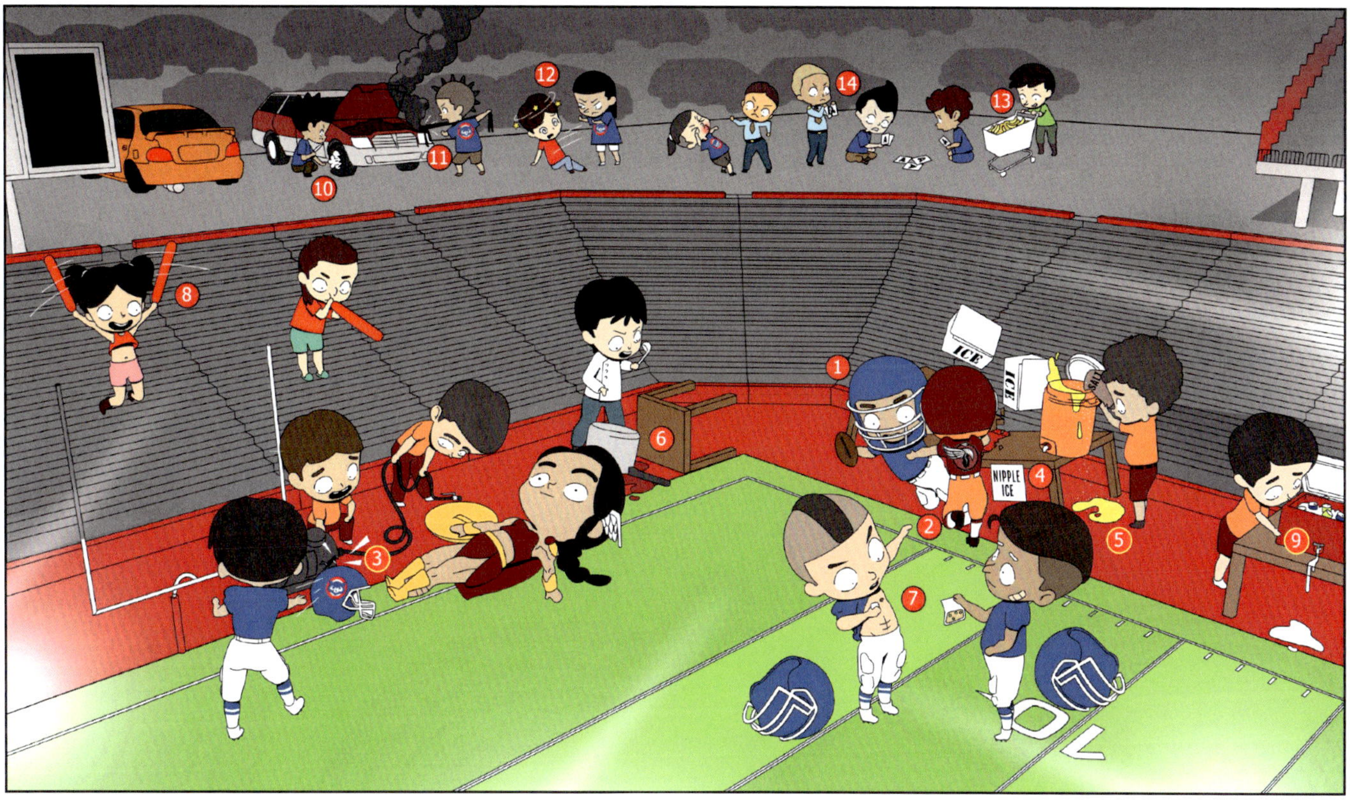

1. Sacked quarterback: Sacubitril

2. Valkyrie team player sacking quarterback: Always used with valsartan

3. Cheerleaders blowing up balloon while Cubs member throws helmet at pump and puts crack in it: Used for heart failure with reduced ejection fraction (HFrEF)

4. "Nipple Ice" Sign on knocked over table: Blocks neprilysin

5. Yellow drink with salt spilling on floor from table: Reduced neprilysin → increased BNP and ANP → increased natriuresis

6. Fallen pressure cooker: Give valsartan with sacubitril in order to prevent hypertension

7. Player icing his chafed nipples with pea powder substance: Neprilysin blockade prevents degradation of substance P

8. Valkyries fans with red and long inflatable stadium noisemakers: The sacubitril-valsartan combination drug causes vasodilation (sacubritil alone would cause vasoconstriction)

9. Waterboy draining excess water from cooler full of drinks: Sacubitril decreased ECF volume

10. Fan stabbing holes into tire in parking lot: Can cause hypotension

11. Fan coughing from smoking engine: Can cause cough

12. Valkyrie fan dizzy from being thrown on ground in parking lot: Can cause dizziness

13. Banana vendor with banana cart: Can cause hyperkalemia

14. Cops tearing up Ace card and punching Cubs fan in face causing a fat lip: Contraindicated when used alongside ACE inhibitors due to angioedema

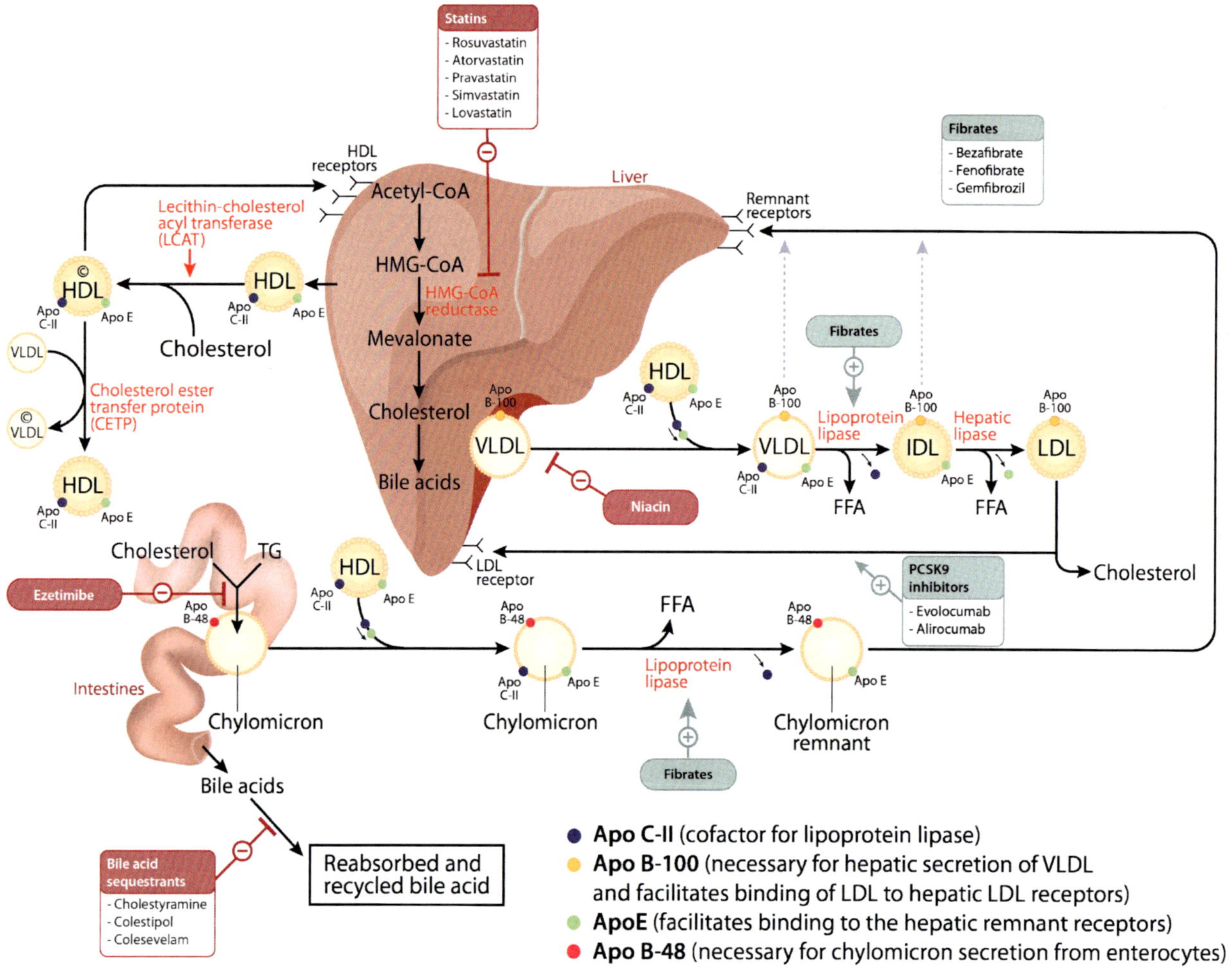

Figure 9.7.5 - Mechanisms of Lipid-Lowering Medications

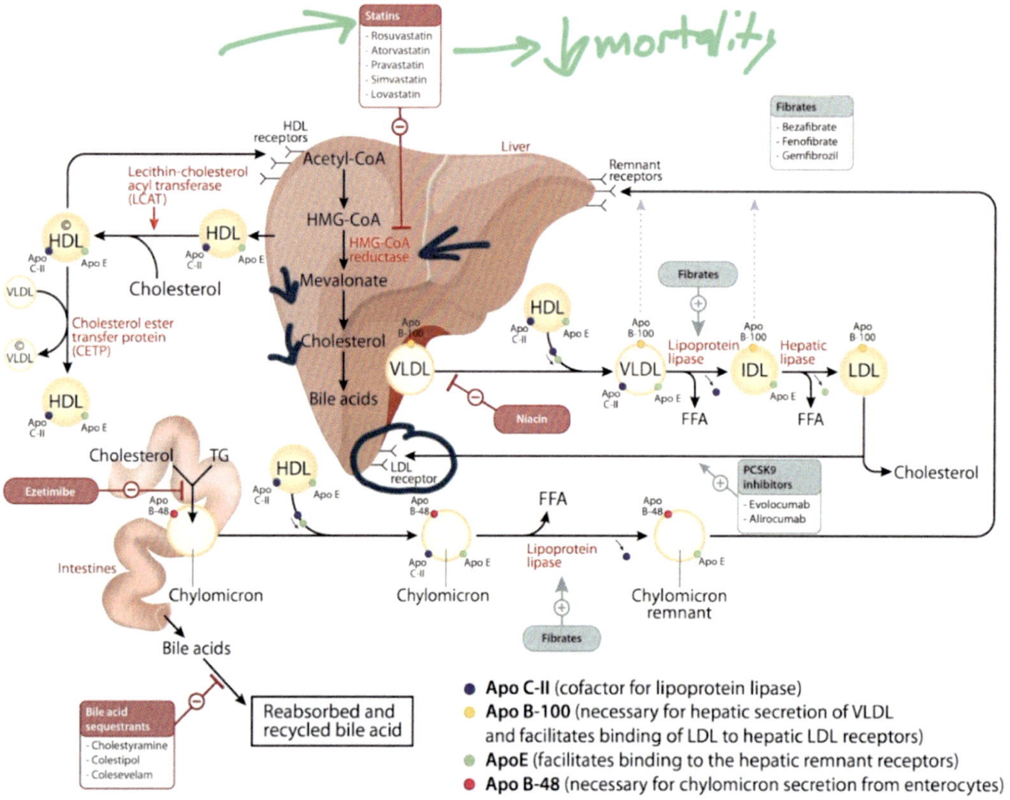

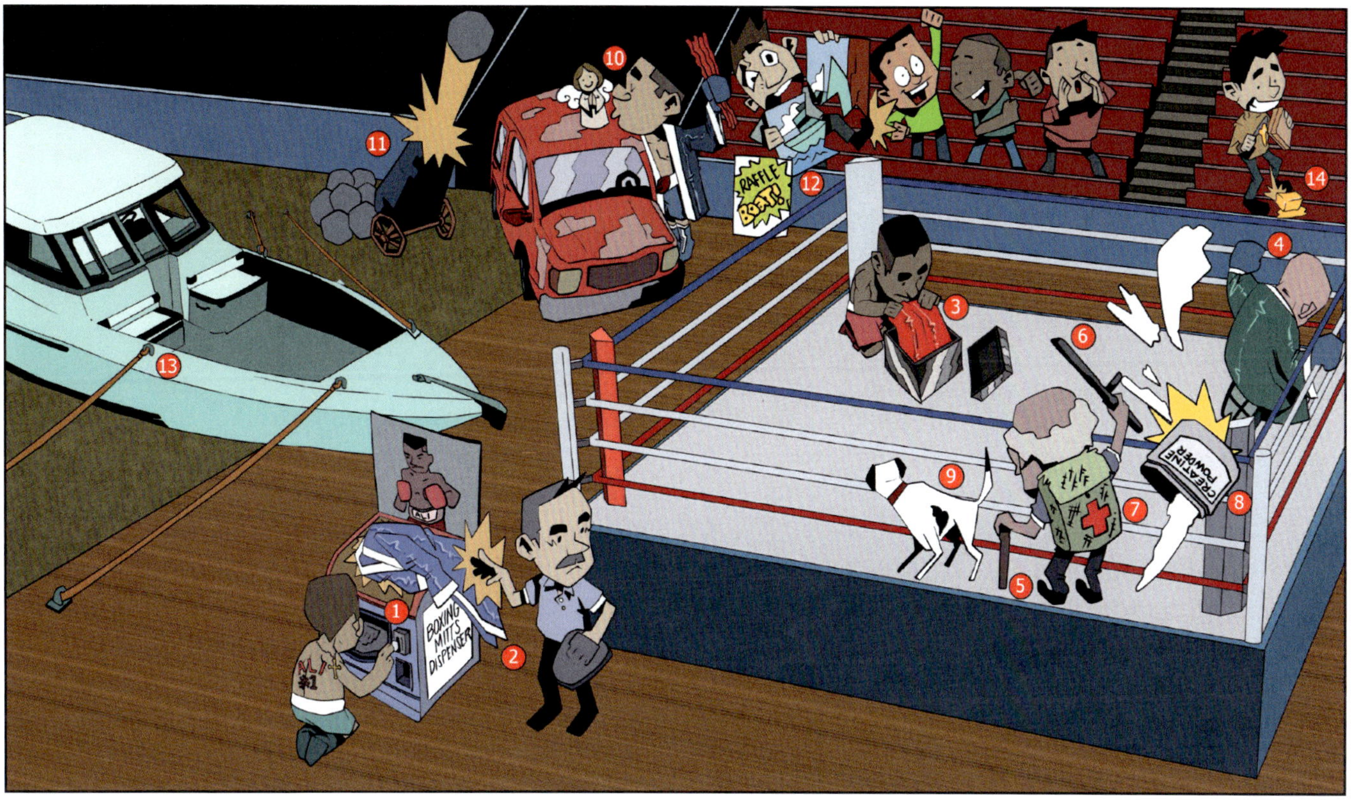

1. Boxer paying homage to Muhammad Ali mitt machine: HMG CoA reductase produces mevalonate

2. Satin robe thrown onto mitt machine stopping production: Statins

3. Boxer putting his satin robe in chrome box: Most statins are metabolized by cytochrome P-450

4. Boxer in satin robe praying in ring: Pravastatin is not metabolized by CYP450, therefore it is the drug of choice if patients are taking other drugs that interact with CYP450

5. Old legend boxer with cane: Statins can cause myopathy

6. Old man trainer with nightstick: Myopathy can worsen with niacin

7. Old guy with fibrous burlap medical kit: Myopathy can worsen with fibrates

8. Old man knocks over jar of creatine powder with nightstick: Myopathy can be measured using serum creatine kinase (CK)

9. Liver-spotted dalmatian who can sniff out drugs: Can cause hepatotoxicity and increased LFTs

10. Boxer in satin robe with licorice kissing angel on car: Decreases mortality in coronary artery disease (CAD) patients

11. Dense cannonballs fired high in the air every hour: Increases good cholesterol (HDL)

12. Broken boat poster in crowd: Decreased bad cholesterol (LDL)

13. Ropes securing boat: Increases LD receptor density

14. Fan dropping stick of butter: Decreased TGs

See Figure 9.7.5 - Mechanisms of Lipid-Lowering Medications (Cardiac Pharmacology, Section 9, Page 129)

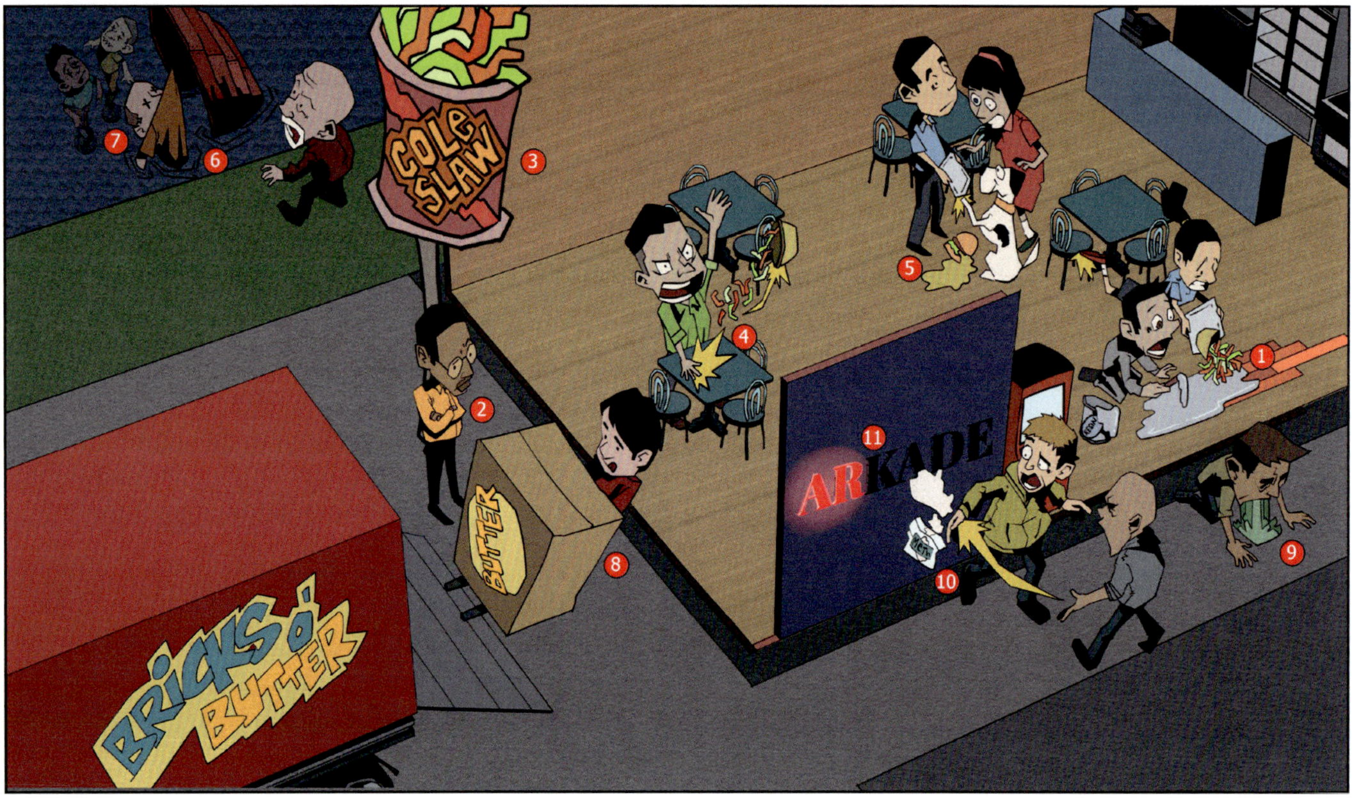

1. Waitress spilling coleslaw on resin floor: Bile acid resins

2. "The Coleslaw Tyrant": Cholestyramine

3. "Coleslaw" bucket sign: Colestipol

4. Guy slamming his hand on table throwing his coleslaw: Colesevelam

5. Liver-spotted dog hitting cholesterol burger on floor, spilling grease: Prevent intestinal reabsorption of bile acids → liver metabolizes cholesterol stores to make more bile

6. Low density boat starting to sink with dead body attached: Decreases LDL

7. High density ball and chains holding dead bodies at bottom of lake: Slightly increases HDL

8. Delivery truck with butter: Slightly increases triglycerides

9. Man vomiting after eating coleslaw: Can cause GI upset

10. Man smacking meth out of other man's hands before he could snort it: Can decrease the absorption of other drugs

11. "Arkade" sign with only "A" and "R" lit: Can decrease absorption of fat soluble vitamins (A, D, E, and K)

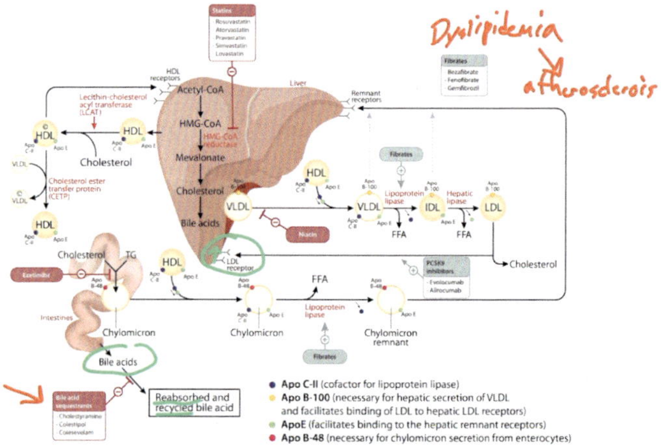

See Figure 9.7.5 - Mechanisms of Lipid-Lowering Medications (Cardiac Pharmacology, Section 9, Page 129)

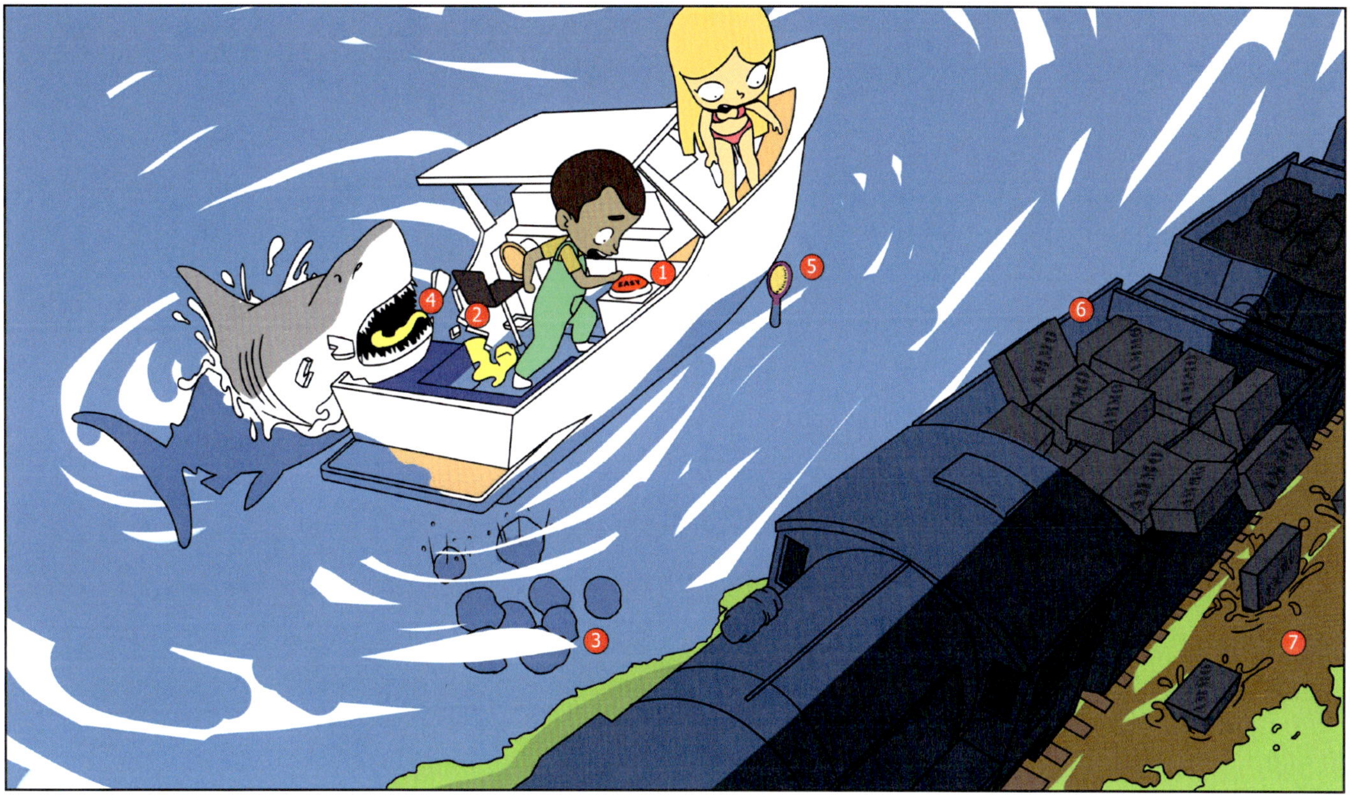

1. EASY button on boat: Ezetimibe

2. Boat being destroyed: Decreases LDL

3. Dense, heavy weights sinking to ocean floor: Increase HDL

4. Butter being eaten and destroyed by shark: Decreases triglycerides

5. Brush with yellow bristles dropped by woman and falling into ocean: Prevents cholesterol absorption at small intestine brush border

6. Train with excess ammo: Can cause an increase in LFTs

7. Mud: Can cause diarrhea

See Figure 9.7.5 - Mechanisms of Lipid-Lowering Medications (Cardiac Pharmacology, Section 9, Page 129)

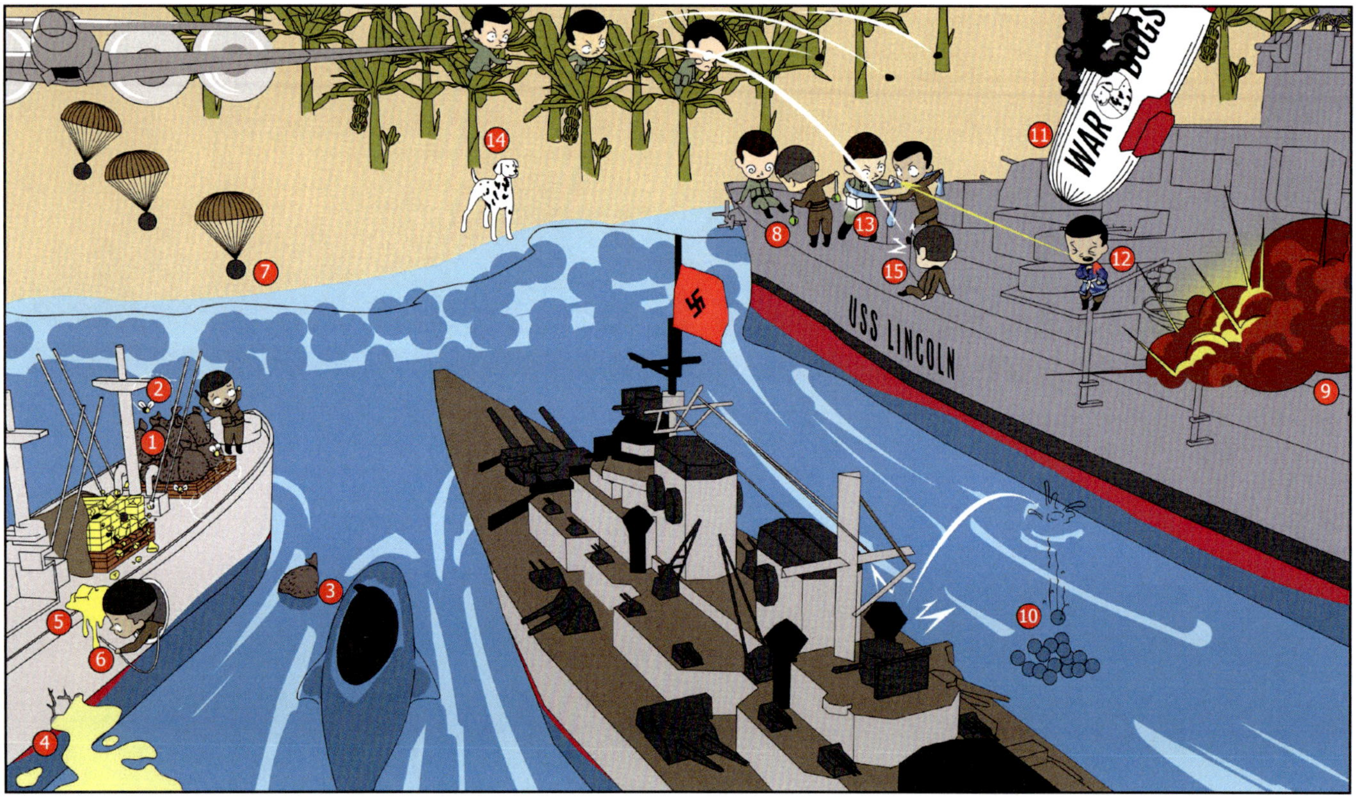

1. Fibrous burlap sacks: Fibrates

2. Bees buzzing around honey filled burlap sacks: Bezafibrate

3. Orca investigating fallen burlap sack only showing dorsal fin: Fenofibrate

4. Yellow colored oil spill: Used to treat dyslipidemia

5. Damaged butter: Decreases triglycerides

6. Liposuction tool used to suck up butter: Upregulates LPL (lipoprotein lipase) → increased TG clearance

7. Cannonballs with parachutes being shipped to boat: Activates peroxisome proliferator-activated receptor alpha (PPAR-alpha) → induced HDL synthesis

8. Hypnotist using green gem on fibrous string: Gemfibrozil

9. Boat damaged by bomb: Decreases LDL

10. Heavy, dense cannonballs accumulating in ocean: Increases HDL

11. Blimp with liver-spotted dog logo crashing into ground: Reduces hepatic VLDL production

12. Captain in satin pajamas holding painful arm: Can cause myopathy

13. Soldiers fighting over ornate chrome boxes while being hypnotized: Inhibits cytochrome P-450

14. Guys throwing rocks from banana trees with liver-spotted dalmatian: Can cause hepatitis

15. Guy with burger gets hit by rock from banana tree, dropping burger: Can cause cholesterol gallstones

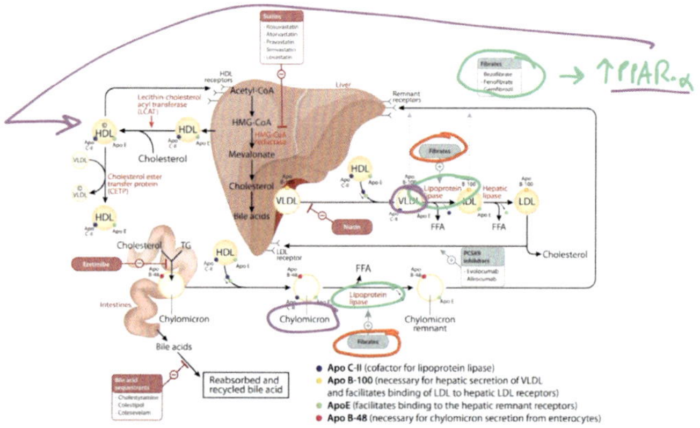

See Figure 9.7.5 - Mechanisms of Lipid-Lowering Medications (Cardiac Pharmacology, Section 9, Page 129)

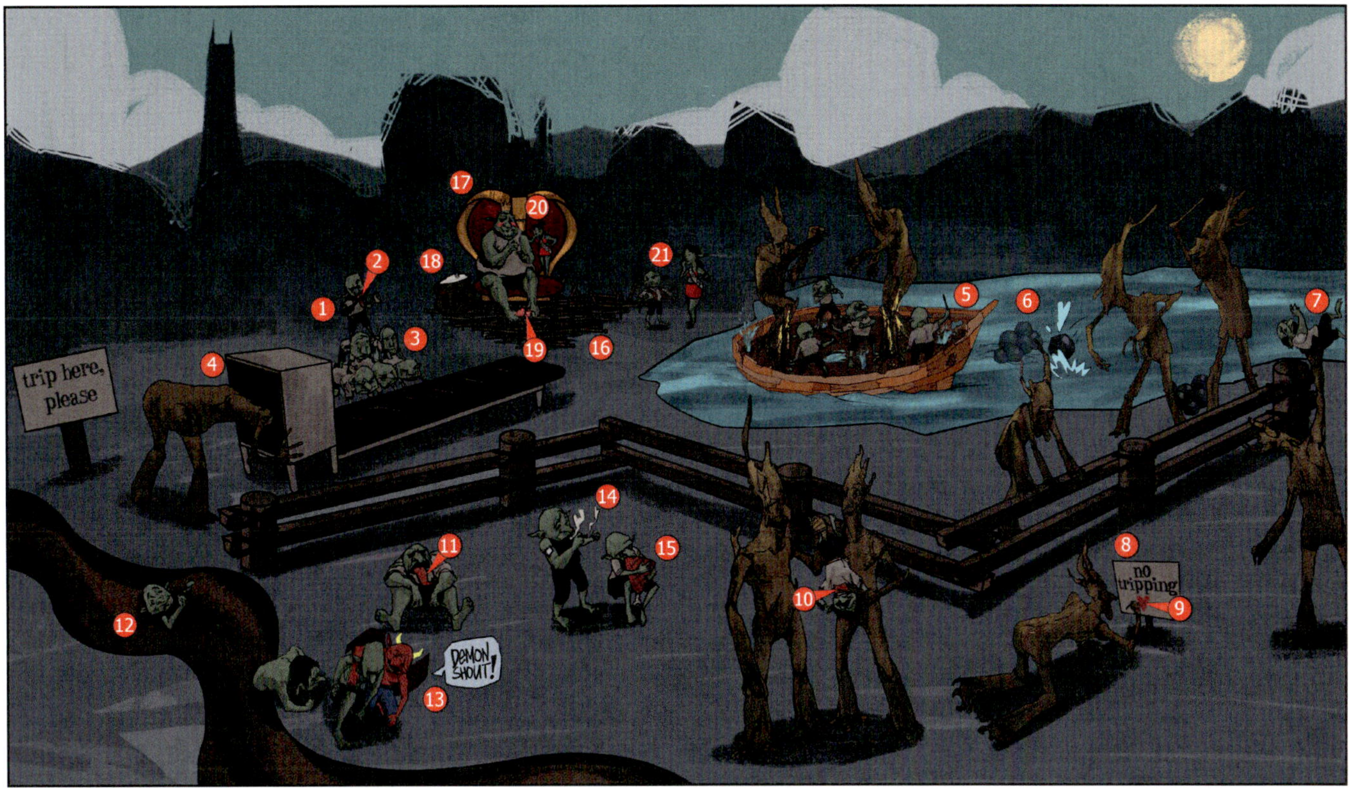

1. Goblins making nightsticks: Niacin

2. Goblin tasting flavorful nightstick: Niacin production requires riboflavin

3. 6 Goblin pyramid: Niacin production requires pyridoxine (B_6)

4. Tree guy tripping into machine: Niacin is derived from tryptophan

5. Sinking boat: Niacin treats dyslipidemia by lowering LDL

6. Dense, sunken balls accumulating in river: Niacin treats dyslipidemia by increasing HDL

7. Nightstick-less goblin with hyperpigmented limbs from sun: Niacin deficiency causes hyperpigmentation of sun-exposed limbs

8. "No tripping" sign: Low tryptophan can cause niacin deficiency

9. Hear ton "no tripping" sign: Low tryptophan can be caused by Hartnup disease

10. Redness collar around nightstick-less goblin's neck: Niacin deficiency causes dermatitis in a collar-like distribution

11. Nightstick-less goblin's splintered tongue: Niacin deficiency causes glossitis

12. Nightstick-less goblin in muddy river: Niacin deficiency can cause diarrhea

13. Confused and disoriented demon goblin yelling, "Demon shout!": Niacin deficiency causes dementia

14. Nicotine patch on goblin's arm: Treat niacin deficiency with nicotinic acid supplementation

15. Goblin comforting himself with ham: Treat niacin deficiency with a high protein diet to obtain more tryptophan

16. Excess pile of nightsticks: Niacin excess

17. B3-shaped throne on top of nightstick pile: Niacin = vitamin B_3

18. Fat king with pile of sugar on nightstick pile: Hyperglycemia

19. King's red, swollen toes: Hyperuricemia

20. Prostitute causing king to blush: Facial flushing induced by prostaglandins

21. Non-blushing goblin with asp: Prevent facial flushing with aspirin

See Figure 9.7.5 - Mechanisms of Lipid-Lowering Medications (Cardiac Pharmacology, Section 9, Page 129)

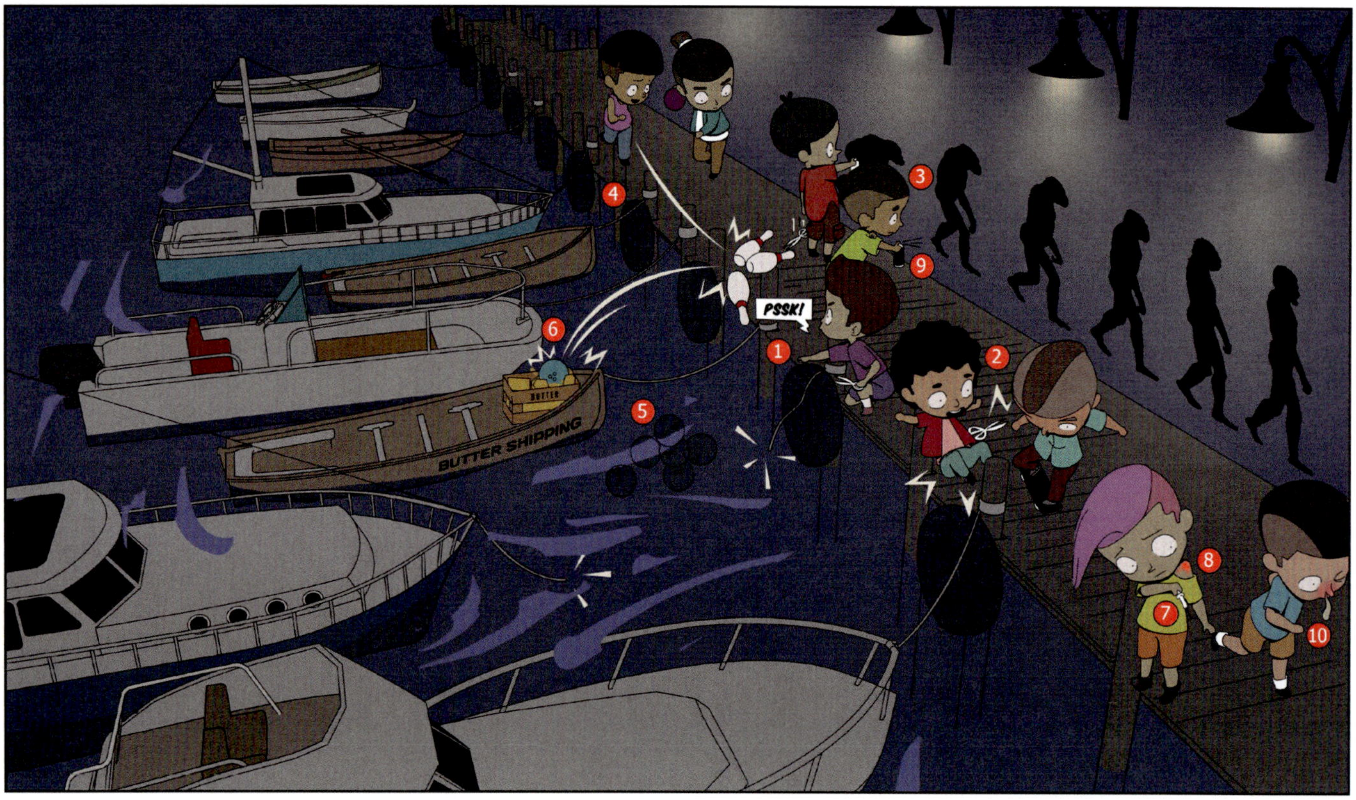

1. Kid saying, "Pssk!" cutting one of the nine boat lines: PCSK9 normally degrades LDL receptors

2. Ollie knocked the scissors to the ground, preventing the kid from cutting mooring lines with "Pssk!" kid: Alirocumab

3. Spray painted evolution mural with dropped scissors nearby: Evolucumab

4. Most of the boats are tied to the doc: Decreases LDL

5. Bowling balls at bottom of ocean: Increased HDL

6. Ball destroyed crate of butter on butter shipping boat: Decreases triglycerides

7. Junkie shooting up through his shoulder: Administered subcutaneously

8. Junky's red and irritated shoulder: Can cause skin rash at injection site

9. Graffiti artist in green shirt with arm pain: Can cause myalgias

10. Kid with irritated red nose: Can cause nasopharyngitis

See Figure 9.7.5 - Mechanisms of Lipid-Lowering Medications (Cardiac Pharmacology, Section 9, Page 129)

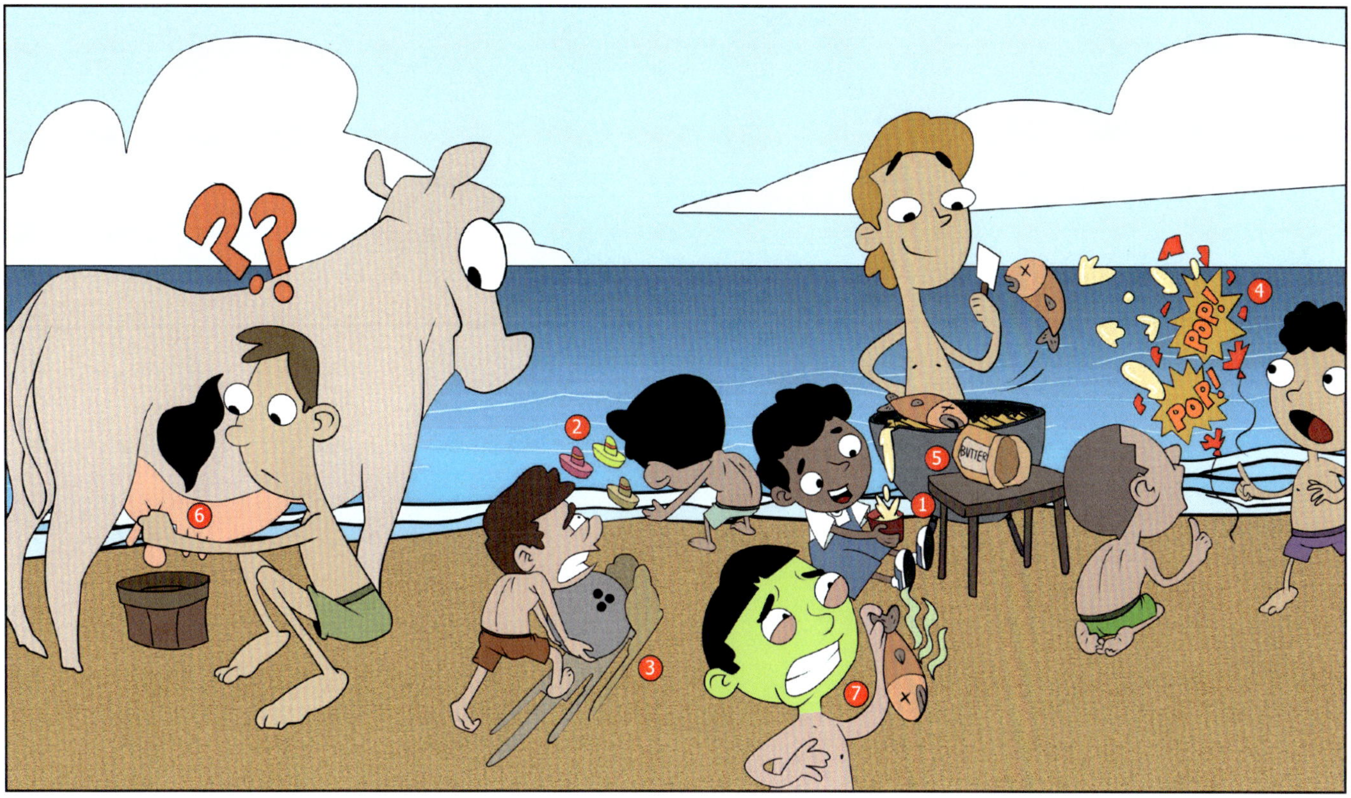

1. Kid collecting fish oil drippings from grill: Fish oil and marine omega-3 fatty acids

2. Toy boats floating on top of ocean water: Slightly increases LDL

3. Heavy bowling ball sinking into sand: Slightly increases HDL

4. Fish oil popping low density balloons: Antagonizes VLDL cholesterol secretion

5. Empty butter container next to grill: Decreases triglycerides at high doses

6. Liver-spotted cow not producing milk: Decreases activity of TG-synthesizing enzymes

7. Nauseous kid with green face unable to eat fish: Can cause nausea and fish-like taste

See Figure 9.7.5 - Mechanisms of Lipid-Lowering Medications (Cardiac Pharmacology, Section 9 Page 129)

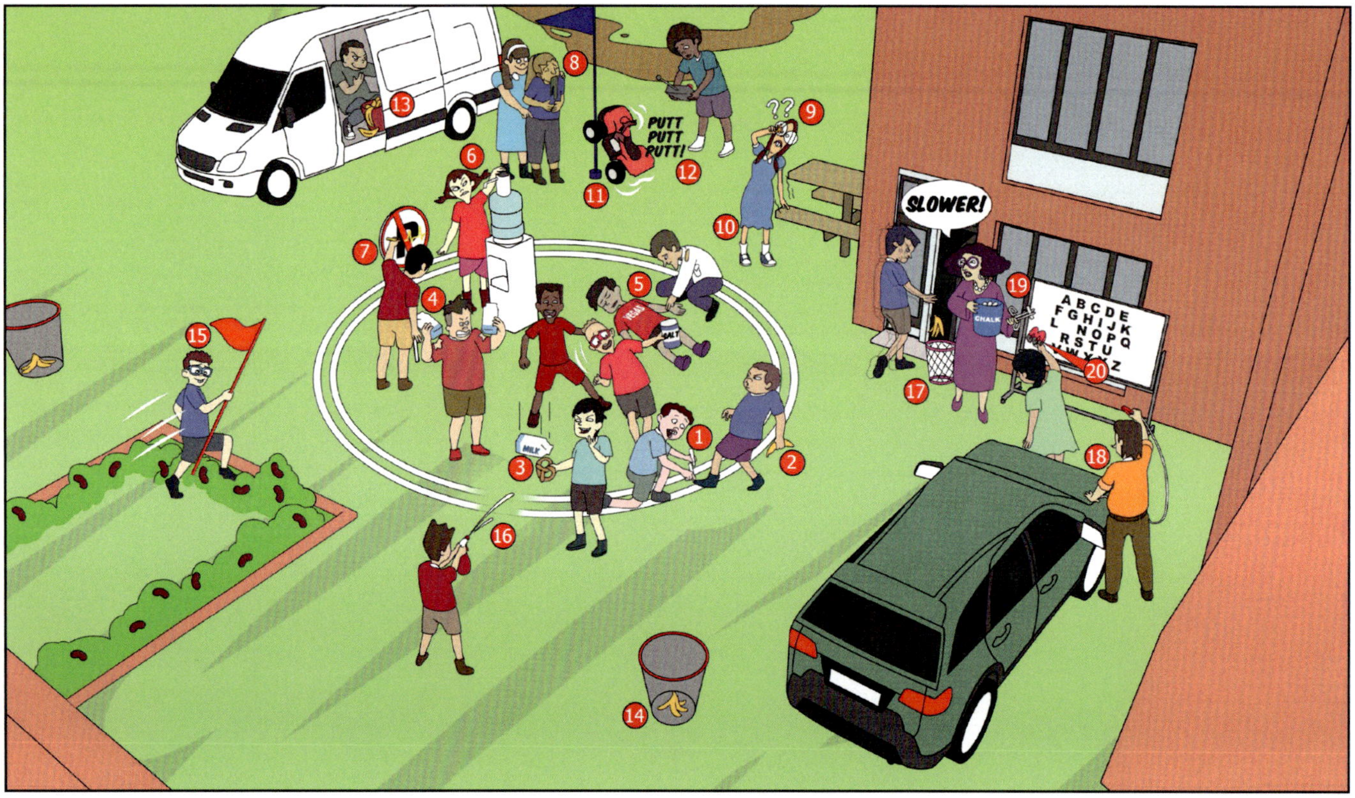

1. Kid with two chalks or "di chalks": Digoxin

2. Prisoner with salt shaker inside of the prison, trying to trade for guard's banana but can't: Direct inhibition of sodium/potassium ATPase → higher intracellular sodium

3. Prison guard with pretzel trying to trade the prisoner's milk but prisoner bumped by prisoner with salt: Higher intracellular sodium indirectly inhibits sodium/calcium exchanger → higher intracellular calcium

4. Prisoner flexing his muscles with milk: Higher intracellular calcium causes positive entropy (increased contractility)

5. Guard checking pulse of sleeping prisoner in "Vegas" shirt: Stimulates vagus nerve which decreases heart rate

6. Broken water pump on water cooler: Clinical use includes HF

7. Prisoner drawing ECG scribbles on no parking sign: Clinical use includes atrial fibrillation

8. Guard vomiting next to muddy water: Can cause nausea, vomiting and diarrhea

9. Guard picking dandelions and rubbing yellow pollen her glasses: Can cause blurry and yellow vision

10. Fatigued, confused guard with pollen on her glasses: Can cause fatigue, weakness, and confusion

11. Rattling, broken toy ATV: Can cause life-threatening arrhythmias

12. Broken ATV car blocked by the flagpole: Can cause AV block

13. Kidnapper in white van with bananas: Can cause hyperkalemia (indicates a poor prognosis)

14. Banana peels in waste baskets: Toxicity is more likely in patients with hypokalemia (the potassium binding site is more available for digoxin to bind)

15. Kid trampling kidney bean plants between waste baskets with banana peels: Toxicity is more likely in patients with renal failure (decreased digoxin clearance)

16. Kid trying to erase chalk outline: Toxicity is more likely in patients taking drugs that can displace digoxin from binding properly to tissues (e.g. verapamil, amiodarone, quinidine)

17. Slow moving kid throwing away banana being yelled at, "Slower!": Antidote to digoxin toxicity includes slowly normalizing serum potassium

18. Parent with broken down car and jumper cables: Antidote to digoxin toxicity includes using a cardiac pacer

19. Teacher using antibody-like tongs to collect chalk: Antidote to digoxin toxicity includes administering anti-digoxin antibodies (Fab fragments)

20. Teacher picking up magnetic "M": Antidote to digoxin toxicity includes administering magnesium (magnesium decrease arrhythmia)

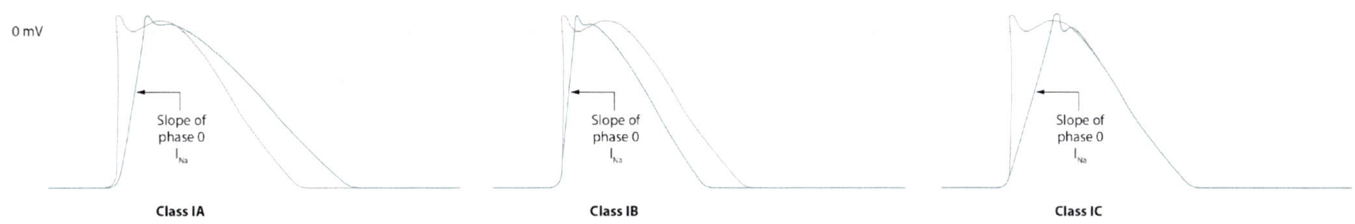

Figure 9.7.6 - Effects of Class I Antiarrhythmics on Cardiac Myocytes

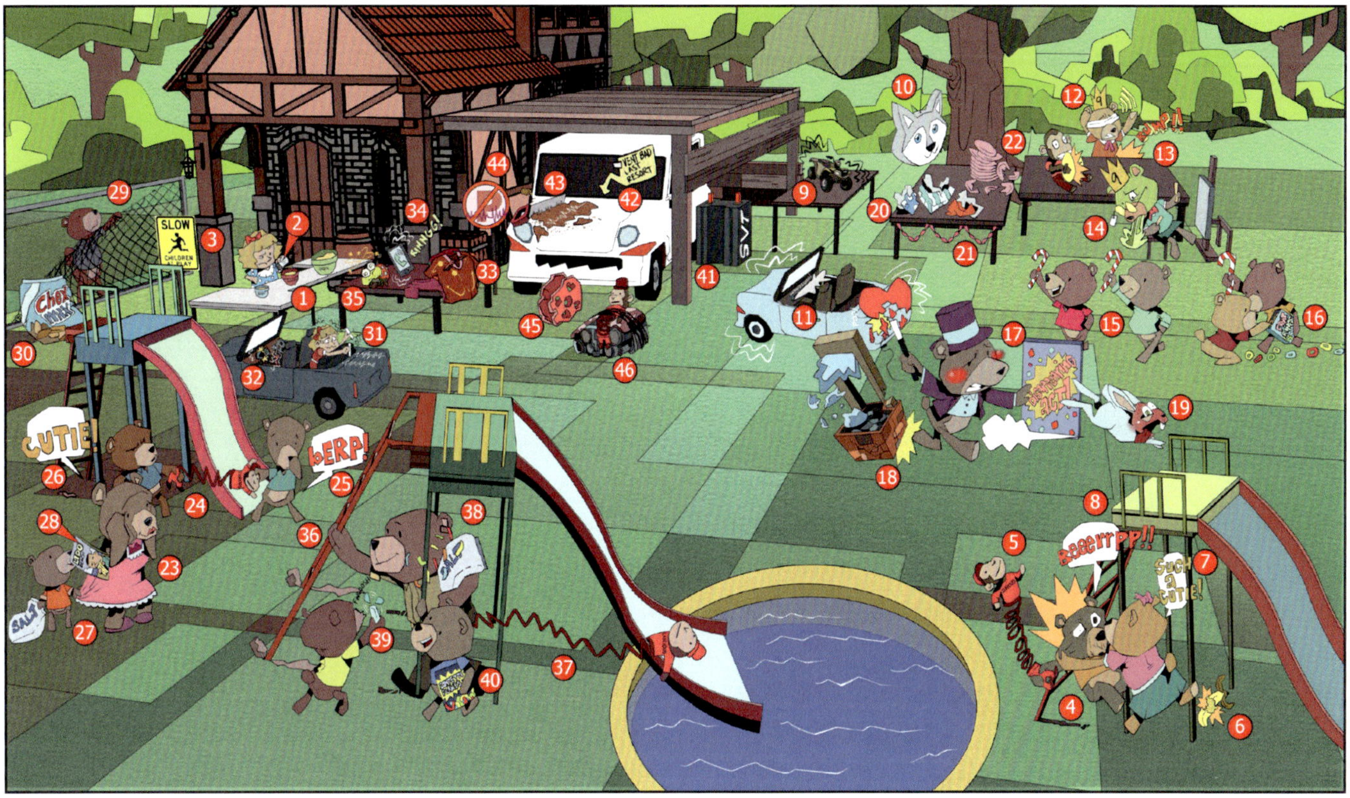

1. Baby bear, mama bear and papa bear bowls on "1" shaped table: Class I antiarrhythmics

2. Salt shaker little girl is shaking is taped closed: Blocks sodium channels

3. "Slow children at play" sign near "1" shaped table: Use dependence, (i.e. the drug's slowing effects on ECG are best appreciated at higher heart rates)

4. Baby bear pushing slide ladder backwards: Class IA antiarrhythmics decrease the slope of phase 0

5. Baby bear's stretched Curious George slinky: Prolongs QRS

6. Crushed bananas next to baby bear's slide: Blocked potassium channels

7. Girl bear saying, "Such a cutie!" stretching out baby bear's cheeks on top of bananas: Blocked potassium channels → prolonged QT

8. Baby bear's "Berp!!!" sound: Prolonged ERP

9. Rattling ATV toy owner by baby bear: Use for both atrial and ventricular arrhythmias

10. Wolf pinata on tree: Use for Wolff-Parkinson-White (type of SVT)

11. Rattling AC vent in baby bear's toy car: Use for ventricular tachycardia

12. Little queen bear wearing the "9" crown: Quinidine

13. Little queen bear blindfolded holding her head while monkey's cymbals ring: Quinidine can cause cinchonism

14. Green face queen bear wearing "9" crown holding the two chalks while vomiting: Quinidine can enhance digitalis toxicity

15. Marching line of bears proudly holding candy canes: Procainamide can cause reversible SLE-like syndrome

16. Little bear's box of froot loops in candy cane procession: Procainamide can cause reversible SLE-like syndrome

17. Magician bear performing disappearing magic trick: Disopyramide

18. Disappearing magician bear popping heart shaped balloon and breaking water pump: Disopyramide can exacerbate heart failure because it has negative inotropic effects

19. "Hot as a hare, dry as a bone, red as a beet, and mad as a hatter" magician's rabbit: Disopyramide can cause anticholinergic effects

20. Torn up wrapping paper on table next to pinata: Adverse effects of class IA

21. Twisted streamers hanging off of table: Torsades de pointes

22. Broken plates on table: Thrombocytopenia

23. Mama bear next to ladder with slide pushed back: Class IB antiarrhythmics minimally decrease the slope of phase 0

24. Two bears stretching out Curious George Slinky: Prolong QRS

25. Little bear letting out short burp: Shorten ERP

26. Mama bear squishing cheeks together exclaiming, "Cutie": Shorten QT interval

27. Little bear's weak attachment to bag of salt: Class IB antiarrhythmics have weak attachment to receptors (i.e. easy fast dissociation)

28. Lido beach brochure with kids chewing sugar cane: Lidocaine

29. Bear putting up fence: Phenytoin

30. Chex Mix: Mexiletin

31. Shaking girl drawing with two chalks: Use for digoxin-induced (digitalis arrhythmias)

32. Rattling car vent: Use for acute ventricular arrhythmias especially after an MI

33. Cut thread on V neck shirt: Can cause AV conduction block

34. Ringing phone: Can cause seizures

35. Dizzy, sick bug: Can cause dizziness and nausea

36. Ladder getting pushed way back: Class IC antiarrhythmics drastically decrease the slope of phase 0 (i.e. prolonged depolarization)

37. Papa bear's stretched out Curious Georgeg slinky: Prolonged QRS

38. Papa bear strongly carrying salt bag: Strong binding

39. Fan propeller: Propafennone

40. Confetti flakes: Flecainide

41. Special Vehicle Tracking device: Use for paroxysmal SVT

42. "Vent bad last resort" note: Used for ventricular tachycardia as a last resort

43. Sawdust pattern: Use for atrial flutter

44. No parking sign: Use for atrial fibrillation

45. Dented, beaten up pink rim: Contraindicated in patients with structural and ischemic heart disease

46. Stretched out Curious George slinked benign changed to car engine: QRS prolongation puts the patient at high risk of cardiac arrest

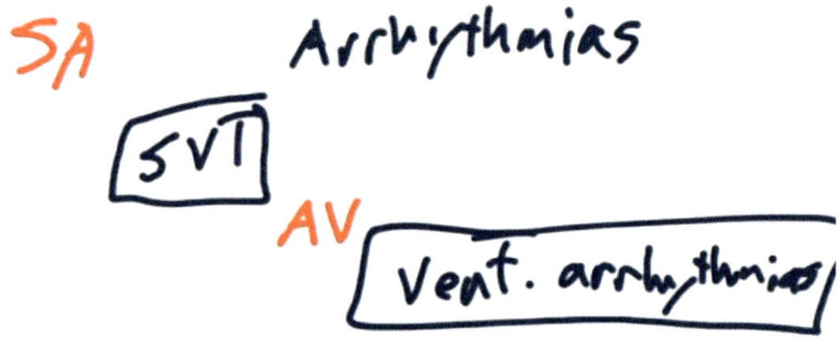

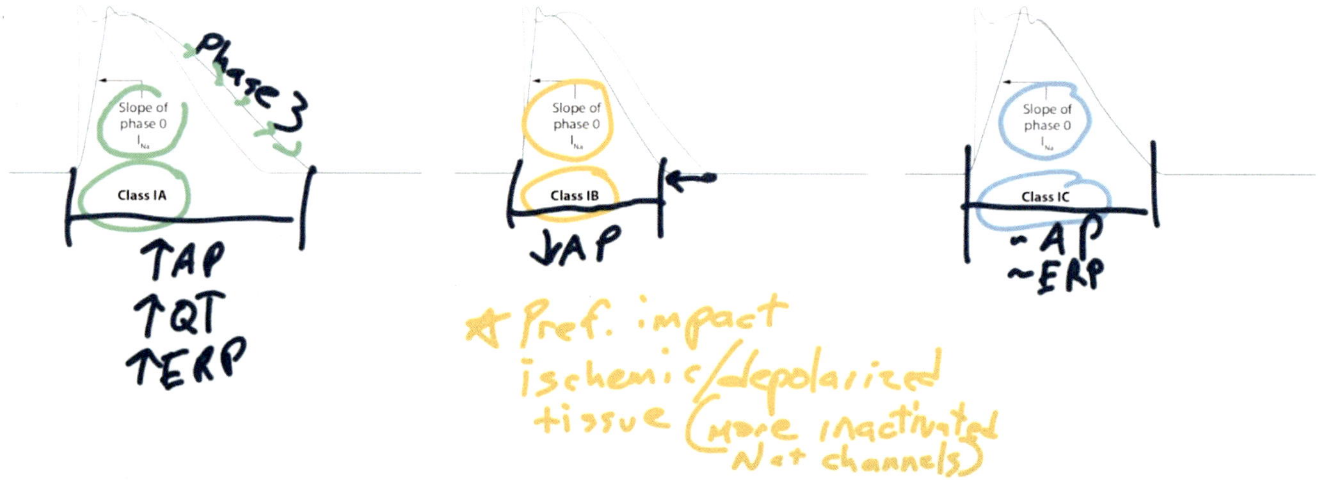

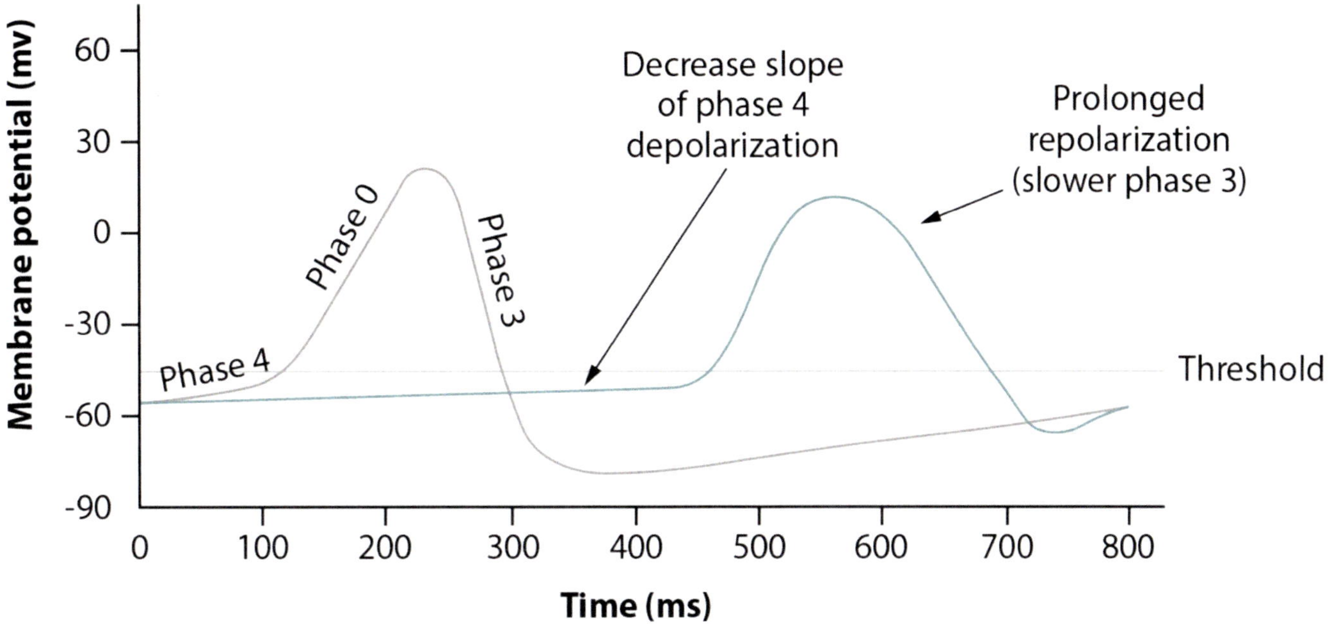

Pacemaker cell action potential

Figure 9.7.7 - Effects of Class II Antiarrhythmics on Cardiac Pacemaker Cells

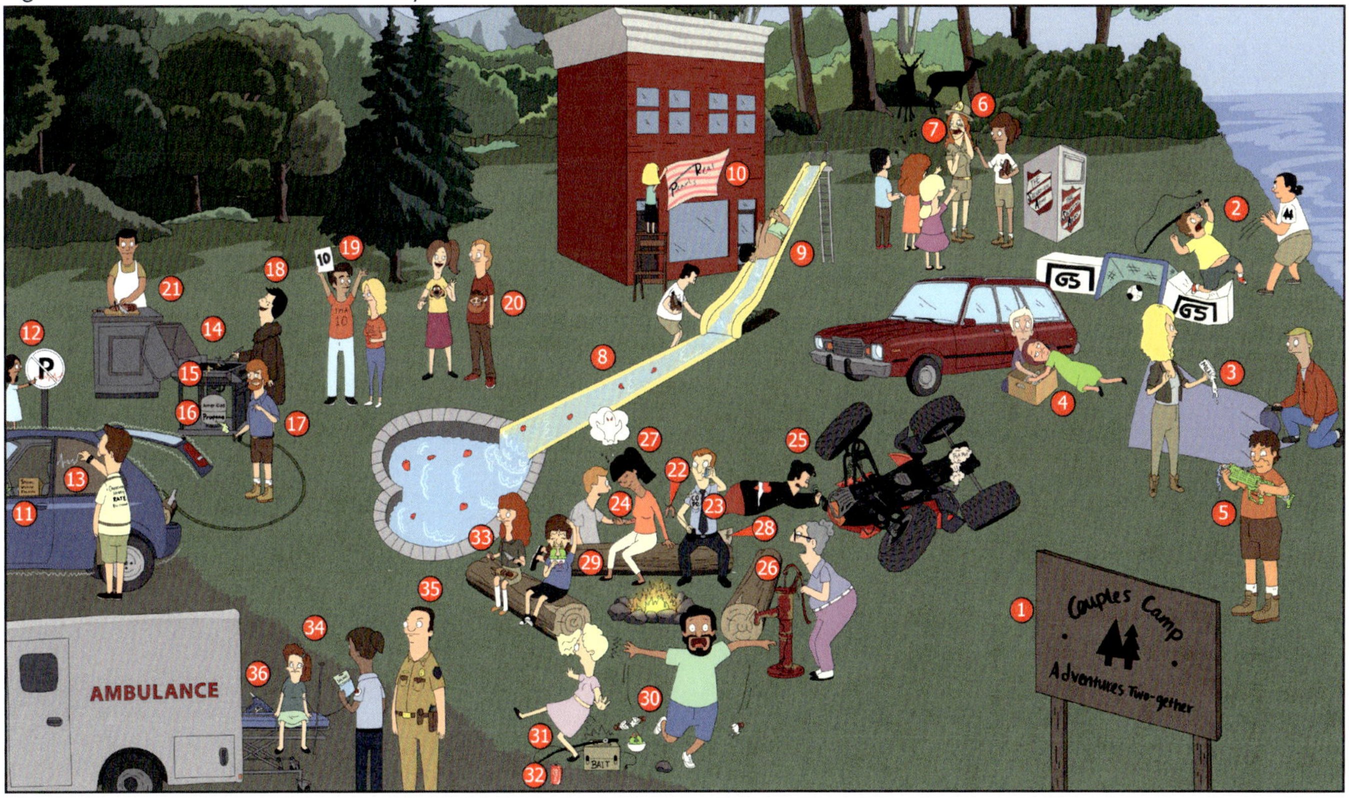

1. Couple camp slogan, "Adventure Two-gether": Class II Antiarrhythmics

2. Camp guest with fishing pole being blocked and crushing the Gs goal station: Blocks β_1 receptors → inhibits Gs

3. Couple taking down tent with empty bottle of milk: Decreased cAMP and Ca^{2+}

4. Exhausted lady trying to pick up box with empty water bottles and husband checking her pulse next to car: Decreases entropy and heart rate

5. Weak shooting water gun: Decreases CO

6. Metronome being held next to salvation Army donation box and employee that work in Antelope Valley: Act on pacemaker cells (AV and SA nodes)

7. Sensitive Antelope Valley employee placing hand on heart: The AV node is particularly sensitive to class II antiarrhythmics

8. Downhill slope of phase 4 section of slip 'N slide: Decrease the slope of phase 4 (slows depolarization) in pacemaker cells

9. Employee with metronome moving slide towards pool for guest crushing bananas: Block phase 3 (repolarization) by inhibiting If K^+ → prolonged repolarization at AV node

10. "Pearl is Real" shop banner being stretched: Prolong PR interval

11. Special Vehicle Tracking, SVT, device with rattling car AC vent: Use for supraventricular tachycardia (SVT)

12. No parking sign with ECG scribbles and girl wearing Fitbit pointing to it: Use for ventricular rate control in atrial fibrillation

13. Saw pattern in car window next to man wearing Fitbit: Use for ventricular rate control for atrial flutter

14. Metal probe on grill: Metoprolol

15. Oil dripping from metal probe: Metoprolol can cause dyslipidemia

16. Propane tank under grill: Propranolol

17. Person clutching their chest next to propane tank and garden hose being squeezed: Propranolol can exacerbate vasospasm in vasospastic angina

18. Laughing eskimo cooking on grill: Esmolol

19. "I'm a 10!" shirt worn by man and wife's matching "LOL" shirt: Atenolol

20. Timone shirt worn by woman laughing out loud: Timolol

21. Man carving meat at grill: Carvedilol

22. Flimsy hot dog near campfire: Class II antiarrhythmics can cause impotence

23. COPD cop with inhaler from campfire: Can exacerbate COPD and asthma

24. Girl's pulse is being checked while she is sleeping next to campfire: Can cause bradycardia

25. Overturned and broken ATV causing rider's jacket to rip in middle of heart logo: Can cause AV block

26. Old lady is too weak to pump the broken water pump: Can cause heart failure due to decreased inotropy

27. Sleeping lady disturbed by her nightmare: Can cause sedation and sleep disturbances

28. Cop hiding empty bag of sugar/chocolate: May mask hypoglycemia

29. Lady sitting next to fire sweating, plae, shaking and holding head while eating ice cream: Use during pheochromocytoma surgical removal

30. Man breaking dessert tray with two alpha shaped handles and teacup with one after tripping over ice cream: Prior to surgical removal of pheochromocytoma, administer an α blockade (α-blockade → β_1 blockade → surgical removal)

31. Man who fell caused lady to crush beta tackle box and fishing pole: blockers are only administered after administering an α blockade (α-blockade → β-blockade → surgical removal)

32. Coke can next to falling lady near beta tackle box and fishing pole: Can use → β-blockers for cocaine intoxication to reduce blood pressure and tachycardia

33. Confused woman eating carved meat next to sweating lady: Carvedilol does not cause unopposed α_1 activity because it also blocks α receptors

34. Lady being hooked up to IV saline near ambulance: Treat β-blocker overdose with saline

35. State trooper near ambulance: Treat β blocker overdose with atropine (stops bradycardia)

36. Glue gun next to lady on ambulance: Treat β-blocker overdose with glucago

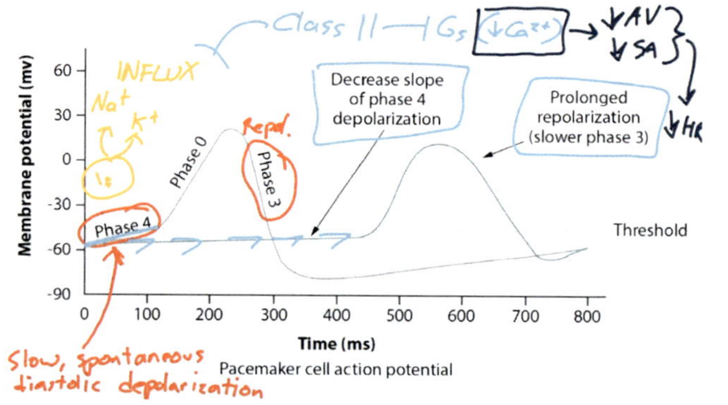

Pacemaker cell action potential

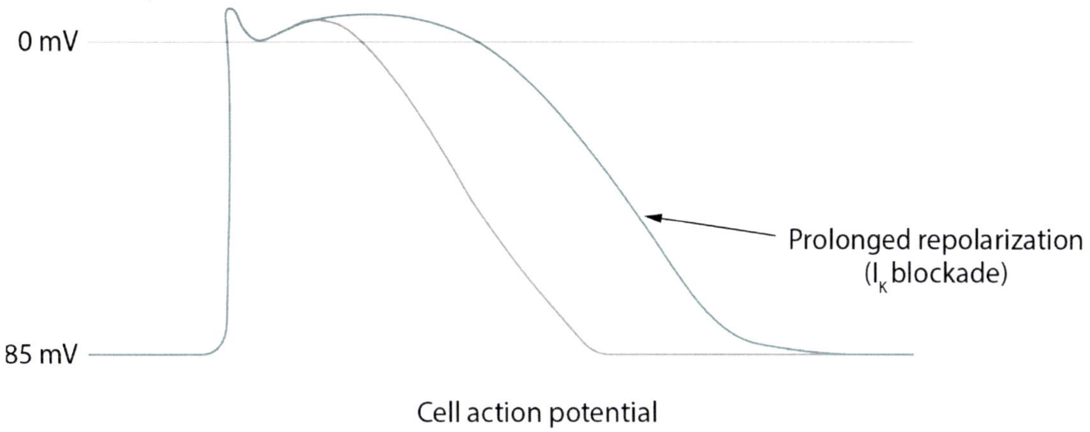

Figure 9.7.8 - Effects of Class III Antiarrhythmics on Cardiac Myocytes

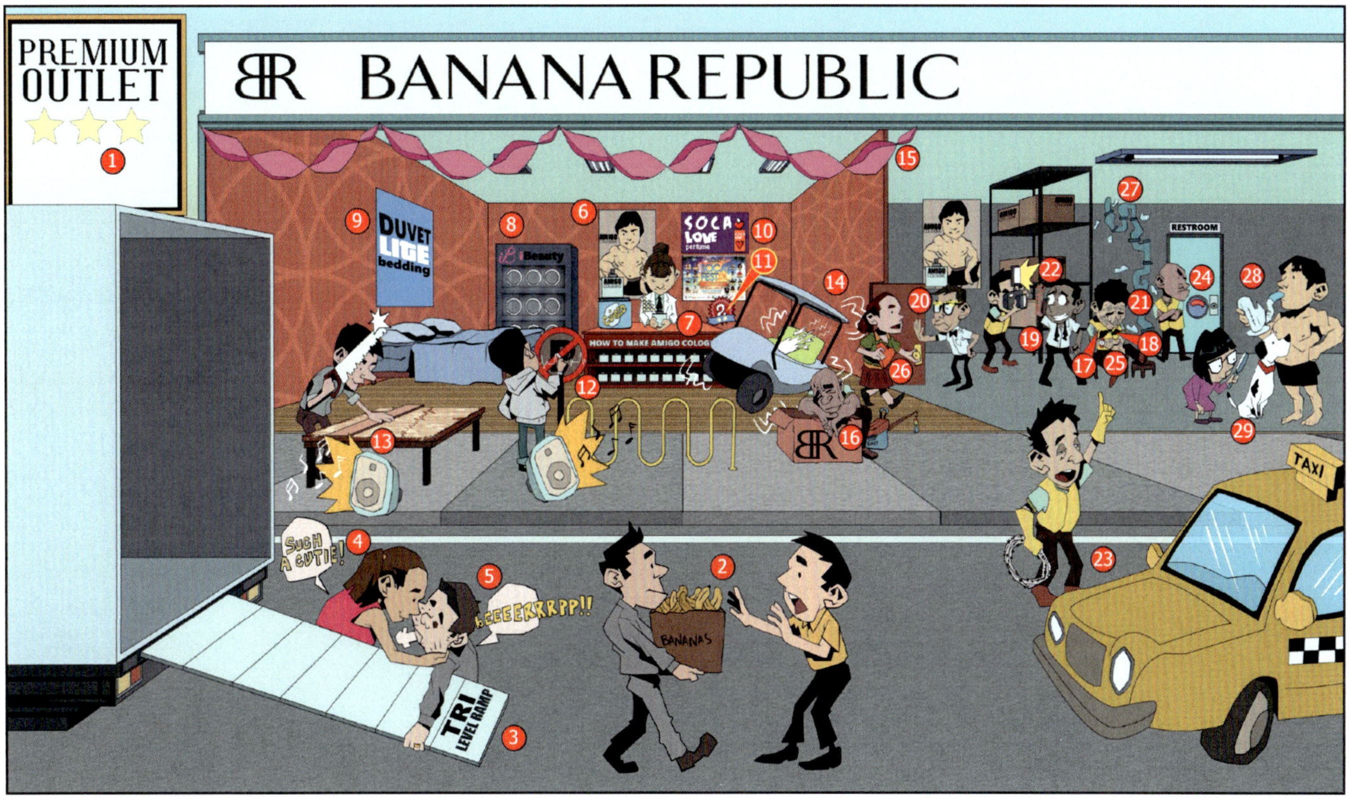

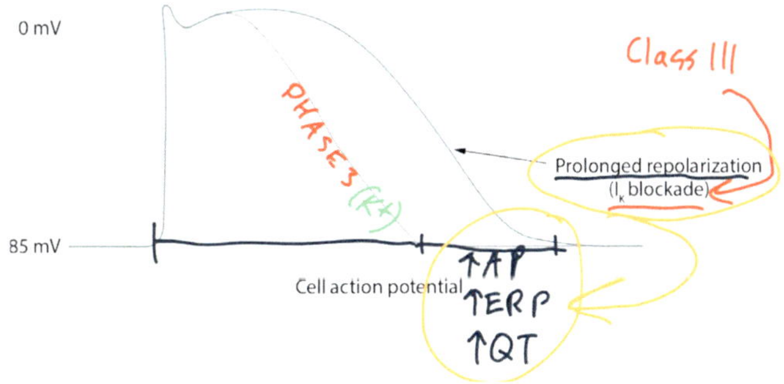

1. Three star premium outlet: Class III antiarrhythmics

2. Manager stopping delivery worker from leaving truck with box of bananas: Potassium channel blockers

3. Worker extending "TRI" level ramp: Increased duration of phase 3 of cardiac action potential (prolonged repolarization)

4. Smitten woman stretches cheeks of worker and saying "Such a cutie!": increase QT interval

5. Long burp from worker extending ramp: Increase effective refractory period (ERP)

6. Amigo cologne poster in store: Amidoarone

7. Fragrance maker with four rows of stars on coat and Crisco in front of amigo cologne poster: Amiodarone is lipophilic and has all class properties (class I, II, III, and IV

8. iBeauty Lite: Ibutilide

9. Duvet lite bedding: Dofetilide

10. "Soca love" perfume poster: Sotalol

11. Soca festival two out of five star review: Sotalol also has class II properties

12. No parking sign with EKG reading and music coming out of speakers on sidewalk: Use class III antiarrhythmics for atrial fibrillation

13. Construction worker using saw on table next to rhythmic music coming out of speakers: Use class III antiarrhythmics for atrial flutter

14. Rattling vent on golf cart in front of amigo cologne and soca love ads: Amiodarone and sotalol can be used for ventricular tachycardia because these drugs can also control rate (unlike dofetilide and ibutilide which only control rhythm)

15. Twisted streamers on roof of stone: Class III antiarrhythmics can cause torsades de pointes (amiodarone is far less comm)

16. Weak guy checking pulse while resting on tackle box and fishing pole: Sotalol can cause excessive beta blockade which can lead to bradycardia and decreased entropy

17. Lung-shaped yellow mesh safety vest in stockroom filled with amigo cologne: Amiodarone can cause pulmonary fibrosis

18. Liver-shaped stain on yellow vest: Amiodarone can cause hepatotoxicity

19. Two storage managers with bow ties tied and untied: Amiodarone can cause hyper or hypothyroidism

20. Yellow clumps of pollen on storage manager's glasses next to cologne: Amiodarone can cause corneal deposits

21. Blue/gray discoloration on yellow vested worker's face and arms: Amiodarone can cause blue gray skin deposits

22. Bright flash from camera causing manager's red and splotchy arms: Amiodarone can cause photodermatitis

23. Drunk yellow vested worker with socks and gloves holding barbed wire calling for taxi: Amiodarone can cause neurologic effects (e.g. ataxia, peripheral neuropathy)

24. Worker in yellow vest waiting long time from bathroom: Amiodarone can cause constipation

25. Worker with discoloration checking his radial pulse: Amiodarone can cause bradycardia

26. Lady with heart shaped perfume walking to storage room blocked by manager: Amiodarone can cause heart block

27. Broken pump in storage room: Amiodarone can cause heart failure

28. Edna Mode and Amigo Cologne, wearing bowtie, using incentive spirometer: Check pulmonary function tests and thyroid function tests when using amiodarone

29. Edna inspecting dalmatian's liver-spot: Check liver function when using amiodarone

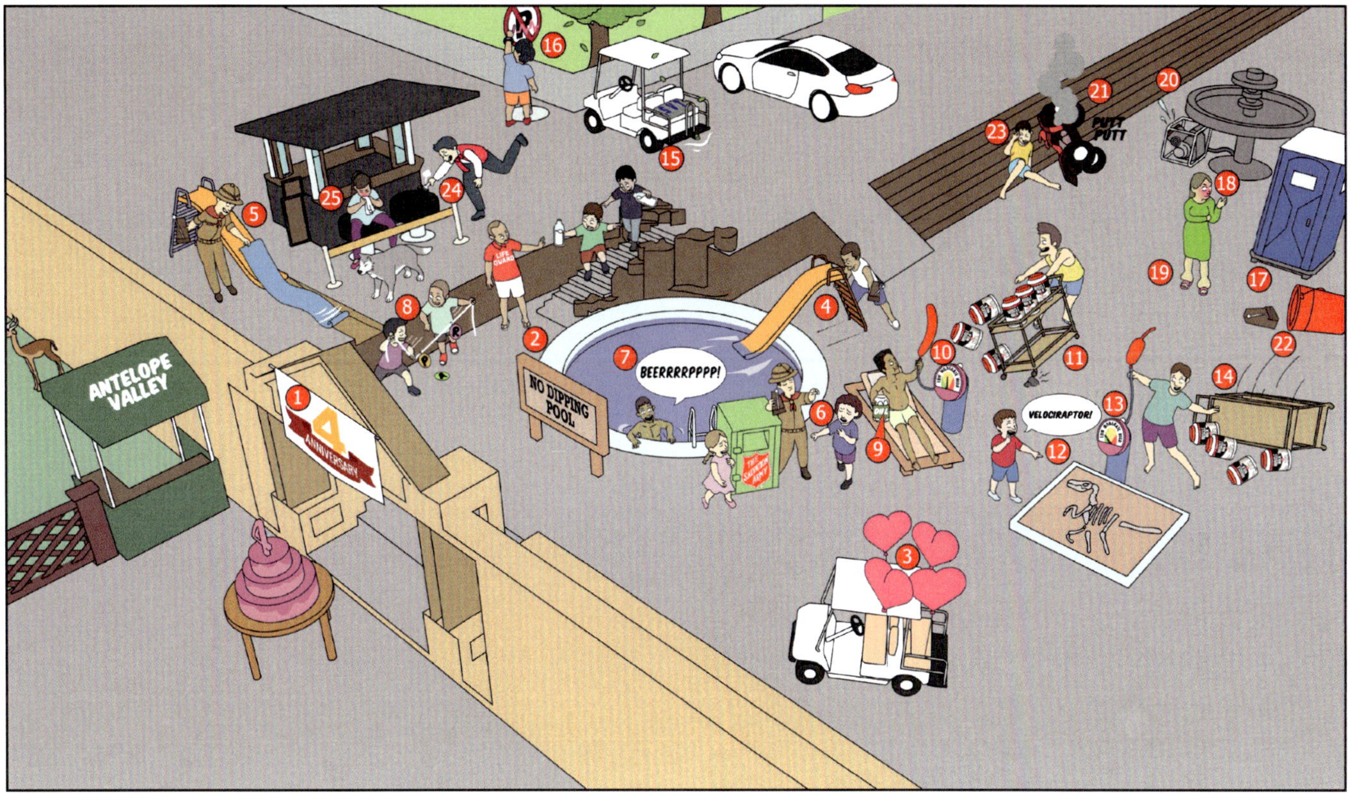

1. 4th anniversary banner and "4" on anniversary cake: Class IV antiarrhythmics

2. Kids trying to sneak milk into the no dipping pool: Nondihydropyridine calcium channel blockers

3. Heart balloons on golf cart in park: Primarily act on the heart

4. Ladder getting pushed back by man to make less sleep: Decreased slope of phase 0 for nodal AP (slow rise of action potential)

5. Antelope Valley ranger rolling out the slip N' slide phase 4 section: Decreased slope of phase 4 (prolonged repolarization at AV node)

6. Antelope ranger holding metronome conducting kid singers next to Salvation Army donation box: Slows conduction velocity in the sinoatrial (SA) and atrioventricular (AV) node

7. Man with long burp, "BEERRPP!" in no dipping pool: Increased effective refractory period (ERP)

8. Kids pulling on and stretching banner that has only P and R on it: Increased PR interval → slower heart rate

9. Dill pickle jar eating next to no dipping pool: Diltiazem

10. Dill pickle man blowing up long red balloon with only moderate pressure: Diltiazem is a moderate vasodilator

11. Cart that topples, dripping half of the muscle milk next to dill pickle man: Diltiazem has moderate myocardial depressant activity

12. Velociraptor excavation site next to kid yelling, "Velociraptor!": Verapamil

13. Parent blowing up long red balloon with only low pressure next to velociraptor: Verapamil is a less potent vasodilator compared to diltiazem

14. Every muscle milk falling off of cart next to velociraptor: Verapamil is a potent myocardial depressant

15. Golf cart with special vehicle tracking device, SVT: Use for supraventricular tachycardia (SV)

16. No parking sign with EKG reading crossed out by kid wearing Fitbit: Use for rate control in atrial fibrillation

17. Person waiting for the porta potty: Can cause constipation

18. Guest in green dress with red face: Can cause flushing

19. Guest in green dress with visibly swollen legs: Can cause edema

20. Broken water pump next to porta potty: Can cause heart failurc

21. Broken, overturned ATV next to green dressed guest: Can cause AV block

22. Salvation Army donation box and metronome falling on ground: Can cause sinoatrial (SA) node depression

23. Guest holding his head in pain: Class IV antiarrhythmics can cause headaches

24. Deflating tire seat at bar: Can cause systemic hypotension

25. Sneezing guest blowing nose at bar: Can cause sick sinus syndrome

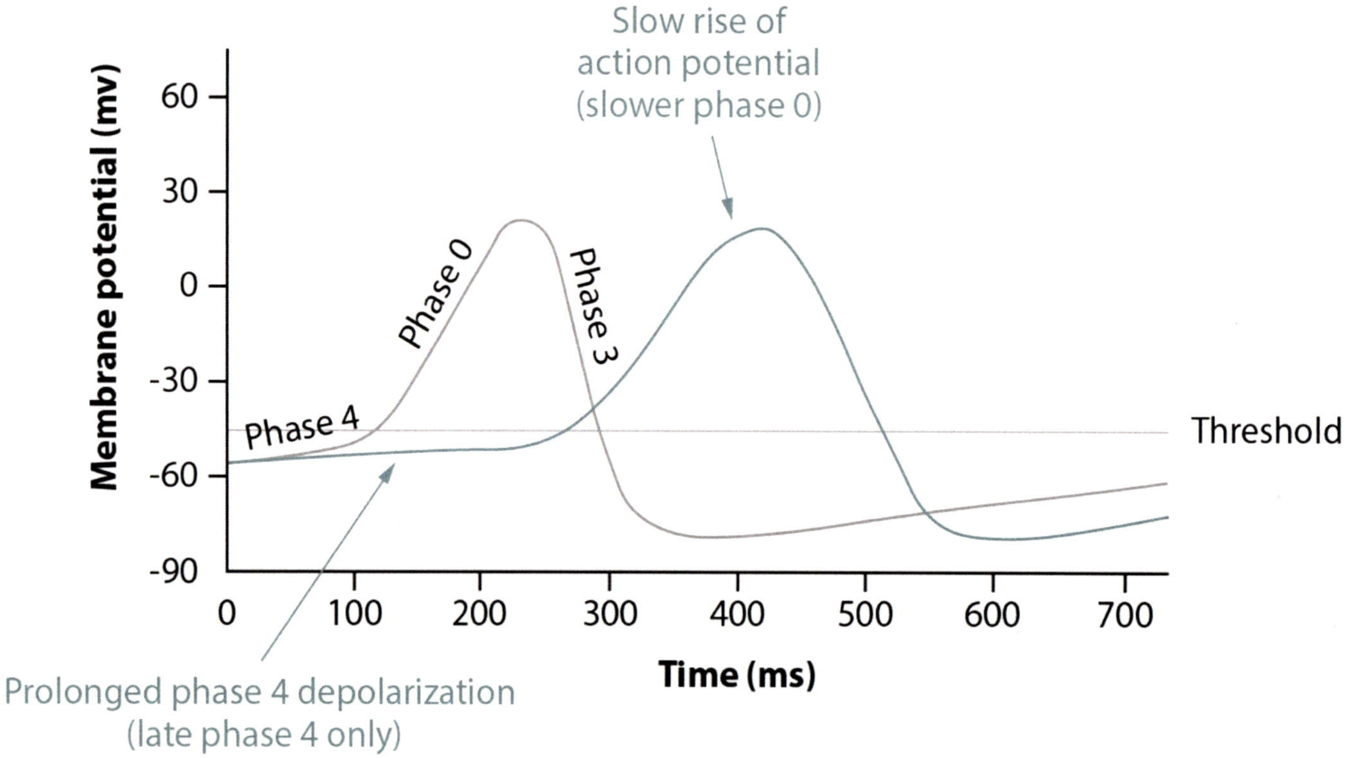

Figure 9.7.9 - Effects of Class IV Antiarrhythmics on Cardiac Pacemaker Cells

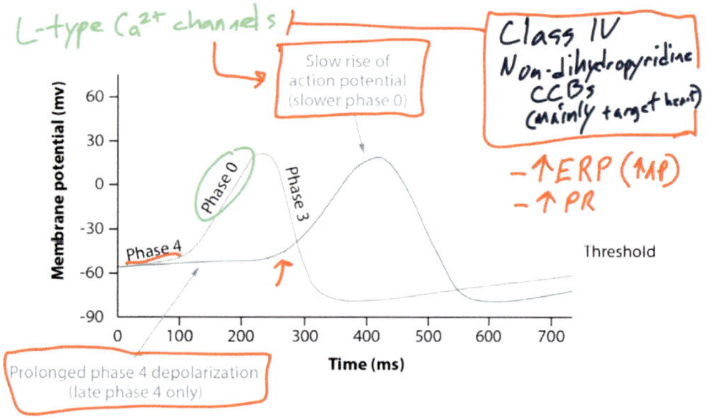

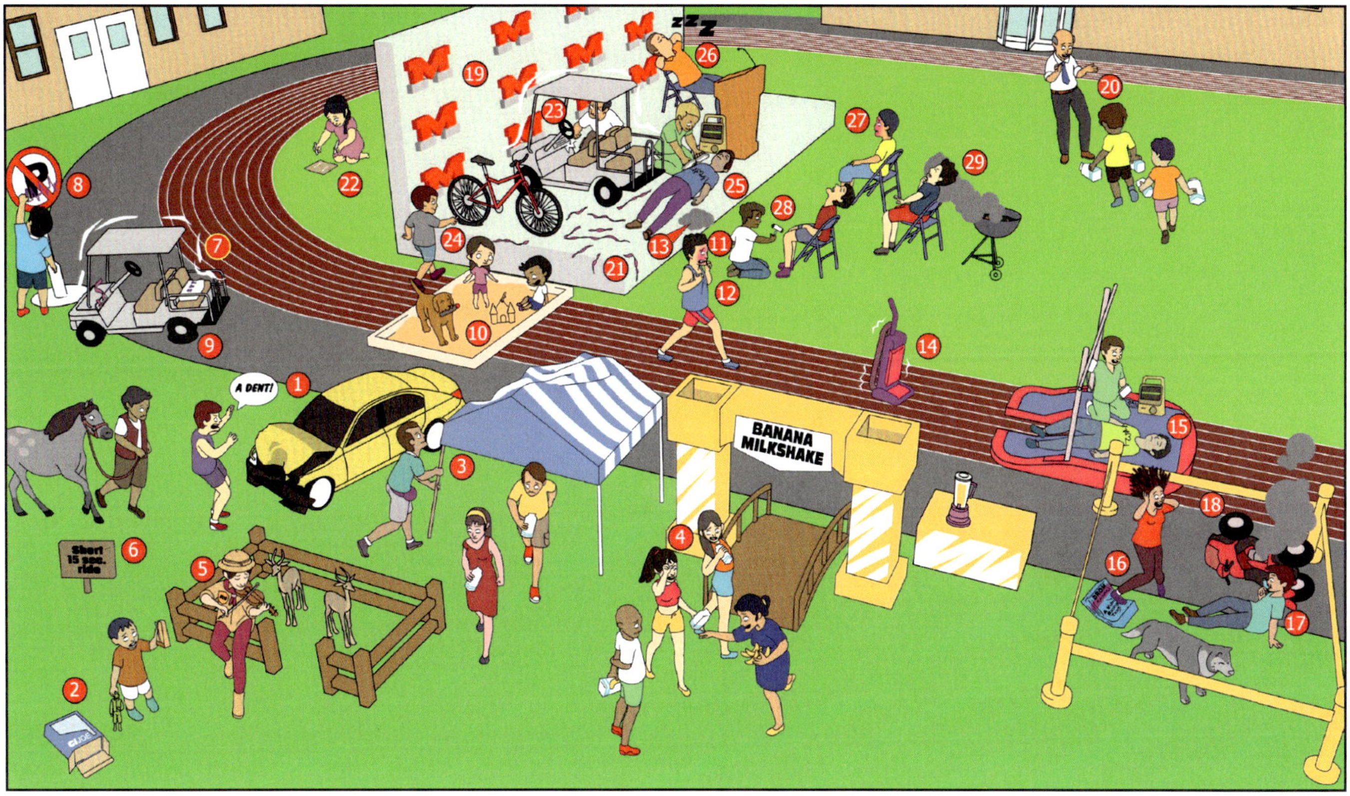

1. A dent in the yellow car next to a man screaming, "A dent!": Adenosine

2. Kid taking GI Joe action figure out of box: Activates Gi protein

3. Dad taking down fundraising tent: $\downarrow$cAMP

4. Customer with "L" hand on forehead is angry because mom collecting bananas and not taking milk: Deactivation of L-type calcium channels and activation of K$^+$ channels → $\downarrow$CA^{2+} and $\uparrow$K$^+$ entry

5. Sister in Antelope Valley outfit with is practicing while her brother is trying to shop her metronome: Transient AV node block

6. "Short 15 sec. ride" sign next to dented car: Very short acting (about 15 seconds)

7. Special Vehicle Tracking device, SVT, and rattling AC vent of golf cart: Drug of choice in diagnosing and terminating certain forms of SVT (e.g. orthodromic AVRT or AVNRT)

8. No parking sign with EKG reading along with golf cart with the special vehicle tracking device: Adenosine use for diagnosis of underlying atrial fibrillation in SVT

9. Flat tire of golf cart: Adenosine can cause hypotension

10. Toddlers sticking stick in sand of sand box while dog holds blunt dog toy: Effects of adenosine and blunted by methylxanthines (i.e. caffeine, theophylline)

11. Red face runner: Adenosine can cause flushing

12. Runner grabbing chest in pain: Adenosine can cause chest pain

13. Runner is anxious with gray cloud over his head: Adenosine can give patients a sense of impending doom

14. Shaking vacuum behind banana milkshake stand: Adenosine can cause bronchospasm

15. Passed out person behind banana milkshake stand with asystole rhythm: Adenosine can cause asystole

16. Excited mom stepping on "A Video Racing Team" with video game with pet wolf in yellow taped area: Adenosine is contraindicated with preexcitation syndromes (e.g. antidromic AVRT, WPW)

17. Man puffing inhaler in caution tape area: Adenosine is contraindicated in asthma

18. Broken, overturned ATV in yellow taped area: Adenosine is contraindicated in AV block

19. M-shaped magnets on stage and podium: Magnesium sulfate

20. Gym teacher stopping students from bringing milk into gym: Decreases calcium influx which prevents afterdepolarizations

21. Twisted streamers on podium: Use magnesium for torsades de pointes

22. Girl with two chalk sticks drawing behind podium: Use magnesium for digoxin toxicity

23. Staff trying to fix rattling AC vent on podium: Use magnesium for refractory ventricular tachyarrhythmias

24. Deflating bike tire on podium: Use magnesium for hypotension

25. Passed out speaker with visible asystole rhythm on defibrillator: Use magnesium for asystole

26. Upcoming speaker sleeping on podium: Use magnesium for drowsiness

27. Red-faced audience member: Magnesium can cause flushing

28. Sleeping audience member's leg does not move after staff with reflex hammer hits it: Magnesium can cause a loss of reflexes

29. Man in audience choking on smoke: Magnesium and cause respiratory depression

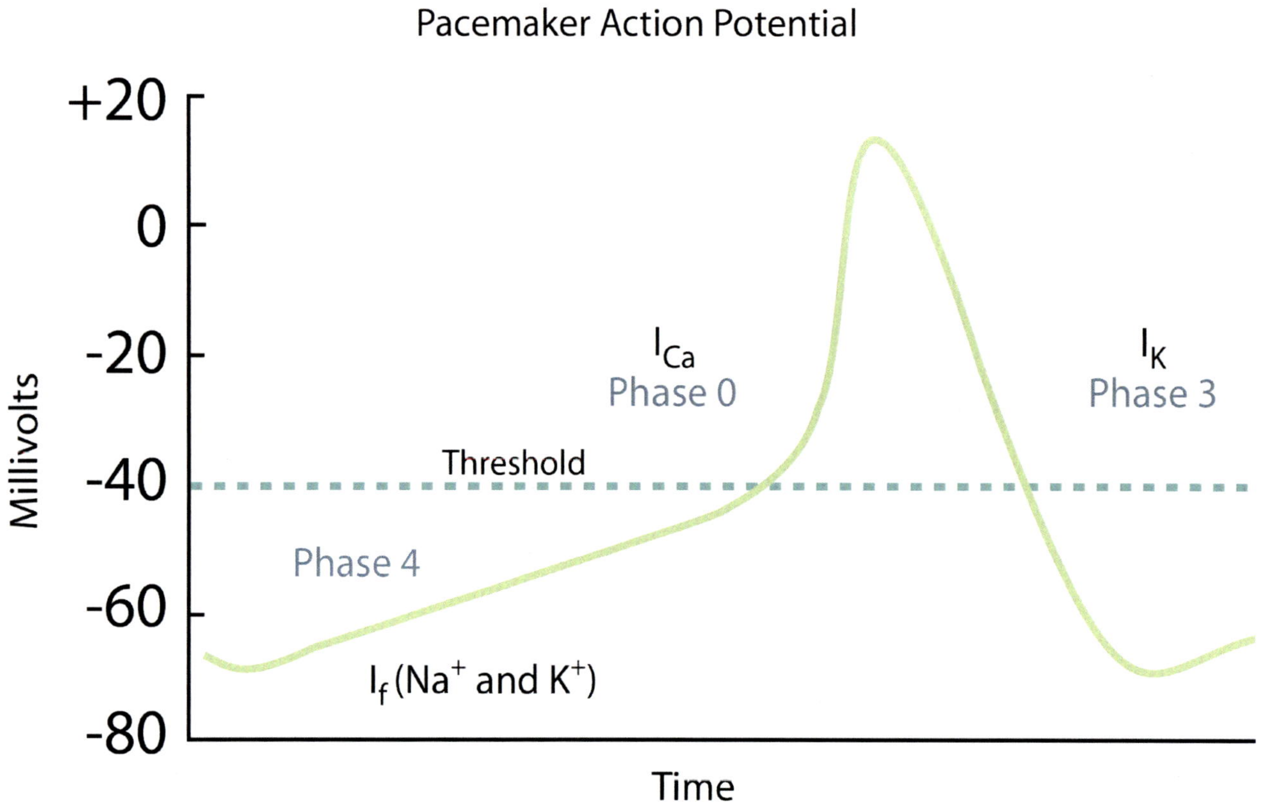

Figure 9.7.10 - Effects of Other Antiarrhythmics (Adenosine and Magnesium) on Cardiac Pacemaker Cells

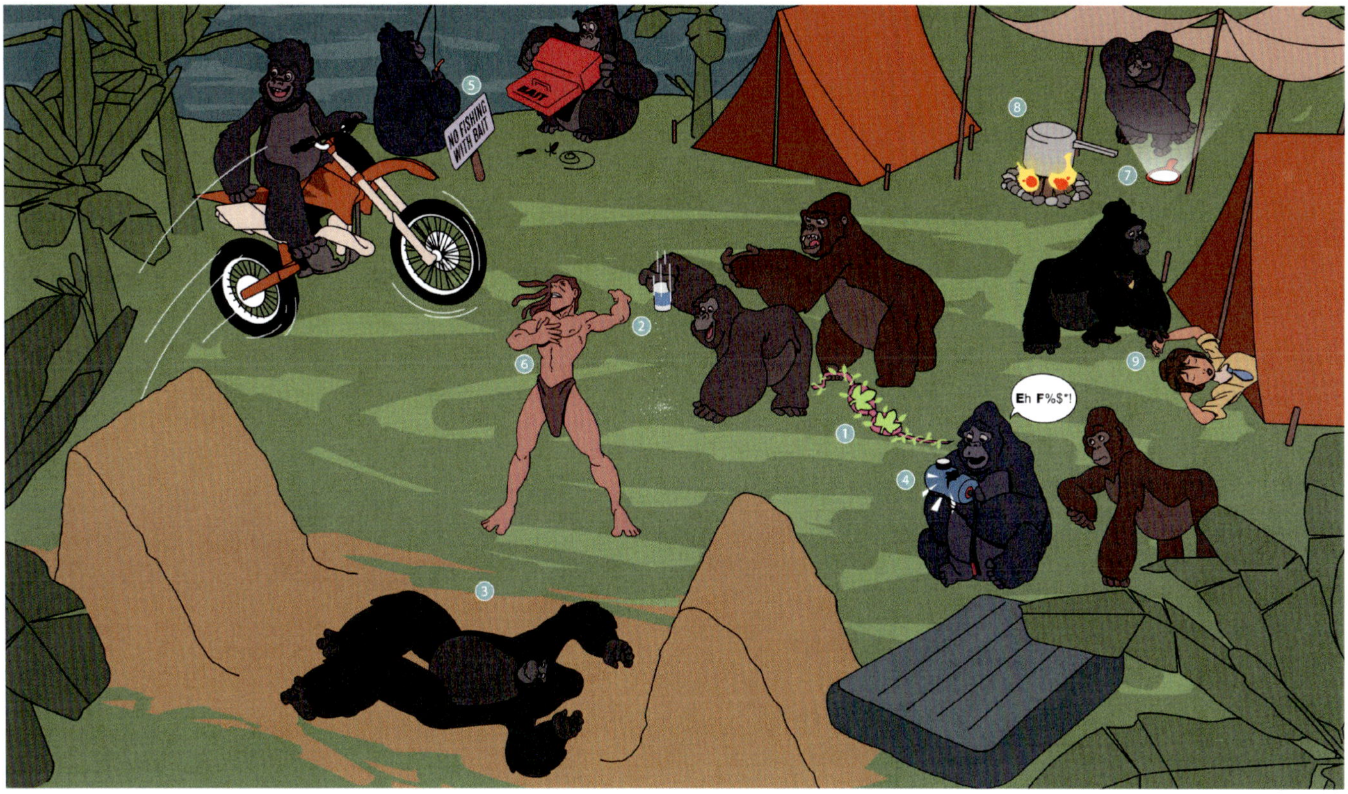

1. Ivy bra next to gorillas: Ivabradine

2. Tarzan acting funny while mother gorilla smacks younger gorilla in the head while using a salt shaker: Bocks sodium "funny" channels (If) in pacemaker cells of SA node

3. Ape stretched across phase 4 of action ramps: Prolongs phase IV of depolarization

4. Gorilla breaking air pump and cussing "Eh F%$!" near thumbs down: Use for heart failure with reduced ejection fraction (HFrEF)

5. Ape fishing with worm next to sign that reads, "No fishing with bait": Used for patients who can't take beta-blockers

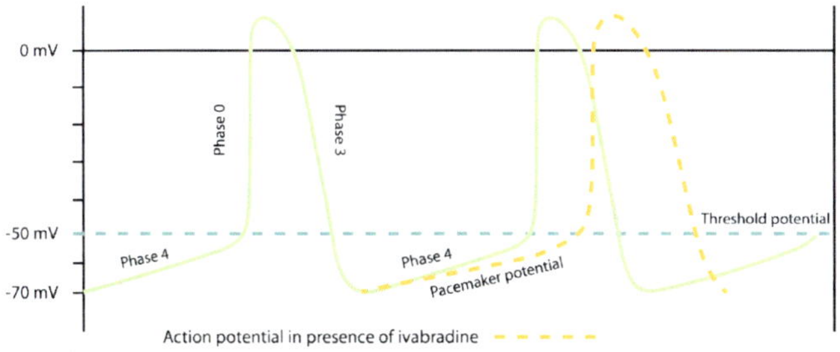

Figure 9.7.11 - Effects of Ivabradine on Pacemaker Action Potential

6. Tarzan holding his chest while stable to ground: Use for stable angina

7. Gorilla being blinded by reflection from mirror: Can cause "phosphene" (visual brightness)

8. Pressure cooker on fire: Can cause hypertension

9. Gorilla checking radial pulse of Jane while she sleeps: Can cause bradycardia

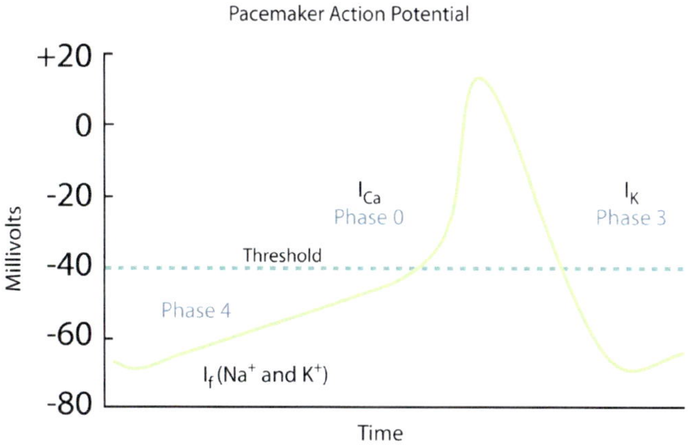

Figure 9.7.12 - Pacemaker Action Potential

Section 1 - Insulin Preparations

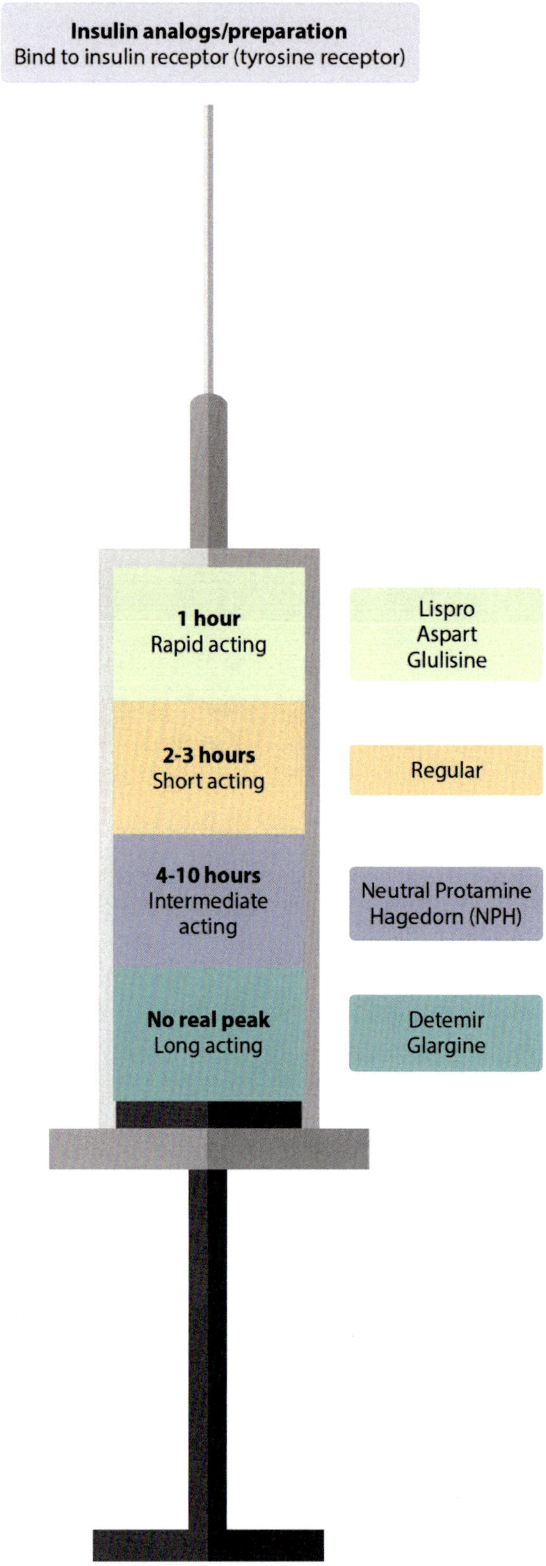

Figure 9.8.1 - Insulin Categories

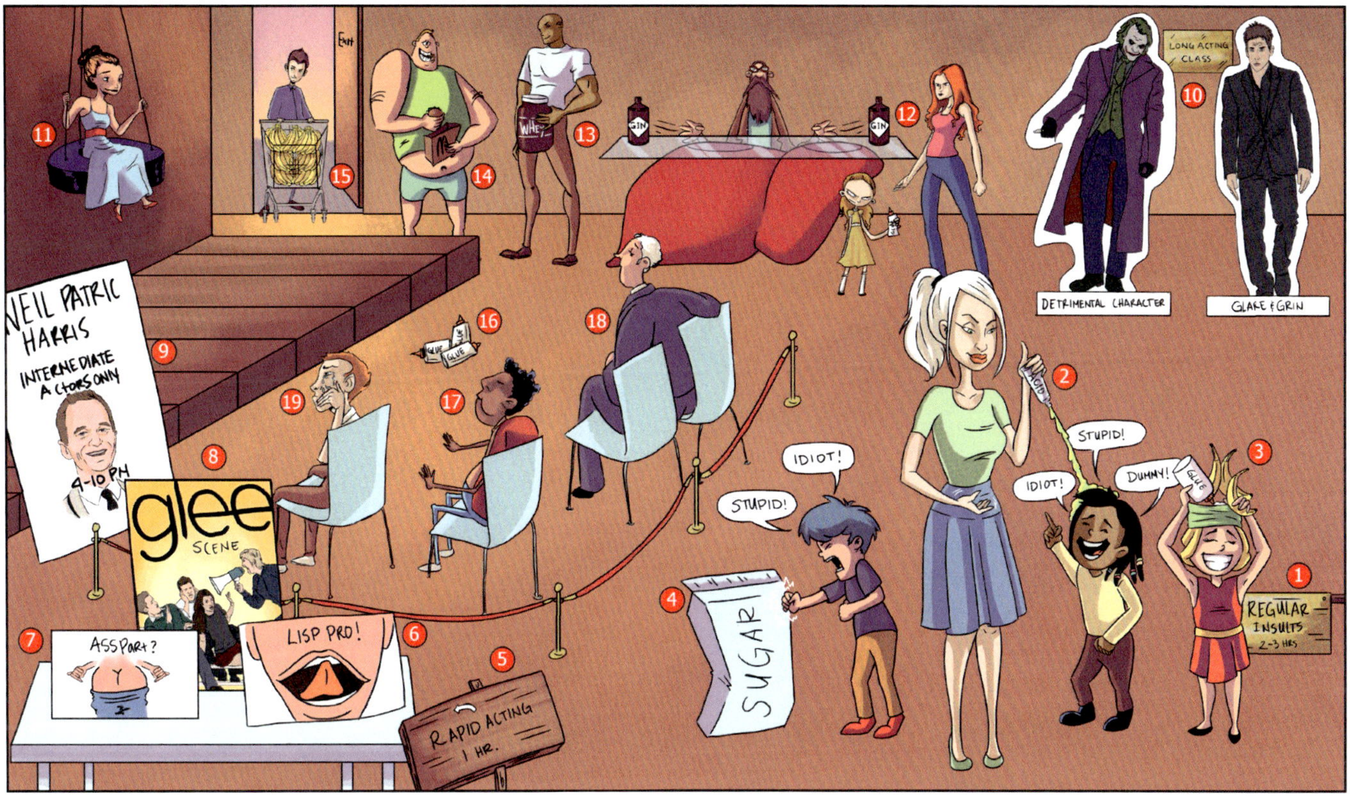

1. Short actor insulting his acting coach with regular insults for 2-3 hours: Regular insulin, short acting (2-3 hr peak)

2. Teachers squirting acid on student's dreadlocks with dyed beads: Use insulin for diabetic ketoacidosis (DKA)

3. Actor is using glue to make a banana hat: Use regular insulin for hyperkalemia

4. Stressed actor punching a bag of sugar: Use regular insulin for stress hyperglycemia

5. "Rapid acting 1 hour" class sign: Rapid acting preparations have a 1 hr peak

6. "Lisp Pro!" poster: Lispro is rapid acting

7. "Ass Part?" poster: Aspart is rapid acting

8. "Glee scene" poster: Glulisine is rapid acting

9. Neal Patrick Harris intermediate acting session from 4-10 pm poster: NPH is intermediate acting and has a 4-10 hr peak

10. Joker and Zoolander, long acting class cutouts, with "detrimental" and "glare and grin" advertisements: Long acting preparations are detemir and glargine

11. Kind actress on tire swing: Binds to insulin receptor (tyrosine kinase receptor)

12. Girl gets glue from liver-shaped bar with gin: Increases glucose stored as glycogen in the liver

13. Fit actor by the liver-shaped bar holding whey protein receiving gin: Increased glycogen and protein synthesis in the muscle

14. Fat guy eating McDonalds: Increased triglyceride storage in fat

15. Stagehand entering through the backdoor with cart of bananas: Increased potassium uptake in cells

16. Empty glue bottles on floor: Can cause hypoglycemia

17. Producer with buffalo hump, round face, and thin limbs: Can cause lipodystrophy

18. Fat producer sitting on two chairs: Can cause weight gain

19. Smitten producer: Can rarely cause hypersensitivity reactions

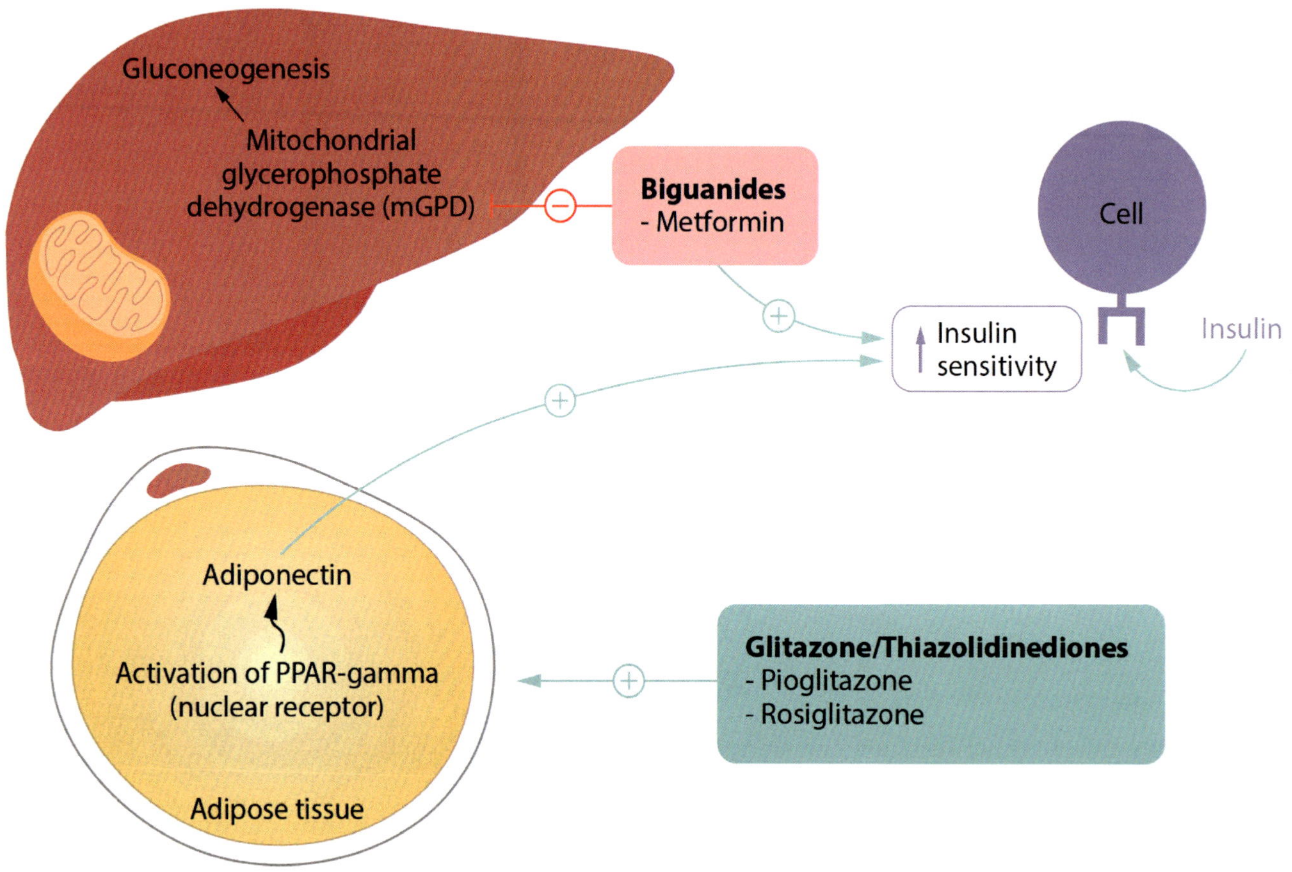

Figure 9.8.2 - Insulin-Related Pharmacology

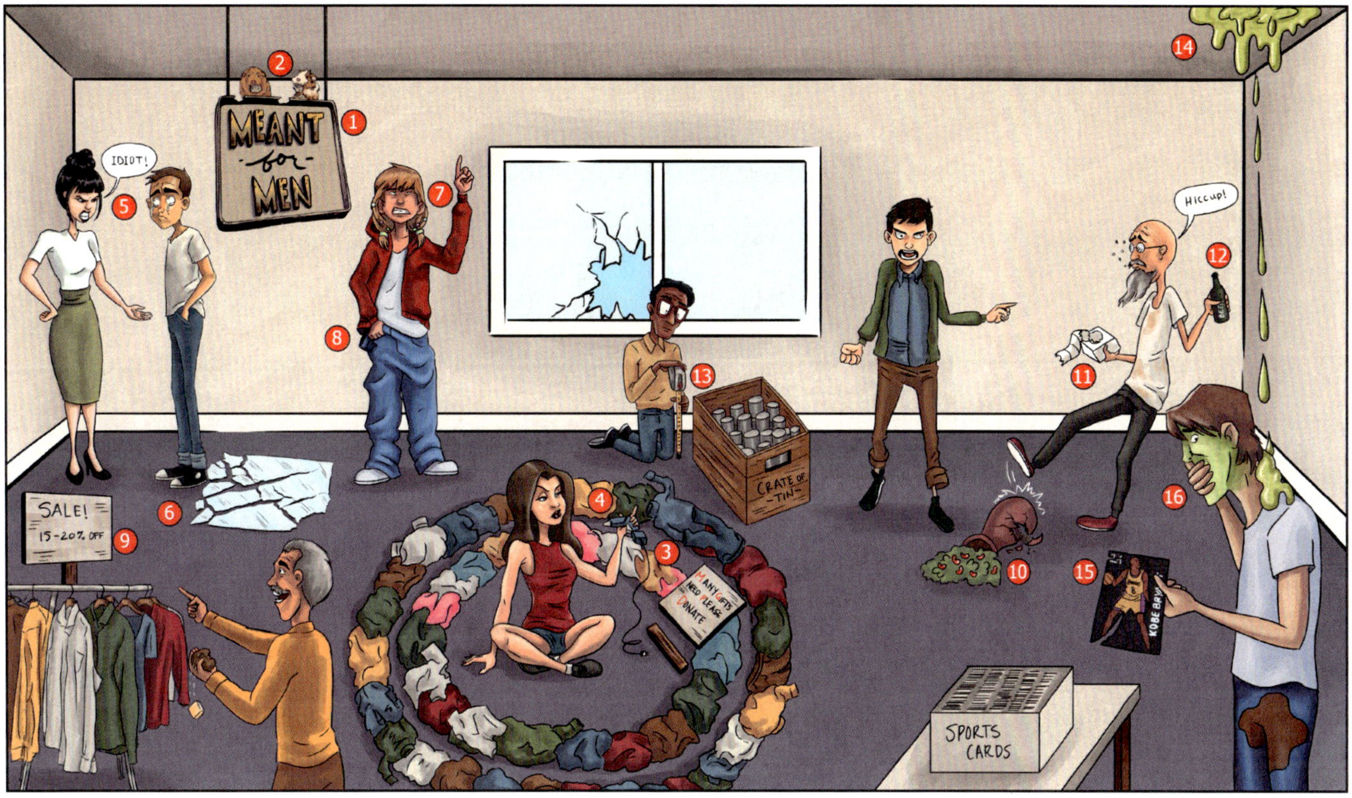

1. "Meant for Men" sign: Metformin

2. Two guinea pigs on "Meant for Men" sign: Metformin is a biguanide

3. Employee sitting inside two layers of clothing and is finishing "Many Gifts need Please Donate" sign with broken glue gun: Inhibits mitochondrial glycerol-3-phosphate dehydrogenase (mGPD)

4. Broken glue gun: Inhibits hepatic gluconeogenesis and glucagon activity

5. Manager insulting hypersensitive employee: Increases insulin sensitivity

6. Broken glass dropped by hypersensitive employee: Increased glycolysis

7. Customer with two dyed beads in hair holding up one finger: First line treatment for type II DM

8. Dyed bead hair guy holding up huge old pants: Promotes weight loss

9. Customer's butter melts off of roll after getting distracted by "Sale! 15-20% Off" sign: Triglycerides are decreased 15-20%

10. Customer who destroyed kidney bean plant and is being told to leave: Avoid in patients with renal failure

11. Customer holding replacement pump being told to leave: Avoid in patients with heart failure

12. Drunk customer being told to leave: Avoid in patients with alcoholism

13. Employee measuring crate of tin: If used in patients with renal insufficiency assess renal function with creatinine measurements

14. Customer soaked in diarrhea and acid: Can cause lactic acidosis

15. Tom Kobe Bryant card: Can cause cobalamin (B_{12}) deficiency

16. Customer soaked in acid nearly vomits: Can cause GI distress

See Figure 9.8.2- Insulin-Related Pharmacology (Endocrine Pharmacology, Section 2, Page 151)

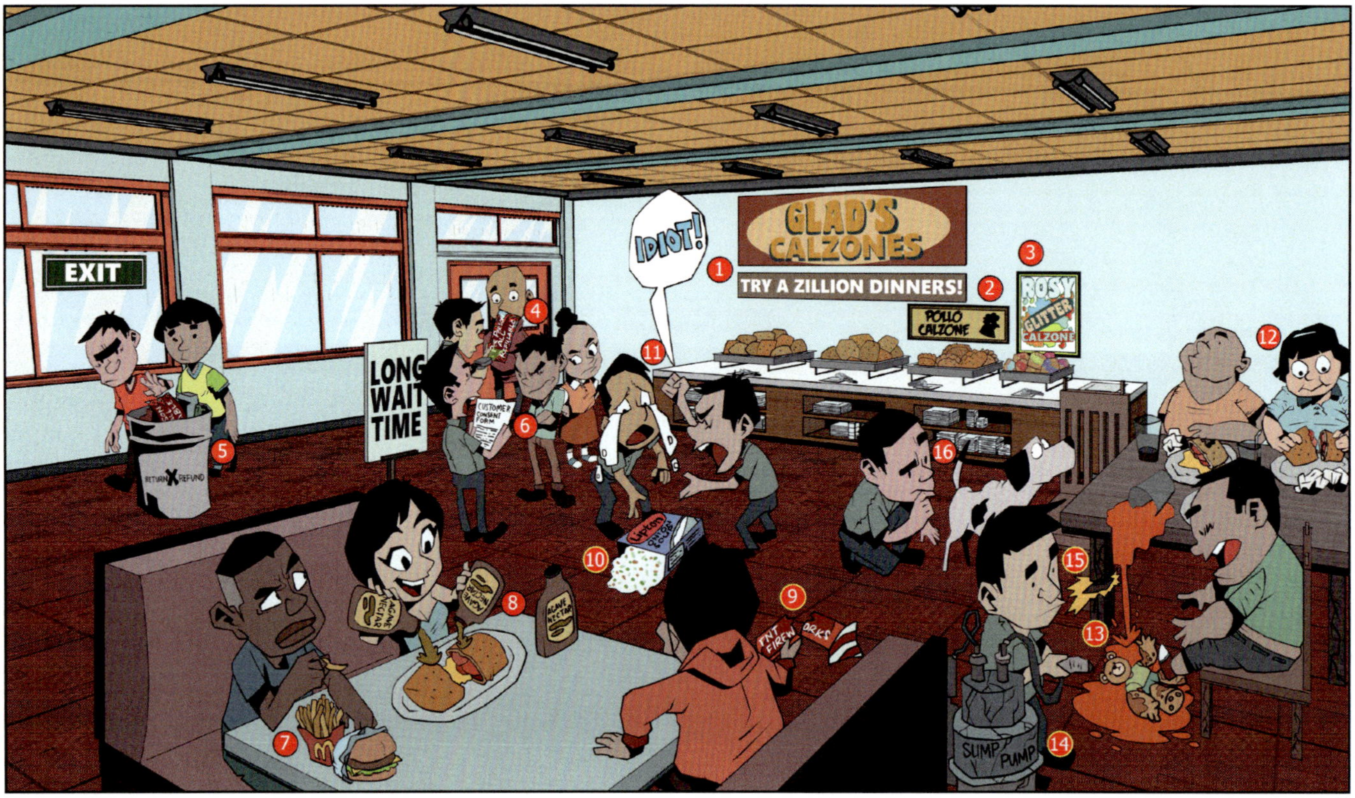

1. Glad's Calzones motto, "Try a zillion dinners": Glitazones and Thiazolidinediones

2. Pollo calzones: Pioglitazone

3. Rosy glitter calzones: Rosiglitazone

4. "Per person, all refillable" passes being scanned by green laser: Activation of PPAR-$_{\gamma}$ in the nucleus

5. "Return X Refund" garbage can to toss drink passes: PPAR-$_{\gamma}$ binds to a retinoid X receptor (RXR) → together they form a heterodimer → upregulated gene transcription

6. Annoyed customers hearing employee read a transcript that takes a long time: Delayed onset of action because time is required for transcription and translation

7. Fatty fast food: Increased fatty acid uptake

8. Girlfriend pouring agave nectar on calzone: Increased adiponectin production

9. Broken TNT firework brought by girlfriend's brother: Decreased TNF-α production

10. Split lipton onion soup: Decreased leptin

11. Manager insulting sensitive employee: Increased insulin sensitivity

12. Fat customers: Can cause weight gain

13. Swollen stuffed animal: Can cause edema

14. Broken sump pump: Can exacerbate heart failure

15. Broken table leg: Can increase risk for fractures

16. Manager inspecting liver-spotted service dalmatian: Monitor liver function with all thiazolidinediones

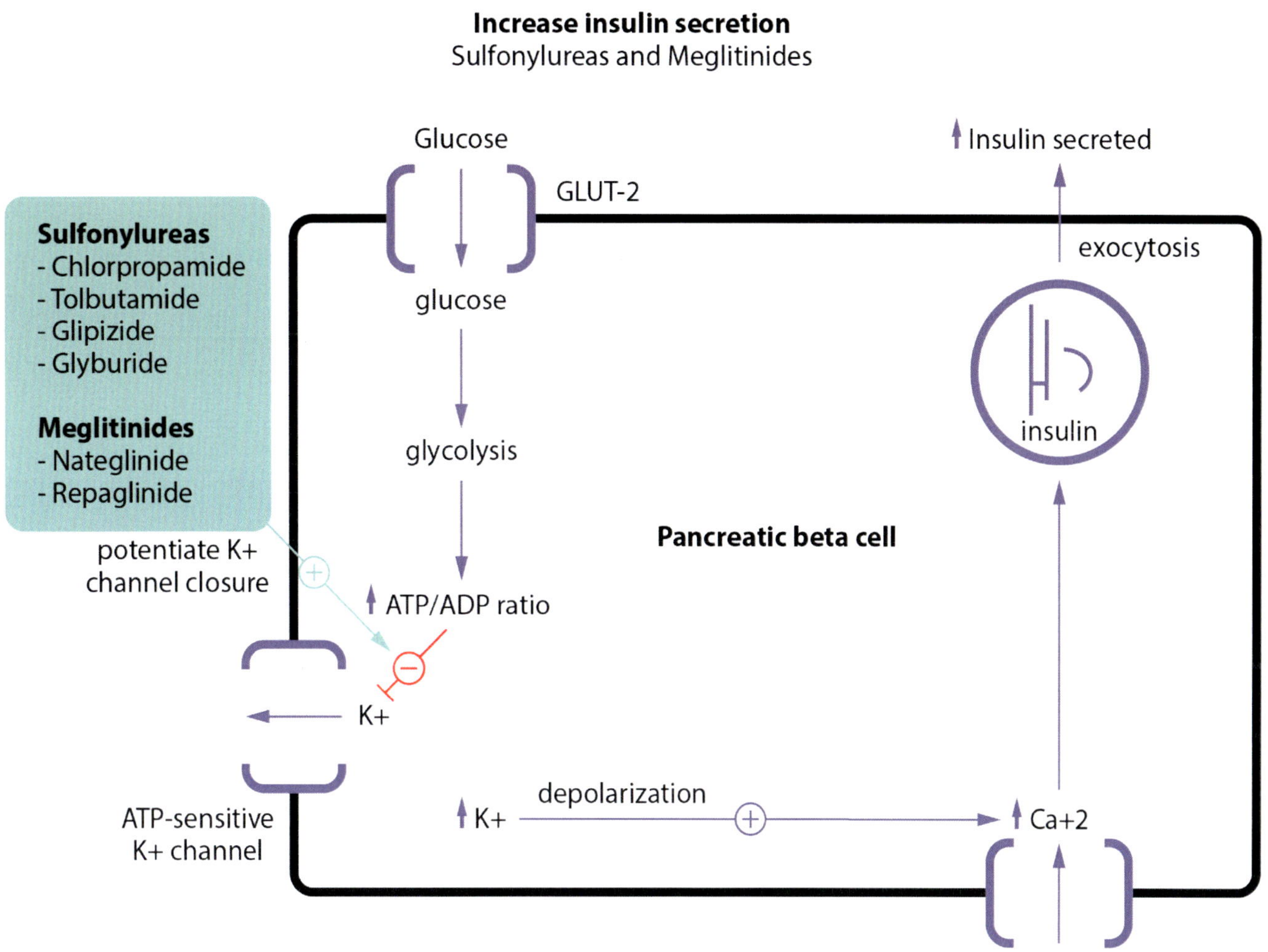

Figure 9.8.3 - Insulin-Related Pharmacology in Beta Cells

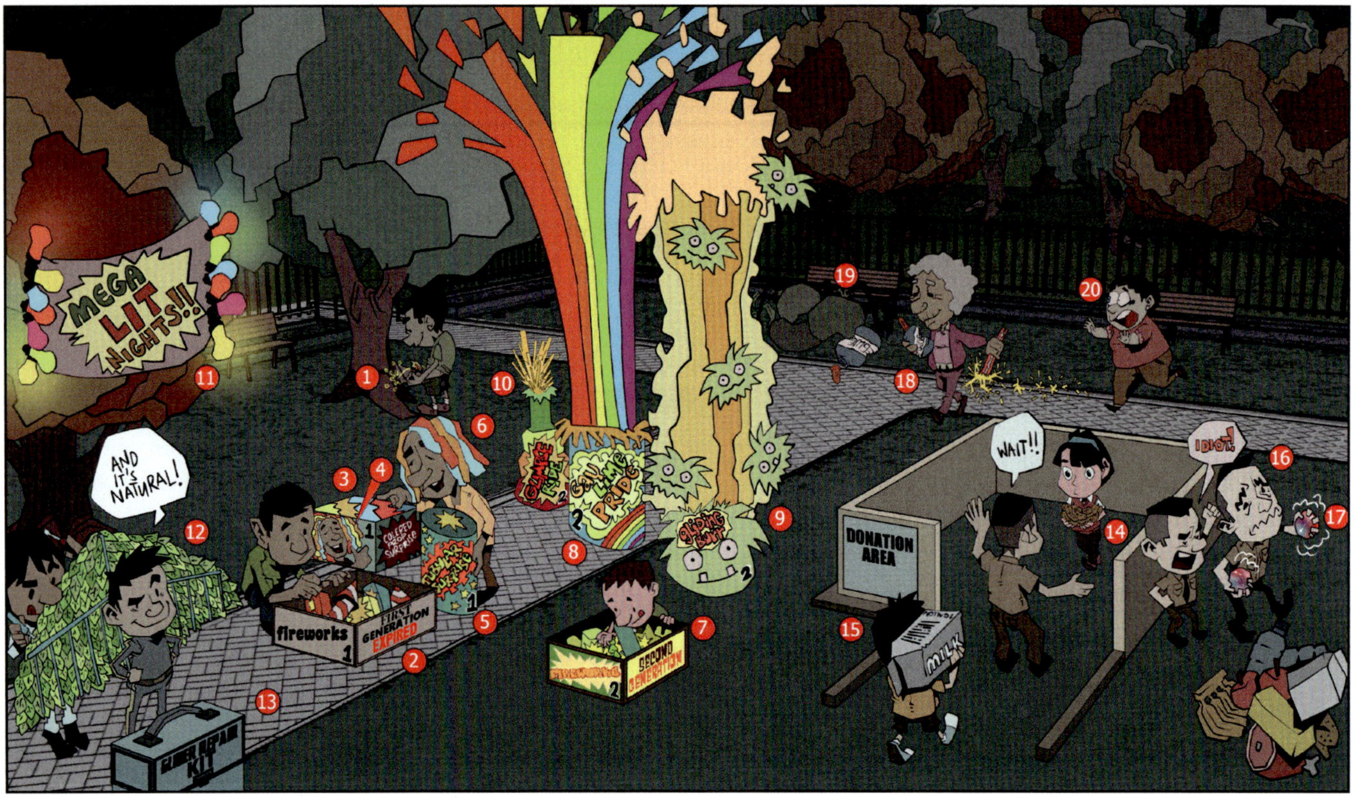

1. Kid urinating on match: Sulfonylureas

2. Firework box with "first generation, expired" sticker: 1st generation sulfonylureas

3. Colored prop surprise box: Chlorpropamide

4. Guy with dyed hair on colored box: Chlorpropamide can cause disulfiram-like reactions

5. "Tubular surprise" firework: Tolbutamide

6. Dyed hair guy carrying "tubular surprise" firework: Tolbutamide can cause disulfiram-like reactions

7. Son with firework box labeled, "second generation": 2nd generation sulfonylureas

8. Large, rainbow firework called, "gay lime pride": Glimepride is long acting

9. The "gliding burr" large firework: Glyburide is long acting

10. The "glimpse ride" small firework: Gliplzide is short acting

11. "Mega Lit Nights" banner: Meglitinides

12. Natural leaf glider: Nateglinide

13. Glider repair kit: Repaglinide

14. Woman being denied to take bananas out of donation area: Meglitinides and sulfonylureas work by closing potassium channels in pancreatic beta cells → increased intracellular potassium

15. Huge carton of milk entering donation area: Increased intracellular potassium → depolarization → influx of calcium

16. Guy insulting another by calling him an idiot outside of donation area: Influx of calcium → increased insulin release

17. Insulted guy squeezing two dyed stress balls:Since viable pancreatic beta cells are required, meglitinides and sulfonylureas only treat type II DM

18. Empty glue bottle: Meglitinides and sulfonylureas can cause hypoglycemia

19. Empty glue bottle by dead kidney bean plant: Risk of hypoglycemia is increased in renal failure

20. Large woman running: Meglitinides and sulfonylureas can cause weight gain

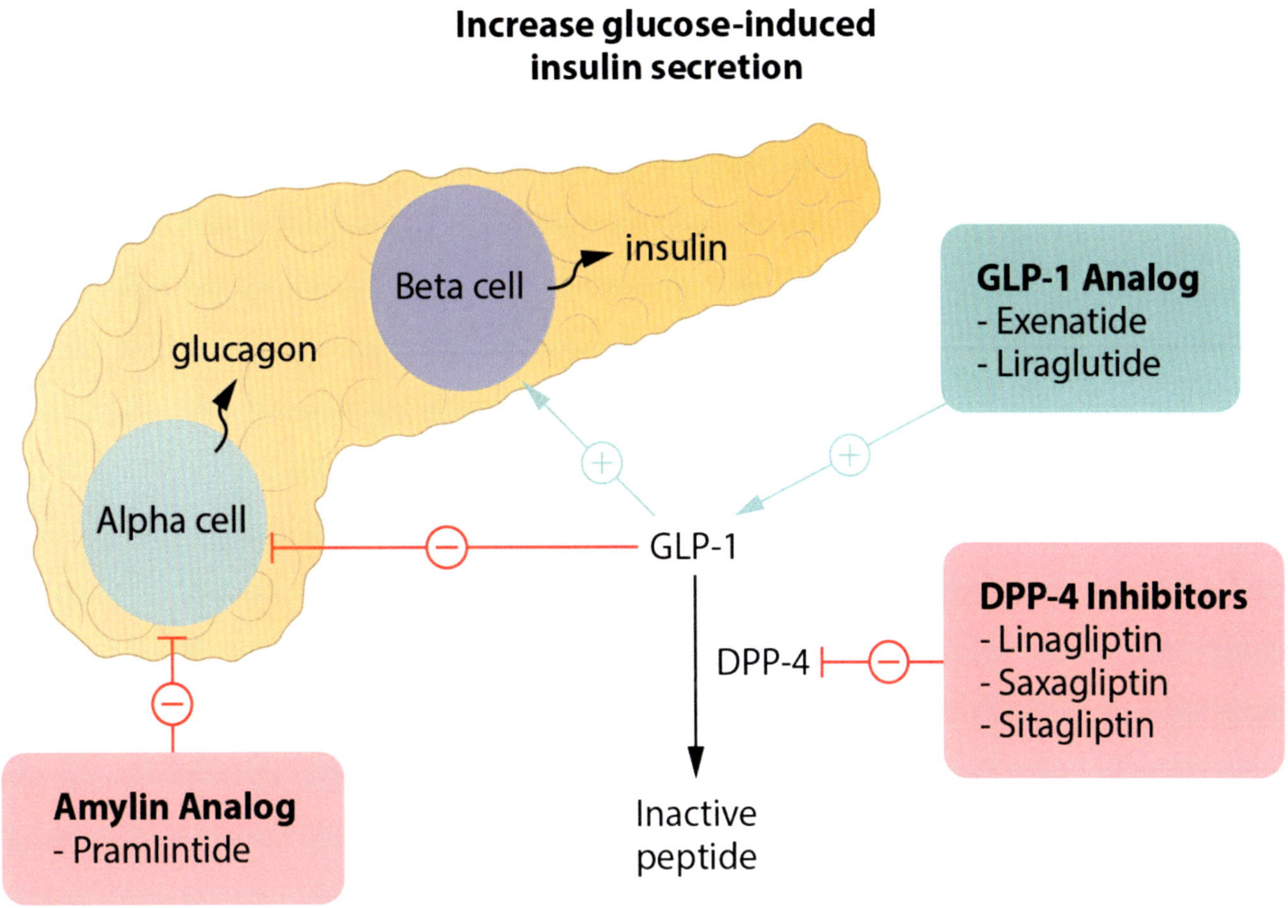

Figure 9.8.4 - Insulin-Related Pharmacology in the Pancreas

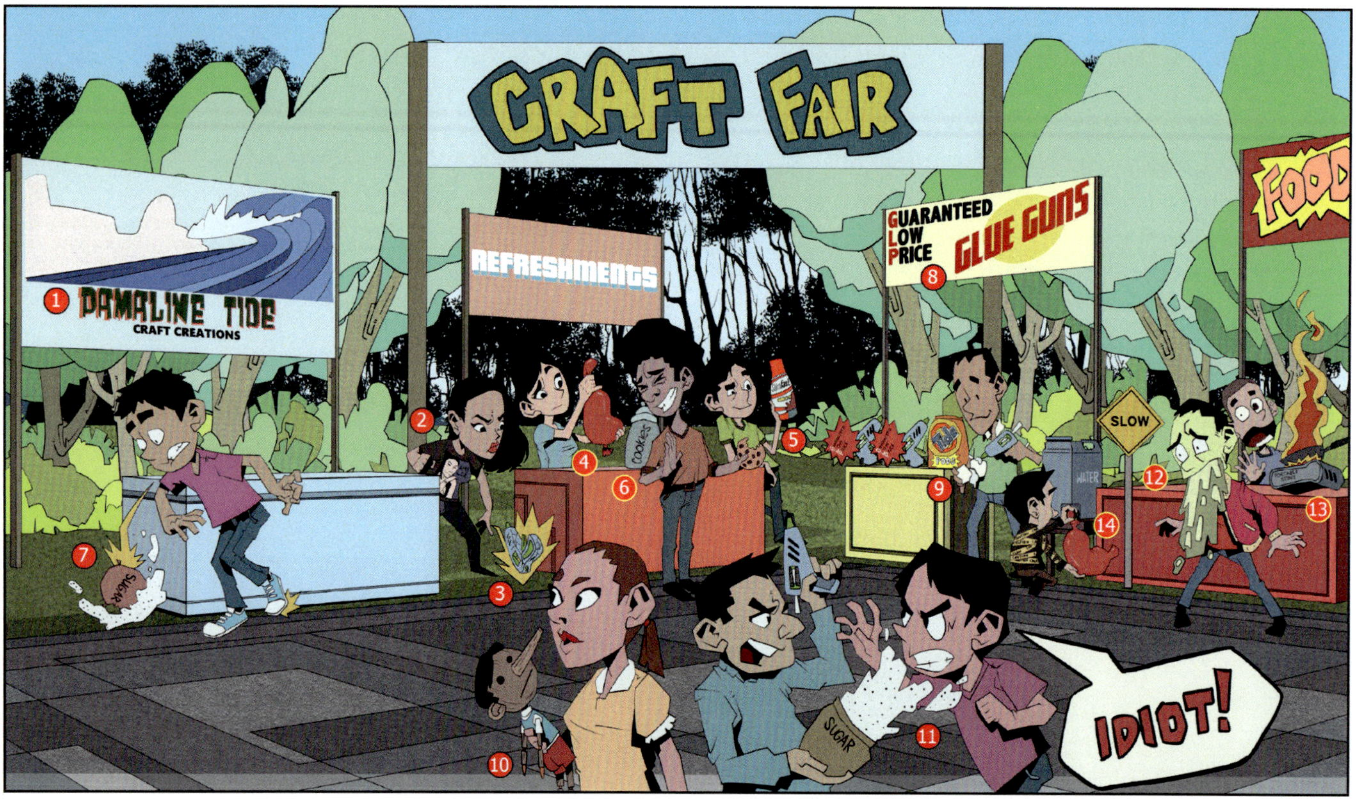

1. "Pamaline tide" booth: Pramlintide

2. Amy Lee fan: Amylin analog

3. Amy Lee fan throwing broken glue gun: Decreased glucagon release

4. Woman squeezing and rolling stomach-shaped balloon: Decreased gastric emptying

5. Skinny guy selling slim fast shakes: Promote weight loss

6. Full guy who did not want to eat his free cookie: Increased satiety

7. Sugar spilling from pamaline tide booth on ground: Can cause hypoglycemia

8. "Guaranteed low price" booth: GLP-1 analogs

9. Tide pod glue gun demonstration: Exenatide

10. Pinocchio doll with long, liar's nose and round glutes: Liraglutide

11. Guys who are fighting over glue gun exchange insults while other throws sugar: Increased glucose-dependent insulin release

12. Guy vomiting next to glue guns: Can cause nausea and vomiting

13. Flaming pan next to glue guns: Can cause pancreatitis

14. Boy wearing caution tape shirt, filling stomach-shaped balloon next to glue guns and "slow" sign: Contraindicated in patients with gastroparesis

See Figure 9.8.4 - Insulin-Related Pharmacology in the Pancreas (Endocrine Pharmacology, Section 5, Page 156

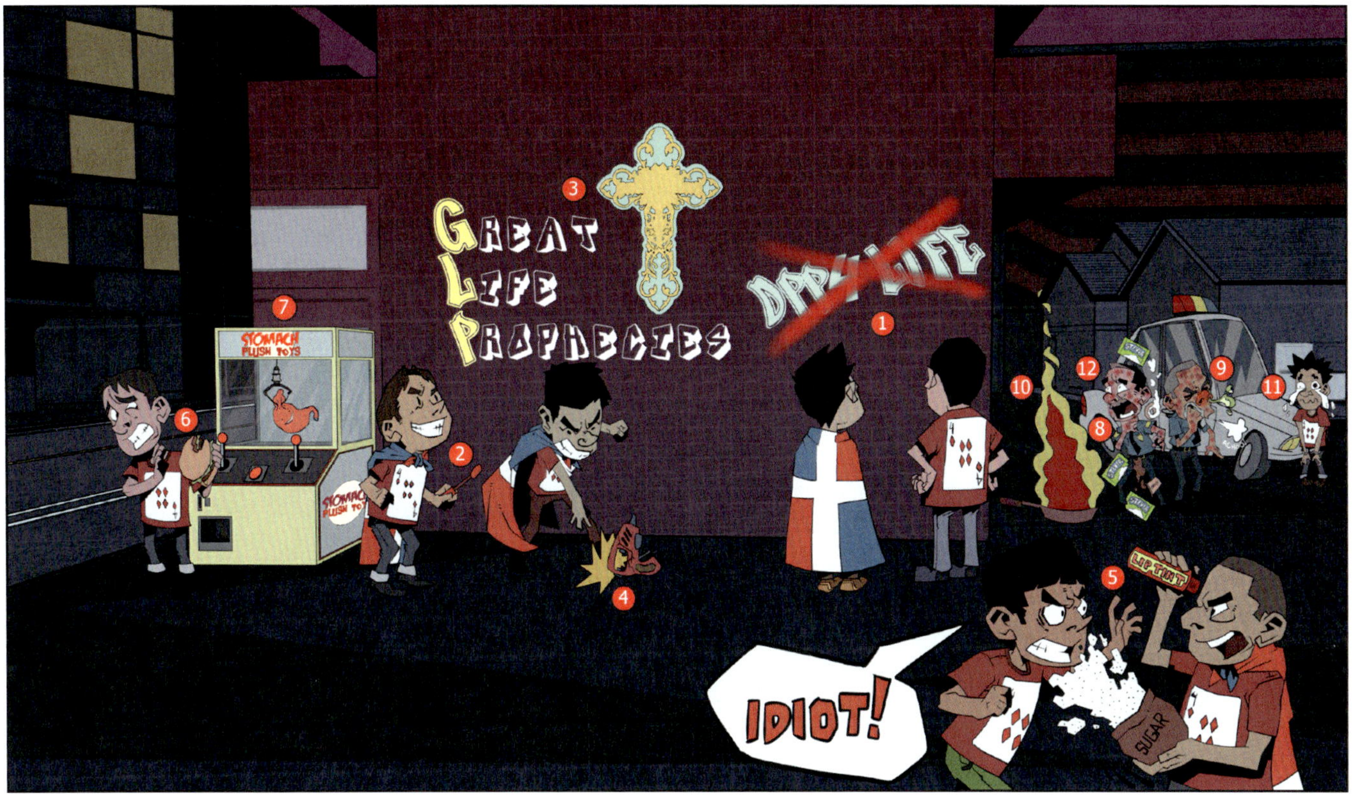

1. Dominican poker player with 4 diamonds shirt and crossed out gang tag: Inhibition of DPP-4

2. Lip tint: "-Liptin" is the common suffix

3. "Great Life Prophecies" tag and cross symbol: Leads to increased GLP-1

4. DPP gang throwing glue gun to ground: Leads to less glucagon release

5. DDP gang insulting each other over sugar holding lip tint: Increased glucose-dependent insulin release

6. Full gang member rejecting hamburger: Increased satiety

7. Empty claw machine squeezing toy stomach: Decreased gastric emptying

8. Cop with coffee on crotch and choking on donut powder: Can cause mild urinary or respiratory infections

9. Cop with allergies sneezing with red nose: Can cause nasopharyngitis

10. Flaming pan near cops: Can cause pancreatitis

11. Hypersensitive DDP gang member near police car: Can cause hypersensitivity reaction

12. Cop's red and splotchy skin: Can cause Stevens-Johnson syndrome

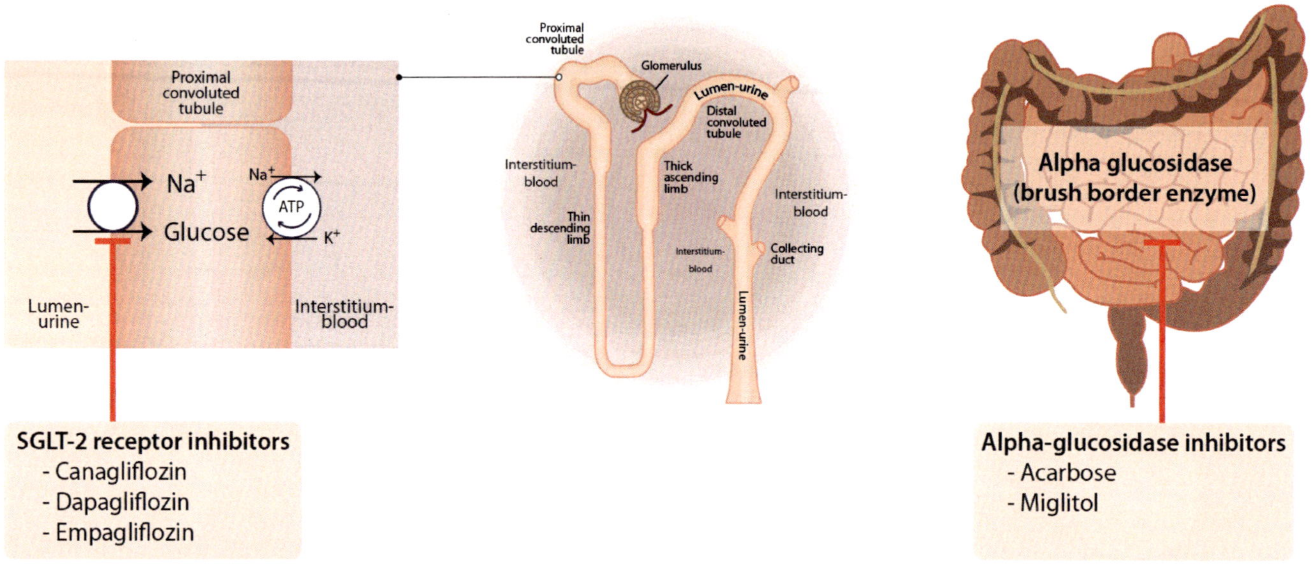

Figure 9.8.5 - Medications to Decrease Glucose Absorption

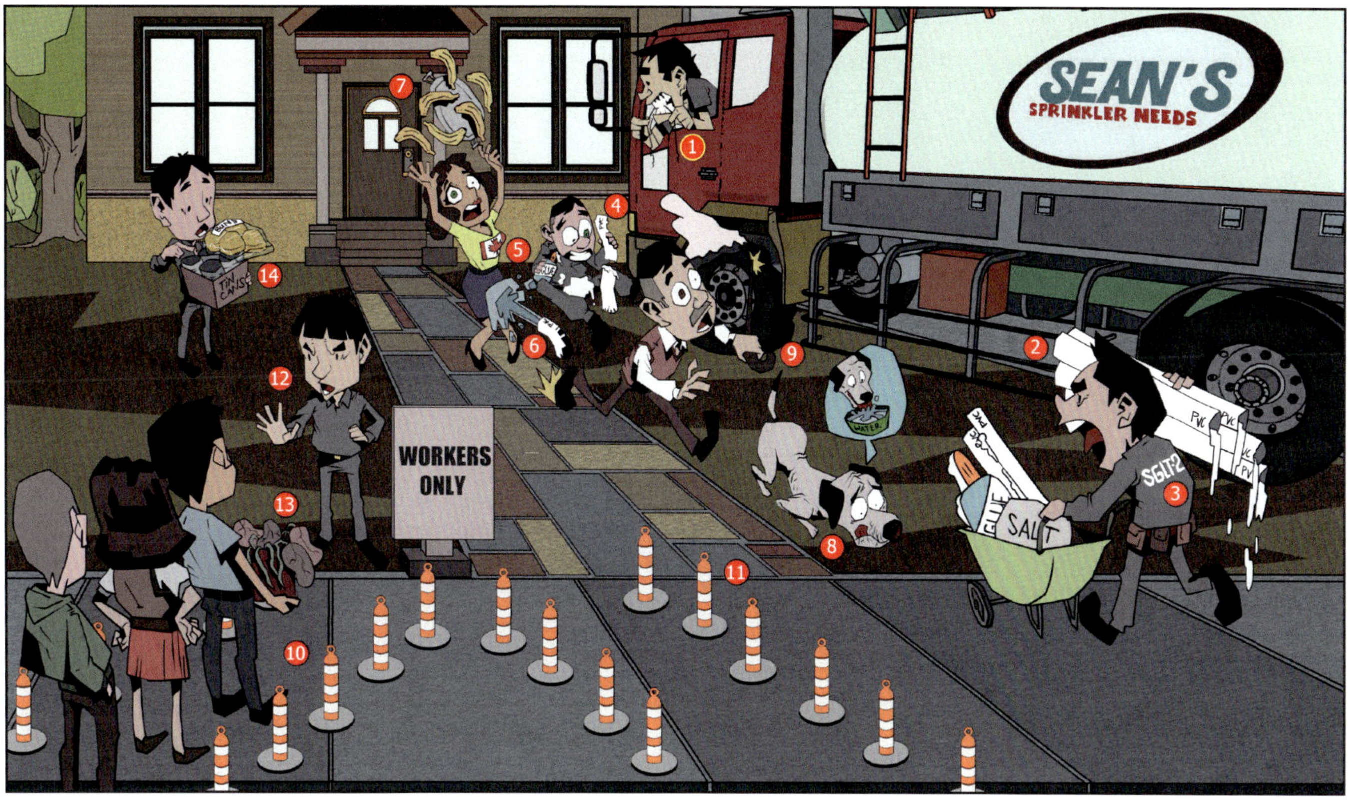

1. Driver flossing teeth: Canagliflozin, dapaliftozin, and empagliflozin ("flozins")

2. Driver blocked where glued PVC pipes were going: Flozins block glucose reabsorption in the PCT

3. "SGLT-2" shirt: Flozins block the sodium-glucose cotransporter 2 ($SGLT_2$) in the PCT

4. Glue gets on crotch of worker: Glucosuria

5. Woman with Canadian shirt near the guy with glue on his crotch: Glucosuria increases risk of vaginal candidiasis

6. Sprinkler sprays woman in crotch: Glucosuria increases risk of UTI

7. Woman tossing bananas upward: Flozins can cause hyperkalemia

8. Thirst and malnourished dog: Flozins can cause dehydration and weight loss

9. Father with cane poking holes in deflating tire: Dehydration can lead to orthostatic hypotension

10. Cones funneling people: Afferent arteriole

11. Right lane exit cones: Efferent arteriole

12. Worker blocking people from entering: Decreased efficacy with decreased GFR

13. Dying kidney bean plants block by worker: Not recommended if kidney function is impaired

14. Worker counting wooden crate with tin cans: Evaluate kidney function with BUN and creatinine

See Figure 9.8.5 - Medications to Decrease Glucose Absorption (Endocrinology Pharmacology, Section 7, Page 159)

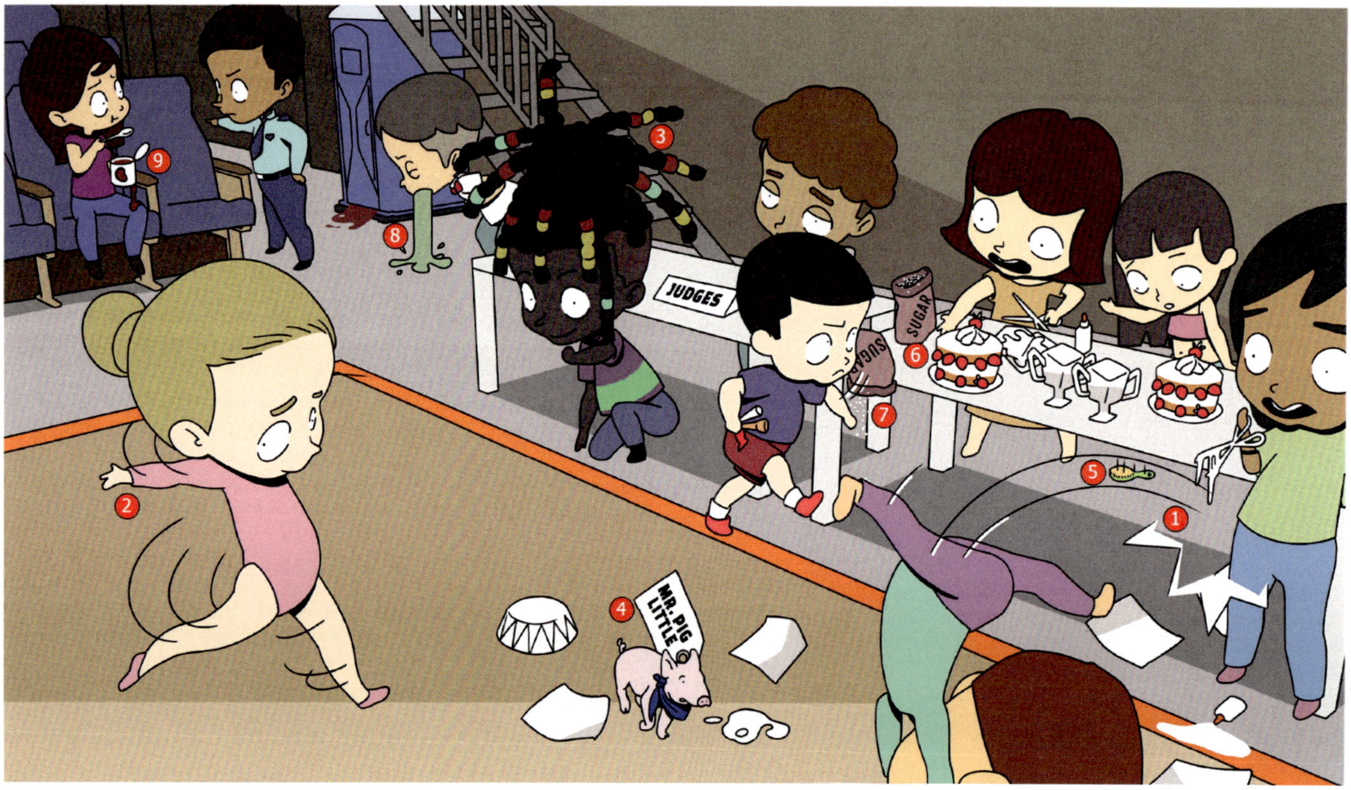

1. Crafty mom with scissors and glue on the side of her leg hit by cartwheeling kid: α-glucosidase inhibitors

2. Acrobatic child: Acarbose

3. Coach with dyed beads in dreads: Use for diabetes mellitus management

4. Mr. Pig Little running through paper and glue: Miglitol

5. Girl dropping her brush: α-glucosidase inhibitors inhibit intestinal brush-border α-glucosidases

6. Chubby kid being denied treats that will be served later: Results in delayed carbohydrate hydrolysis and glucose absorption

7. Chubby kid, who already ate, knocks over sugar: Results in decreased postprandial hyperglycemia

8. Vomiting judge near a bathroom leaking diarrhea: Can cause GI upset and diarrhea

9. Lady eating a can of kidney beans with hole in can: Not recommended if kidney function is impaired

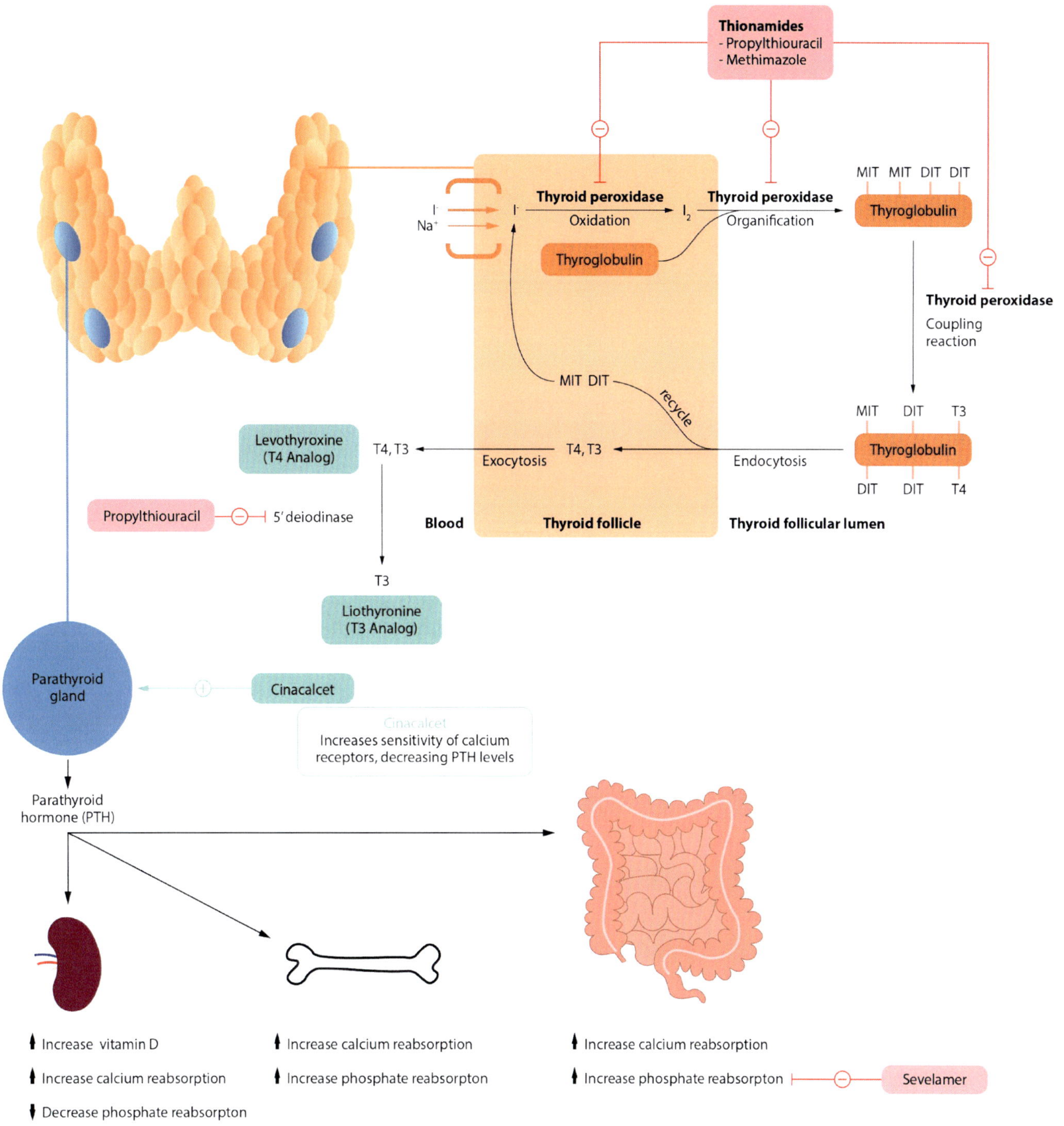

Figure 9.8.6 - Pharmacologic Interactions with Thyroid and Parathyroid

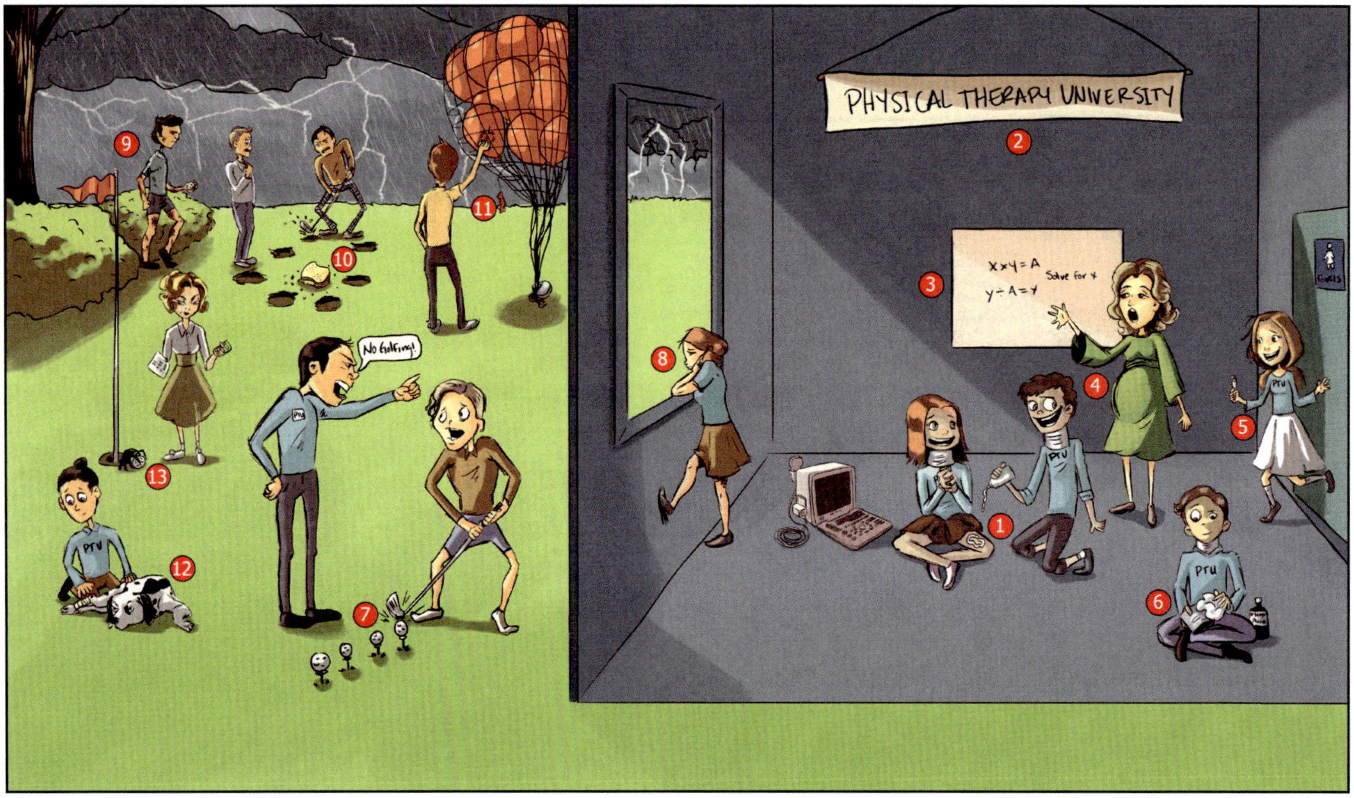

1. Boy draws "o" on girl's thigh with gel: Thioamides

2. "Physical Therapy University" banner: Propylthiouracil (PTU)

3. Math on whiteboard: Methimazole

4. Professor in final stages of pregnancy: Methimazole is used during second and third trimesters of pregnancy

5. Student who found out she's pregnant: PTU is used during the first trimester of pregnancy

6. Guy using hydrogen peroxide to clean neck guard that protects his thyroids: PTU and methimazole blocks thyroid peroxidase inhibiting the oxidation of iodide as well as the organification and coupling of iodine → inhibition of thyroid hormone synthesis

7. Manager with PTU badge won't let golfer who set up 4 tees hit 1 ball: PUT blocks 5'- deiodinase →↓ peripheral conversion of T_4 to T_3

8. Bored student looking at a brewing storm: Thionamides treat hyperthyroidism

9. Scraped up golfer retrieving his ball: Thionamides can cause a skin rash

10. Angry golfer smashing holes and throws sandwich on ground while his friend tugs at collar: Thionamides can cause agranulocytosis which can lead to ulcerative pharyngitis

11. Kid popping red helium balloons in large net: Thionamides can cause aplastic anemia

12. Student with PTU shirt is with a liver-spotted dalmatian with broken leg: PTU can cause hepatotoxicity

13. Golfer in early pregnancy doing math that has a tarantula blocking golf hole by her: Methimazole is a teratogen by causing aplasia cutis

See Figure 9.8.6 - Pharmacologic Interactions with Thyroid and Parathyroid (Endocrine Pharmacology, Seciton 9, Page 164)

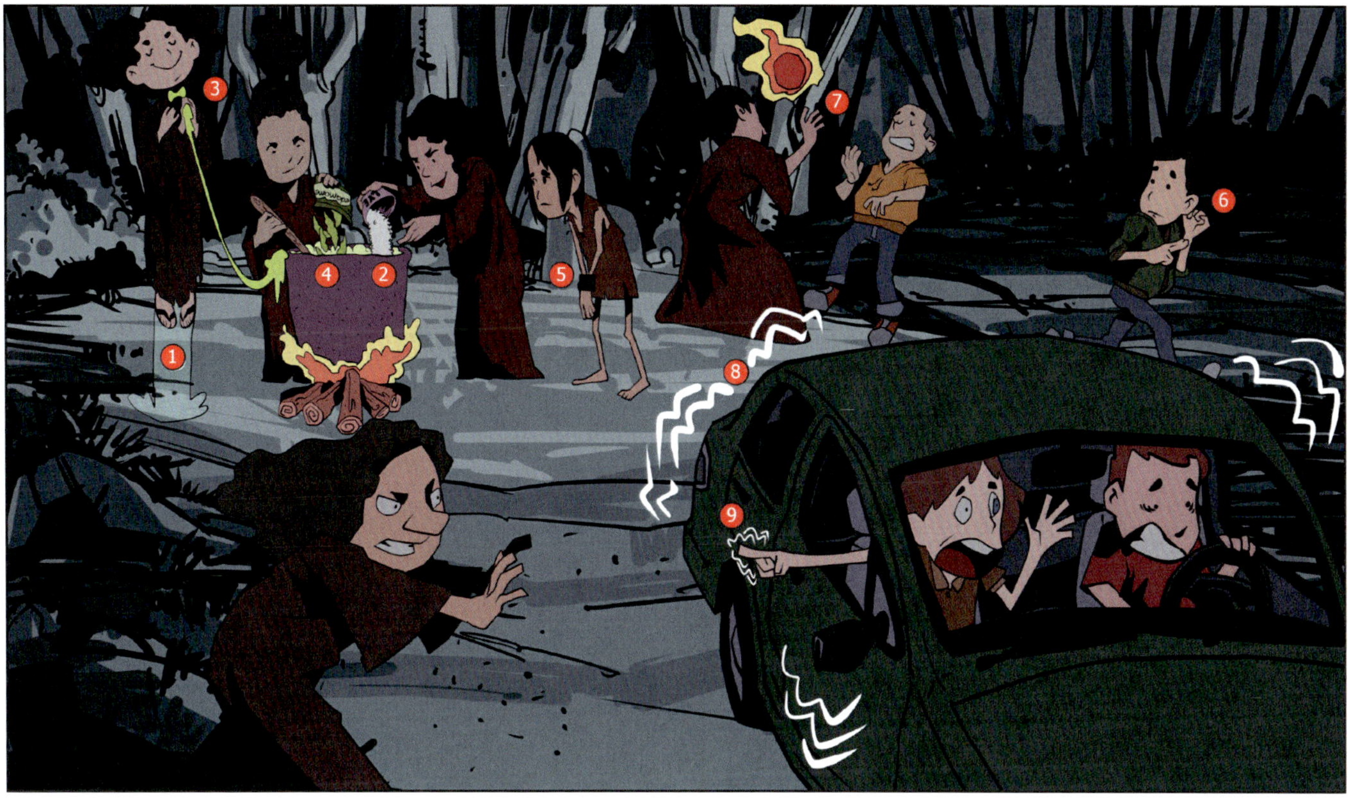

1. Witch practicing levitation: Levothyroxine (synthetic thyroxine T_4)

2. Witch adding lye to potion: Liothyronine (synthetic triiodothyronine/T_3)

3. Levitating witch rubbing potion on neck and making thyroid-shaped smear: Used to treat hypothyroidism

4. Witch mixing edamame into potion: Used to treat myxedema coma

5. Starved, emaciated prisoner captured by witches: May be abused for weight loss

6. Scared man checking his pulse while running away from witches: Can cause tachycardia

7. Witch casting fireball spell on second man: Can cause heat intolerance

8. Third man trying to escape in violently shaking car: Can cause arrhythmias

9. Girl inside car pointing at witch with trembling hand: Can cause tremors

See Figure 9.8.6 - Pharmacologic Interactions with Thyroid and Parathyroid (Endocrine Pharmacology, Seciton 9, Page 162)

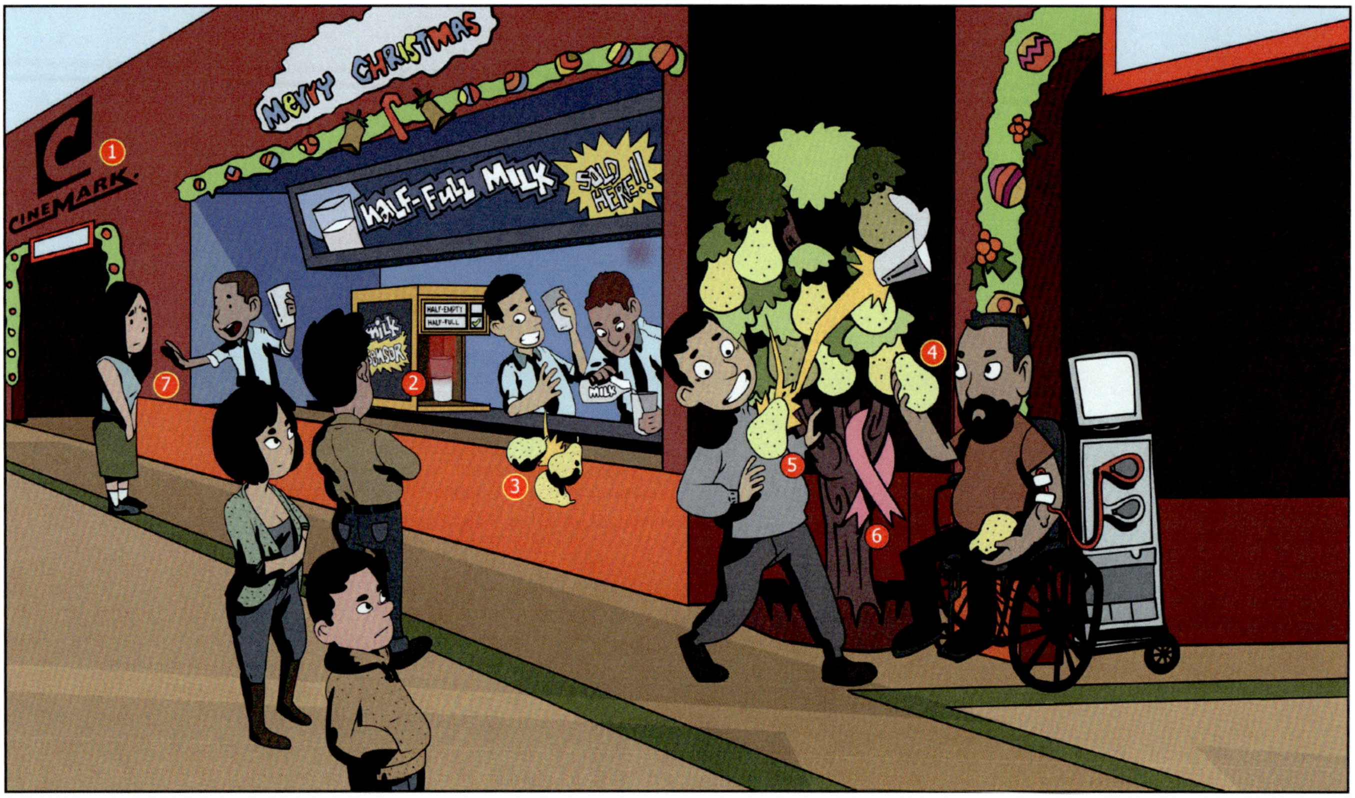

1. Cinemark movie theater: Cinacalet

2. Calcium milk censors: Cinacalcet increases the sensitivity of calcium-sensing receptors (CaSR) in the parathyroid gland

3. Knocked over pears: Increased CaSR sensitivity → decreased PTH secretion

4. Man on dialysis holding two pears from primary pear tree: Used for 2° hyperparathyroidism

5. Falling pear from tree knocks milk high out of man's hand: Used for hypercalcemia in 1° hyperparathyroidism

6. Pink cancer ribbon around pear tree: Used for parathyroid carcinoma

7. Lady being denied glass of milk: Can cause hypocalcemia

See Figure 9.8.6 - Pharmacologic Interactions with Thyroid and Parathyroid (Endocrine Pharmacology, Seciton 9, Page 162)

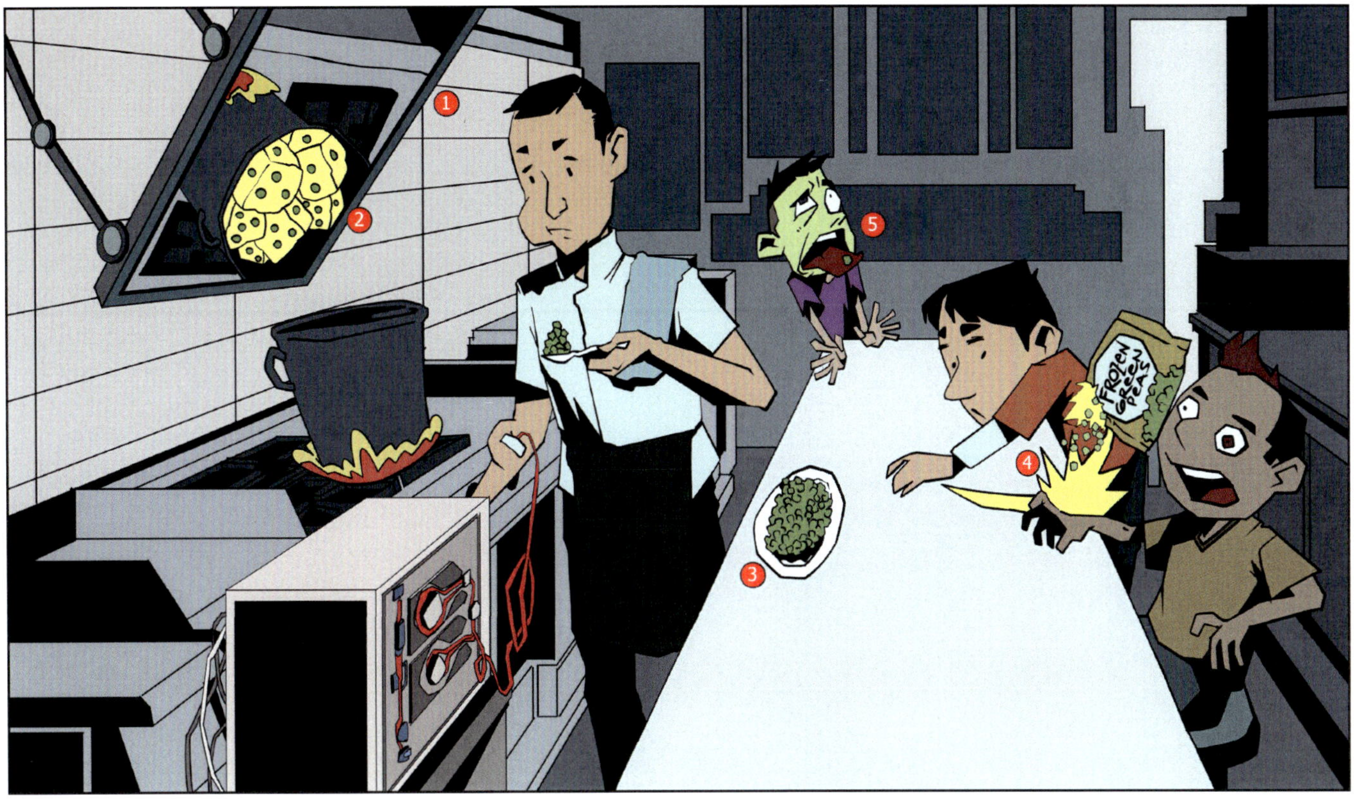

1. Silver mirror: Sevelamer

2. Sponges and peas stuck in a circular pot: Binds phosphate

3. Chef on dialysis eating large amount of peas: Can treat hyperphosphatemia in chronic kidney disease

4. Knocked over falling peas: Can cause hypophosphatemia

5. Student is dramatically sick after trying peas: Can cause GI upset

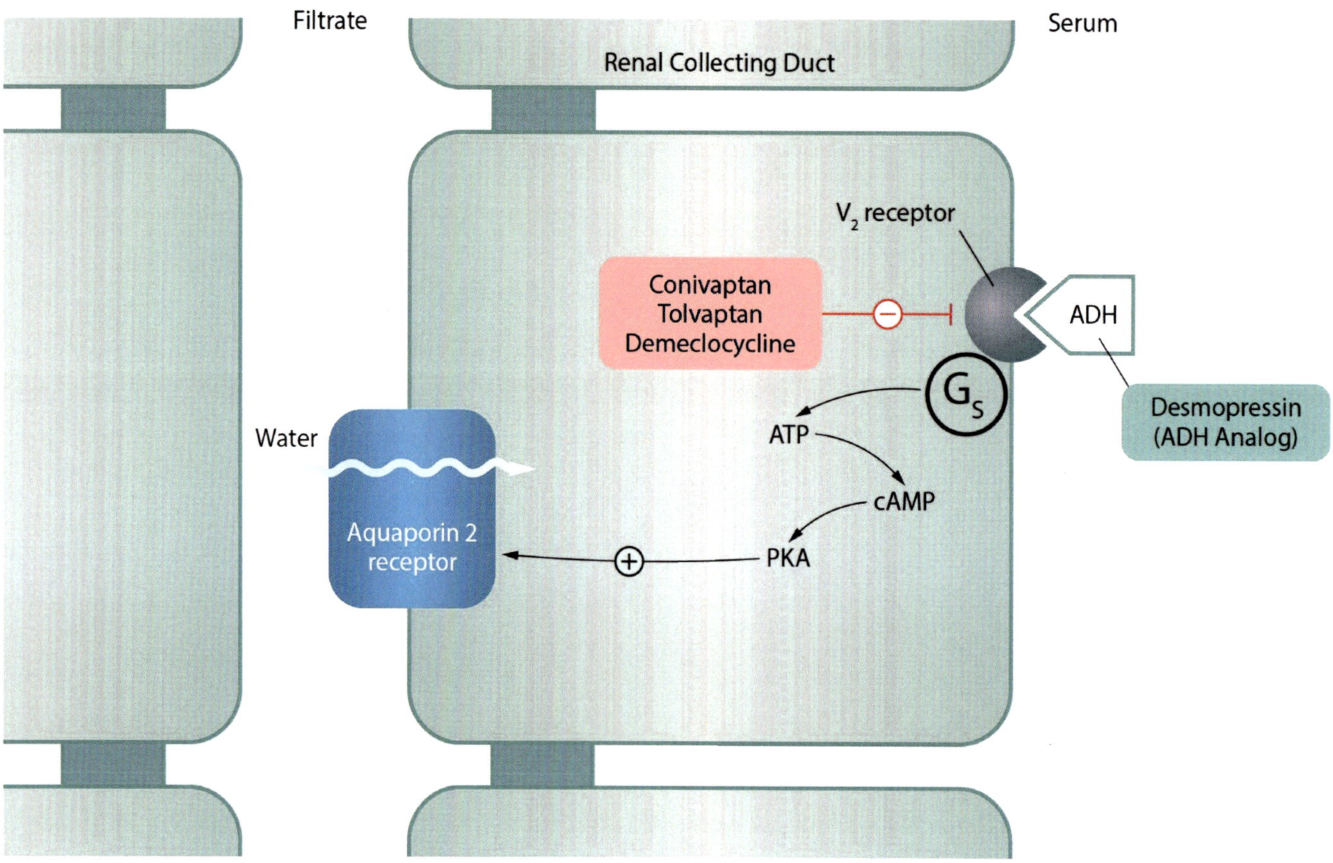

Figure 9.8.7 - Overview of ADH-Related Drugs

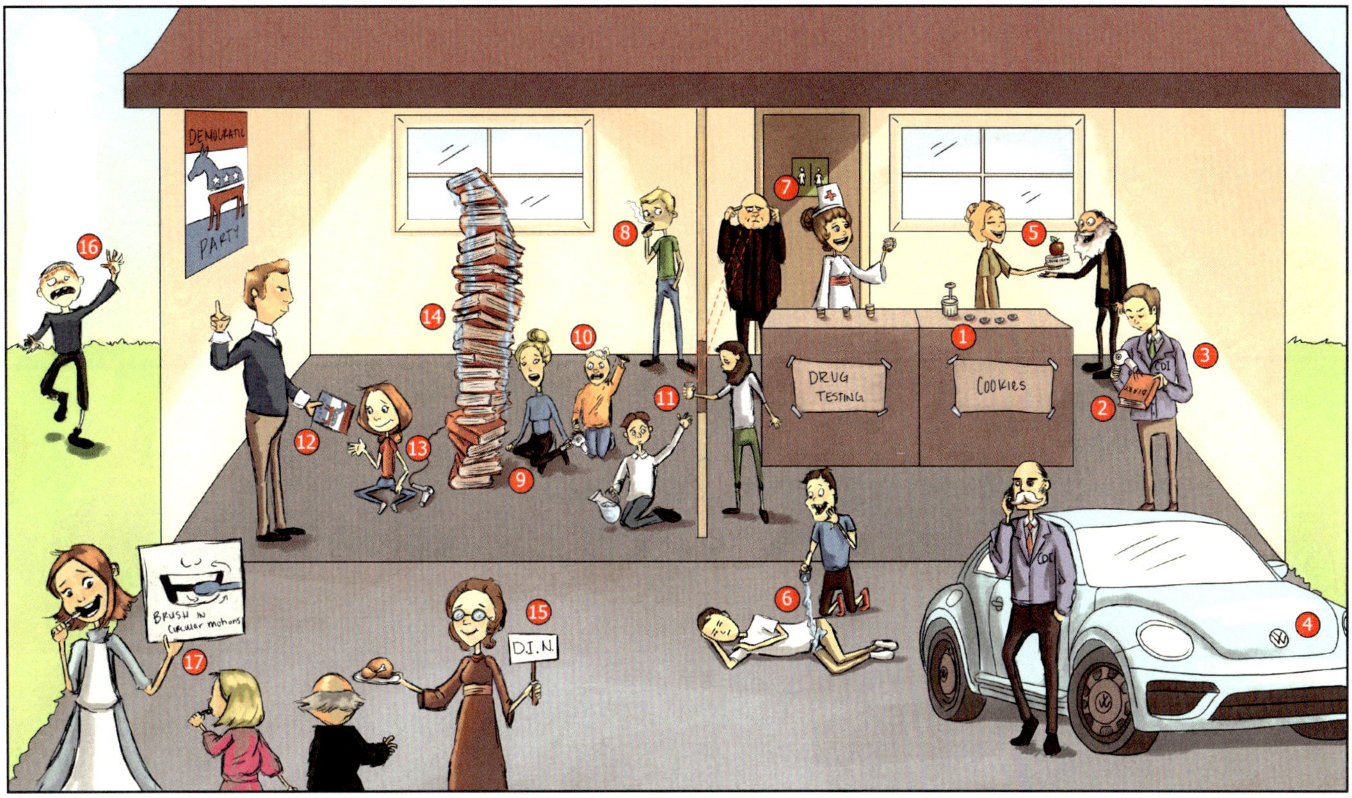

1. Dessert press: Desmopressin

2. Hair dryer used to dry off drug lord's diary: Desmopressin is an ADH analog

3. CDI on investigator's jacket: Desmopressin is used to treat central diabetes insipidus (CDI)

4. Volkswagen (VW): Desmopressin is used to treat von Willebrand disease

5. Philadelphia cream cheese cookie apple: Desmopressin is used to treat hemophilia A

6. Friend pours water on sleeping homeless guy's crotch: Desmopressin is used to treat sleep enuresis

7. Concentrating drug lord takes urine drug test: Desmopressin concentrates the urine

8. Drug lord's right-hand-man vaping: Conivaptan and tolvaptan

9. Large stack of soaked diaries being dried with a hairdryer: Conivaptan and tolvaptan are used for SIADH

10. Minion smashing hair dryer with two vape pens: Conivaptan and tolvaptan are ADH antagonists

11. Minion mixing water in drug lord's urine sample: Conivaptan and tolvaptan dilute the urine

12. Democratic candidate: Demeclocycline

13. Worker stops drying diaries to take democrat's pamphlet: Demeclocycline is an ADH antagonist

14. The large stack of diaries is between the democrat and vapers: Demeclocycline can be used to treat SIADH

15. "DIN" sign used to help democratic candidate: Democlycline can cause nephrogenic DI

16. Homeless man with skin blisters and burns from sun: Demeclocycline can cause photosensitivity

17. With of the democratic candidate teaching oral hygiene: Demeclocycline can cause abnormalities of bone and teeth

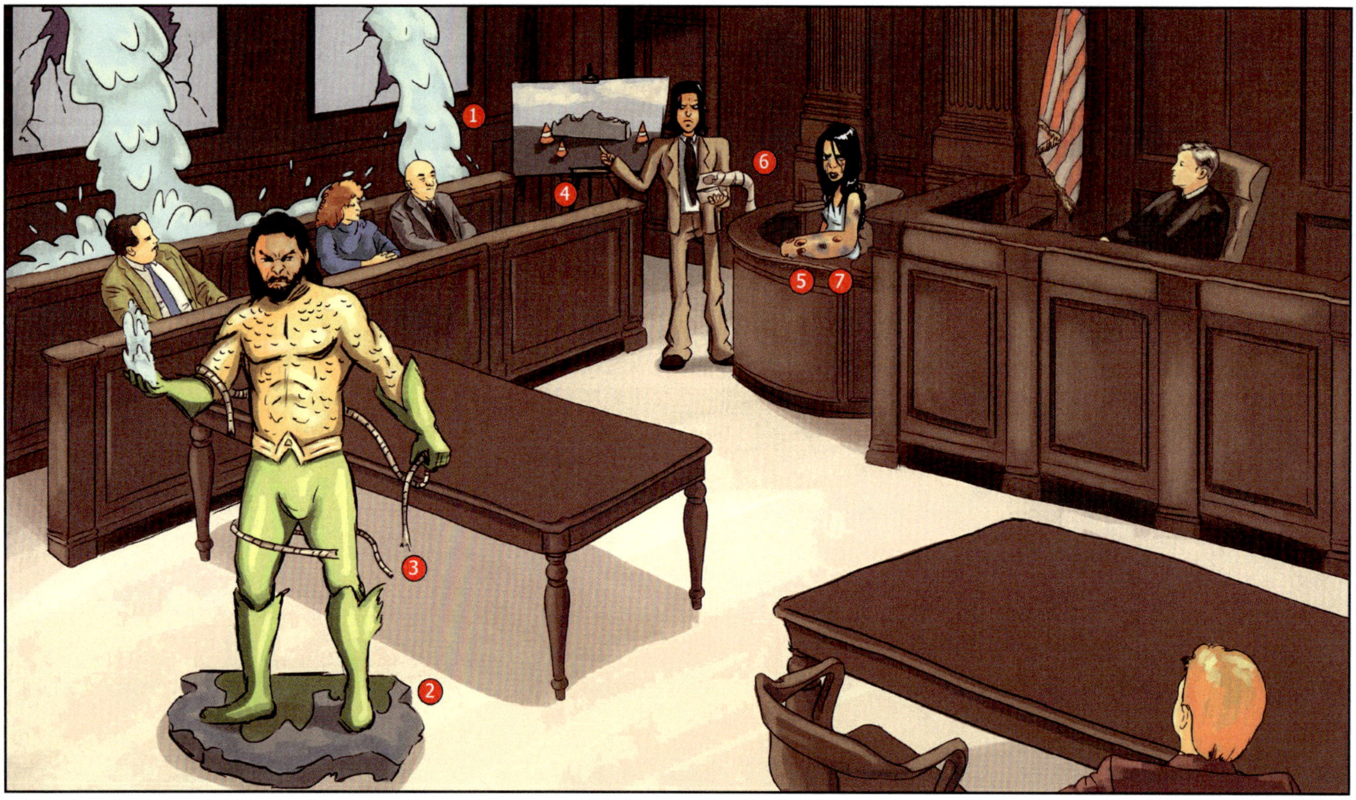

1. Aquaman flooding a courtroom: Fludrocortisone

2. Aquaman on old stone: Aldosterone analog

3. Few broken glued cords: Few glucocorticoid effects

4. Orange adrenal shaped barrier cones in picture: Mineralocorticoid replacement in 1° adrenal insufficiency

5. Witness with swollen arm: Can cause edema

6. Broken water pump held by prosecutor: Can cause exacerbation of heart failure

7. Bruised and wounded witness: Can cause hyperpigmentation

GASTROINTESTINAL PHARMACOLOGY

Section I - Histamine-2 (H₂) Blockers

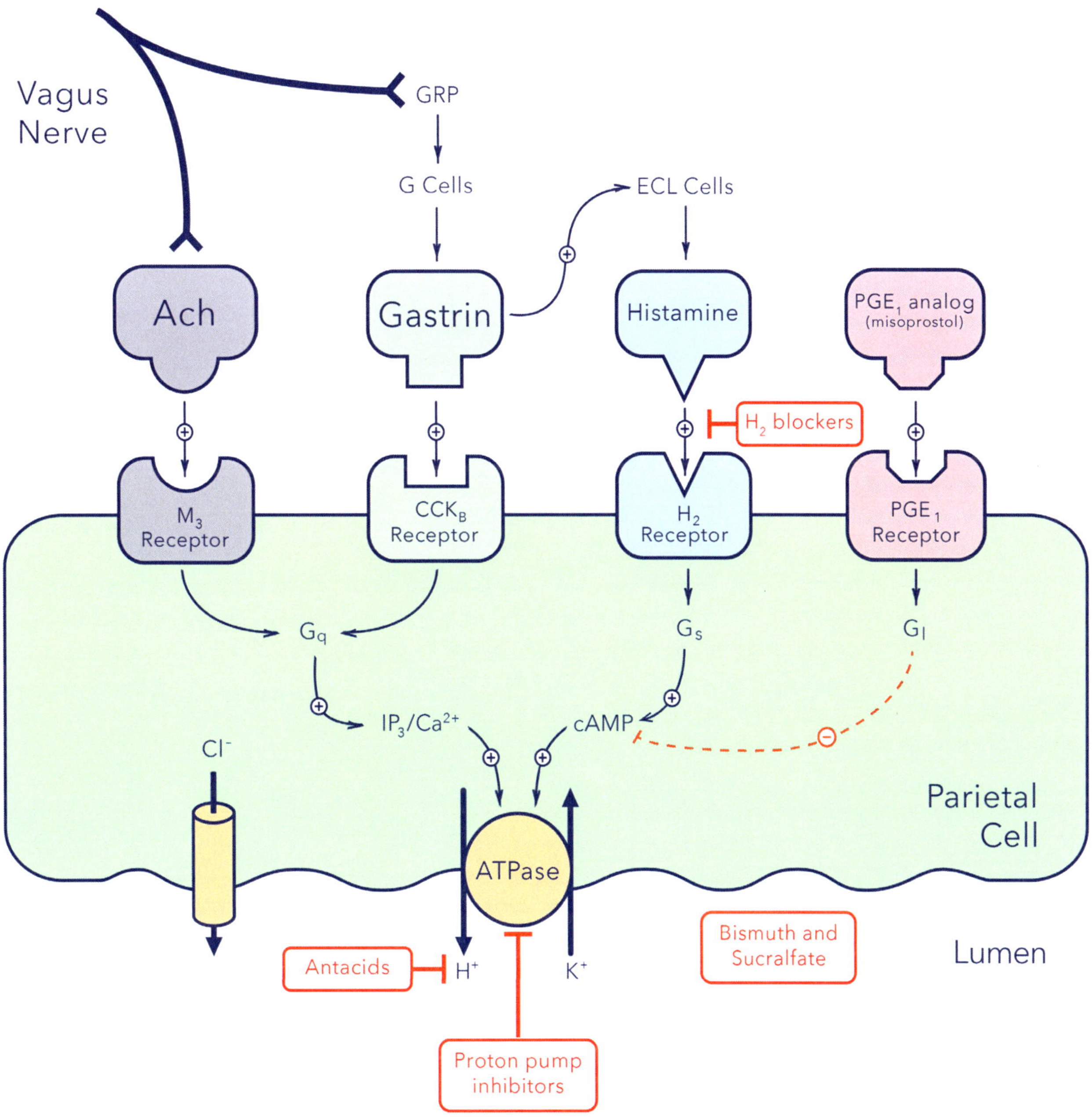

Figure 9.9.1 - Acid Suppression Therapies

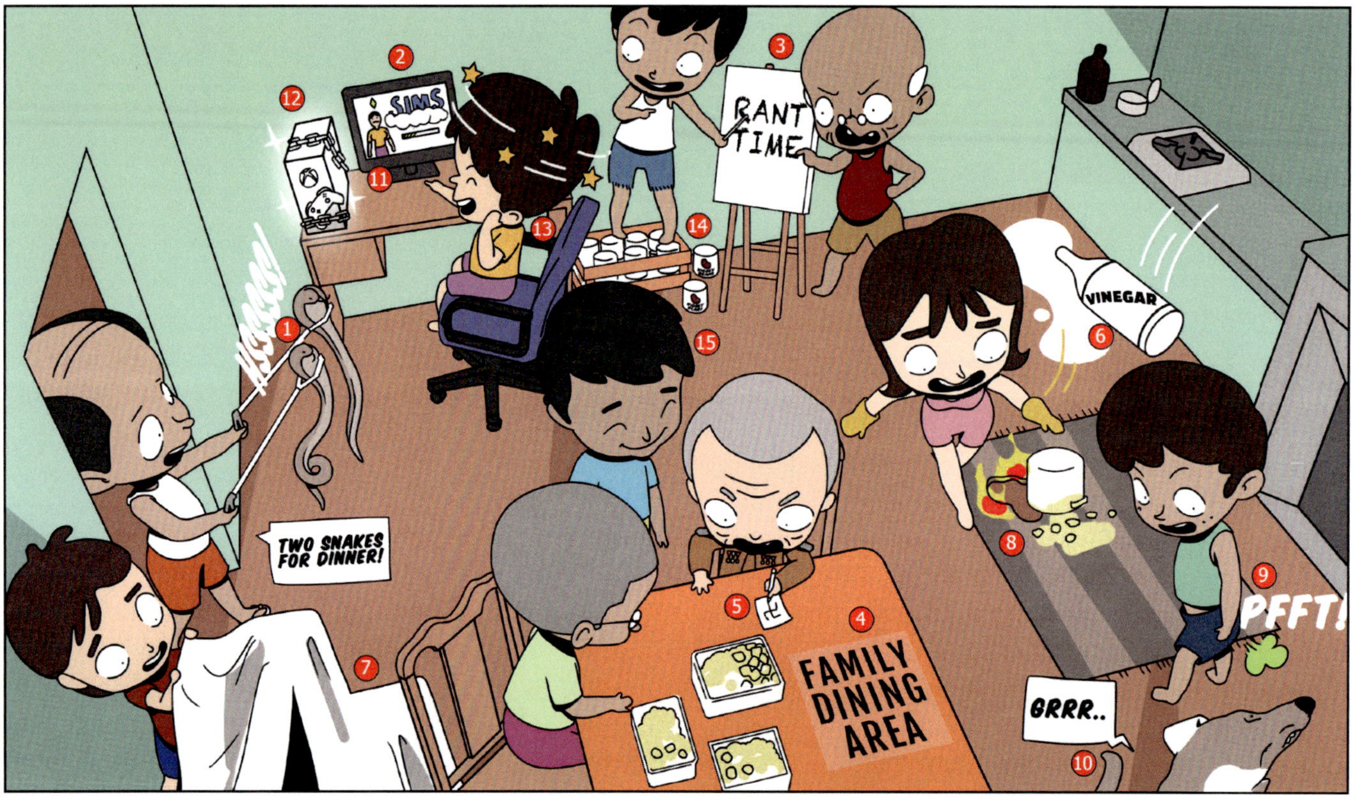

1. Two caught hissing snakes: Histamine-2 (H_2) blockers

2. SIMS game on computer: Cimetidine

3. "Rant Time" sign: Ranitidine

4. "Family dining area" table: Famotidine

5. Grandpa drawing Nazi swastika: Nizatidine

6. Bottle of acidic vinegar shattering: H2 blockers cause decreased H^+ secretion from parietal cells

7. Kid pretending to camp: Upregulate cAMP when stimulated

8. Ulcer-lookinghole in carpet: Use to treat peptic ulcers

9. Gassy teenager: Used to treat gastritis

10. Growling dog: Used to treat esophageal reflux (GERD)

11. Kid making androgynous SIMS avatar: Cimetidine can cause antidrogenic effects

12. Chained up chrome video console next to computer with SIMS: Cytochrome P-450 inhibitor

13. Kid confused that SIMS isn't loading: Can cause confusion, dizziness and headaches

14. Crate of tin cans of kidney beans between ranting grandpa and SIMS game: Cimetidine and ranitidine can decrease renal excretion of creatinine

15. Happy kid standing next to grandpa drawing Nazi swastika: Famotidine and nizatidine don't have any adverse effects

See Figure 9.9.1 - Acid Suppression Therapies (Gastrointestinal Pharmacology, Section 1, Page 170)

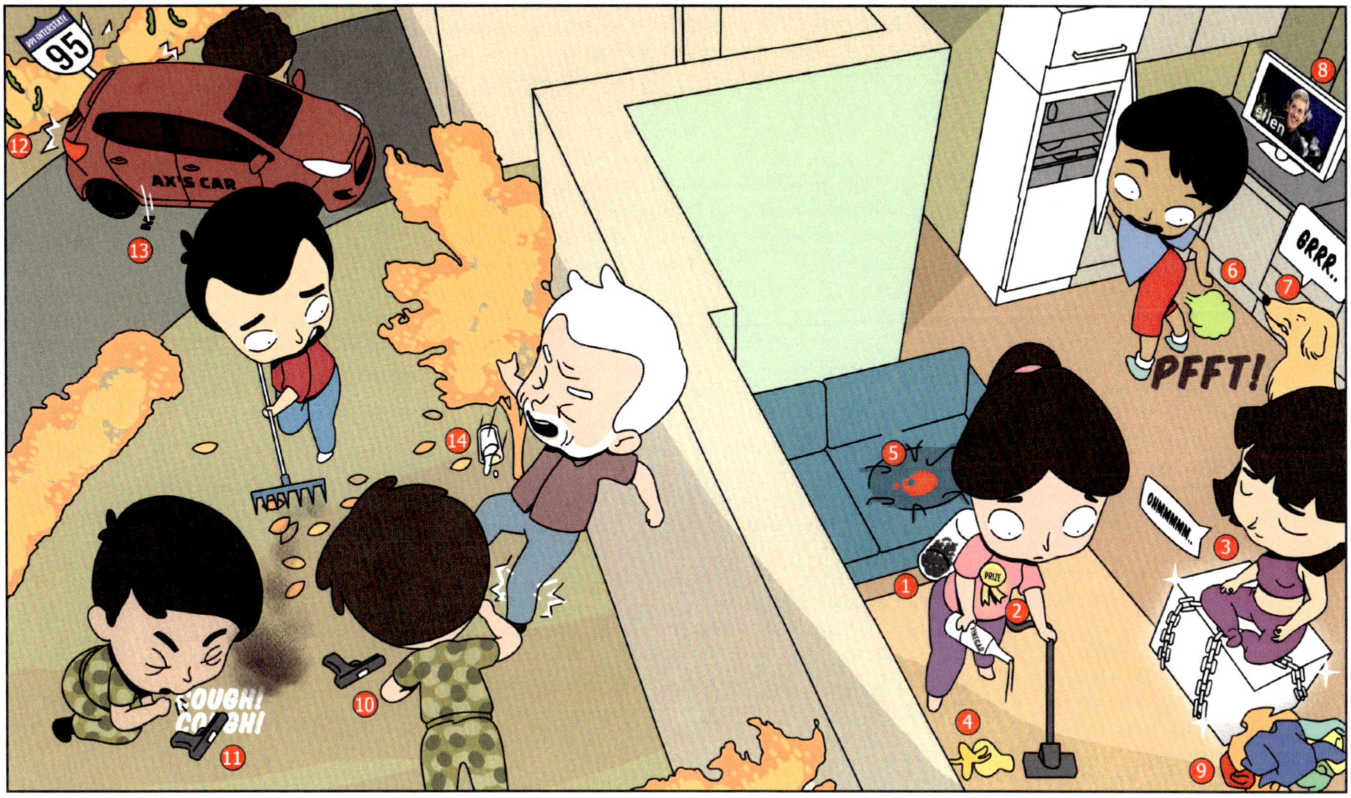

1. Vacuum pump: Proton pump inhibitors

2. Prize ribbon on woman's shirt: All drugs end with "prazole"

3. Meditating girl chanting "ohmmm" on chained chrome box: Omeprazole is a cytochrome P-450 inhibitor

4. Cleaning mom unable to remove banana stain with vinegar: Irreversibly inhibit H^+/K^+ ATPase in stomach parietal cells

5. Ulcer-like indent on couch: Used for peptic ulcer and stress ulcer prophylaxis

6. Gassy teenage boy: Used for gastritis

7. Dog growling, "Grr": Used for gastroesophageal reflux disease (GERD)

8. Ellen on TV in kitchen: Used to treat Zollinger-Ellison syndrome

9. Pile of dirty laundry on floor: Component of therapy for *H. pylori*

10. "Difficult" boot camp soldiers: Adverse effects include increased risk of *C. difficile* infection

11. Coughing soldier: Adverse effects include pneumonia

12. Car backing into interstate sign and destroying kidney bean plant: Adverse effects include acute interstitial nephritis

13. "M" magnet falling to the ground from a car: Adverse effects include ↓ serum Mg^{2+} with long term use

14. Grandpa breaking his leg and dropping milk: Adverse effects include decreased Ca^{2+} absorption and increased risk of fracture in elderly

See Figure 9.9.1 - Acid Suppression Therapies (Gastrointestinal Pharmacology, Section 1, Page 170)

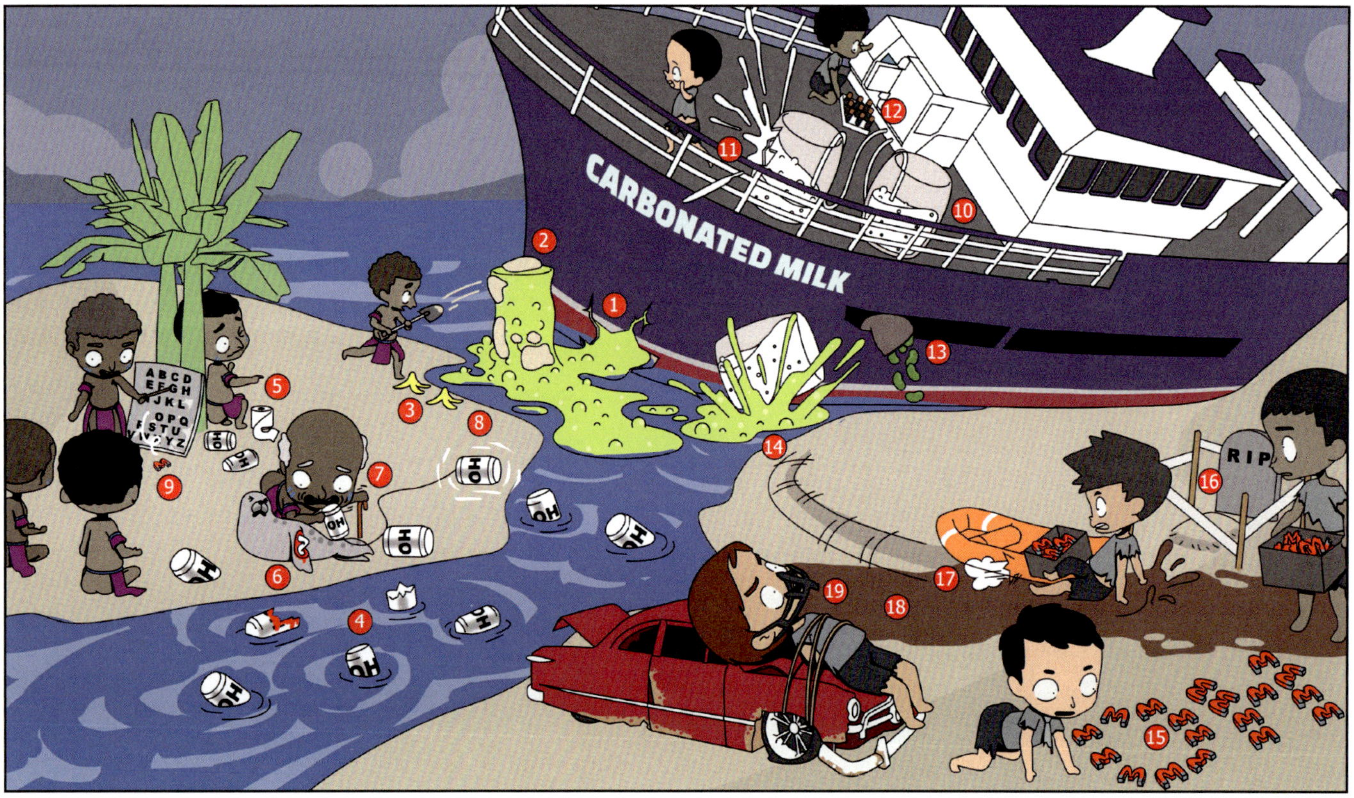

1. Boat crashing into island, spilling acid: Antacids work by neutralizing the H^+ in the stomach

2. Cylindrical shape covered in acid: Antacids can minimize the symptoms of reflux esophagitis (heartburn)

3. Two discarded banana peels: All antacids cause hypokalemia

4. Aluminum cans of "Oh" soda: Aluminum hydroxide

5. Constipated man that drank "OH" soda: Aluminum hydroxide can cause constipation

6. Seal's bone being mangled because of aluminum cans: Aluminum hydroxide can cause osteodystrophy

7. Frail, shaky old man with cane helping seal: Aluminum hydroxide can cause proximal muscle weakness

8. Shaking aluminum can of "OH" soda: Aluminum hydroxide can cause seizures

9. Fallen magnetic "M" on teacher's board: Aluminum hydroxide can cause low magnesium

10. Carbonated milk on boat deck: Calcium carbonate

11. Carbonated milk explosion: Calcium carbonate can cause hypercalcemia

12. Tray full of alkaline batteries about to go into the carbonated milk machine: Calcium carbonate can cause metabolic alkalosis and kidney disease

13. Spoiled kidney beans spilling from boat: Calcium carbonate can cause kidney damage

14. Barrel of carbonated milk falling into acid-filled water: Calcium carbonate can cause rebound increase in stomach acid production

15. "OH" spelled in "M" magnets: Magnesium hydroxide

16. Shipmate holding "M" magnets, avoiding grave: Avoid magnesium hydroxide in myasthenia gravis patients

17. Raft popping and flying towards magnets: Magnesium hydroxide can cause hypotension

18. Box of magnets falling into muddy intel: Magnesium hydroxide can cause diarrhea

19. Criminal tied and arrested on car: Magnesium hydroxide can cause cardiac arrest

See Figure 9.9.1 - Acid Suppression Therapies (Gastrointestinal Pharmacology, Section 1, Page 170)

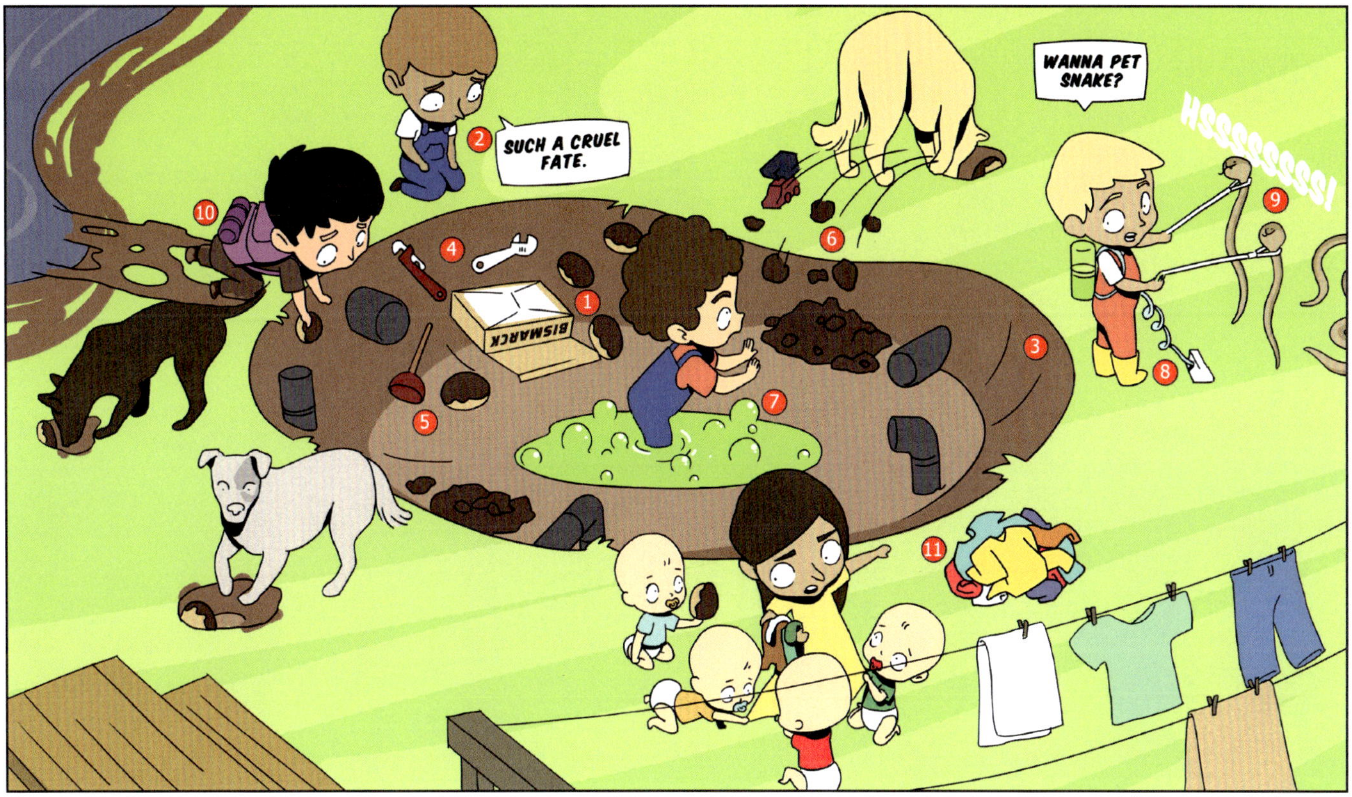

1. Bismarck donut box: Bismuth

2. "Such a cruel fate." speech bubble from plumber: Sucralfate

3. Ulcer shaped hole: Use bismuth and sucralfate to increase ulcer healing

4. Donut box and cruel fate textbox are located inside hole: Bismuth and sucralfate bind to the base of the peptic ulcer

5. Donuts and tools covering the ground in hole: Bismuth and sucralfate form a protective coat around the ulcer

6. Digging dog propelling glued toy cars and dirt into hole: Protective coat allows HOC_3- to reestablish an appropriate pH to the mucosa

7. Plumber with no donuts, cruel fate, standing in acid in hole: Sucralfate needs an acidic environment to work

8. Plumber not wanting to work with weird vacuum pump: Don't administer sucralfate with PPIs (sucralfate needs an acidic environment)

9. Two hissing snakes held by guy with weird vacuum: Don't administer sucralfate with histamine-2 blockers (sucralfate needs an acidic environment)

10. Traveler crawling out of muddy river and grabbing donut: Use bismuth for traveler's diarrhea

11. Mom hanging pile of laundry with quadruplets: Use bismuth to treat H. pylori as part of quadruple therapy

See Figure 9.9.1 - Acid Suppression Therapies (Gastrointestinal Pharmacology, Section 1, Page 170)

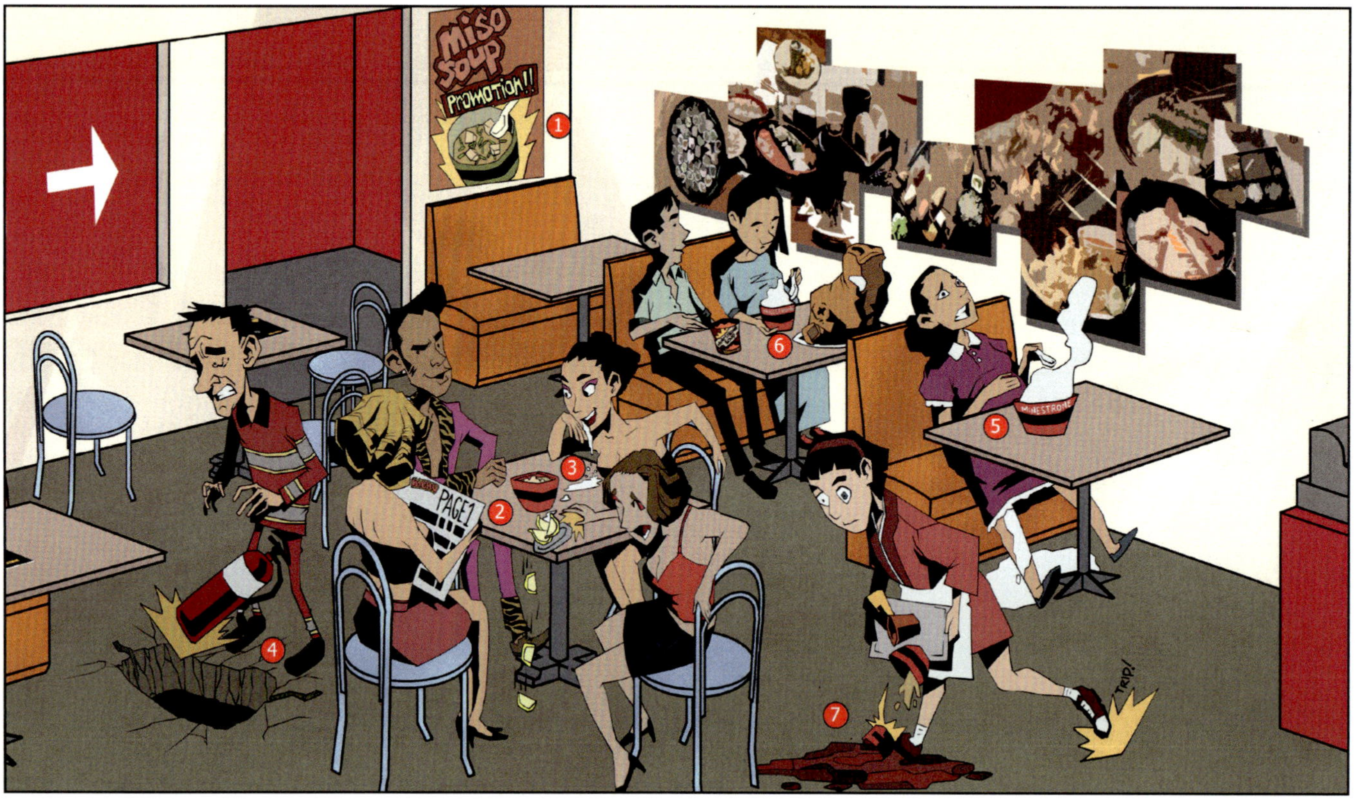

1. "Miso Promotion" advertisement: Misoprostol

2. Page 1 of the menu: PGE 1 analog

3. One prostitute drooling, causing the other prostitue to drop lemons on the floor: Decreases acid production by increasing gastric mucous production

4. Dropped fire extinguisher creates ulcer hole in ground: Used to prevent NSAID-induced peptic ulcers

5. Pregnant woman going into labor from miso soup: Used for labor induction (use cautiously in women of child-bearing age)

6. Pregnant lady with a boar's head and friend with minestrone soup, eating together: May be combined with mifepristone to perform medical abortion

7. Teriyaki sauce spilled onto ground: Can cause diarrhea

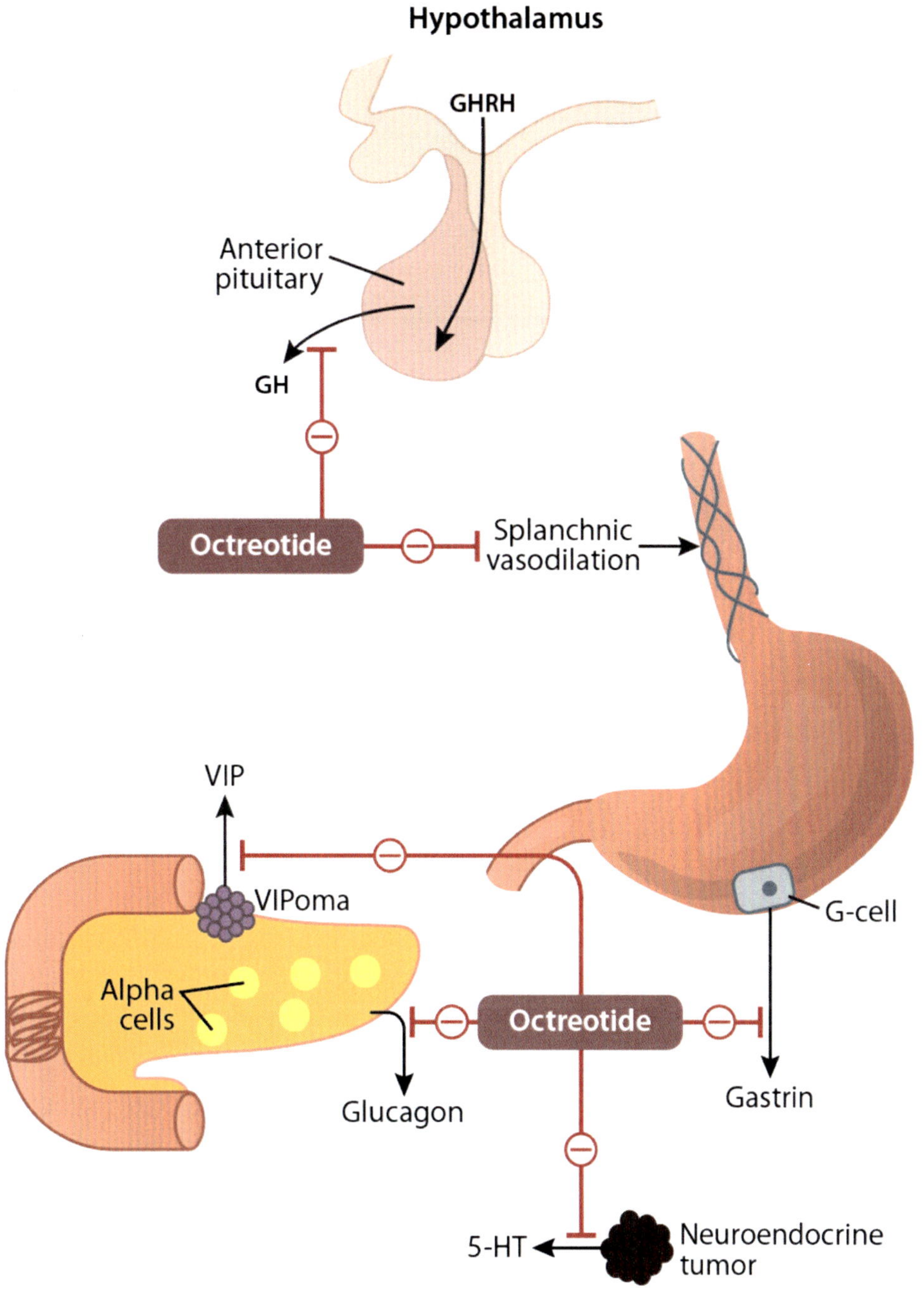

Figure 9.9.2 - Mechanism of Octreotide

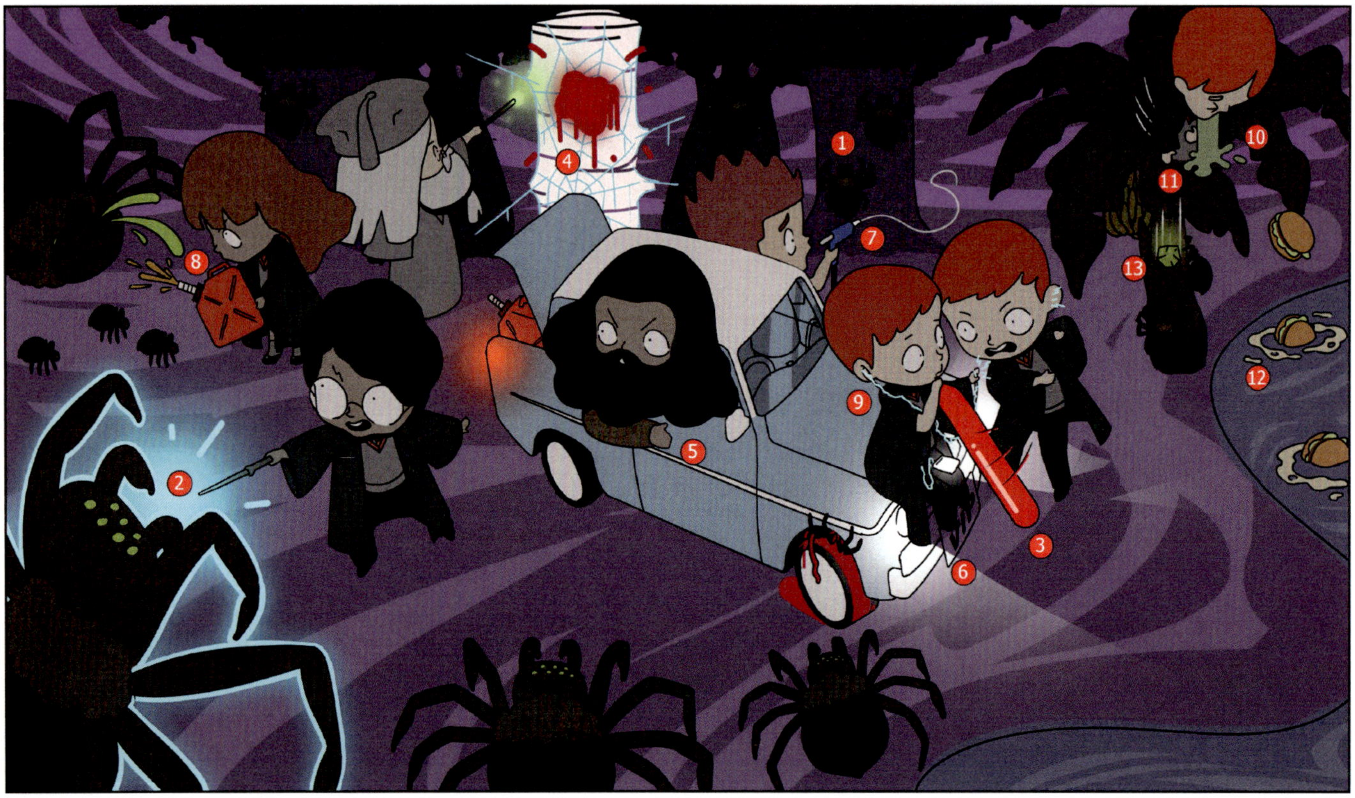

1. Spiders with eight legs on trees: Octreotide

2. Harry casting stasis spell on spider: Long lasting somatostatin analog

3. Twin with a long, red balloon smacked by other twin on top of car with squished spider guts: Inhibits the secretion of various splanchnic vasodilatory hormones

4. Cylindrical, blue webs that held a spider that bursted into a cloud of blood: Can be used for acute variceal bleeds

5. Giant not fitting in car: Used for acromegaly

6. "VIP" license plate on car: Used to treat VIPomas

7. Shooting glue gun by terrified kid: Used for glucagonomas

8. Spider spitting acid at girl with gas can: Can be used to treat gastrinomas

9. Twins sharing tunes and shock of electricity on car: Can be used to treat carcinoid tumors

10. Boy in banana tree vomiting: Adverse effects include nausea

11. Boy in tree holding belly in pain: Adverse effects include cramps

12. Fatty burgers in water: Adverse effects include steatorrhea

13. Green stone falling out of banana tree: Increases the risk of choleithiasis due to CCK inhibition

Section VII - Sulfasalazine

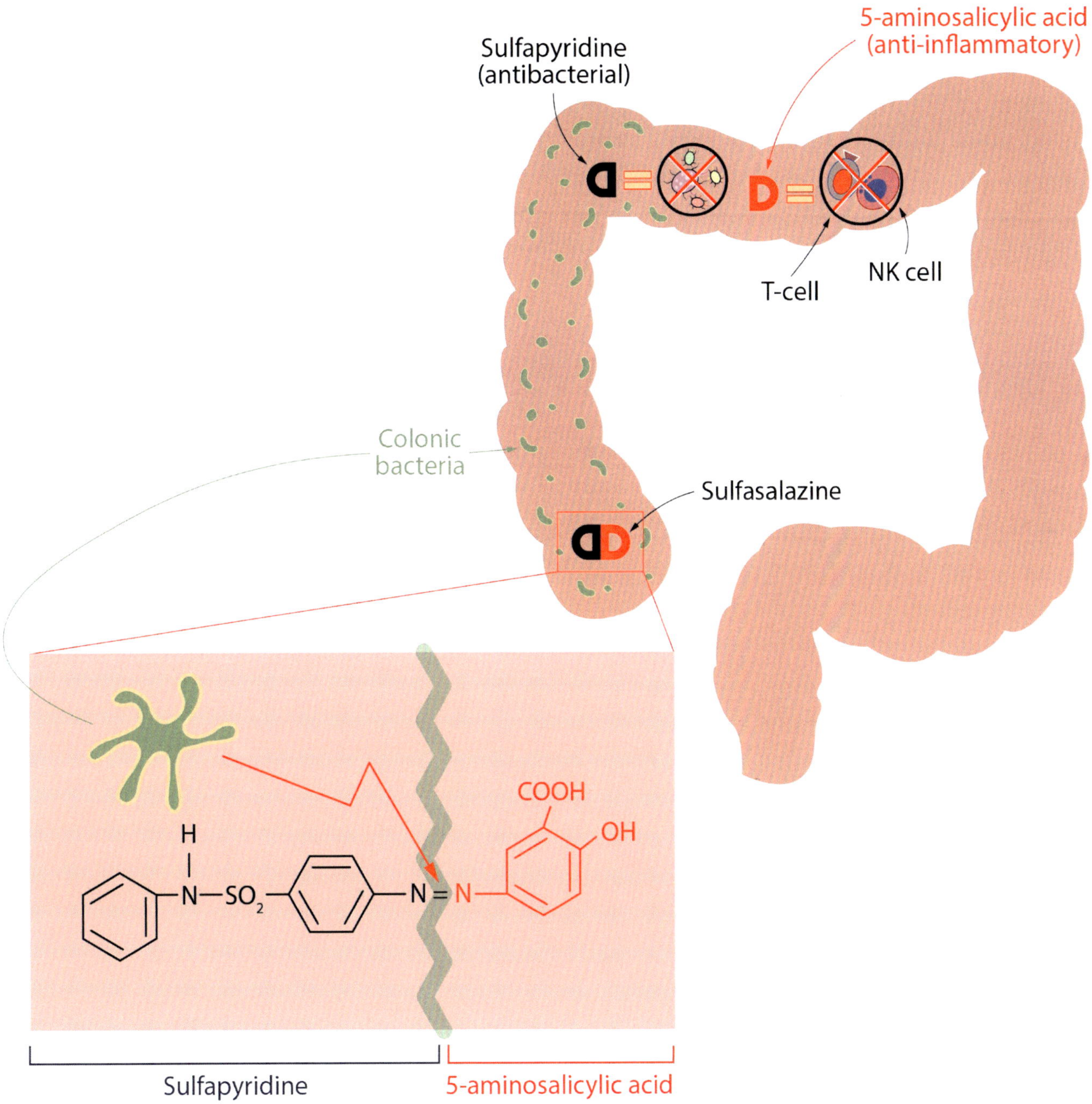

Figure 9.9.3 - Sulfasalazine Mechanism

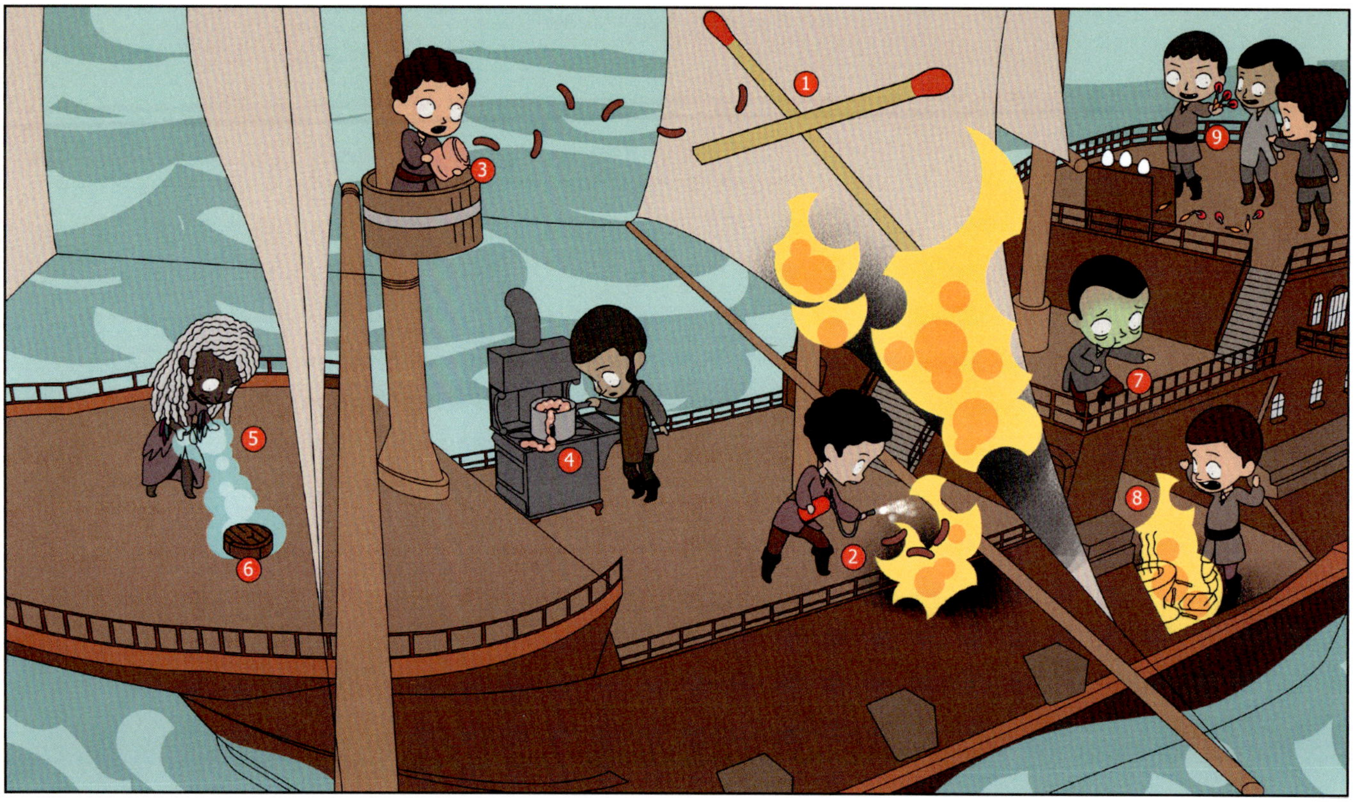

1. Crossed sulfur matches on sail: Sulfasalazine

2. Pirate extinguishing fire and discarding old hot dogs: Sulfasalazine is a combination (antibiotic) of sulfapyridine and 5-aminosalicylic acid (anti-inflammation)

3. Pirate holding hofstra-shaped bucket, tossing bacteria-shaped hot dogs towards the sulfur match sail: Activated by colonic bacteria

4. Cook cooking ulcerated intestines: Used for ulcerative colitis

5. Old magical crone: Use for Crohn's disease

6. Roomba: Use for rheumatoid arthritis

7. Seasick pirate: Can cause malaise and nausea

8. Sulfur matches lighting the bathroom on fire: Can cause sulfonamide toxicity

9. Pirates throwing few darts at eggs: Can cause reversible oligospermia

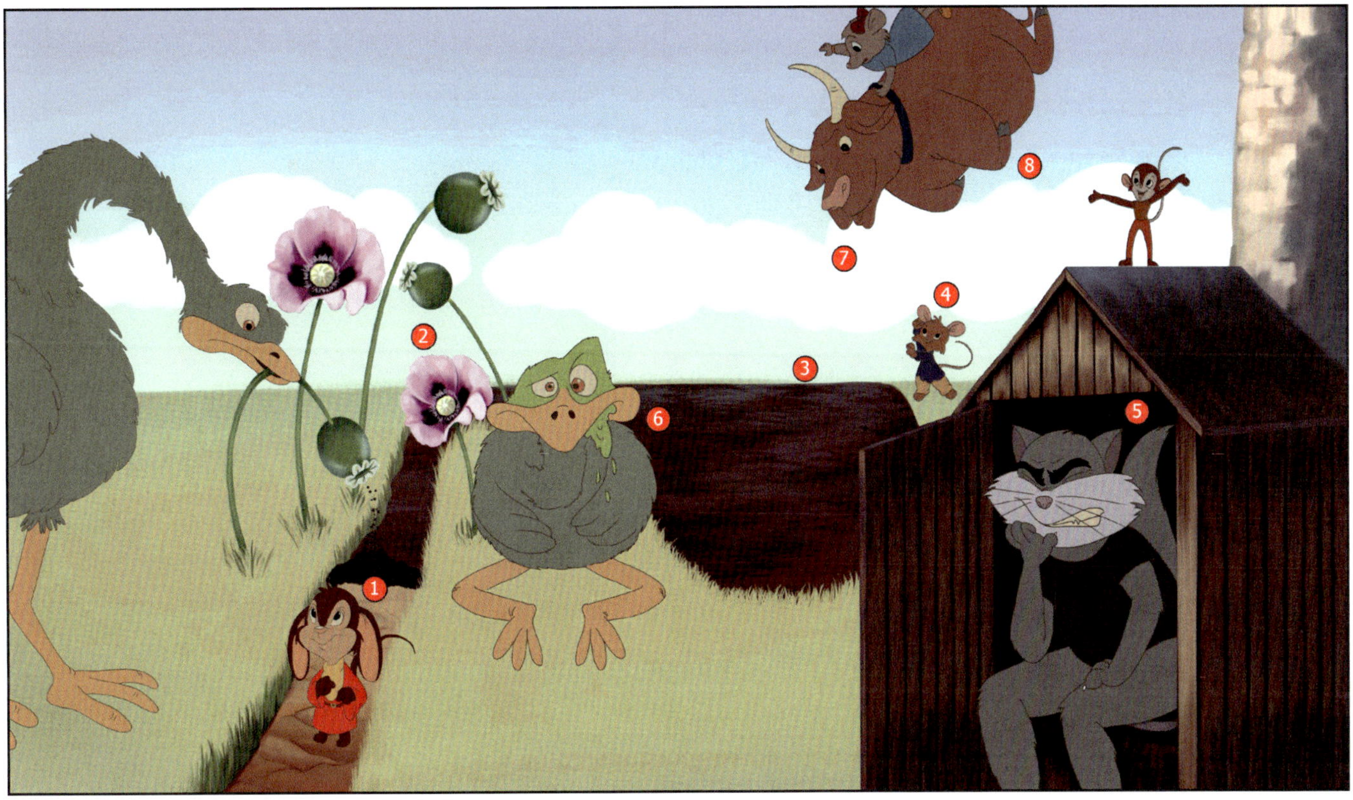

1. Lop-eared mouse: Loperamide

2. Emu shaking seeds out of poppy plant creating a dam: Slows gut motility by binding to mu (μ) opioid receptors in the gut

3. Muddy river: Use for diarrhea symptom control

4. Lop-eared mouse in blue shirt unable to reach above clouds: Loperamide does not easily cross the blood-brain barrier → low opioid addictive potential

5. Constipated cat on portable toilet: Can cause constipation

6. Vomiting emu: Can cause nausea

7. Lop-eared mouse riding driving ox: Diphenoxylate is much like loperamide

8. Diving ox above clouds: Diphenoxylate does not cross the blood-brain barrier → opioid addictive potential

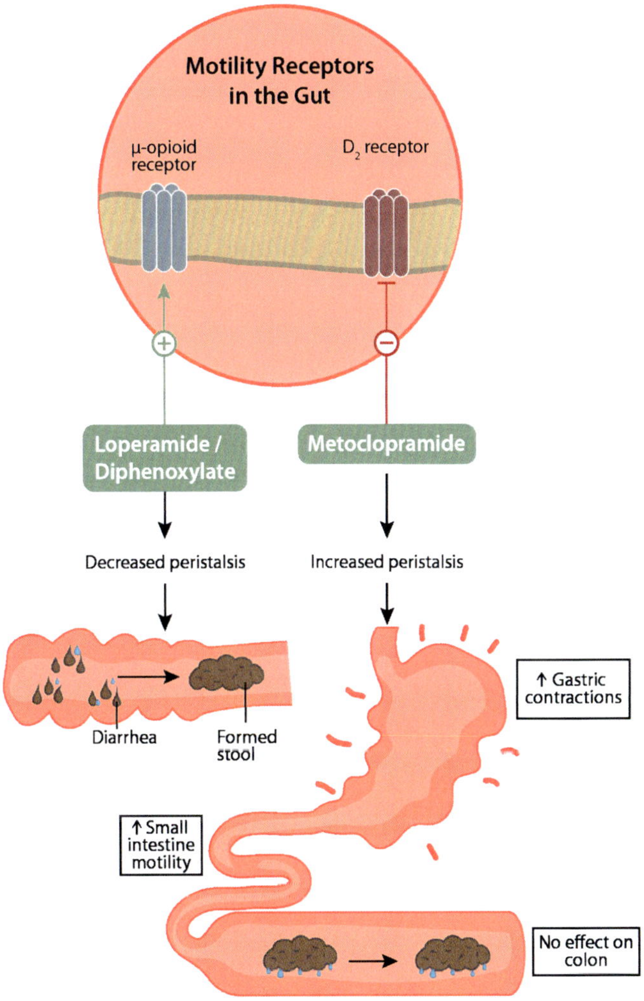

Figure 9.9.4 - Pharmacologic Effects on GI Motility

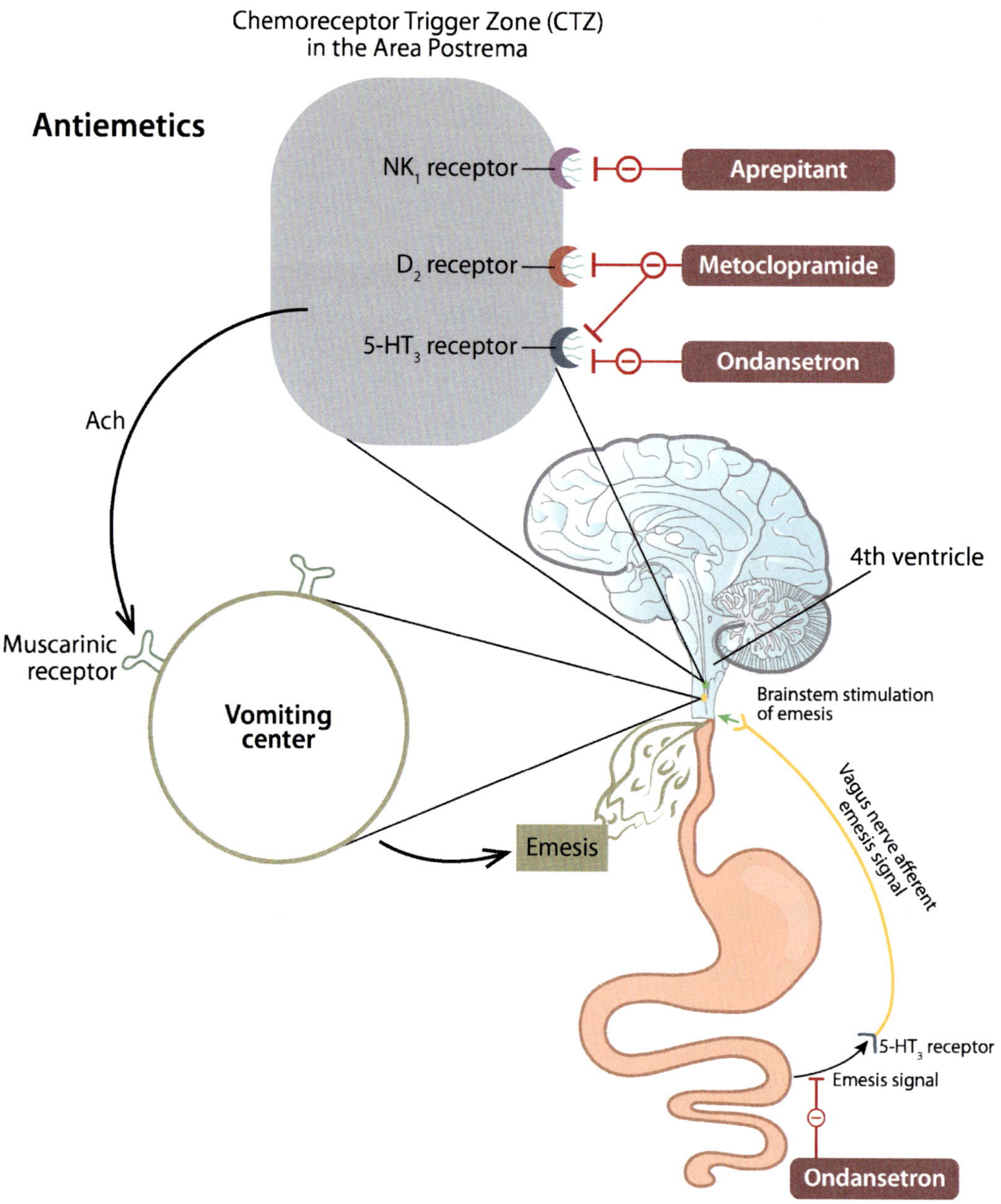

Figure 9.9.5 - Antiemetic Mechanisms

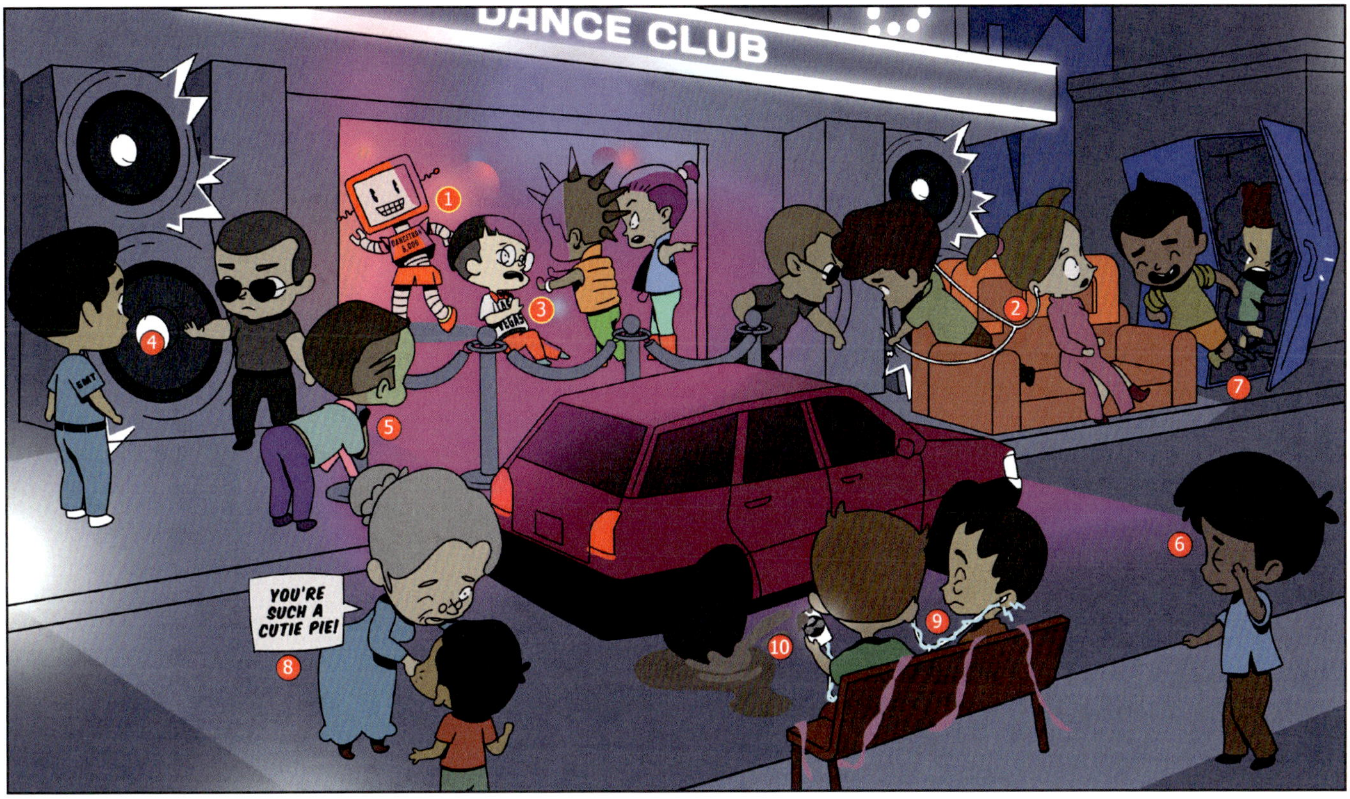

1. Dancetron 5000 robot dancing in club: Ondansetron

2. Couple outside of club trying to share a tune on "3"-shaped couch, but bouncer punches man's plug away: 5-HT_3 antagonist

3. Man in "Las Vegas" shirt being pushed to the ground in club: Decreases vagal stimulation

4. Anti-medic bouncer preventing EMT from joining club: Powerful central-acting antiemetic

5. Nauseous man with pink cancer ribbon with green face, but not puking outside of club: Controls vomiting in patients undergoing cancer chemotherapy

6. Man with headache outside of club: Can cause headaches

7. Constipated man in porta potty: Can cause constipation

8. Grandma stretching kid's cheeks saying, "You're such a cutie pie!": Can cause QT interval prolongation

9. Two men sharing a tune getting shocked by headphones on bench outside of club: Can cause serotonin syndrome

10. Two men sharing a tune sitting on bench with streamers on it: Can cause Torsades de pointes

See Figure 9.9.4 - Pharmacologic Effects on GI Motility (Gastrointestinal Pharmacology, Section 8, Page 180)

See Figure 9.9.5 - Antiemetic Mechanisms (Gastrointestinal Pharmacology, Section 9, Page 181)

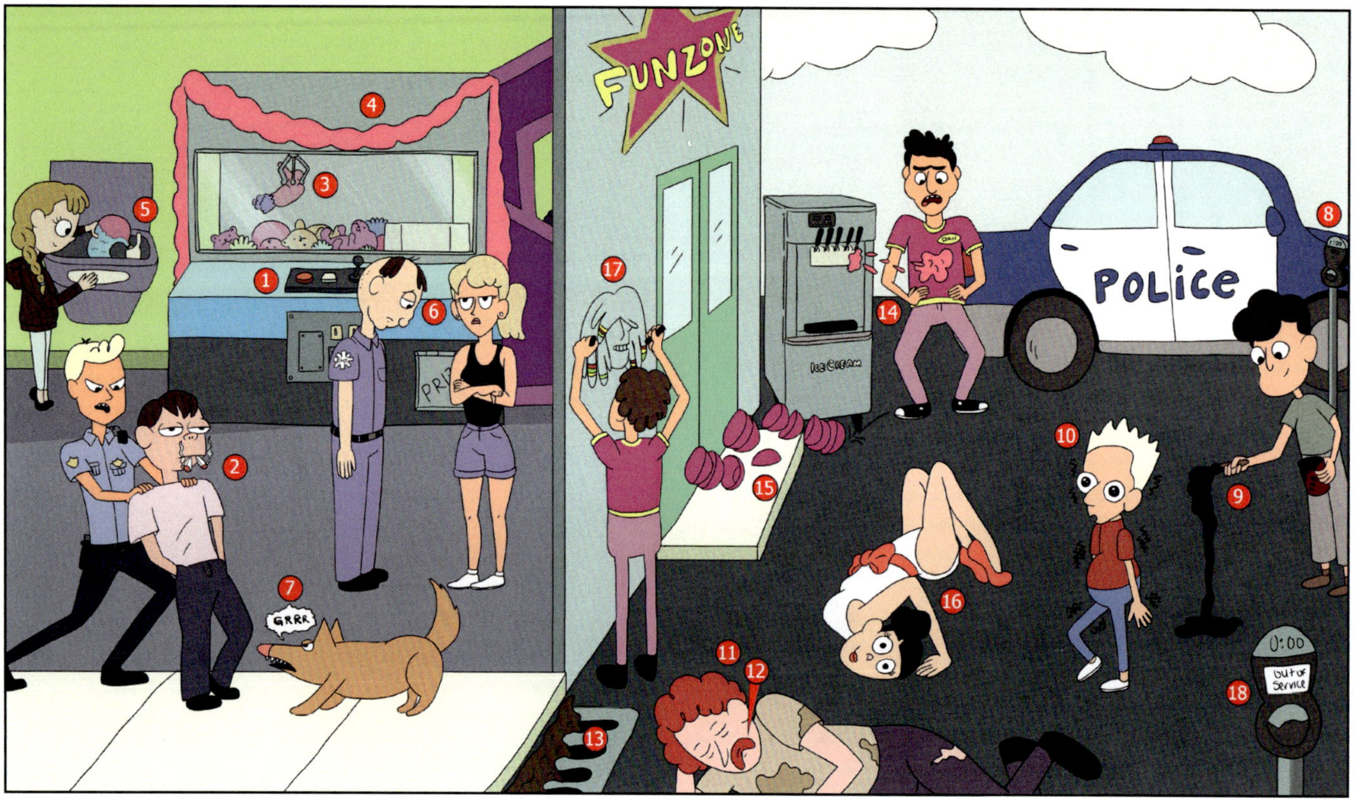

1. Metal claw machine: Metoclopramide

2. Dope smoking teenager pushed out of arcade: Dopamine (D_2) receptor antagonist

3. Claw with stomach plush with seams torn: Causes increased resting tone, contractility, LES tone, motility and gastric emptying

4. Colon-shaped tubing around claw machine: Does not influence colon transport time

5. Girl filling up stomach water balloon to full capacity: Used for diabetic gastroparesis and postoperative gastroparesis

6. Medic being rejected by anti-medic girl: Antiemetic

7. Dog growling who won't move: Used for persistent GERD

8. Police car parked by meter: Can cause parkinsonian effects

9. Person filling asphalt cracks with tar: Can cause tardive dyskinesia

10. Jittery kid outside of store: Can cause restlessness

11. Homeless man sleeping in parking lot: Can cause drowsiness and fatigue

12. Sad homeless man with painted frown: Can use depression

13. Brown water: Can cause diarrhea

14. Ice cream machine spraying ice cream on guy's chest: Can cause hyperprolactinemia which can cause galactorrhea

15. Small bowls blocking the door: Metoclopramide is contraindicated in patients with small bowel obstruction

16. Contortionist: Can cause acute dystonia

17. Employee drawing Bob Marley with two pieces of chalk: Can cause drug interaction with digoxin and diabetic agents

18. Out of service parking meter: Contraindicated in Parkinson disease

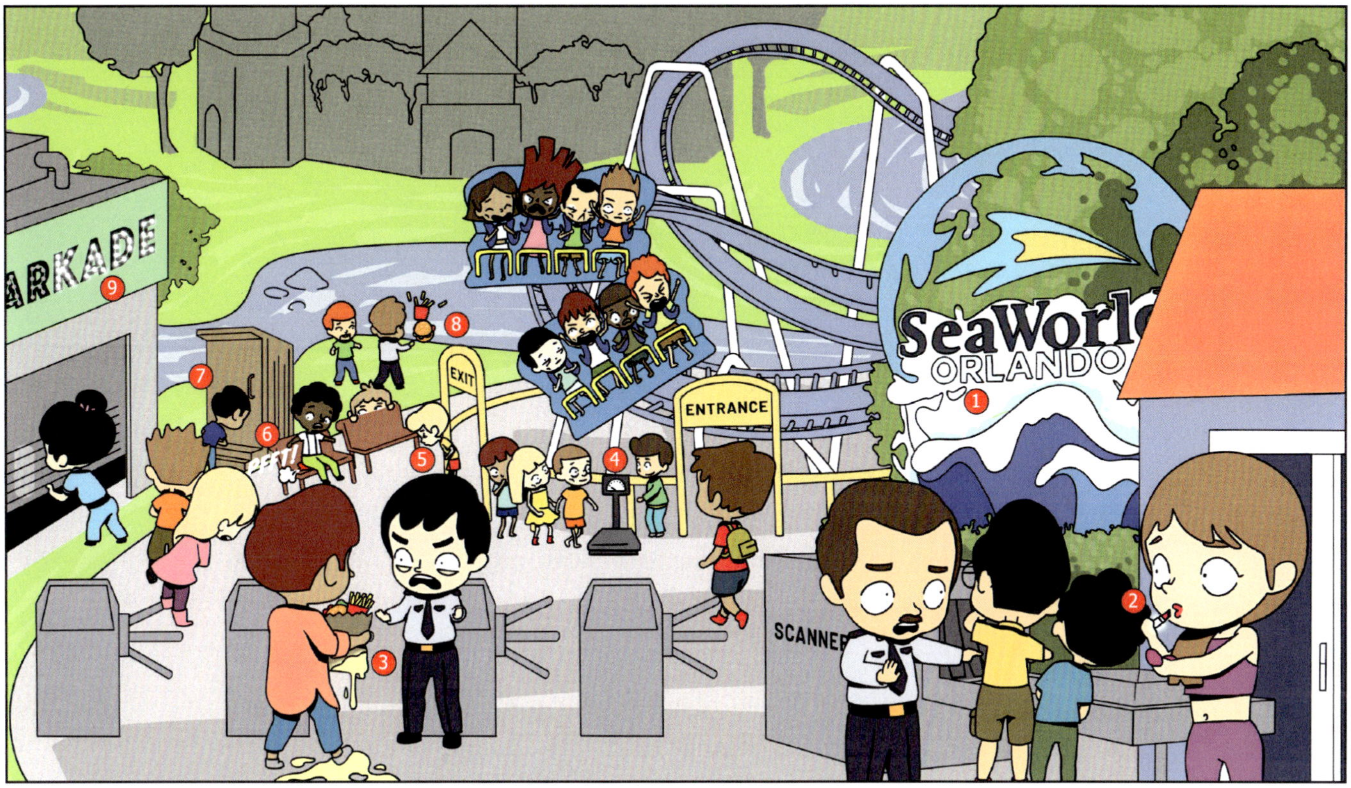

1. SeaWorld Orlando sign: Orlistat

2. Girl being rejected from entering with lipstick: Inhibits gastric and pancreatic lipase

3. Fat and grease falling down from fast food that will not be permitted to the park: Decreases the breakdown and absorption of dietary fats

4. Scale measuring skinny little people by ride: Use for weight loss

5. Little guy with hurt stomach near exit sign: May cause abdominal pain

6. Kid farting on bench: May cause flatulence

7. People in line for the portable toilet: May cause frequent bowel movements

8. Greasy food thrown in river: May cause steatorrhea

9. "Arkade" lights with KADE lit: May result in malabsorption of fat soluble vitamins (K, A, D, E)

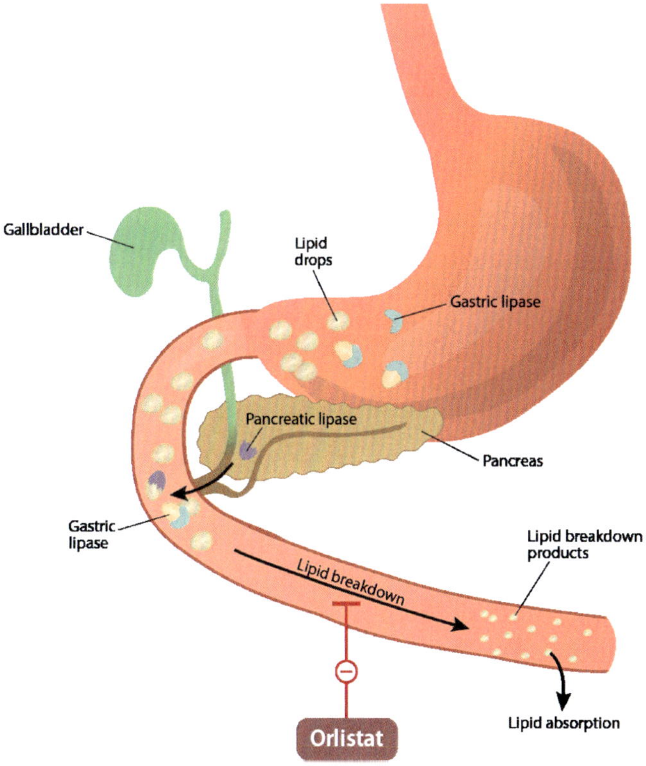

Figure 9.9.6 - Effects of Orlistat on GI Absorption

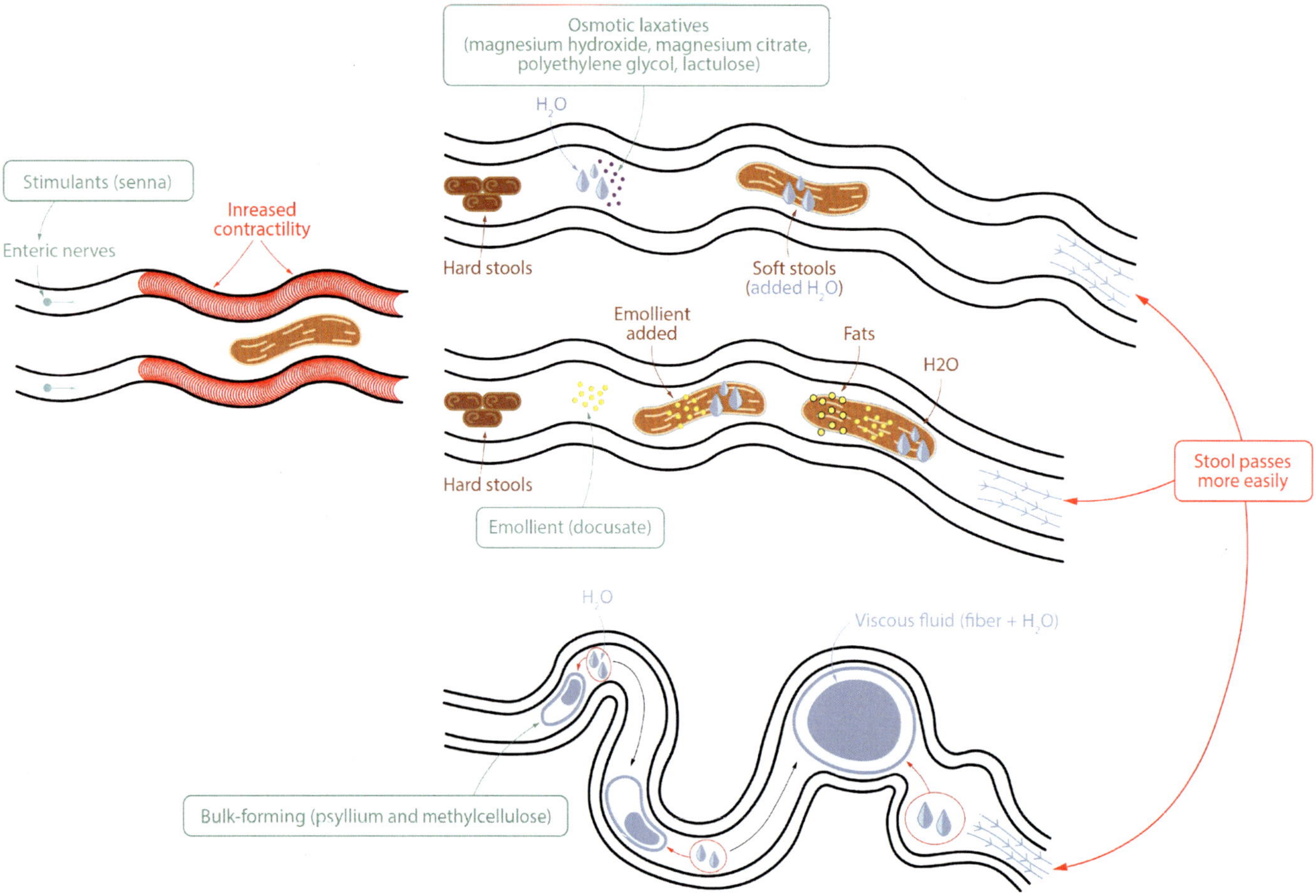

Figure 9.9.7 - Laxatives Overview

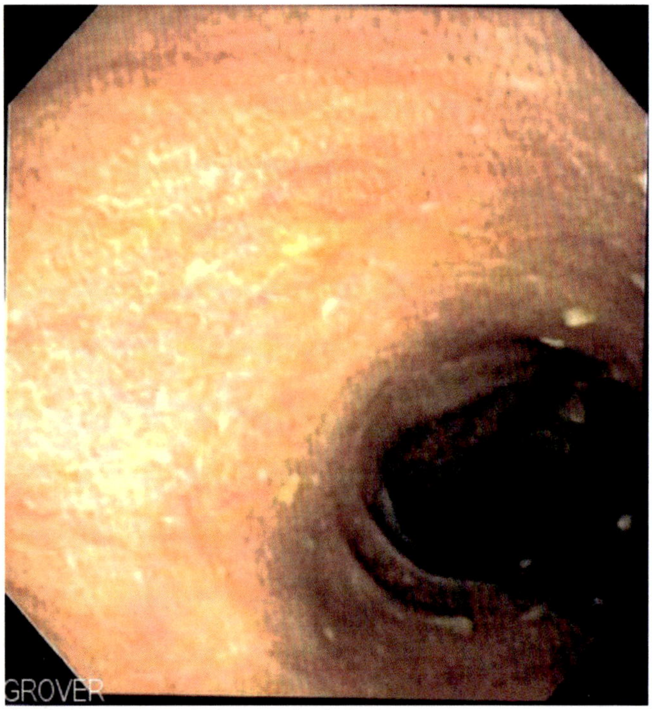

Figure 9.9.8 - Melanosis Coli

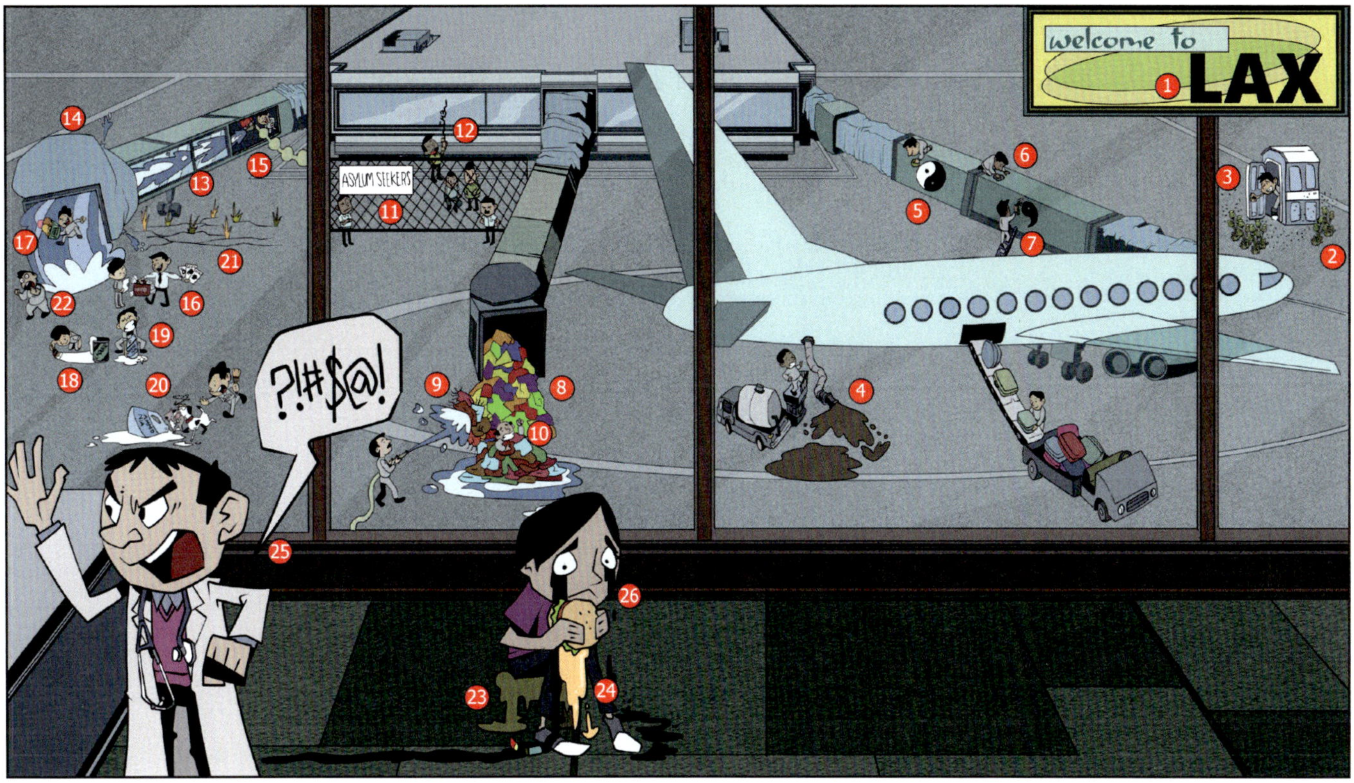

1. "Welcome to LAX" sign at airport: Laxatives

2. Opium plants and seeds blowing off LAX sign: Used for patients on opiates

3. Constipated guy in porta potty near opioid seeds: Use for patients with constipation

4. Brown waste all of tarmac: Can cause diarrhea

5. Zen sign on jet bridge: Seena

6. Zen jet bridge scrubbed clean by men from outside: Stimulant laxatives (e.g. senna) work by stimulating enteric nerves, causing the colon to contract and pass stool

7. Partial finished yin yang symbol on jet bridge: Can cause melanosis coli

8. Large extrusion of clothes coming out of the jet bridge and being sprayed with water: Bulk-forming laxatives draw water into the stool, making it easier to pass

9. Loose fibers on clothing that is being blasted with water: Bulk-formers are soluble fibers

10. Pile of clothes swelling with water: Bulk-formers can cause bloating

11. "Asylum Seekers" sign: Psyllium is a bulk-forming laxative

12. Long antenna attached to cell phone: Methylcellulose is a bulk-forming laxative

13. Workers spraying inside of the jet bridge: Osmotic laxatives draw more water into the GI lumen

14. Water pressure causing flexible opening at the end of the jet bridge to bulge: By bringing more water into the lumen, it's easier for stool to pass

15. Worker holding firehose and "M" magnets inside jet bridge: Magnesium (e.g. magnesium citrate or magnesium hydroxide) is an osmotic laxative

16. Insurance salesman selling different types of insurance: Polyethylene glycol is an osmotic laxative

17. Man flying out of slide holding sorbet: Sorbitol is an osmotic laxative

18. Man applying a thick coat of lacquer: Lactulose is an osmotic laxative

19. Glued bottle of ammonia to ground by lacquer: Lactulose binds to ammonia

20. Liver-spotted dog sniffed out ammonia in stuffed elephant toy: Lactulose can also treat hepatic encephalopathy which is caused by high NH_2 in the blood

21. Dehydrated weeds: Osmotic laxatives can cause dehydration

22. Bulimic man: Osmotic laxatives can be abused by bulimics

23. Emo kid sitting on melted soft stool: Emollients (aka, stool softener)

24. Grease falling out of burger held by emo kid: Emollients help add water and fat into the stool

25. Cursing doctor: Docusate is an emollient

26. Mascara on and running around emo kid: Emollients can cause diarrhea

See Figure 9.9.5 - Antiemetic Mechanisms (Gastrointestinal Pharmacology, Section 9, Page 181)

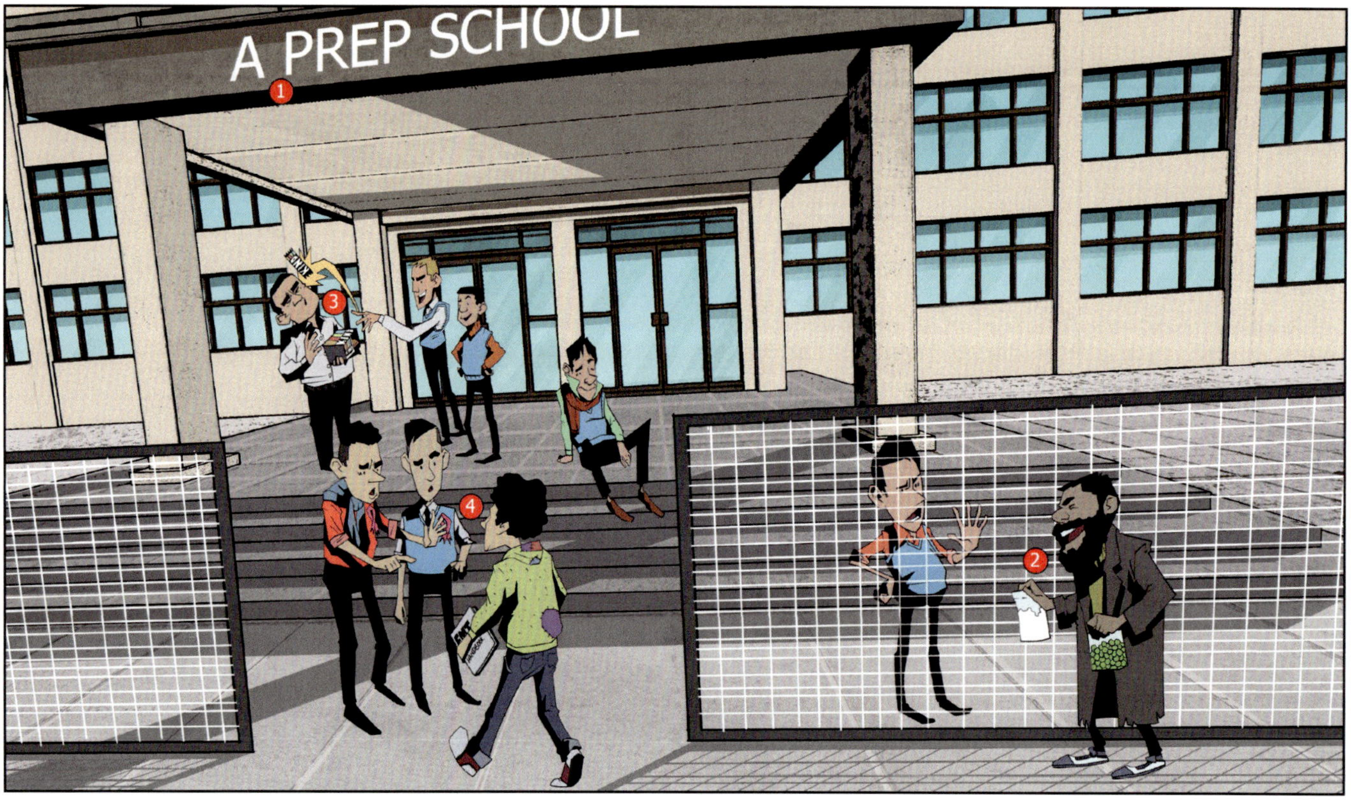

1. Prep school and student with scarf around his neck: Aprepitant

2. Guy selling peas and fake substance as drugs and prep student rejecting him: Substance P antagonist

3. Kids throwing Kind bars at salesman's head: Blocks NK_1 (neurokinin-1) receptors in the brain

4. Kids with pink cancer ribbons sending EMT aspired kid away: Antiemetic for chemotherapy-induced nausea and vomiting

HEMATOLOGY & ONCOLOGY PHARMACOLOGY

Section 1 - Heparin, LMWHs, and Fondaparinux

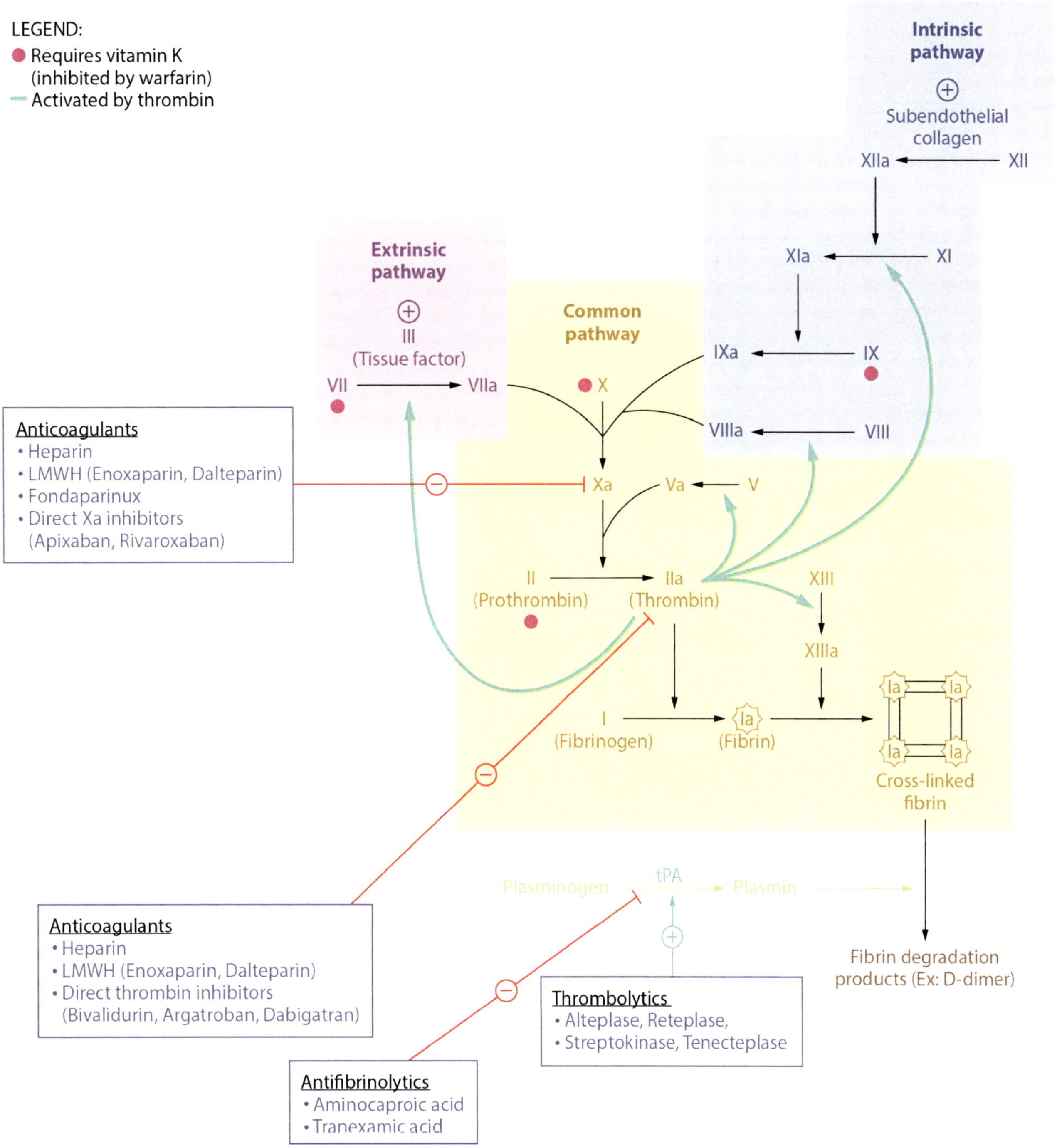

Figure 9.10.1 - Mechanism of Anticoagulants that Interact with Secondary Hemostasis

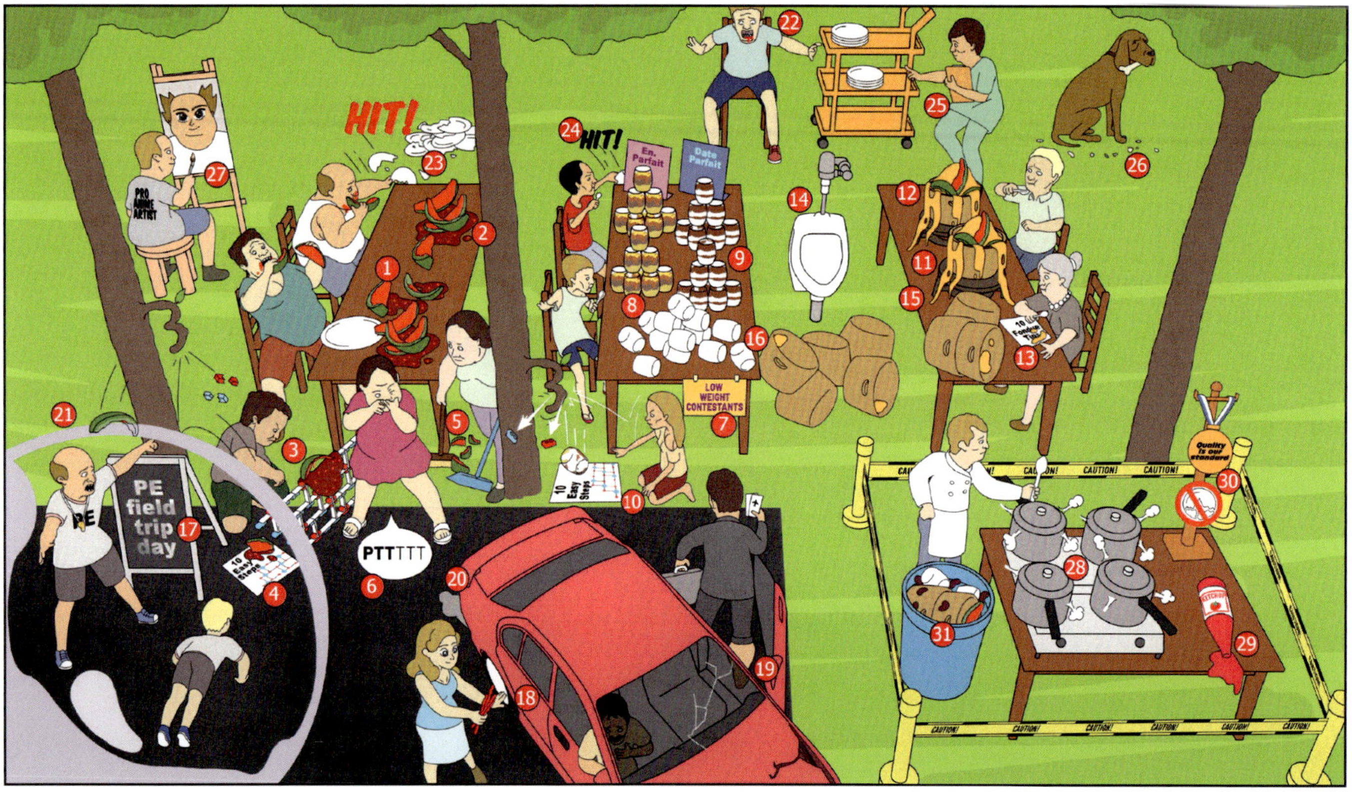

1. Fat, high weight people in eating competition next to heaps of rinds: Heparin

2. Red, runny watermelon remnants on rinds: Heparin is an anticoagulant

3. Boy throwing and breaking two Lego blocks against tree branch shaped like a "3" after heap of rind falls onto Lego set of cross-linked structure: Heparin activates antithrombin III → lower action of factor IIa (thrombin)

4. Heap of rinds falling onto "10 easy steps" Lego instructions: Heparin activates antithrombin III → lower action of factor Xa

5. Boy's mom quickly clearing away half of rinds on grass: Short half-life

6. Girl making "PTTTTT" sounds like pretend gun: Monitor PTT

7. "Low weight contestants" sign: Low molecular weight heparins (LMWHs)

8. "En. Parfaits" sign next to enchilada parfait: Enoxaparin

9. "Date parfait" sign next to date parfait: Dalteparin

10. Dad throwing parfait container that bounces off "3" shaped tree branch and falls onto girl's "10 easy steps" instructions without breaking: LMWHs bind to antithrombin III in a way that causes inhibition of factor Xa (minimal factor IIa inhibition) → decreased fibrin meshwork

11. Fondue and nuts: Fondaparinux

12. Fondue pot filled with heaps of rinds and synthetic Velveeta cheese: Fondaparinux is a synthetic heparin

13. Lady spilling fondue cheese on "10 fondue tips" instruction paper: Fondaparinux inhibits factor Xa only

14. Open-air urinal between skinny contestant table and fancy fondue table: LMWHs and fondaparinux are renally excreted

15. Lots of food available at skinny and fondue tables versus less food at fat table: LMWHs and fondaparinux have better bioavailability than unfractionated (regular heparin)

16. Large piles of discarded parfaits and fondue pots on skilly fondue tables versus small heaps and rinds on fat table: LMWHs and fondaparinux have a longer half life (2-4x heparin)

17. Kid immediately stating to do push-ups during PE: Use heparins for immediate anticoagulation for pulmonary embolism (PE)

18. Teenager in red car and cute girl offering him licorice: Use heparins for acute coronary syndrome

19. Parent with swollen leg getting out of car after long trip: Use heparin for deep venous thrombosis (DVT)

20. Car's clogged exhaust pipe: Use heparins for myocardial infarction (M)

21. Clear plastic dome protecting spectators from messy heaps of rinds: Use heparins during pregnancy since heparins do not cross placenta

22. Contestant with bleeding gums after eating too quickly: Heparins can cause bleeding

23. Fat man breaking plates near heaps of rinds and making loud "HIT!" sound: Heparins can cause thrombocytopenia (i.e. HIT, heparin-induced thrombocytopenia)

24. Skinny guy trying to break the plate, but only making small cracks and weak "HIT!" sound compared to fat people: LMWHs are less likely to cause HIT

25. Medical personnel monitoring number of plates consumed: Heparin treatment requires regular monitoring of platelet count, especially for unfractionated heparin, even before starting treatment

26. Dog eating bone and scattering bone fragments: Heparins can cause osteoporosis

27. Artist in "pro anime artist" shirt painting reverse of actual situation at fat table: Rapidly reverse heparin-induced bleeding using protamine sulfate

28. Four pressure cookers to prepare contest food inside yellow caution tape: Heparins are contraindicated in severe uncontrolled hypertension

29. Spilled ketchup bottle behind yellow caution tape: Heparins are contraindicated with an uncontrolled active bleed

30. Sign banning serving food on broken plates: Heparins are contraindicated with a history of HIT

31. Trash cans of parfaits and fondue mixed with kidney beans behind yellow caution tape: LMWH and fondaparinux are contraindicated in kidney disease because these are renally excreted

See Figure 9.10.1- Mechanism of Anticoagulants that Interact with Secondary Hemostasis (Hem/Onc Pharmacology, Section 1, Page 188)

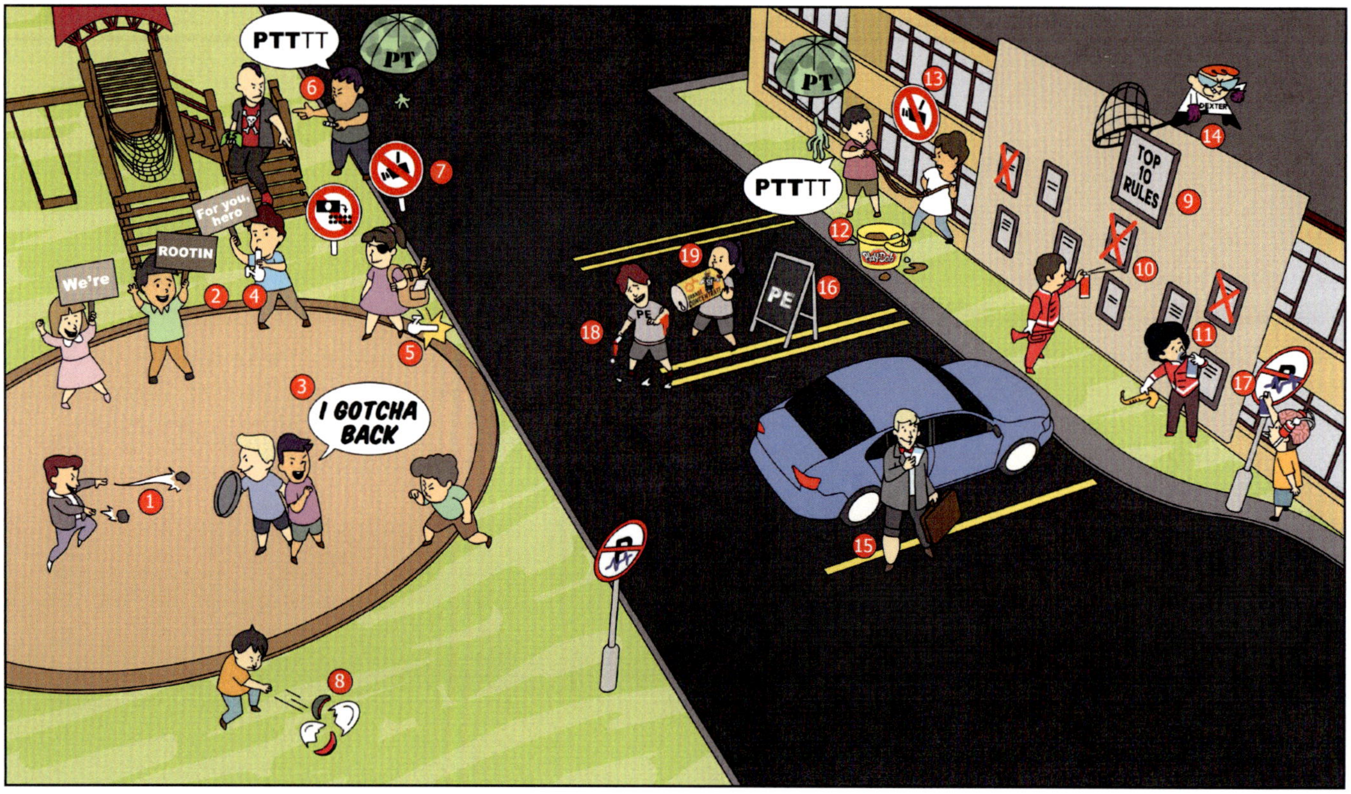

1. Bullying victim blocking two thrown rocks with bin lid: Direct thrombin (IIa) inhibitors

2. Kids rooting for victim as hero of story: Some drug names have the suffix "rudin" (e.g. desirudin and bivalirudin)

3. Kid saying "I gotcha back" to victim: Argatroban (IV administration)

4. Kid dabbing weed through mouth: Dabigatran (oral administration)

5. Girl with eyepatch and rucksack knocking over smoking kid's extra bong: Reverse dabigatran with idarucizumab

6. Paratrooper toy making "PTT" sound next to weed dealer with "no charge" sign: Direct thrombin (IIa) inhibitors do not change PT or PTT

7. "No surveillance" sign next to dealer: Direct thrombin (IIa) inhibitors do not require lab monitoring

8. Kid breaking plate with heap of fruit rinds on grassy section of playground: Use direct thrombin (IIa) inhibitors in the treatment of heparin-induced thrombocytopenia (HIT)

9. "Top ten rules" poster on wall of school to prevent kids from misbehaving: Direct factor Xa inhibitors

10. Band member X-ing out rules he doesn't like: Direct factor Xa inhibitors have the suffix "xaban" (e.g. apixaban, rivaroxaban, edoxaban)

11. Band member spraying paint in mouth to get high: Direct factor Xa inhibitors are oral medications

12. Brown Play-Doh machine gun and Play-Doh paratrooper being stretched out by squabbling kids: Direct factor Xa inhibitors prolong PT and PTT

13. "No surveillance" sign next to rules poster: Direct factor Xa inhibitors do not require lab monitoring

14. Dexter trying to get rid of "top 10 rules" sign by using net: Reverse factor Xa inhibitors with andexanet alfa

15. Parent getting out of car with swollen leg after long trip: Use direct factor Xa and direct thrombin (IIa) inhibitors for deep vein thrombosis (DVT)

16. PE teacher's parking sign: Use direct factor Xa and direct thrombin (IIa) inhibitors for pulmonary embolism (PE)

17. Kid wearing helmet with brain pattern and clogged straws and crossing out "no parking" with EKG-like squiggles: Use direct factor Xa and direct thrombin (IIa) inhibitors for atrial fibrillation stroke prophylaxis

18. Kid bleeding after getting cut: Both classes cause bleeding

19. Girl giving bleeding friend juice concentration from juice box with picture of quarterback throwing ball and complex molecular structures: Life-threatening bleeding caused by either drug class can be reversed using prothrombin complex concentrate (PPC)

See Figure 9.10.1- Mechanism of Anticoagulants that Interact with Secondary Hemostasis (Hem/Onc Pharmacology, Section 1, Page 188)

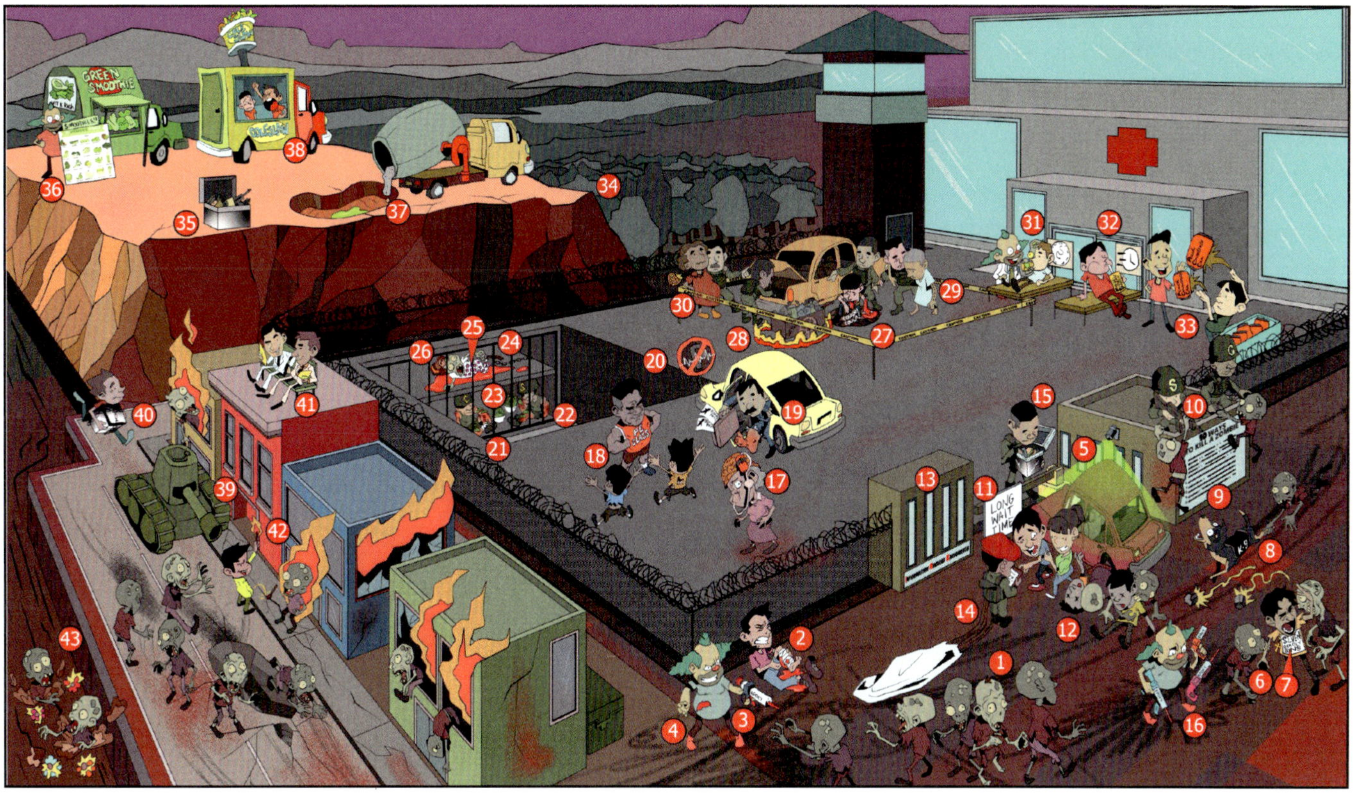

1. Zombies vs. humans war: Warfarin

2. Human bleeding out despite gauze: Anticoagulant

3. Krusty the Klown with epoxy gun: Warfarin inhibits hepatic epoxide reductase

4. Krusty the Klown with liver-shaped blood stain on shirt: Warfarin decreases hepatic synthesis of the reduced form of vitamin K (active vitamin K)

5. Zombies interfering with gamma ray toll booth for cars: Warfarin interferes with γ-carboxylation factors

6. Human who failed to reach gamma ray booth in time, throwing two rocks at zombies: Decreased γ-carboxylation results in decreased factor II (thrombin)

7. Man wearing "7 deadly sins" shirt unable to reach gamma toll booth: Decreased γ-carbonylation results in decreased factor VII

8. K-9 dog unable to return to gamma ray toll booth: Decreased γ-carboxylation results in decreased factor IX

9. "10 ways to kill a zombie" sign on toll booth: Decreased γ-carboxylation results in decreased factor X

10. Corporal with "C" helmet and sergeant with "s" helmet on top of gamma ray booth being attacked by zombies: Warfarin interferes with the regular γ-carboxylation of anti-clotting proteins C and S

11. "Long wait time" sign with line of people, half of whom have been killed by zombies: Warfarin's onset relles on the half-lives of normal clotting factors (i.e. factors II, VI, IX and X are initially present in the serum at normal levels)

12. Long line of people: Long half-life (days)

13. Thin windows into prison complex: Narrow therapeutic index

14. Paratrooper (PT) monitoring each person as they go through the "information Nuclear Radiometer" (NR) for inspection: Patients' PT/NR need to be monitored

15. Open chrome box at entrance to prison complex: Metabolized by cytochrome P-450

16. Krusty the Klown's varying epoxy guns with varying efficacy against zombies: Polymorphisms in the gene for vitamin K epoxide reductase complex ($VKORC_1$) affect warfarin efficacy and metabolism

17. Elderly teacher wearing brain-pattern helmet with built-in straws unable to drink because straws are clogged: Used as chronic prevention of ischemic stroke (e.g. from an embolus)

18. PE class inside prison complex: Use patient with a pulmonary embolism

19. Parent getting out of car with swollen leg after long trip: Use in patients with a deep vein thrombosis

20. "No parking" sign with EKG-like graffiti squiggles: Use in patients with atrial fibrillation

21. Corporal with "C" helmet and sergeant with "s" helmet in underground prison: Proteins C and S are the first proteins to decrease when patients first start warfarin therapy

22. Corporal with "C" helmet and sergeant with "S" helmet who have been bitten by zombies developing skin lesions: Low proteins C and S can cause initial hypercoagulation and skin necrosis

23. Heap of fruit rinds that corporal with "C" helmet and sergeant with "S" helmet are rubbing into their wounds and skin lesions: Employ "heparin bridging": Administer heparin alongside initial warfarin regimen → reduced risk of skin/tissue necrosis or recurrent venous thromboembolism

24. Pool of blood around zombie: Warfarin can increase bleeding risk

25. Zombie wearing purple polka dot clothes: Warfarin can cause hemorrhagic blisters and painful purpura

26. Tarantula crawling around zombie: Warfarin is teratogenic

27. Soldiers saving actively bleeding guy sitting in ulcer-shaped ditch within yellow caution tape area: Contraindicated in patients with active bleeding, have a high risk of bleeding, or ulcer-related GI bleeding

28. Cart catching fire while soldier loads people and weapons into getaway car within yellow caution tape area: Contraindicated in patients with pericarditis or endocarditis

29. Person in hospital gown with surgical scar within yellow caution tape area: Contraindicated in patients with recent surgery

30. Pregnant woman holding mechanical heart-shaped watch winin yellow caution tape area: Contraindicated in pregnancy unless the pregnant patient has a mechanical heart valve

31. Krusty the Klown administering antidote to zombie, who slowly turns back into human: Slow warfarin reversal (non-urgent reversal) is achieved via vitamin K administration

32. Fresh frozen peach slushie antidote working quickly: Achieve rapid warfarin reversal with fresh frozen plasma (FFP)

33. Two Peach Concentrate Cans being thrown to hospital worker: Achieve rapid reversal with prothrombin complex concentrate (PCC)

34. Area with decreased war and zombies: There are substances that can decrease warfarin's anticoagulant effects

35. Open chrome box in decreased war area: Cytochrome P-450 inducers → decrease warfarin effect

36. Food truck with vitamin K rich foods: Foods rich in vitamin K → decreased warfarin effect

37. Cement being poured to neutralize acid in stomach-shaped hole: Gastric acid inhibition → decreased warfarin effect

38. Tyrant boss inside food truck: Cholestyramine → decreased warfarin effect

39. Zombie wearing purple polka dot clothes: Warfarin can cause hemorrhagic blisters and painful purpura

40. Chained up, locked chrome box: Cytochrome P-450 inhibitors → increased warfarin effect

41. Rich men in roof seat watching war: Acetaminophen → increased warfarin effect

42. Guy preparing to light zombies on fire by urinating on sulfur match: Sulfonamides and sulfonylureas → increased warfarin effect

43. Zombies crushing flowers in muddy brown river: Damage to the gut flora (e.g. antibiotic therapy) → increased warfarin effect

See Figure 9.10.1- Mechanism of Anticoagulants that Interact with Secondary Hemostasis (Hem/Onc Pharmacology, Section 1, Page 188)

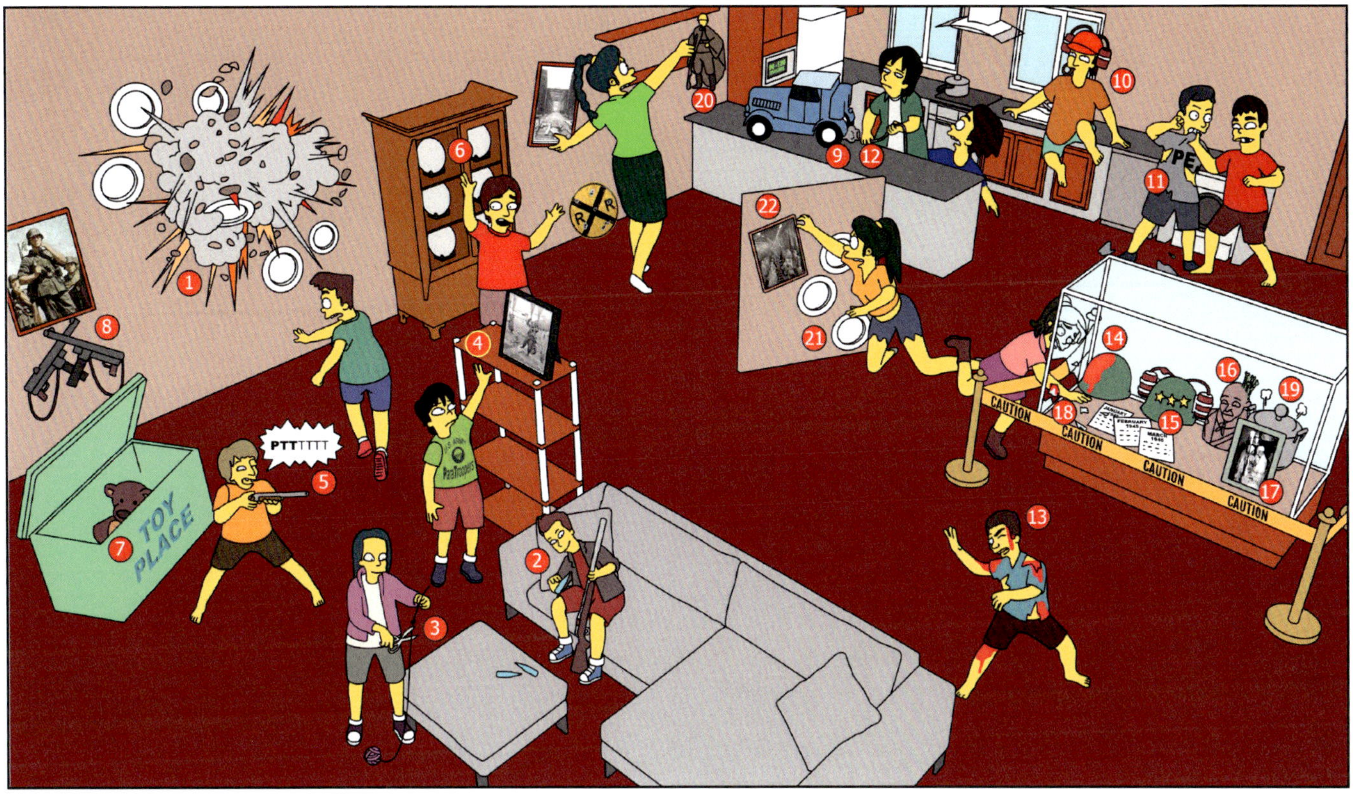

1. Plates broken by thrown grenade: Thrombolytics

2. Kid loading plastic ammo into BB gun to make active weapon: Directly or indirectly aid in conversation of plasminogen to plasmin

3. Scissors cleaving big knots of fibrous yarn: Cleave fibrin clots

4. Pictures of dad as paratrooper (PT) located high on shelf: Increase PT

5. Kid saying "PTTTTTT" while pretending to shoot gun: Increase PTT

6. Son guarding plates to prevent any more from being broken: No changes to platelet count

7. "Toy place" label on box of toys in corner: Several thrombolytics have the suffix "teplase" (alteplase, reteplase, and tenecteplase)

8. Two crossed strap-on guns on wait next to picture of soldier from King's African Rifles regiment: Streptokinase is another thrombolytic

9. Clogged exhaust pipe of toy car on counter: Use early for an MI

10. Kid wearing helmet with built-in cups and straws, but unable to drink through clogged straws: Use early for ischemic stroke

11. Kid wearing tattered PE shirt: Use for direct thrombolysis of severe pulmonary embolism (PE)

12. Older kid snaking clogged exhaust pipe near oven timer set to 90 minutes: Use as an alternative to percutaneous coronary intervention (PTCA) in a STEMI if PTCA cannot be performed within 90-120 minutes

13. Kid covered in blood after breaking glass case: Can cause hemorrhage

14. Old, blood-stained battle helmet in glass case: Contraindicated in patients with a history of hemorrhagic strok

15. New, bloodless collector's helmet decorated with three stars next to three months' worth of calendar pages: Contraindicated in patients with a history of nonhemorrhagic stroke within 3 months

16. Soldier head chia pet with growth on only one side of head and cancer ribbon around neck: Contraindicated in patients with intracranial neoplasm

17. WWII operating room picture in memorabilia case: Contraindicated in patients with recent surgery

18. Bleeding kid reaching across yellow caution tape: Contraindicated in patients with a known bleeding disorder

19. Pressure cooker inside yellow caution tape: Contraindicated in patients with severe hypertension

20. Sister putting soldier figurine with ammo and cape out of reach next to pictures of railroad crossing and train crossing sign: Reverse thrombolytics with antifibrinolytics (e.g. aminocarproic acid and tranexamic acid)

21. Sister hanging more decorative plates on wall to replace broken ones: Reverse thrombolytics with platelet transfusions

22. Crooked factory picture straightened by sister: Reverse thrombolytics with factor corrections (e.g. cryoprecipitate, FFP, PCC)

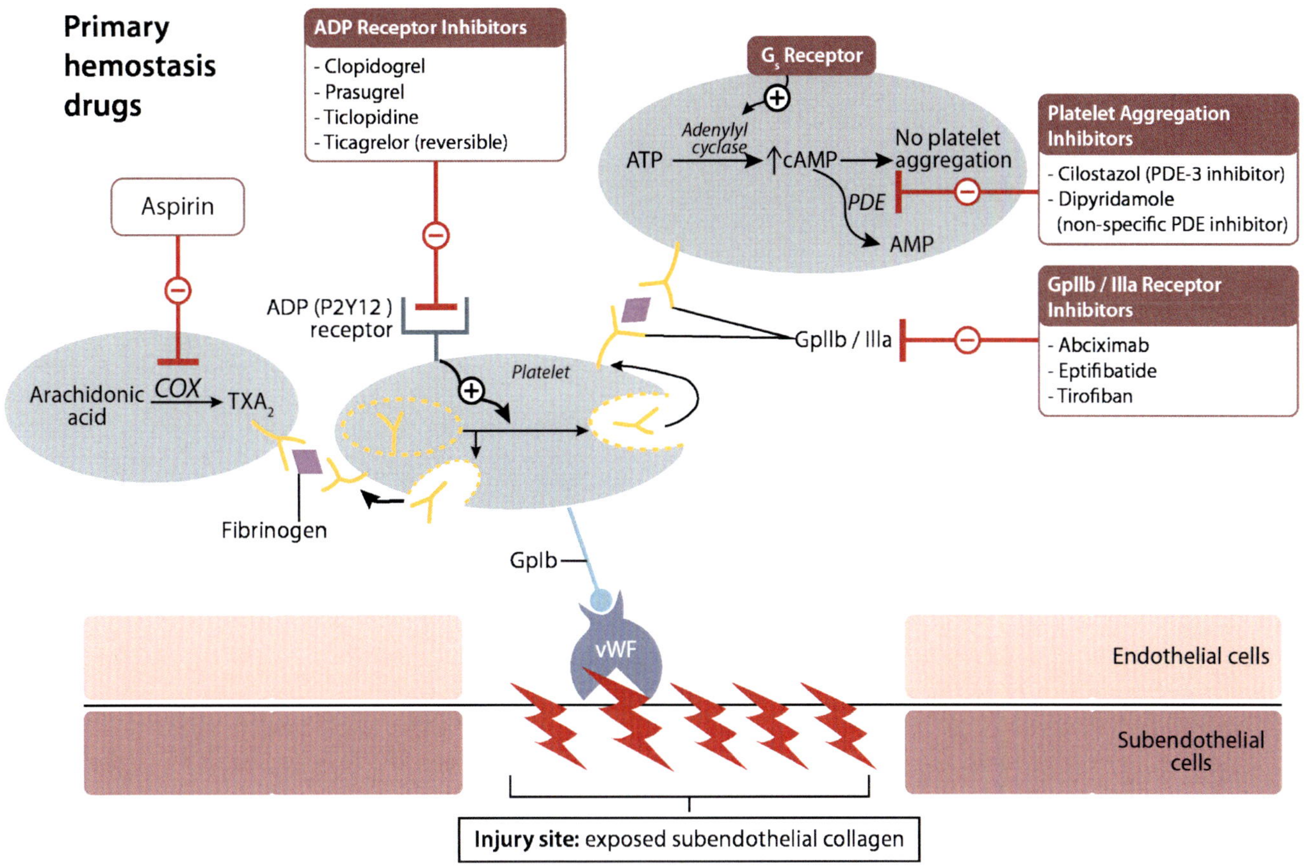

Figure 9.10.2 - Primary Hemostasis Drug Mechanisms

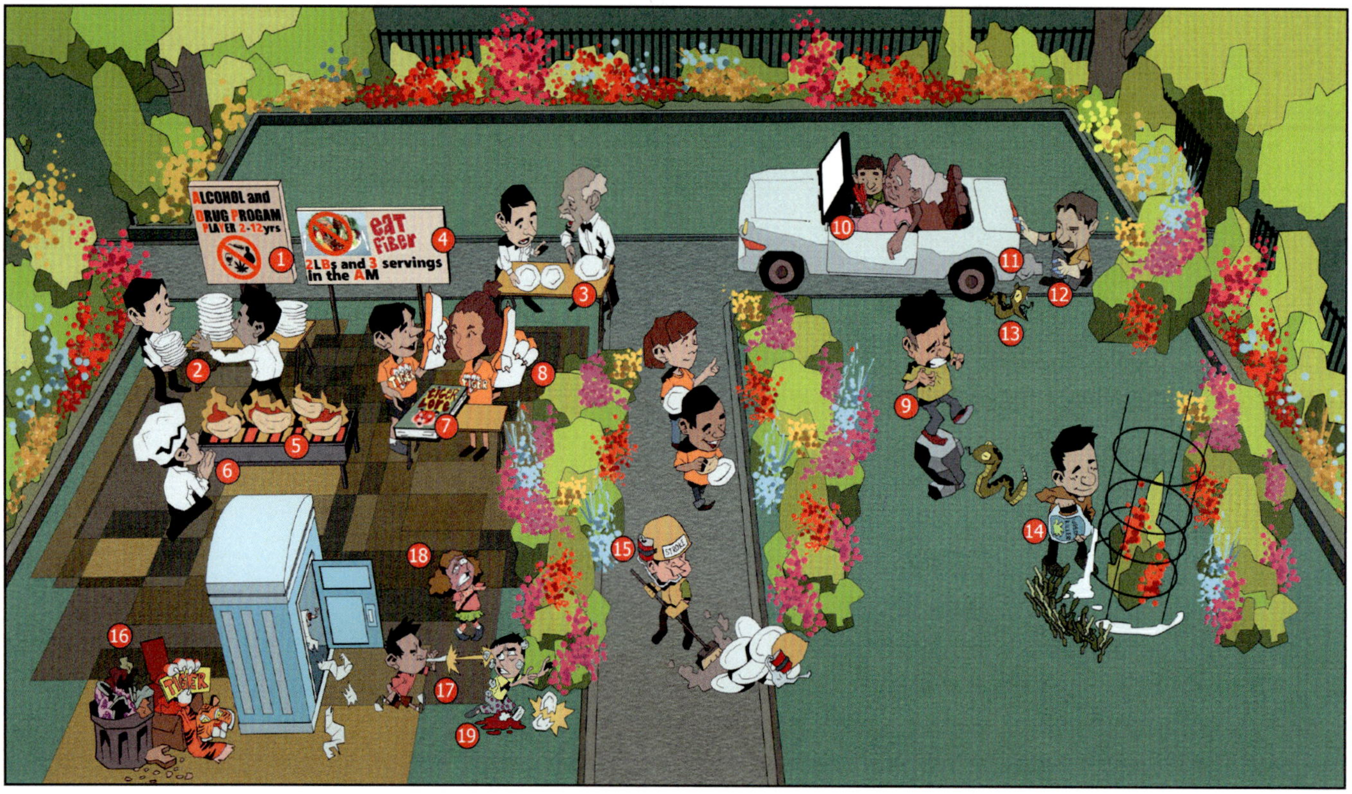

1. "Alcohol and Drug Program" sign targeted towards "Players 2-12 Yrs": ADP inhibitors irreversibly block ADP (P2Y12) receptors

2. Server being prevented from setting out more plates: Considered antiplatelet drugs

3. Supervisor preventing server from putting plates too close together: Prevent platelet aggregation

4. "Eat Fiber" poster reading, "2 LBs and 3 servings in the AM": Prevent the expression of glycoproteins IIb/IIa on platelet surface

5. Garlic cloves on grill: Clopidogrel

6. Grill chef praying food isn't burned: Prasugrel

7. "Tiger Lore" book on lunch table: Ticagrelor

8. Basketball team wearing jerseys with tiger claw logo: Ticlopidine

9. Guy clutching chest in terror while balancing on unstable rock with asp on ground nearby: Use for unstable angina/NSTEMI (usually in combination with aspirin)

10. Grandma sitting inside car, shaking red licorice to distract grandson from scary snake: Use for acute coronary syndrome

11. Clogged muffler on grandma's car: Use to treat myocardial infarction (MI)

12. Guy wearing gloves with blue fingertips to unclog muffler: Use for symptomatic peripheral arterial disease (PAD)

13. Grandma's car crushing asp: Use as an alternative to aspirin

14. Gardener spraying weed killer around structural cages that help guide plant growth: Used with coronary stents to prevent platelet clots forming around stent

15. Worker wearing helmet with built-in cups and straws clearing clumps of platelets from ground: Can decrease incidence and recurrence of thrombotic stroke

16. Tattered tiger claw sign next to garbage can containing purple polka-dotted turtle shell with old bread and grains: Ticlopidine can cause neutropenia and agranulocytosis

17. Little brother wearing purple polka dot pants dropping plate after being pelted with spitball clots: ADP inhibitors can cause thrombotic thrombocytopenic purpura (TTP)

18. Girl with allergic reaction developing rash and struggling to breathe: ADP inhibitors can cause an allergic reaction (e.g. rash, pruritus, anaphylaxis)

19. Little brother falling and getting bloody knee: ADP inhibitors can cause hemorrhage

See Figure 9.10.2 - Primary Hemostasis Drug Mechanisms (Hem/Onc Pharmacology, Section 5, Page 198)

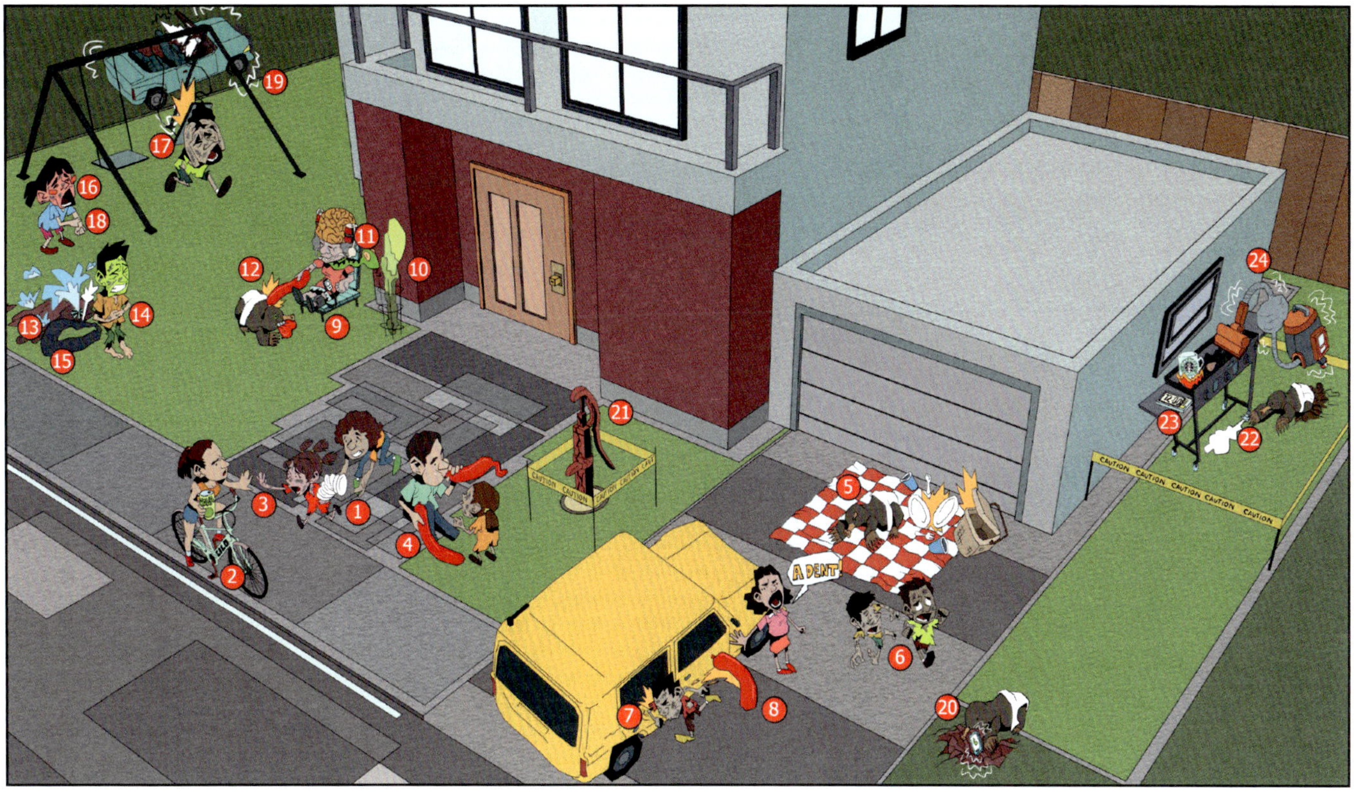

1. Mom blocking foster girl and taking plates from her so they don't fall: Antiplatelet PDE inhibitors

2. Big sister riding Cilo brand bike and drinking Zola energy drink: Cilostazol

3. Big sister blocking foster sister from getting on bike: Cilostazol is a phosphodiesterase 3 inhibitor that inhibits platelet aggregation

4. Dad blowing up long red balloons: Cilostazol is a direct arterial vasodilator

5. Mole wearing diaper: Dipyridamole

6. Angry mole in diaper scattering plates everywhere: Dipyridamole is a nonspecific phosphodiesterase inhibitor that inhibits platelet aggregation

7. Kid running away from mole in diaper runs into car and makes dent: Dipryidamole increases adenosine (blocks adenosine reuptake into platelets)

8. Kid running away from mole in diaper dropping long red balloon: Dipyridamole causes higher adenosine → vasodilation

9. Nanny wearing blood pressure cuff: Use cilostazol and dipyridamole to alleviate intermittent claudication

10. Hollow lumen formed by structural cage used to guide plant growth: Use cilostazol and dipyridamole with coronary stents to prevent platelet clots forming around stent

11. Nanny wearing helmet with brain pattern and built-in straws and cups, but unable to drink through clogged straws: Use cilostazol and dipyridamole in ischemic stroke or TIA prevention (alongside aspirin)

12. Diapered mole by nanny's feet grabbing heart-shaped stress ball while she hits it with long red balloon: Dipyridamole can be used in cardiac stress testing (due to coronary vasodilation)

13. Muddy brown water near nauseated kid: Dipryidamole and cilostazol can cause nausea and diarrhea

14. Kid grabbing belly in pain: Dipyridamole and cilostazol can cause abdominal pain

15. Deflating toy tire: Dipryidamole and cilostazol can cause hypotension

16. Running kids's red face: Dipyridamole and cilostazol can cause facial flushing

17. Kid holding head in pain after being hit by swing: Dipyridamole and cilostazol can cause headaches

18. Running kid checking pulse: Dipryidamole and cilostazol can cause tachycardia

19. Rattling AC vent in toy car: Ventricular arrhythmias (most common and severe side effects for PDE-3 inhibitors)

20. Diapered mole burying dad's ringing cell phone: Dipyridamole can cause neurotoxicity at high levels (e.g. seizures)

21. Broken water pump behind yellow caution tape near Cilo bike: Cilostazol is contraindicated in heart failure

22. Diapered mole deflating mobile grill's tire behind yellow caution tape: Dipyridamole is contraindicated in hypotension

23. Starbucks coffee cup on top of mobile grill along with twelve-hour timer and diapered mole behind yellow caution tape: Dipryidamole is contraindicated with caffeine within 12 hours

24. Spasming vacuum hose behind yellow caution tape: Dipridamole is contraindicated with bronchospasm (e.g. asthma, reactive airway disease)

See Figure 9.10.2 - Primary Hemostasis Drug Mechanisms (Hem/Onc Pharmacology, Section 5, Page 196)

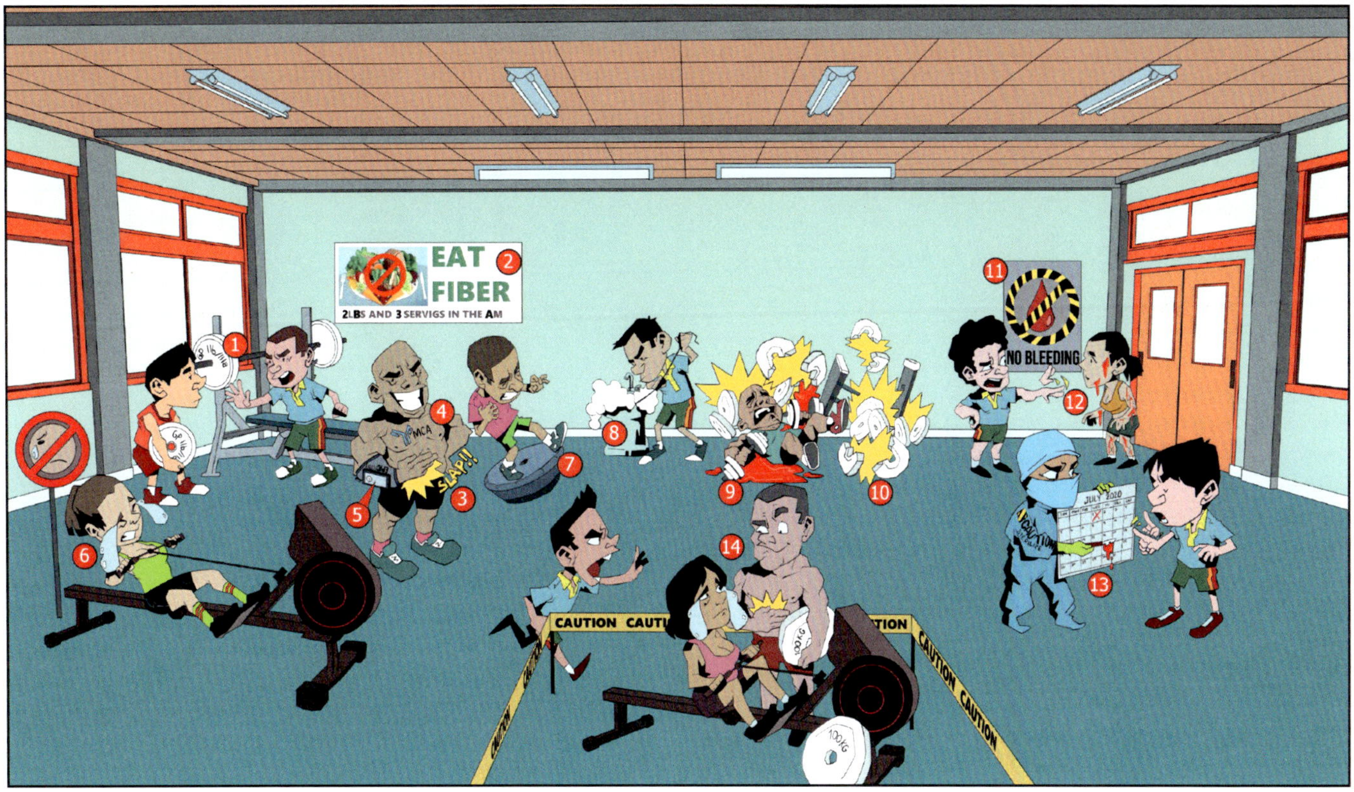

1. Gym employee stopping guest from adding too many weight plates with "GP IIb/IIIa" lettering to bench press: Glycoprotein IIb/IIIa inhibitors

2. "Eat Fiber" poster on wall of gym with "2 lbs and 3 servings in the AM" written on it: Block fibrinogen binding to platelets → prevents proper platelet aggregation and thrombus formation

3. Buff guy slapping his six-pack abs: Abciximab

4. YMCA tattoo with antibody-shaped "Y" on buff guy with six-pack abs: Abciximab is made from monoclonal antibody Fab fragments

5. Buff guy wearing epic Fitbit: Eptifbatide

6. Crying girl on rowing machine, ignoring sign that bans tears in gym: Tirofiban

7. Guy grabbing chest in pain while on unstable balance board: Use for unstable angina

8. Employee snaking overflowing, clogged sink: Use for percutaneous coronary intervention

9. Guy bleeding after weights fall on him: Can cause bleeding

10. Broken weight plates knocked over by bleeding guy: Can cause thrombocytopenia

11. "No Bleeding" sign on wall of gym: Contraindicated with an active bleed

12. Bleeding customer being turned away from gym gy employee: Contraindicated if the patient has a high risk for bleeding

13. Surgeon being turned away from gym near calendar showing 30 days remaining in month: Contraindicated if major surgery or severe trauma occurred within the past 30 days

14. Second buff guy with six-pack abs holding 1000kg weight plate down low while harassing crying girl on rowing machine inside caution tape: Abciximab and tirofiban are contraindicated with platelet counts < 100,000/mm³

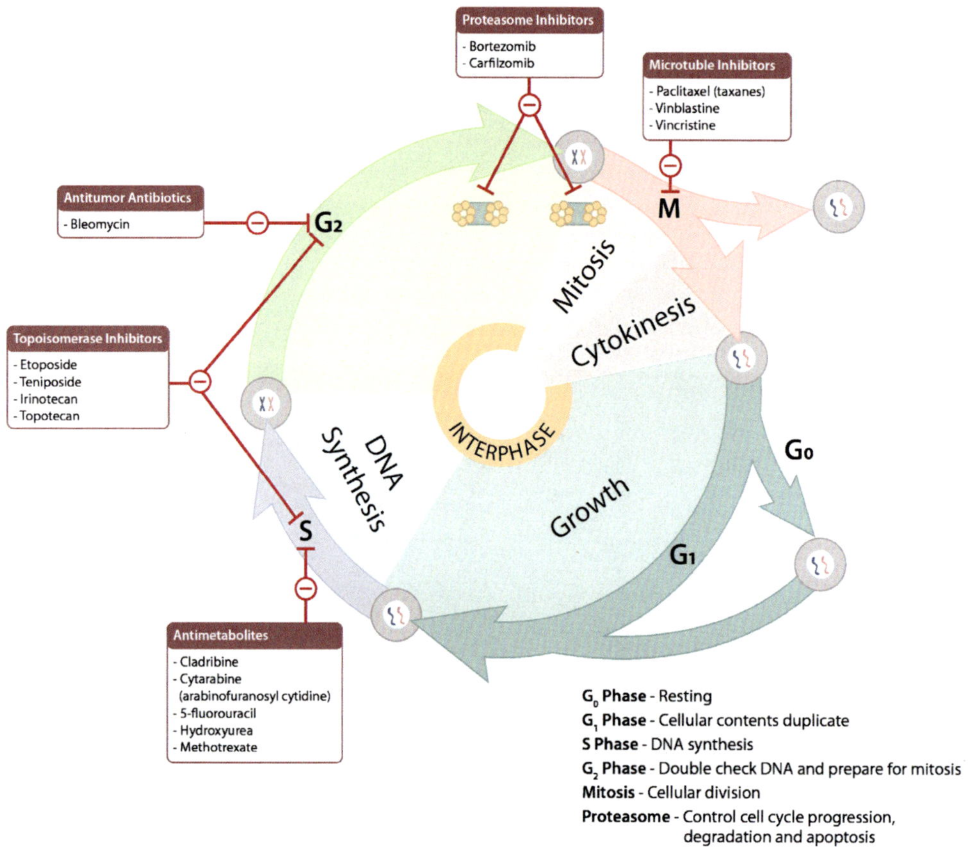

Figure 9.10.3 - Cell Cycle-Disrupting Cancer Drug Overview

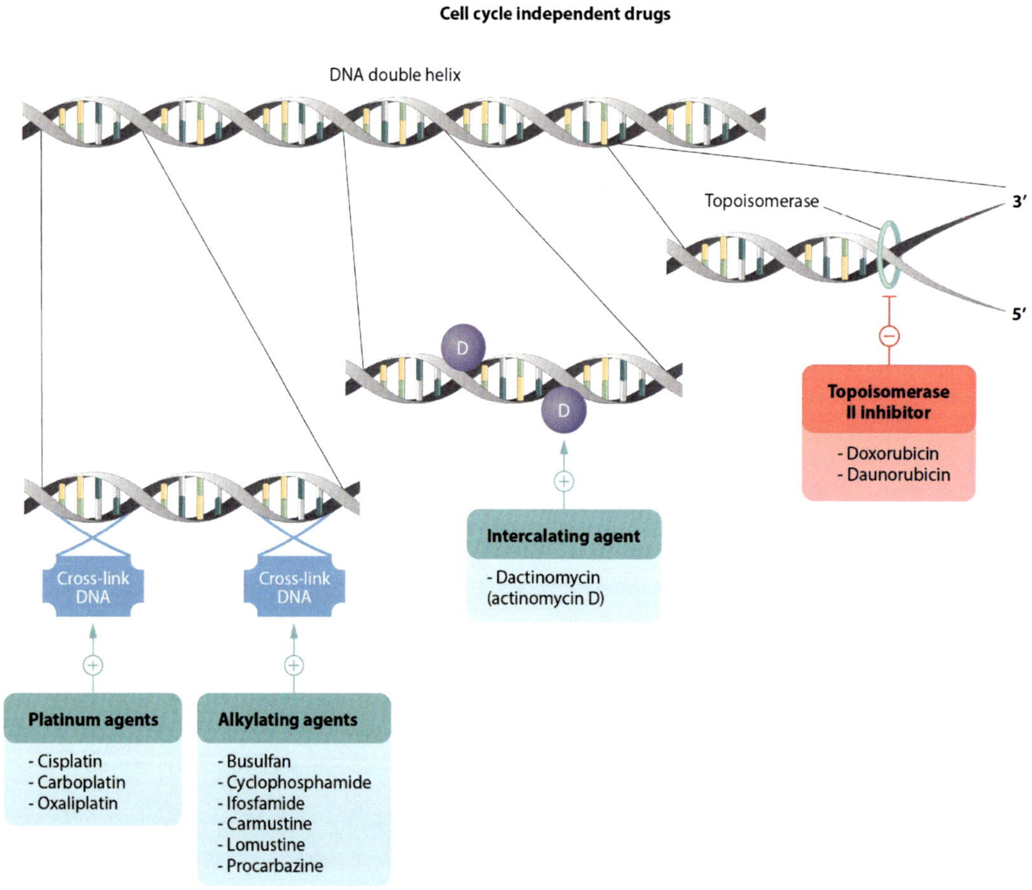

Figure 9.10.4 - Cell Cycle Independent Cancer Drug Overview

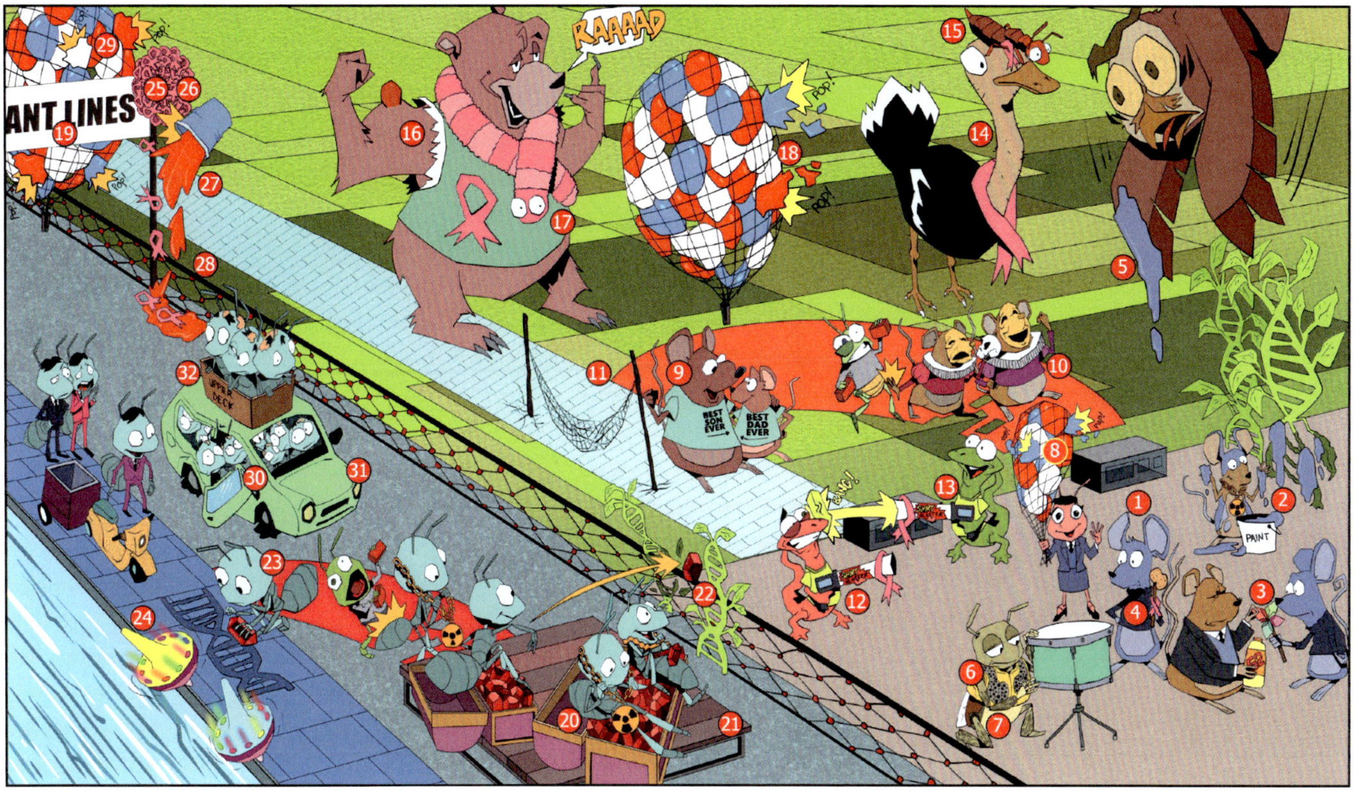

1. Group of blue mice performing at animal concert: Bleomycin

2. Mouse with radiation symbol necklace getting blue paint on DNA-shaped vines and causing them to wither: Bleomycin works by inducing free radical formation → DNA strand breakage

3. Stage manager stopping pinwheel from spinning and holding bottle of G2 Gatorade: Bleomycin arrests the cell cycle at G2 phase

4. Drum stick in testicle shape with pink cancer ribbon tied to it: Use bleomycin for testicular cancer

5. Toxic blue paint splashing into owl's eyes: Use bleomycin for Hodgkin lymphoma

6. Worker wearing lung-shaped mech yellow safety vest: Bleumycin can cause pulmonary fibrosis

7. Worker's splotchy tan skin from applying sunscreen unevenly: Bleomycin can cause hyperpigmentation

8. Blue mice group's agent holding different colored balloons in net, only very few of which have popped: Bleomycin can cause minimal myelosuppression

9. Dad and son mice wearing matching dad/son shirts: Dactinomycin

10. Acting mice about to perform in play wearing sad/happy theater masks with D-shaped mouths: Actinomycin D

11. Long blue path being destroyed by dad and son mice, while worker mouse is unable to finish tiling red path: Dactinomycin (actinomycin D) intercalates into DNA → transcription prevented → RNA synthesis prevented

12. Newt blasting t-shirts out of t-shirt cannon: Use dactinomycin for neuroblastoma

13. Reptile blasting t-shirts out of t-shirt cannon: Use dactinomycin for retinoblastoma

14. Ostrich wearing pink cancer boa around neck: Use dactinomycin for osteosarcoma

15. Earwig wearing pink cancer ribbon: Use dactinomycin for Ewing sarcoma

16. Bear saying "rad" with bump on bicep and pink cancer ribbon: Use dactinomycin for rhabdomyosarcoma

17. Bear saying "rad" with fuzzy pink worm around neck that looks like cancer ribbon: Use dactinomycin for Wilms' tumor

18. Net of multicolored balloons popping in wind: Dactinomycin can cause myelosuppression

19. "Ant lines" banner near audience section reserved for ants: Anthracyclines

20. Ants donning rubies as decoration: Daunorubicin

21. Ants donning rubies on dock near water: Doxorubicin

22. Ant with radiation symbol necklace breaking DNA-shaped vines by throwing rubies through them: Doxorubicin and daunorubicin create free radicals

23. Ants ruining long blue walkway and preventing worker from tiling short red walkway: Doxorubicin and daunorubicin intercalate into DNA → transcription prevented → RNA synthesis prevented

24. Ant interfering with two spinning tops and knocking them off blue path: Interfere with topoisomerase II enzyme

25. Solid ball of pink cancer ribbons: Use for solid tumors

26. Solid ball of pink cancer ribbons on pole holding up "ant lines" banner: Doxorubicin and daunorubicin are used for solid tumors

27. Spilled red Kool-Aid washing small creatures away: Doxorubicin and daunorubicin are used for leukemias

28. Net with large knots between audience members and water: Doxorubicin and daunorubicin are used for lymphomas

29. Net of partly popped multicolored balloons for ant lines: Doxorubicin and daunorubicin can cause myelosuppression

30. Bald ants arriving at concert: Can cause alopecia

31. Weight-down car bulging with ants: Can cause dilated cardiomyopathy

32. Box on top of car labeled "upper deck" and extra room on Razor brand scooter, preventing car from getting too full and breaking down: Give an iron chelator, dexrazoxane to prevent cardiotoxicity

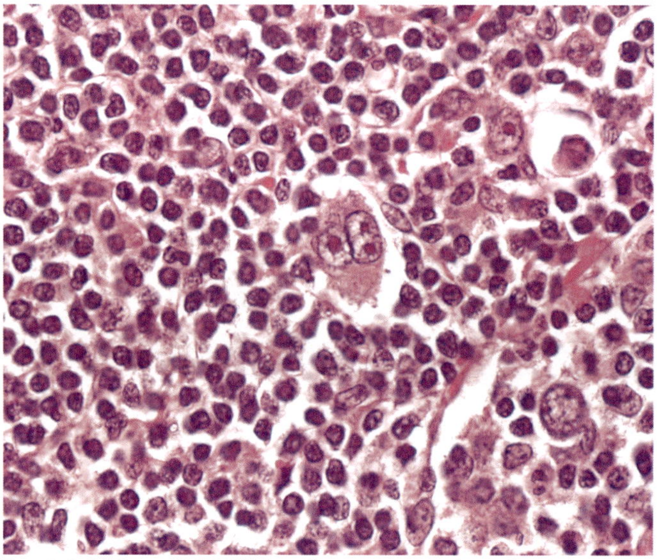

Figure 9.10.5 - Histological Image of Hodgkin Lymphoma

See Figure 9.10.4 - Cell Cycle Independent Cancer Drug Overview (Hem/Onc Pharmacology, Section 8, Page 203)

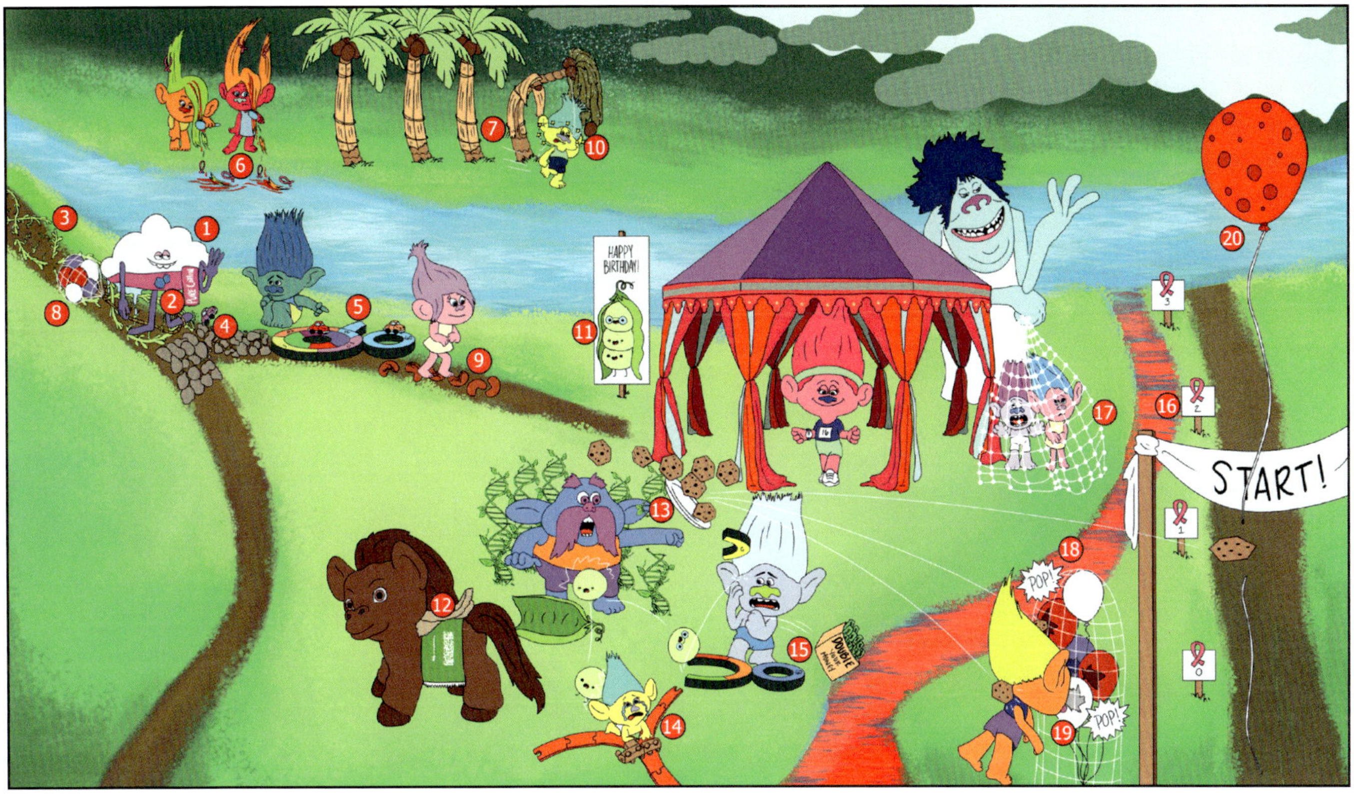

1. Dripping wet cloud character: Cladribine

2. Dripping cloud guy wearing scarf labeled "pure cotton" and purine-shaped button: Cladribine is a purine analog

3. Cloud guy tearing through DNA-shaped vines: Cladribine can directly break DNA strands

4. Cloud guy kicking toy car off forked road: Cladribine inhibits DNA polymerase

5. Cloud guy refusing to play with any part of Hot Wheels track: Cladribine is the only antimetabolite that is cell cycle nonspecific

6. Hair, blood, and pink cancer ribbons floating down river: Use cladribine for hairy cell leukemia

7. Wrapped trees next to partially unwrapped, damaged tree: Use cladribine for relapsing form of multiple sclerosis

8. Cloud guy holding net of multicolored balloons: Cladribine cna cause myelosuppression

9. Kidney bean-shaped stepping stones being trampled: Cladribine can cause nephrotoxicity

10. Dizzy troll holding head with and seeing stars after coconut falls on him: Cladribine can cause neurotoxicity (often manifests as dizziness and headaches)

11. Three bean characters standing on top of each other while squinting due to poor sight: Cytarabine

12. Arabian-themed party with Arabian horse for guests to ride: Cytarabine is also called arabinofuranosyl cytidine

13. Three bean characters knocking over plate of hexagonal pyramid-shaped cookies and tearing through DNA vines: Cytarabine is a pyrimidine analog that leads to DNA chain termination (inhibits S-phase)

14. Baby troll falling out of stroller and knocking toy train off forked track: At higher drug concentrations, cytarabine inhibits DNA polymerase

15. "S phase" portion of Hot Wheels track being dislodged near bookie's "double your money" box being knocked down: Cytarabine is S-phase specific

16. Red trail towards river with pink cancer ribbon mile markers: Use cytarabine for acute myelogenous leukemia (AML)

17. Villain trapping trolls inside net with large knots: Use cytarabine for lymphomas

18. Multicolored balloons trapped inside second net: Cytarabine can cause myelosuppression

19. Guest being hit by cookie sand falling onto balloons, popping some of them: Cytarabine can cause pancytopenia

20. Blood-red moon balloon's string being cut by sharp, pyrimidine-shaped cookie so that it flies away: Cytarabine can cause megaloblastic anemia

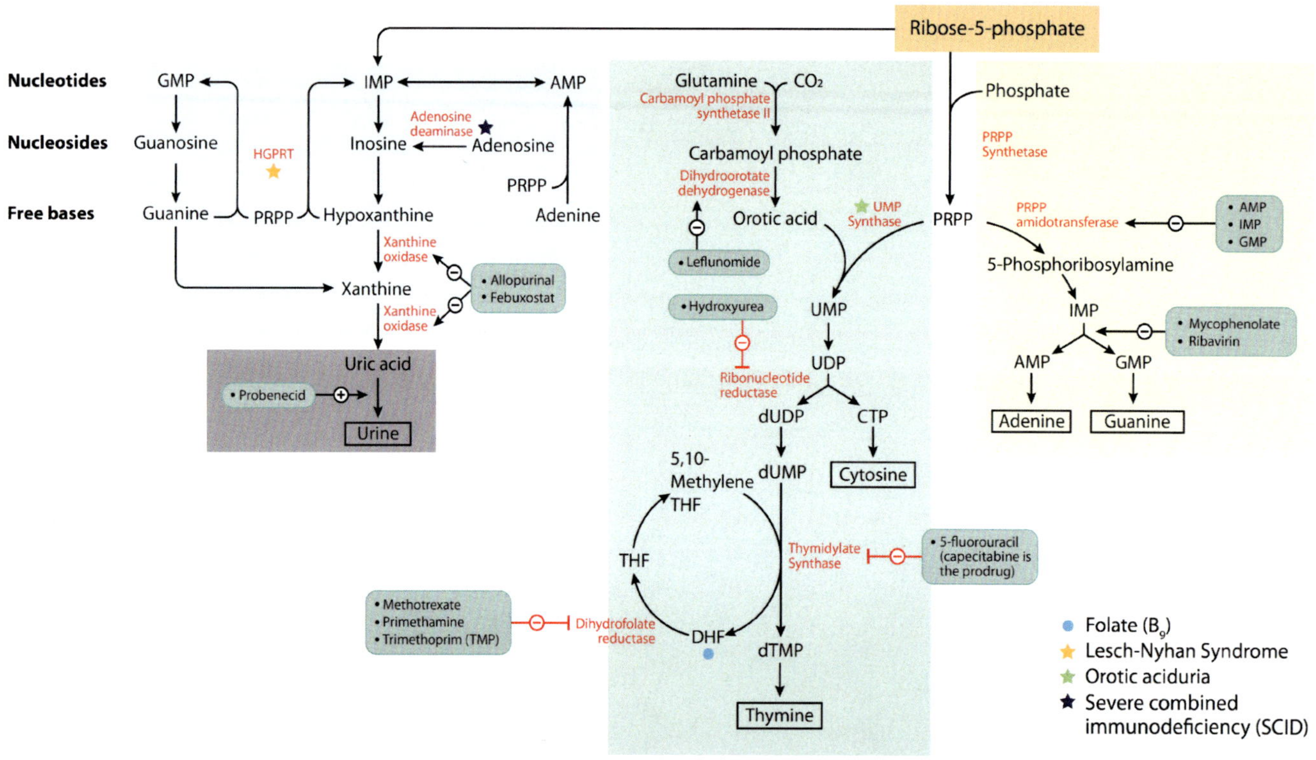

Figure 9.10.6 - Nucleotide Synthesis Overview

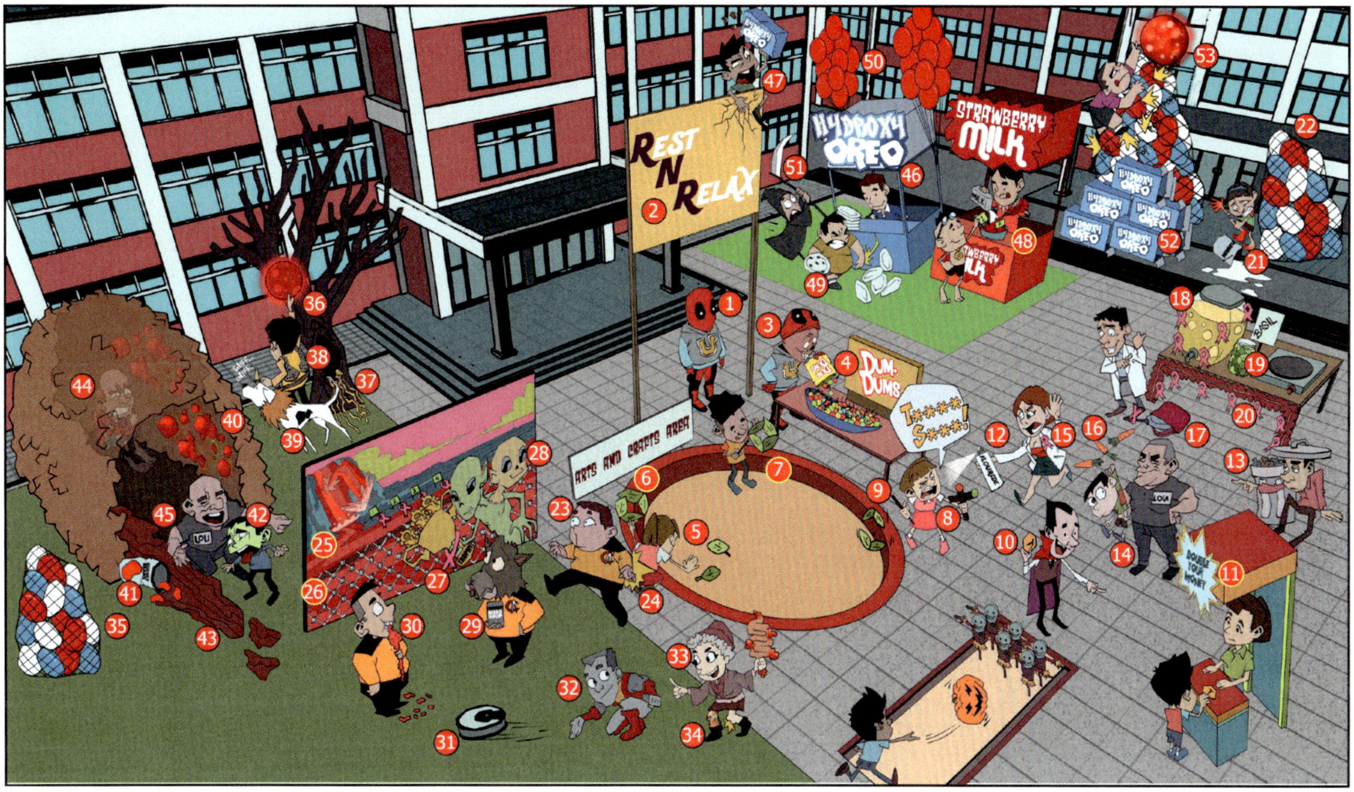

1. College student in Deadpool costume and university sweatshirt with big "U" on it: UDP (uridine monophosphate)

2. "Rest N Relax" sign to welcome guests: Ribonucleotide reductase

3. Second student dressed in Deadpool costume with mask off to show dead tired face from studying: Ribonucleotide reductase converts UDP to dUDP (deoxyuridine monophosphate)

4. Dum-Dum lollipops handed out to trick-or-treaters: dUDP becomes dUMP (deoxyuridine monophosphate)

5. Girl playing with two pieces of foliage in arts and crafts area: Dihydrofolate (DHF)

6. Second girl playing with four pieces of foliage in arts and crafts area: DHF becomes tetrahydrofolate (THF) via dihydrofolate reductase

7. Kid assembling four pieces of foliage with stick: THF acquires a methyl group

8. Girl holding four pieces of foliage with stick in one hand and two T-shaped Dum-Dums in other hand while cursing: Methylated THF and dUMP are substrates of thymidylate synthase

9. Girl's four pieces of foliage splitting into two groups of two while Dum-Dums remain in T-shape on top of licorice sticks: Thymidylate synthase takes a methyl group (i.e. carbon) from the THF and donates it to dUMP → dTMP (deoxythymidine monophosphate) and DHF

10. Man in vampire costume holding tokens with "t" on them: dTMP is the precursor for thymine (a pyrimidine)

11. "Double your money" booth claiming that you can get two tokens back if you enter game for one token and win: Thymine is required for DNA replication (S phase of the cell cycle)

12. Dental hygienist mom spraying fluoride at swearing daughter while holding up five fingers: 5-Fluorouracil (5-FU)

13. Dad with garbage lid on head next to trash bin: Capecitabine is the prodrug of 5-FU

14. Campus bouncer with name tag reading "Lou" assisting mom: Leucovorin helps 5-FU kill cancer cells

15. Dental hygienist mom with large breasts and pink cancer ribbon: Use 5-FU for breast cancer

16. Dental hygienist mom handling out carrots instead of candy: Use 5-FU for actinic keratosis

17. Frying pan with pink cancer ribbon tied to handle: Use 5-FU for pancreatic cancer

18. Bladder-shaped lemonade dispenser with pink cancer ribbons: Use 5-FU for urothelial cell carcinoma

19. Basil leaves to put in lemonade: Use 5-FU for basal cell carcinoma (topical)

20. Colon-like table decoration with pink cancer ribbons: Use 5-FU for colon cancer

21. Girl with red hands and feed due to fluoride: 5-FU can cause palmar-plantar erythrodysesthesia (hand-foot syndrome)

22. Net filled with multicolored balloons: 5-FU can cause myelosuppression

23. Student dressed as character from Star Trek: Methotrexate

24. Trekkie bumping into girl and knocking over foliage project with two and four leaves: Methotrexate competitively inhibits dihydrofolate reductase

25. TV showing red river with geyser blasting upwards suddenly and pink ribbons along bank: Use methotrexate for acute lymphoblastic leukemia (ALL)

26. Robe bridge across river with big knots: Use methotrexate for lymphomas

27. Alien on TV screen holding choir trophy: Use methotrexate for choriocarcinoma

28. Baby alien growing directly out of adult alien's shoulder: Use methotrexate for ectopic pregnancy

29. Student wearing both boar costume and trekkie costume while holding mis soup: Use methotrexate for medical abortion with misoprostol

30. Trekkie eating red licorice rope that's been nibbled and damaged: Use methotrexate for vasculitis

31. Guest sending Roomba vacuum to clean up: Use methotrexate for rheumatoid arthritis

32. Student dressed as silver Colossus character from Marvel Comics: Use methotrexate for psoriasis

33. Student dressed as old crone holding handful of intestine: Use methotrexate for IBD (Crohn's disease and ulcerative colitis)

34. Moldy paper mache leg with extra bony knee: Use methotrexate for sarcomas

35. Multicolored balloons trapped in net: Methotrexate can cause myelosuppression

36. Trekie hanging up blood-red full moon decoration: Methotrexate can cause megaloblastic anemia (due to folate deficiency)

37. Paper mache vines made to look like nerves spilling from tree: By causing a folate deficiency, methotrexate can cause neural tube defects (teratogenic)

38. Trekkie wearing lung-shaped yellow mesh safety est to climb tree: Methotrexate can cause pulmonary fibrosis

39. Dalmatian with liver-shaped spot next to tree: Methotrexate can cause hepatotoxicity

40. Alien cave attraction with rubies near opening: Methotrexate can cause mucositis (mouth ulcers)

41. Damaged kidney beans spilling out of crushed can: Methotrexate can cause nephrotoxicity

42. Trekkie feeling nauseated by kidney beans and vomiting: Methotrexate can cause nausea and vomiting

43. Muddy brown river flowing out of cave: Methotrexate can cause diarrhea

44. Bald hobo hiding in cave: Methotrexate can cause alopecia

45. Bouncer named Lou rescuing nauseated kid: Reduce toxicity to methotrexate by administering leucovorin (folinic acid) "leucovorin rescue"

46. "Hydroxy Oreo" stand selling snacks: Hydroxyurea

47. Kid upset by hydroxy Oreos destroying "Rest N Relax" sign with Oreos: Hydroxyurea inhibits ribonucleotide reductase

48. Kid dressed in Olympic swimmer costume holding mile markers and waiting near strawberry milk stand: Use hydroxyurea for acute and chronic myelogenous leukemia

49. Angry kid breaking essential cookie plates: Use hydroxyurea for essential thrombocytopenia

50. Too many red balloons on hydroxy Oreo stand: Use hydroxyurea for polycythemia vera

51. Boy dressed as grim reaper holding sickle: Use hydroxyurea as prophylaxis for sickle cell crisis

52. Kid popping lots of multicolored balloons in net near mountain of hydroxy Oreo boxes: Hydroxyurea can cause severe myelosuppression

53. Red blood moon decoration at top of hydroxy Oreo mountain: Hydroxyurea can cause megaloblastic anemia

See Figure 9.10.4 - Cell Cycle Independent Cancer Drug Overview (Hem/Onc Pharmacology, Section 8, Page 203)

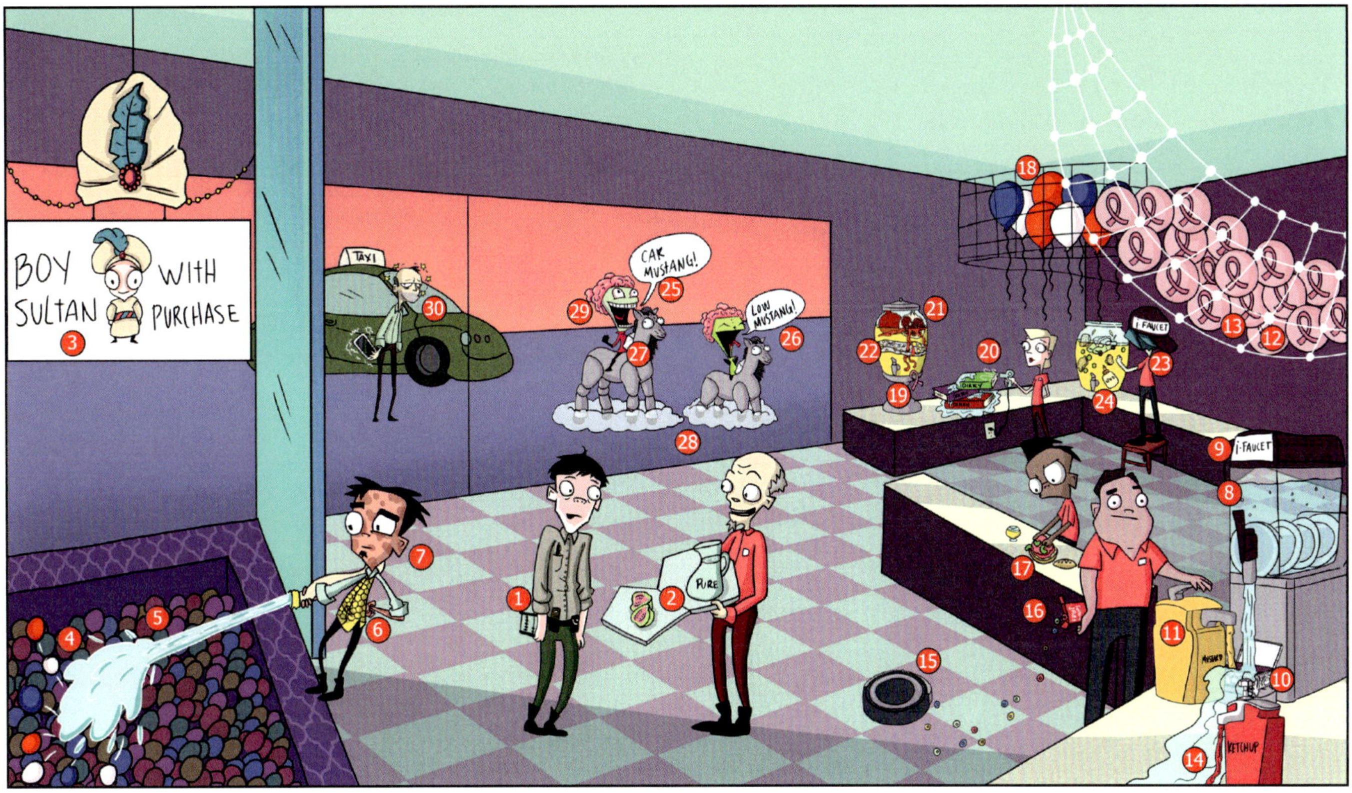

1. Accountant at family entertainment center: Alkylating agents

2. Manager offering accountant guavas and water in jug labeled "pure" on hexagon-shaped tray: Work by cross-linking DNA at guanine leading to impaired DNA synthesis

3. Boy sultan toy advertised near ball pit: Busulfan

4. Worker blasting multicolored balls out of ball pit in boy sultan area: Busulfan is used to ablate patient's bone marrow before bone marrow transplantation

5. Lots of balls being knocked out of ball pit: Can cause severe myelosuppression (very common)

6. Worker wearing lung-shaped yellow mesh safety vest: Busulfan can cause pulmonary fibrosis

7. Worker's splotchy tanned skin due to applying sunscreen unevenly: Busulfan can cause hyperpigmentation

8. Water being churned in cycle by slushie machine before coming out of faucet: Cyclophosphamide

9. iFaucet sticker showing that high-tech slushie machine is made by Apple: Ifosfamide

10. Open chrome box being filled with water from faucet: Cyclophosphamide and ifosfamide require liver bioactivation (CYP-450)

11. Worker squirting mustard into chrome box: Cyclophosphamide and ifosfamide are nitrogen mustards

12. Net of pink cancer ribbon balls that come with child meal: Use cyclophosphamide and ifosfamide for lymphomas

13. Pink cancer ribbon balls are solid: Use cyclophosphamide and ifosfamide for solid tumors

14. Spilled ketchup mixing with water to create red stream: Use cyclophosphamide and ifosfamide for leukemia

15. Roomba vacuum cleaning food area: Use cyclophosphamide and ifosfamide for rheumatoid arthritis

16. Worker eating Froot Loops near water machine: Use cyclophosphamide and ifosfamide for lupus

17. Worker adding kidney beans to hamburger meat to reduce protein per serving: Use cyclophosphamide and ifosfamide for severe nephrotic syndrome

18. Multicolored balloons trapped in net: Cyclophosphamide and ifosfamide can cause myelosuppression

19. Bladder-shaped lemonade dispenser with pink cancer ribbon: Cyclophosphamide and ifosfamide can cause bladder cancer

20. Stack of wet diaries being blow dried: Cyclophosphamide and ifosfamide can cause syndrome of inappropriate antidiuretic hormone (SIADH) secretion

21. Lemonade infused with pomegranate clumps: Cyclophosphamide and ifosfamide can cause hemorrhagic cystitis

22. Mesh sponge preventing pomegranate clumps from coming out of spigot: Prevent hemorrhagic cystitis with Mesna (binds to toxic metabolites) and adequate hydration

23. Employee behaving bizarrely and wearing iFaucet hat: Ifosfamide can cause encephalopathy (neurotoxic)

24. Strange employee putting glue, peas, two toy cars glued together, and chicken nuggets into lemonade: Ifosfamide can cause Fanconi syndrome (glucose, phosphate, bicarbonate, and amino acids enter the urine)

25. Alien riding robotic mustang horse while shouting "Car mustang!": Carmustine

26. Smaller alien riding a shorter robotic mustang horse while shouting "Low mustang!": Lomustine

27. Open chrome boxes on mustang's backs: Require bioactivation by the liver cytochrome P-450

28. Two aliens on mustangs riding above smoke cloud: Nitrosoureas are able to cross the blood brain barrier to enter CNS

29. Two aliens wearing helmets shaped like brains with lots of protuberances: Use carmustine and lomustine for brain tumors

30. Dizzy man with ringing phone getting out of taxi: Nitrosoureas can cause ataxia, dizziness, and seizures

See Figure 9.10.4 - Cell Cycle Independent Cancer Drug Overview (Hem/Onc Pharmacology, Section 8, Page 201)

See Figure 9.10.5 - Histological Image of Hodgkin Lymphoma (Hem/Onc Pharmacology, Section 8, Page 203)

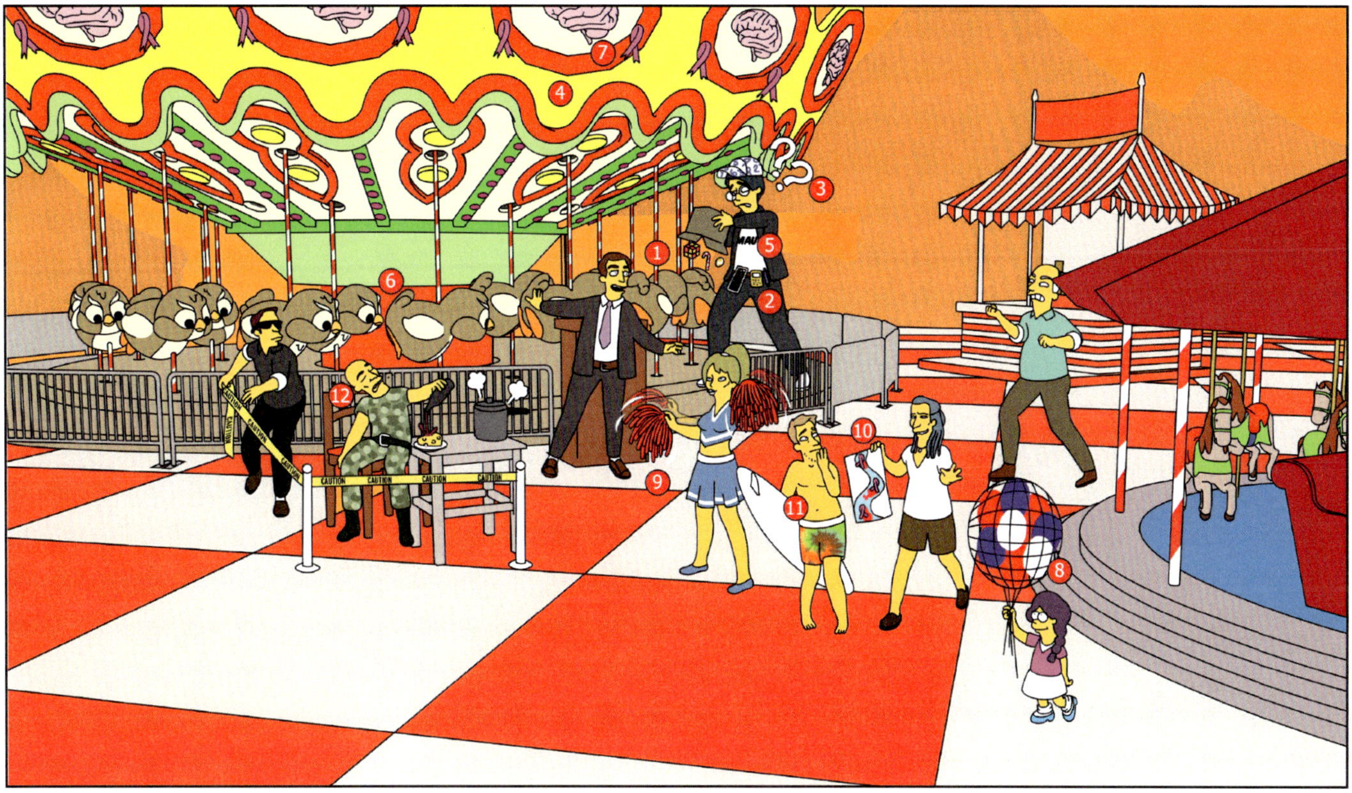

1. Pro carousel breaker sent to break competitor's carousel: Procarbazine

2. Pro carousel breaker is also accounting agent carrying calculator and abacus: Procarbazine is an alkylating agent

3. Accounting agent not knowing what he is doing: MOA unknown

4. Accounting agent stops carousel from spinning: Procarbazine halts the progression of the cell cycle

5. Pro carousel breaker wearing shirt that reads "Maui": Weak MAO inhibitor

6. Owl figurines on carousel: Use for Hodgkin lymphoma (HL)

7. Brain pictures with pink cancer ribbons on top of carousel: Can use for brain tumors

8. Girl with different colored balloons contained inside net: Can cause myelosuppression

9. Cheerleader shaking red pom poms shaped like lungs: Can cause pneumonitis

10. Artist selling painting of red river with pink cancer ribbons: Increased risk of developing leukemia

11. Surfer wearing tie-dye: Can cause a disulfiram-like reaction

12. Marine inside caution tape falling asleep after eating wine and cheese prepared in pressure cooker: Tyramine-induced hypertensive crisis with consumption of tyramine-rich foods

See Figure 9.10.4 - Cell Cycle Independent Cancer Drug Overview (Hem/Onc Pharmacology, Section 8, Page 201)

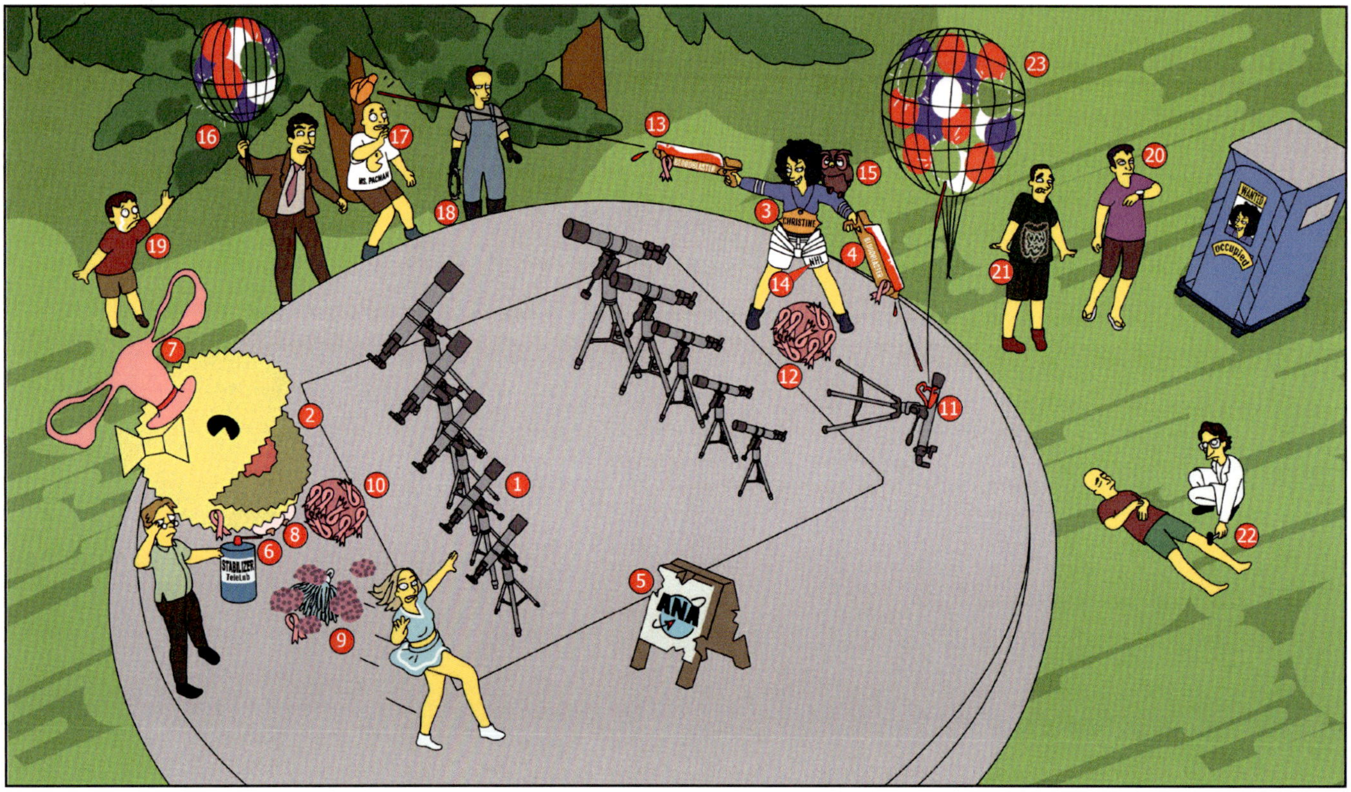

1. Telescopes organized on platform to look like metaphase of mitosis: Microtubule inhibitors stop mitosis

2. GIant, pixelated Ms. Pac-Man: Pacitaxel

3. Evil villain named Christine: Vincristine

4. VIllain holding blasters: Vinblastine

5. Damaged "ANA" sign for "Aeration and Aeronautics": Microtubule inhibitors prevent anaphase of mitosis

6. Ms. Pac-Man preventing astronomers from testing telescope lube marked with "stabilizer" label: Paclitaxel is a taxane that hyper stabilizes polymerized microtubules → mitotic spindle cannot break down (i.e. stuck in metaphase of mitosis)

7. Ms. Pac-Man wearing uterus had with bobbles for ovaries and pink cancer ribbon: Paclitaxel can be used for ovarian carcinomas

8. Ms. Pac-Man has breasts and is wearing pink cancer ribbon: Paclitaxel can be used for breast carcinomas

9. Lung-shaped pom poms decorated with pink cancer ribbons in large (non-small) pile of trash: Paclitaxel can be used for non-small cell lung cancer

10. Solid ball of pink cancer ribbons left onstage: Pacitaxel can be used for many solid tumors

11. Cristine hitting telescope tube with blasting gun: Vincristine and vinblastine are vinca alkaloids → prevent beta-tubulin from polymerizing into microtubules → mitotic spindle unformed → mitosis blocked

12. Solid ball of pink cancer ribbons on stage next to Christine: Use vincristine and vinblastine for solid tumors

13. Christine firing bloody water from blaster and hitting spectator's orange hat: Use vinblastine and vincristine for leukemias

14. Christine wearing NHL jersey: Use vinblastine and vincristine for non-Hodgkin lymphomas (NHL)

15. Christine carrying pet owl on shoulder: Use vinblastine and vincristine for Hodgkin lymphomas

16. Event organizer holding net of multicolored balloons: All microtubule inhibitors can cause myelosuppression

17. Bald man wearing Pac-Man shirt being blasted and losing his hat: All microtubule inhibitors can cause alopecia

18. Construction worker wearing gloves and knee-high boots while holding barbed wire: All microtubule inhibitors can cause peripheral neuropathy

19. Sensitive boy near Ms. Pac-Man crying because he wants balloon: Paclitaxel can cause hypersensitivity

20. Astronomer behind Christine impatiently waiting for bathroom while other astronomer uses it: Vincristine can cause constipation

21. Man paralyzed with fear outside bathroom after seeing "Wanted" poster with Christine's face: Vincristine can cause paralytic ileus

22. Doctor checking reflexes of person who fainted and not getting response: Vincristine can cause neurotoxicity including areflexia (i.e. decreased reflexes)

23. Christine blasting net of multicolored balloons with blaster gun: Vinblastine is used to blast the bone marrow before transplants

See Figure 9.10.4 - Cell Cycle Independent Cancer Drug Overview (Hem/Onc Pharmacology, Section 8, Page 203)

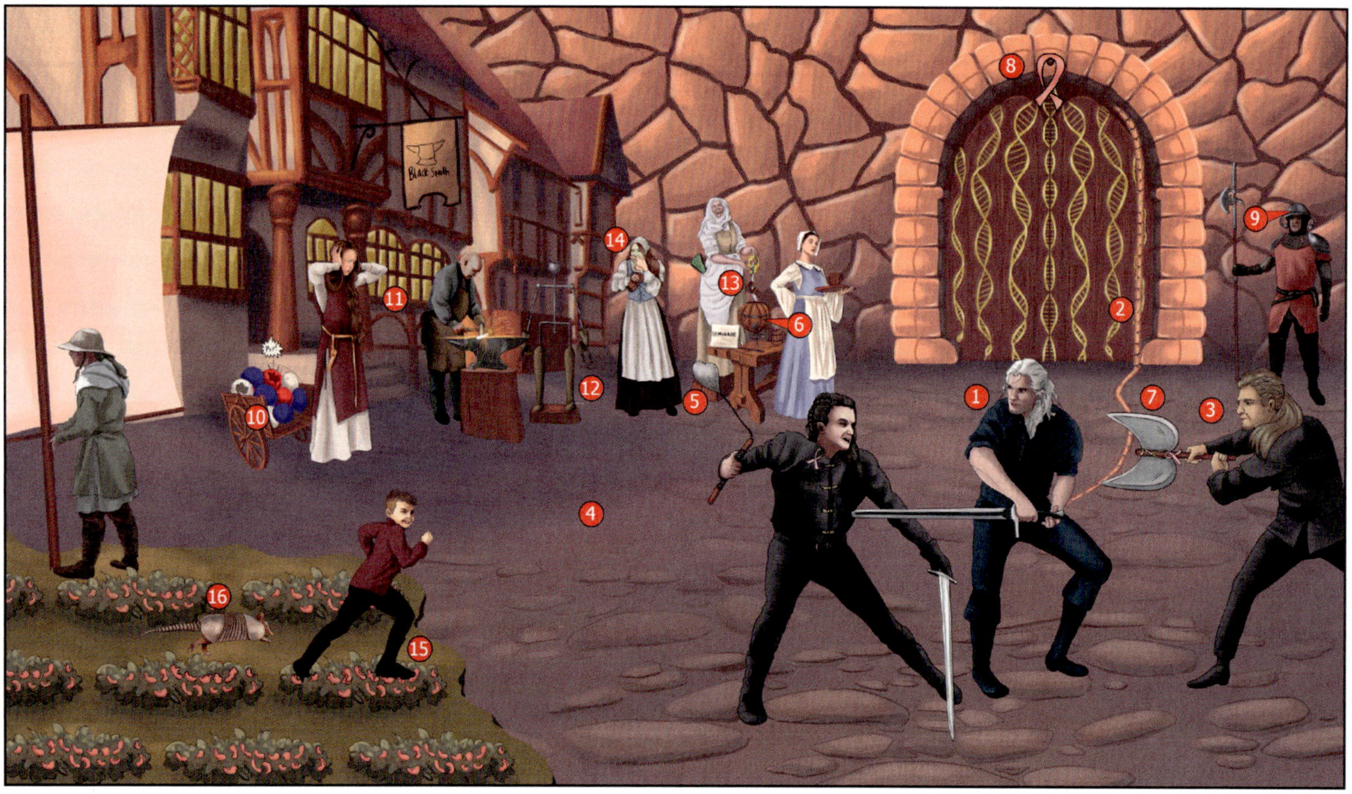

1. Platinum-haired Witcher character: Platinum-based agents

2. Plaited rope tied to door with DNA design to pull door down: Work by cross-linking DNA → decreased DNA replication

3. Puffins' Viking-style plaited hair: Names of platinum agents end with suffix, "-platin" (e.g., cisplatin, carboplatin, oxaliplatin)

4. No cell cycle diagram in image: Cell cycle independent

5. Ruffian wearing pink cancer ribbon and holding testicle-like ball and chain weapon: Use for testicular cancer

6. Lemonade dispenser shaped like a bladder with pink cancer ribbon: Use for bladder cancer

7. Second ruffian wearing pink cancer ribbon and holding lung-shaped ax: Use for lung cancer

8. Castle archway designed like ascending, transverse, and descending colon: Use for colorectal cancer

9. Guard wearing pink cancer ribbon and helmet shaped like uterus and ovaries: Use for ovarian cancer

10. Popped balloons of different colors contained within net: Can cause myelosuppression

11. Villager shielding her ears from blacksmith's loud noises: Can cause ototoxicity

12. Blacksmith's mannequin with gloves, knee-high socks, and crown of barbed wire: Can cause central and peripheral neuropathies

13. Elderly woman mistakenly putting two toy carts glued together, steak, peas, and glue into lemonade dispenser: Can cause Fanconi syndrome (glucose, phosphate, bicarbonate, and amino acids enter the urine)

14. Nauseous villager sick after drinking bad lemonade: Can cause nausea and vomiting

15. Village kid trampling kidney bean plants: Can cause nephrotoxicity

16. Garden owner putting up ship sails and training guard armadillo to protect kidney bean plants from village kid: Nephrotoxicity can be prevented with saline diuresis and amifostine (scavenger of free radicals)

See Figure 9.10.3 - Cell Cycle-Disrupting Cancer Drug Overview (Hem/Onc Pharmacology, Section 8, Page 201)

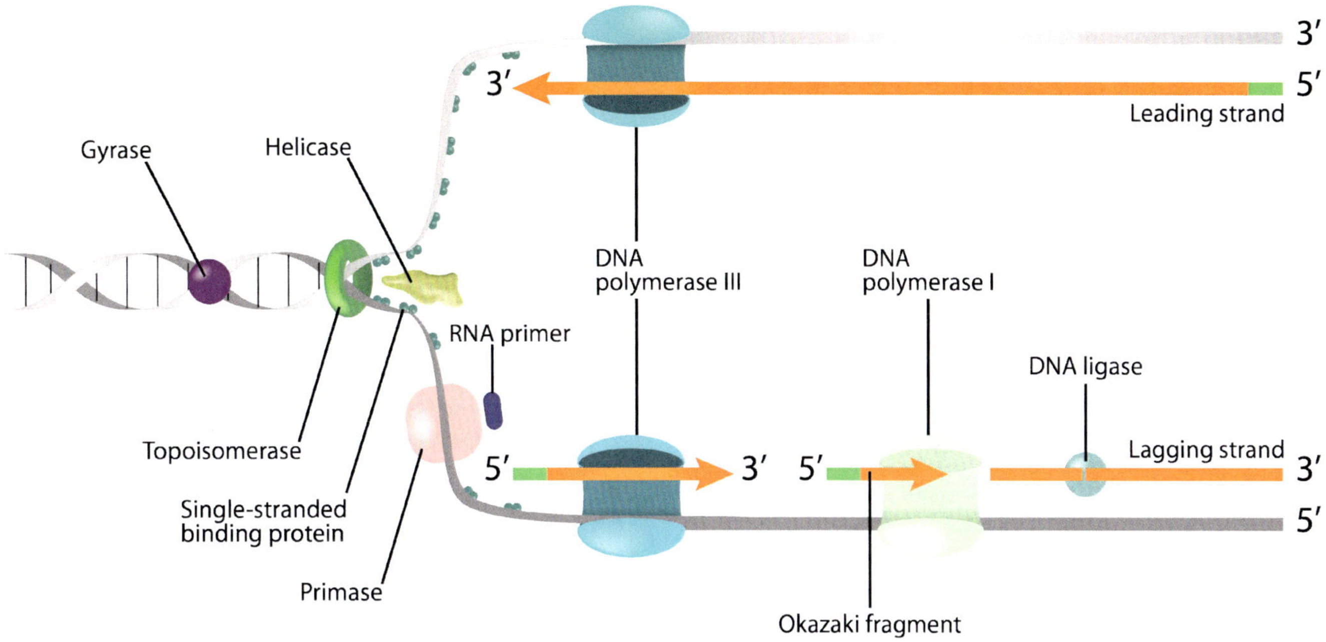

Figure 9.10.7 - DNA Replication

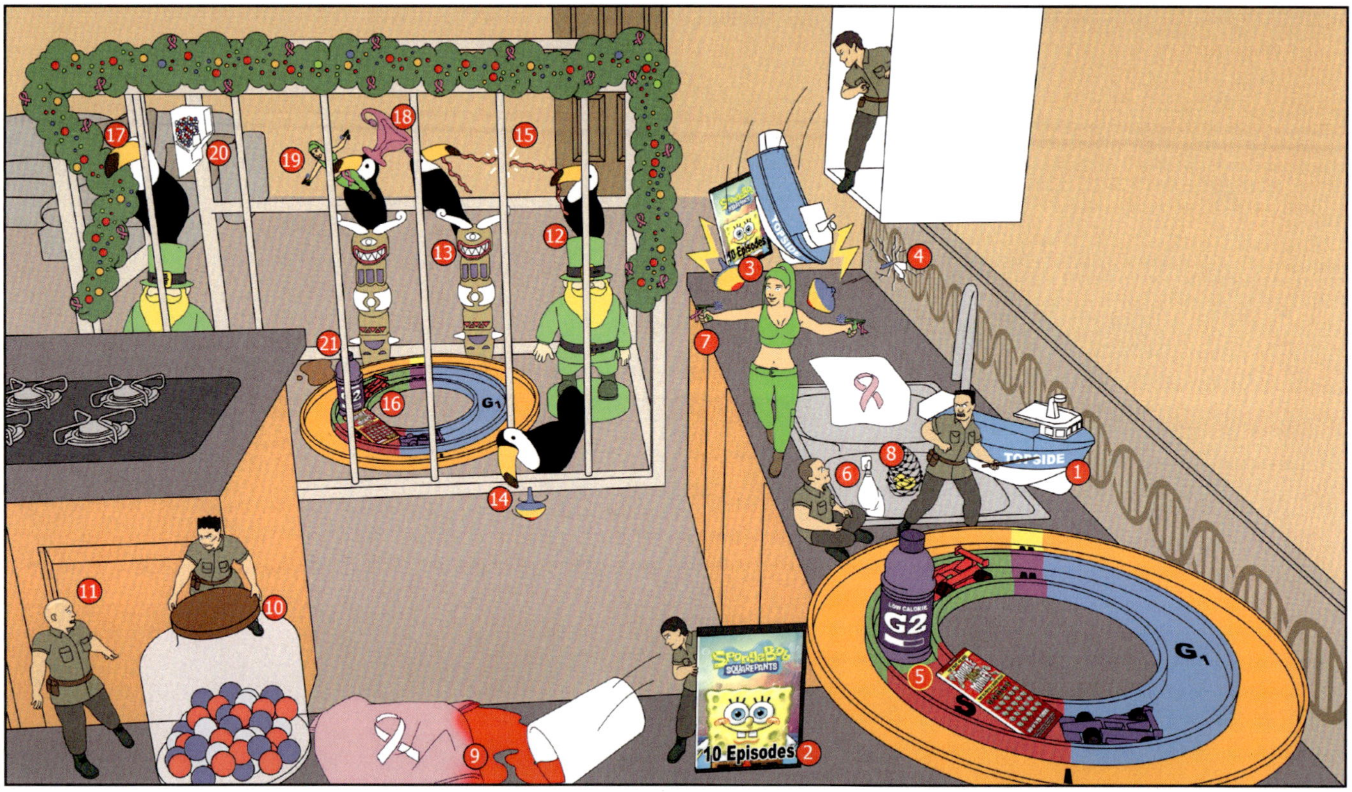

1. Toy ship with top marked "topside": Etoposide

2. Toy army man dragging DVD with ten SpongeBob episodes: Teniposide

3. "Topside" ship and ten episode DVD knocking over two tops and preventing them from spinning: Teniposide and etoposide inhibit topoisomerase II

4. "Topside" ship and ten episode DVD cracking backsplash of kitchen countertop decorated with DNA pattern: Causes dsDNA breaks

5. Hot Wheels racetrack with car stuck behind G2 Gatorade bottle and "double your money" lottery ticket: Causes cell cycle arrest in G2 and S phases

6. Pink cancer ribbon kitchen towel and two sponges hanging in sack like scrotum: Use etoposide and teniposide for testicular cancer

7. Large toy shooting tiny Koosh flingshot decorated with pink cancer ribbons: Use etoposide and teniposide for small cell lung cancer

8. Net with large knots hanging in kitchen sink: Use etoposide and teniposide for lymphomas

9. Red Kool-Aid spilling onto breast cancer awareness shirt: Use etoposide and teniposide for leukemias

10. Toy army man unable to open jar of multicolored candies: Etoposide and teniposide can cause myelosuppression

11. Bald toy soldier: Etoposide and teniposide can cause alopecia

12. Toucan perched on Irish gnome figurine: Irinotecan

13. Toucan perched on totem pole: Topotecan

14. Toucan poling one top and preventing it from spinning: Irinotecan and topotecan inhibit topoisomerase I

15. Two toucans breaking single-stranded necklace: Irinotecan and topotecan work by causing ssDNA breaks

16. Hot Wheels racetrack in toucan cage with toy car stuck behind G2 Gatorade bottle and "double your money" lottery ticket: Causes cell cycle arrest in G2 and S phases

17. Garland arranged like colon with pink cancer ribbons draped over toucan cage while toucan perched on Irish gnome tugs at it: Use irinotecan for colon cancer

18. Toucan perched on totem pole wearing uterus hat with bottles for ovaries and pink cancer ribbon: Use topotecan ovarian cancer

19. Toucan perched on totem pole holding tiny Koosh flingshot and Vicky Grimm figurine: Use topotecan for small cell lung cancers

20. Jammed toucan feeder unable to release multicolored pellets: Irinotecan and topotecan can cause severe myelosuppression

21. Brown puddle in toucan cage: Irinotecan and topotecan can cause diarrhea

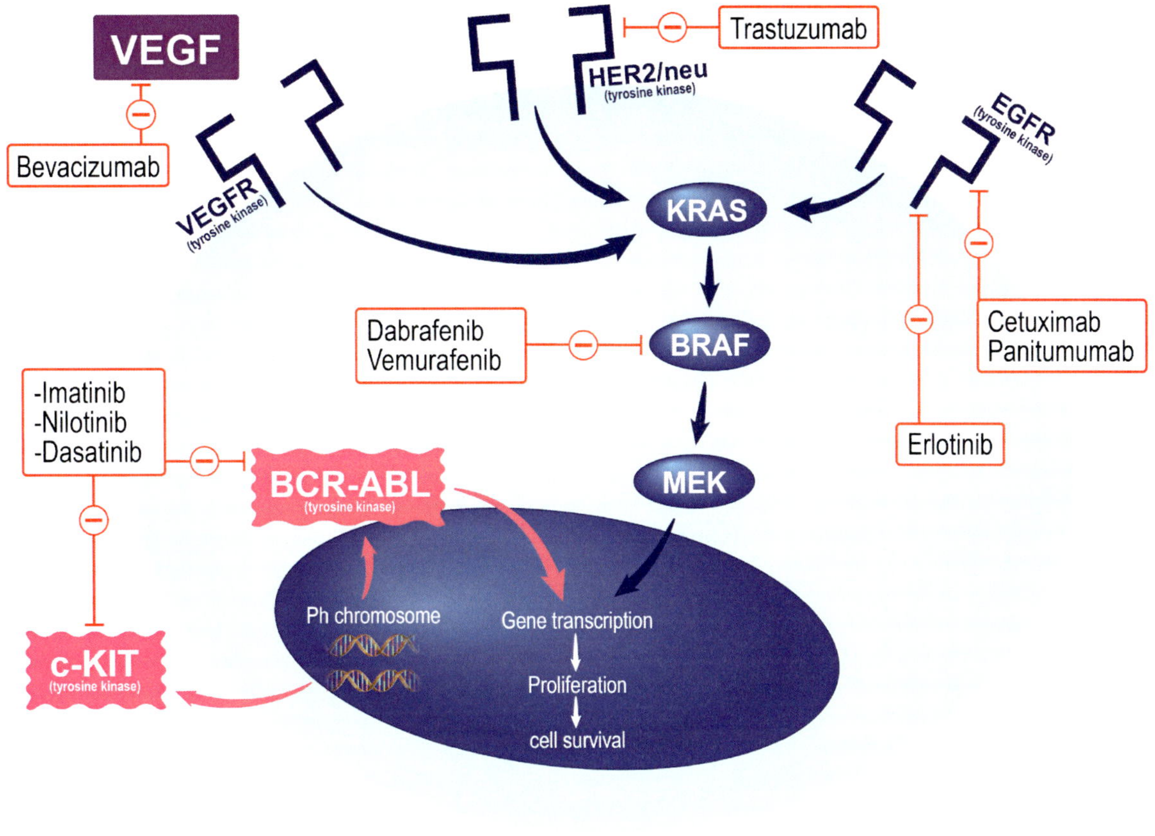

Figure 9.10.8 - Pharmacologic Anti-Cancer Mechanisms Through Tyrosine Kinase Pathway

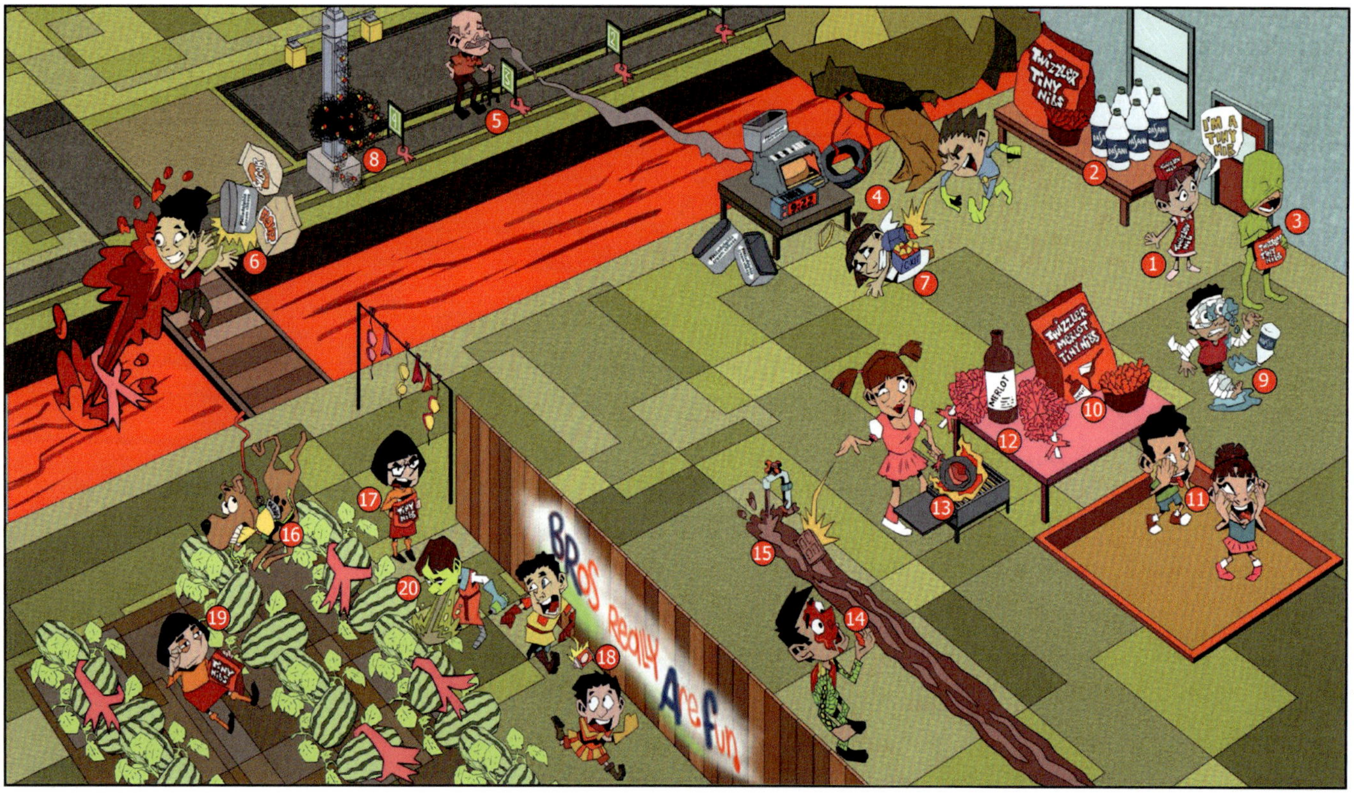

1. Toddler in Twizzler costume saying, "I'm a tiny nib": Imatinib

2. Dasani water bottles on table next to bowl of "tiny nib" candy: Dasatinib

3. Man eating tiny nibs while dressed in nylon suit: Nilotinib

4. Girl being prevented from checking on Easy Bake oven by kid throwing tiny nibs: Imatinib, dasatinib, and nilotinib inhibit the BCR-ABL tyrosine kinase

5. Old man with pink cancer ribbon walking next to river dyed red for Halloween: Use imatinib, dasatinib, and nilotinib for chronic myelogenous leukemia (CML)

6. Cute girl being blasted by fountain in red river while carrying Philadelphia cream cheese: Use imatinib, dasatinib, and nilotinib to treat BCR-ABL (Ph+) acute lymphoblastic leukemia (ALL)

7. Girl dressed as angel dropping candy kit on ground as kid throws tiny nibs at her: Imatinib, dasatinib, and nilotinib inhibit the c-KIT tyrosine kinase

8. Halloween garlands that look like spider webs decorated with candy corns from girl's candy kit: Use imatinib, dasatinib, adn nilotinib for GI stromal tumors (GISTs)

9. Kid dressed as mummy with toilet paper costume soaking up water around eyes and ankles: Imatinib, dasatinib, and nilotinib can cause fluid retention (periorbital and ankle most common)

10. Merlot-flavored tiny nibs: Erlotinib

11. Kids exfoliating faces in sandbox next to table with merlot tiny nibs: Erlotinib is a EGFR inhibitor (EGFRi)

12. Large (not-small) pom poms with pink cancer ribbon: Erlotinib can be used for non-small cell lung cancer (NSCLC)

13. Frying pan decorated with pink cancer ribbon: Erlotinib can be used for pancreatic cancer

14. Guy in snakeskin costume with red paint on face, chest and back eating merlot tiny nibs: Erlotinib can cause xerosis and acneiform rash

15. Brown chocolate stream on ground: Erlotinib can cause diarrhea

16. Dog nibbling on bra with "Debra" name tag: Dabrafenib

17. Twin girls dressed as Velma nibbling on candy: Vemurafenib

18. Twin girl dressed as Velma preventing three hooligans dressed up as medieval "SIRs" from spray-painting "Bros Really Are FUn" on fence: Dabrafenib and vemurafenib are small molecule inhibitors of the BRAF oncogene (a serine-threonine kinase)

19. Twin girl dressed as Velma being woken up by dog nibbling on bra in melon garden: Dabrafenib and vemurafenib can be used for metastatic melanoma

20. Hooligan dressed as medieval "SIR" vomiting at sight of dog: Dabrafenib and vemurafenib can cause nausea and vomiting

See Figure 9.10.8 - Pharmacologic Anti-Cancer Mechanisms Through Tyrosine Kinase Pathway (Hem/Onc Pharmacology, Section 16, Page 216)

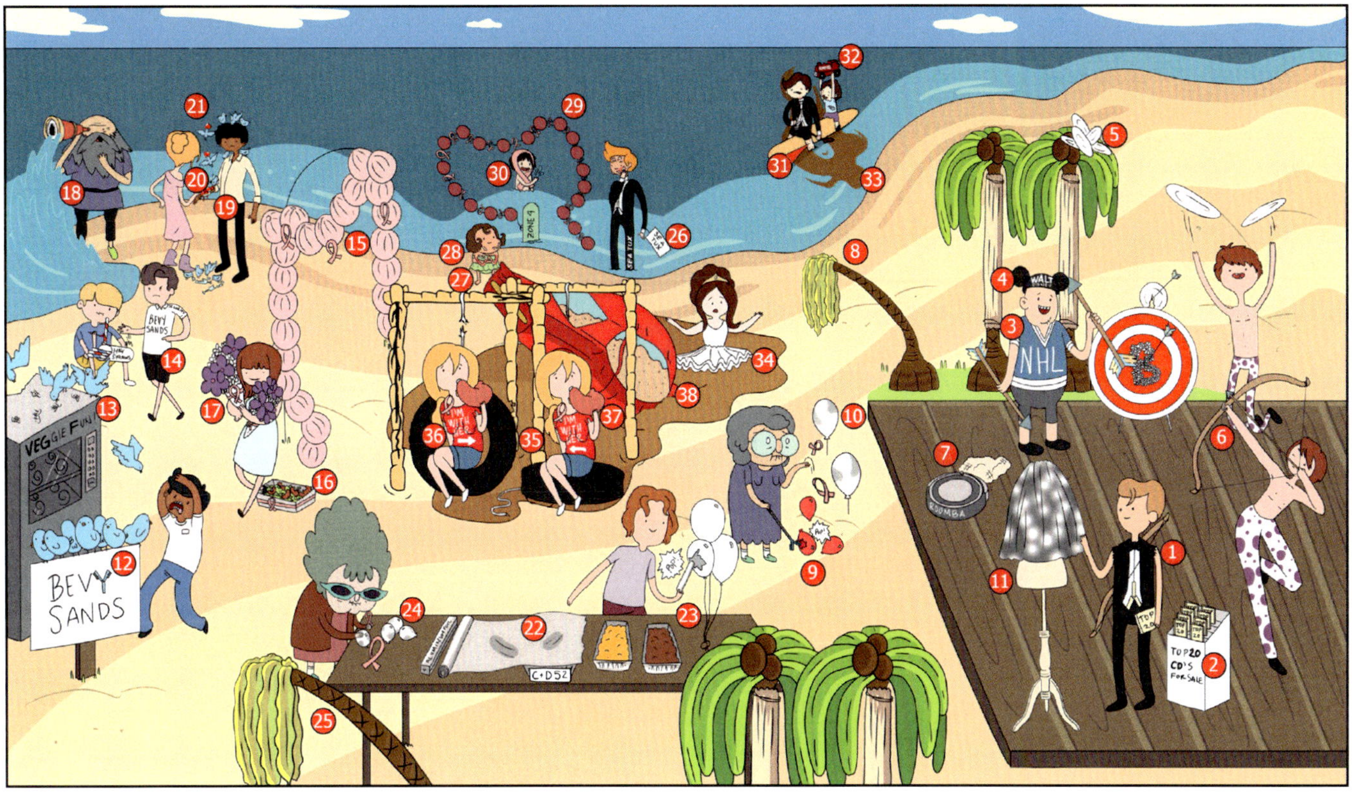

1. Hillbilly groom wearing tux with ripped sleeves: Rituximab

2. Target sign with "B" on it near groom wearing antibody-shaped cummerbund and selling "Top 20" CDs: Rituximab is an anti-CD20 monoclonal antibody (mab) → target B-cells

3. Hillbilly dad wearing NHL jersey and holding large arrows: Use rituximab for non-Hodgkin lymphoma

4. Hillbilly dad wearing Walt Disney World hat and holding large arrows: Use rituximab for Waldenstrom macroglobulinemia (a type of NHL)

5. Broken and stuck plates in tree: Use rituximab for thrombotic thrombocytopenic purpura (TTP)

6. Plate spinning cousin with purple polka dot pants getting plates stuck in tree: Use rituximab for thrombotic thrombocytopenic purpura (TTP)

7. Roomba vacuum on dance floor: Use rituximab for rheumatoid arthritis (RA)

8. Dying palm tree with unwrapped trunk: Use rituximab for multiple sclerosis (MS)

9. Old woman picking up red balloons with tongs and popping them: Use rituximab for autoimmune hemolytic anemia (AIHA)

10. Old lady tying pink cancer ribbons to white balloons with smudged writing on them: Use rituximab for chronic lymphocytic leukemia (CCL)

11. Bride's polka dot veil on mannequin: Rituximab can cause an increased risk of progressive multifocal leukoencephalopathy (PML)

12. "Bevy Sands" bench sign with birds perched on it: Bevacizumab

13. "Veggie Fun" vending machine with birds pecking at it angrily because it's empty: Bevacizumab is a monoclonal antibody (mab) → targets and inhibits vascular endothelial growth factor (VEGF)

14. Bevy Sands enforcer confiscating red and blue straws being sold by kid: Bevacizumab inhibits angiogenesis by inhibiting VEGF

15. Pink cancer balloons arranged like descending colon with pink cancer ribbons: Use bevacizumab for colorectal cancer

16. Kidney beans decorated with pink cancer ribbons dumped on beach: Use bevacizumab for renal cell carcinoma

17. Lung-shaped bouquets of huge flowers with pink cancer ribbons: Use bevacizumab for non-small cell lung cancer

18. Elderly man near ocean whose telescope is destroyed by wave: Use bevacizumab for wet age-related macular degeneration

19. Guest hemorrhaging after cutting arm: Bevacizumab can cause hemorrhage

20. Guest unsuccessfully wrapping bleeding arm while birds peck at wound: Bevacizumab can cause impaired wound healing

21. Bevy Sands birds carrying off bloody clots of gauze from wounded man: Bevacizumab can cause blood clots

22. Tube of aluminum foil on table: Alemtuzumab

23. Kid using aluminum shiv to pop white balloons next to "C D 52" tray (Core Dish 52): Alemtuzumab is a monoclonal antibody (mab) against CD-52 → targets mature lymphocytes

24. Woman decorating table with smudged white balloons and pink cancer ribbons: Use alemtuzumab for chronic lymphocytic leukemia (CCL)

25. Dying, unwrapped palm tree next to table: Use alemtuzumab for multiple sclerosis (MS)

26. Groomsman on beach wearing wetsuit sea tuxedo: Cetuximab

27. Groomsman's daughter in pain from sunburns and wearing tutu: Panitumumab

28. Girl's skin peeling due to sunburns: Cetuximab and panitumumab are monoclonal antibodies (mab) → target epidermal growth factor receptor (EGFR)

29. Safe-swim zone 4 marked with buoys arranged like descending colon and decorated with pink cancer ribbons: Use cetuximab and panitumumab for stage IV colorectal cancer (wild-type KRAS)

30. Kid with pink cancer ribbon towel wrapped around head and neck: Use cetuximab and panitumumab for head and neck cancer

31. Groomsman in sea tux developing rash on uncovered legs: Cetuximab and panitumumab can cause a rash

32. Son holding up toy ammo train with liver-shaped wet spot from seawater on shirt: Cetuximab and panitumumab can cause elevated liver function tests (LFTs)

33. Muddy brown water in ocean: Cetuximab and panitumumab can cause diarrhea

34. Bride trashing tutu-style dress by jumping into mud puddle: Trastuzumab

35. Two women wearing "I'm with her" shirts sitting on two tire swings with one swing broken after bride pulls it down: Trastuzumab is a monoclonal antibody (mab) against the HER-2 (tyrosine kinase receptor)

36. Text on "I'm with her" shirts positioned over woman's breasts: Use trastuzumab for HER-2 + breast cancer

37. Women drinking from stomach-shaped water canteens with pink cancer ribbons on them: Use trastuzumab for gastric cancer

38. Broken-down car bulging with sand: Trastuzumab can cause dilated cardiomyopathy

See Figure 9.10.3 - Cell Cycle-Disrupting Cancer Drug Overview (Hem/Onc Pharmacology, Section 8, Page 203)

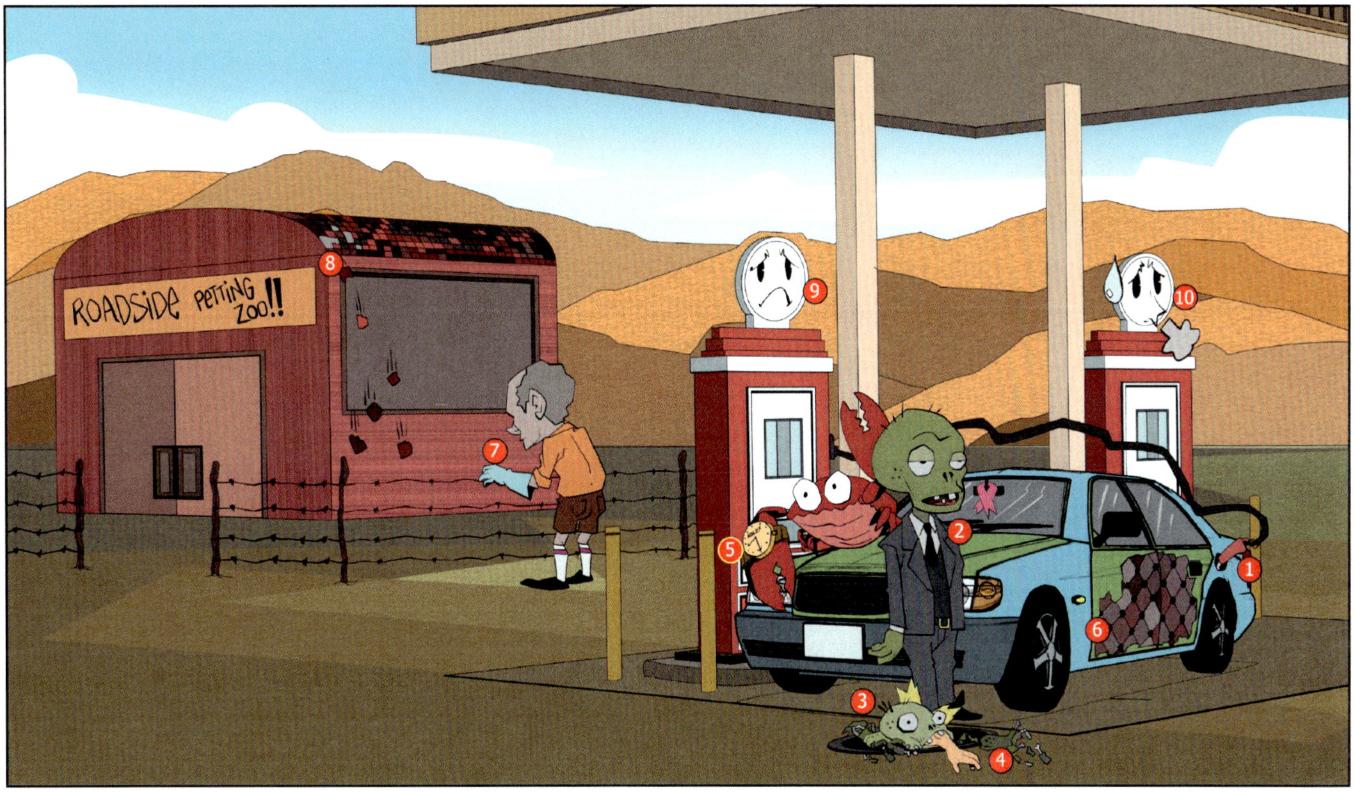

1. Zombie filling car with gas: Carfilzomib

2. Zombie getting bored while waiting for tank to fill up: Bortezomib

3. First zombie stomping on zombie that is crawling out of sewer while digesting muscly, human arm: Proteasome inhibitor

4. Zombie dying in sewer: Arrest cell growth at the G2-M phase and causes apoptosis

5. Zombie's pet crab with Rolex watch: Use for multiple myeloma (CRAB findings: Calcium (elevated), renal failure, anemia, and bone lesions)

6. Net-like car frame with knots exposed by peeling car paint in globe design: Use for mantle cell lymphoma

7. Rancher wearing gloves and knee-high socks to work on barbed wire fence: Can cause peripheral neuropathy

8. Shingles falling off petting zoo rooth: Can cause reactivation of herpes zoster (shingles)

9. Worn out gas pump: Carfilzomib can cause fatigue

10. Second gas pump running out of breath: Carfilzomib can cause dyspnea

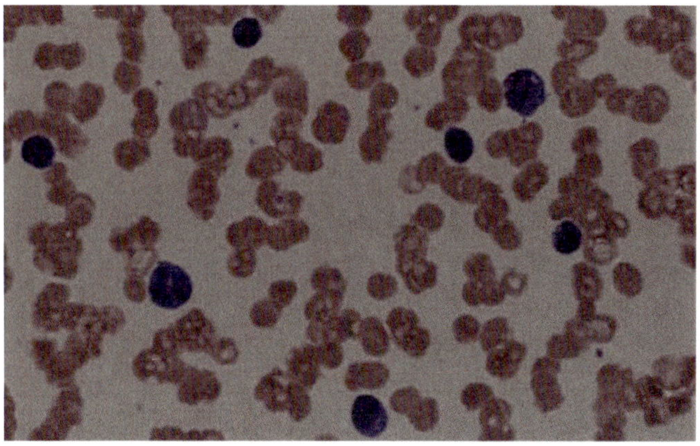

Figure 9.10.9 - Peripheral Blood Smear Showing Rouleaux Formation

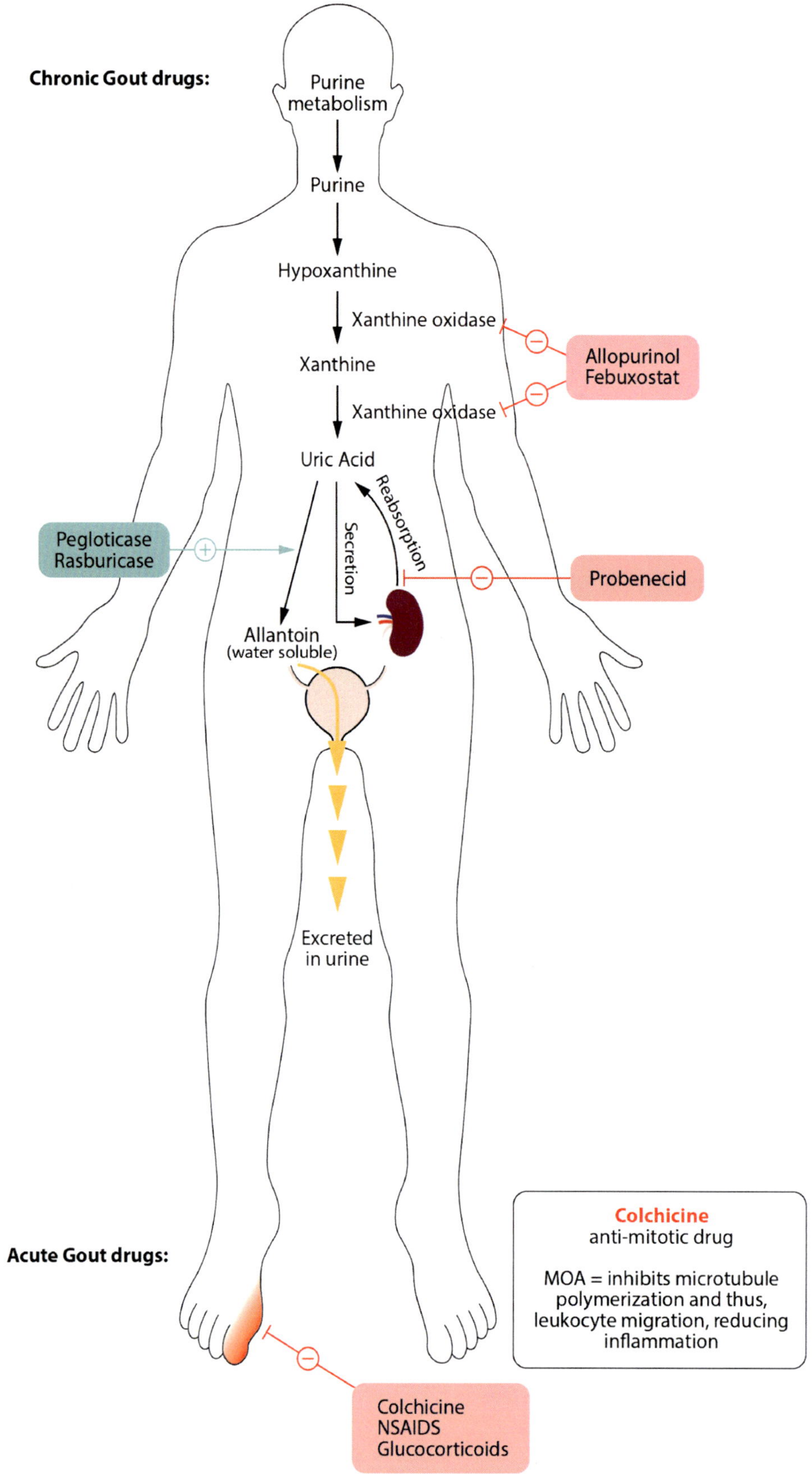

Figure 9.10.10 - Gout and Tumor Lysis Nephropathy Drug Overview

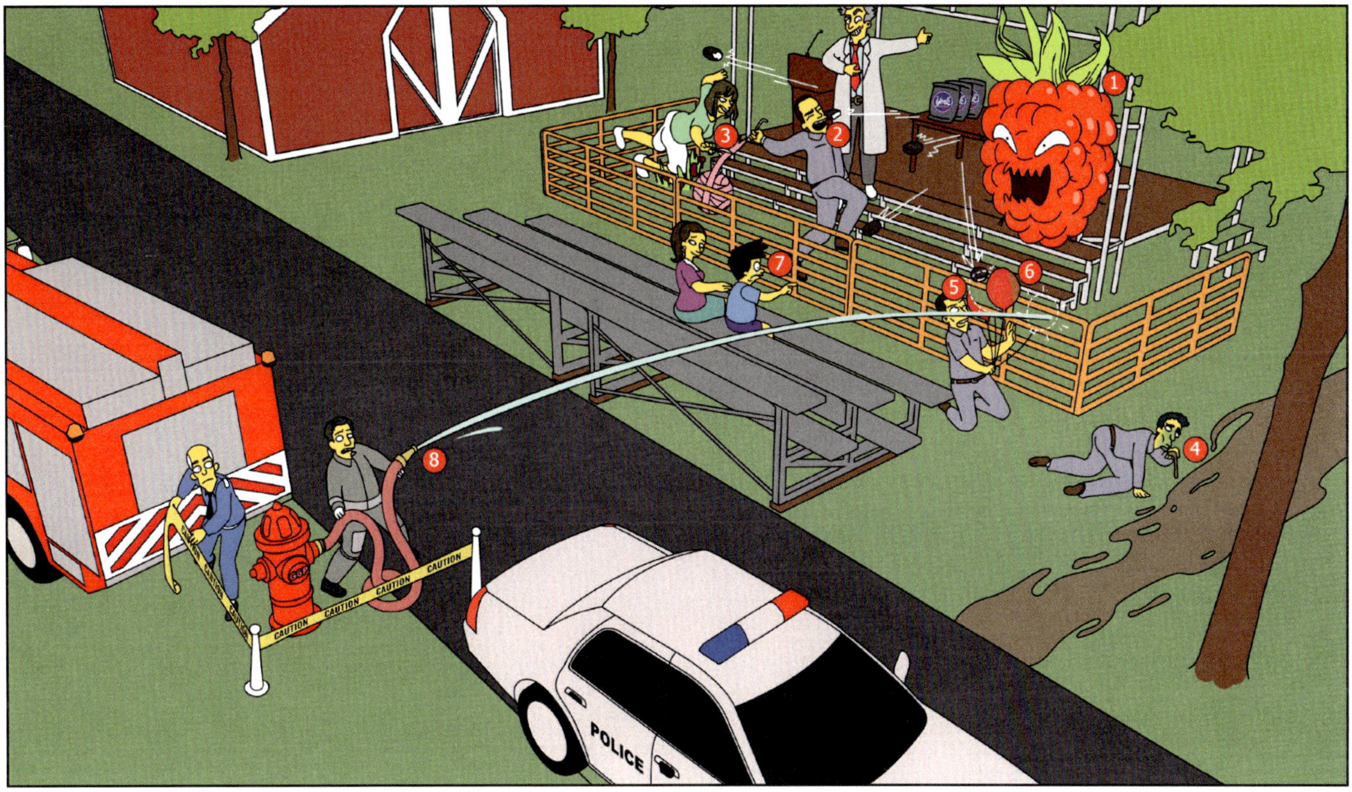

1. Raspberry: Rasburicase

2. Mutant raspberry attacking worker holding Allen wrench by throwing York patties at him: Rasburicase is a recombinant uricase that catalyzes metabolism of uric acid to allantoin

3. Mutant raspberry attacking lady who is cutting pink cancer ribbons from ribbon ball, causing her to crush kidney bean plant: Rasburicase can be used to treat and prevent tumor-lysis nephropathy

4. Worker drinking from muddy brown river and getting sick: Can cause GI toxicity (nausea, vomiting, diarrhea)

5. Raspberry throwing York patties at red balloons and popping them: Can cause hemolysis

6. Worker with balloons bumping into iron fence, causing iron rust to turn balloons brown: Can cause methemoglobinemia

7. Sensitive boy crying: Can cause hypersensitivity reaction

8. Jet of water from fire hydrant behind caution tape, popping red balloon: Avoid in glucose-6-phosphate dehydrogenase (G6PD) deficiency

Section 1 - Acetaminophen

Arachidonic acid pathway and drugs

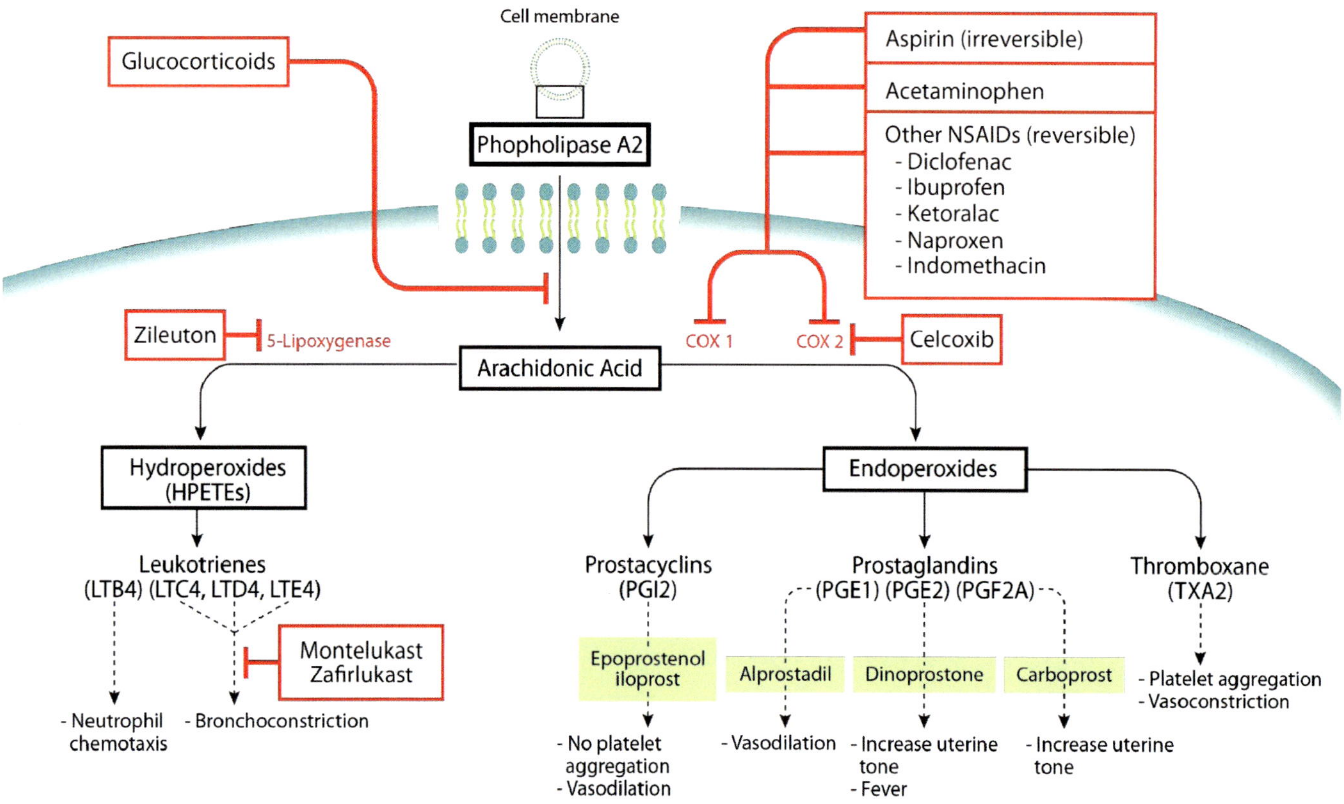

Figure 9.11.1 - Pharmacologic Effects on Arachidonic Acid Synthesis

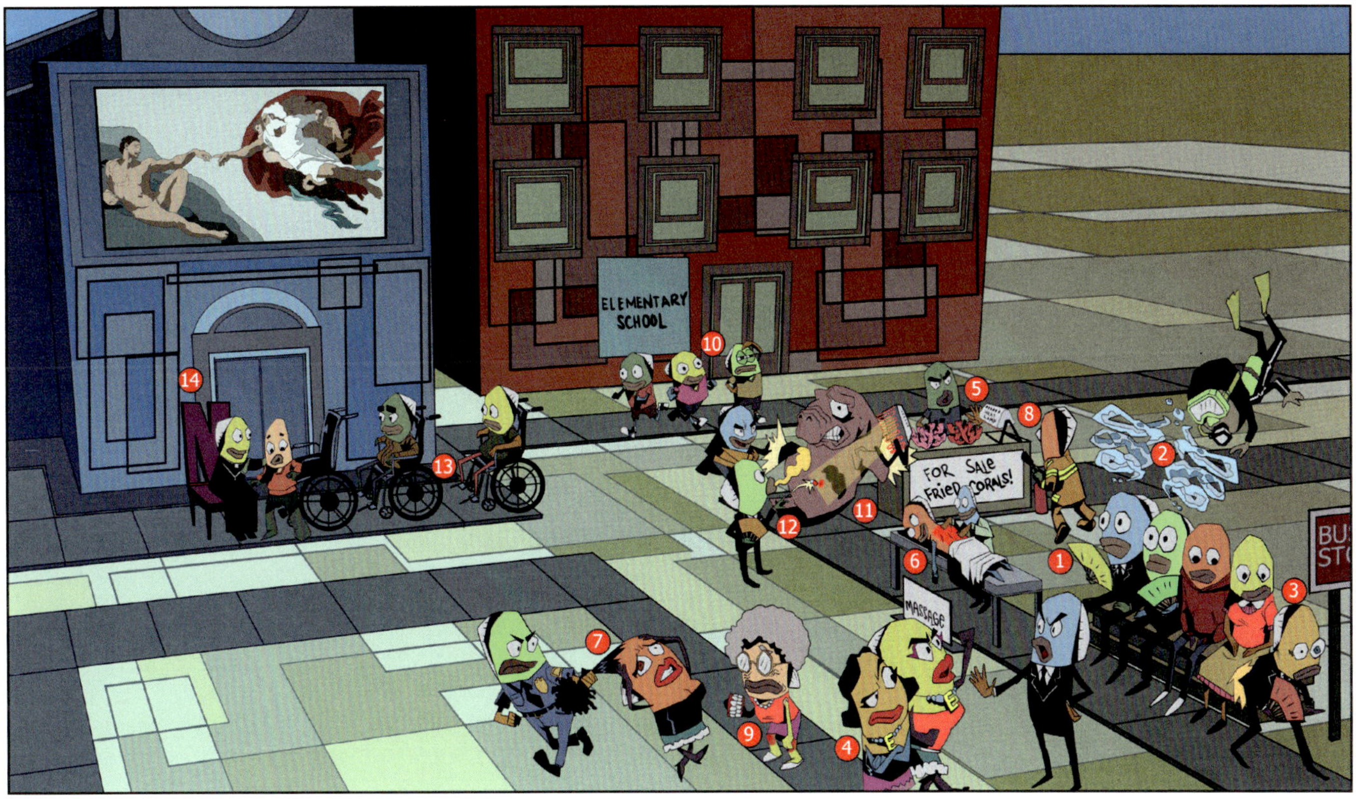

1. Sitting businessmen fanning themselves: Acetaminophen

2. Cyclones from fans block the diver's view: Inhibits cyclooxygenase

3. Guy sitting on bench is pushed aside: Inactive peripherally

4. Two prostitutes wearing big, gold "E" necklace being rejected by businessmen: Decreases synthesis of PGE_2 in the hypothalamus

5. Heat lamp: Used to treat fever

6. Relaxed red guy is getting a massage: Use as an analgesic

7. Prostitute has headache from pulled hair: Used to treat tension headaches

8. Fireman trying to extinguish heat lamp, but it's not working: Not used as an anti-inflammatory

9. Old prostitute with knee pain: Used to treat osteoarthritis

10. Kids not under a ray of sunshine: Does not cause Reye syndrome in children

11. Heat lamp burns sea cow's liver spot, making it black: Side effects of overdose include hepatic necrosis

12. Businessman burns sea cow near his liver spot: Side effects of overdose include forming toxic tissue byproducts in liver

13. Atrophied glutes and thighs of men in wheelchairs: Side effects of overdose include depleted glutathione

14. N-shaped throne sitting underneath copy of the Sistine Chapel: Overdoses are treated with N-acetylcysteine (replenishes glutathione)

See Figure 9.11.1 - Pharmacologic Effects on Arachidonic Acid Synthesis (Musculoskeletal Pharmacology, Section 1, Page 223)

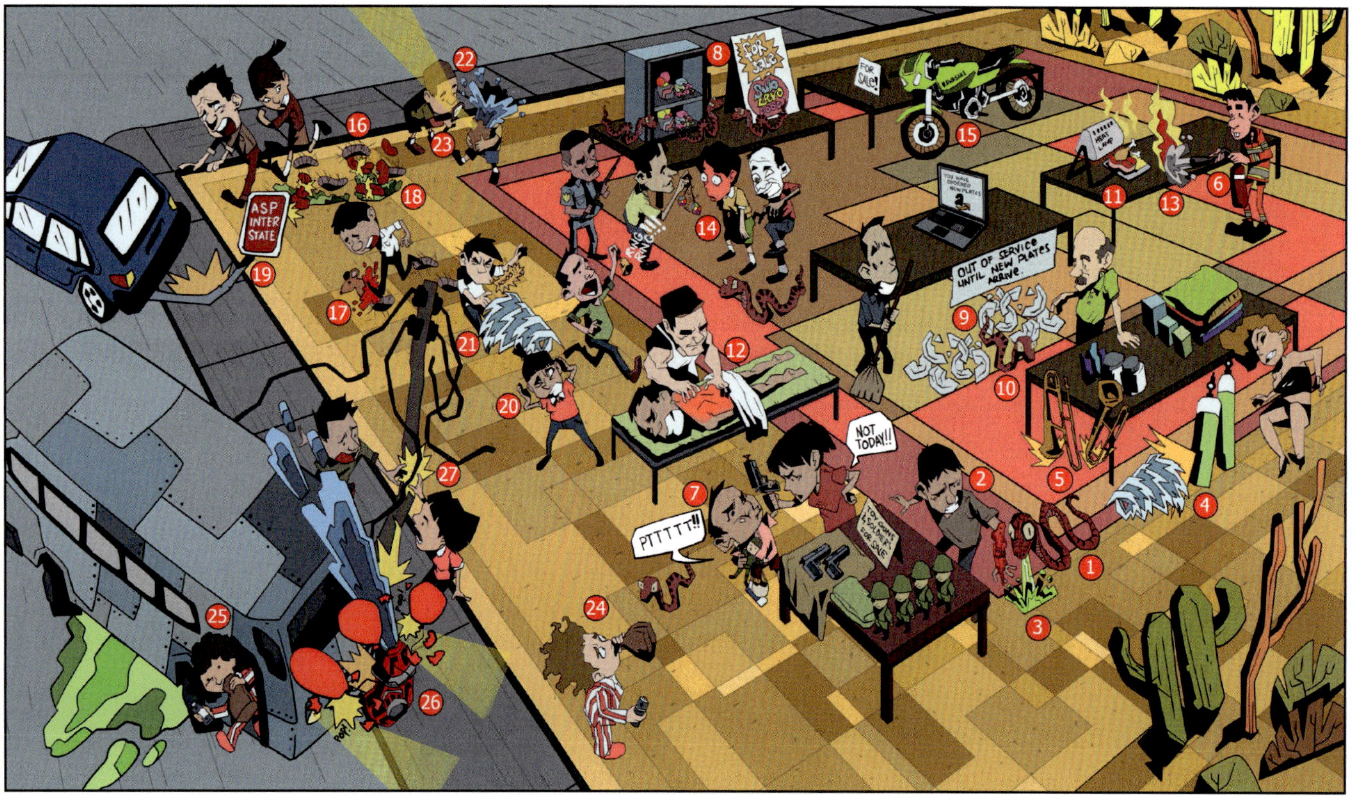

1. Asp: Aspirin

2. Bitten guys' blood from asp bite getting on his watch: Increases bleeding time

3. Asp splitting green acid: Weak acid

4. Cyclone from asp knocks over oxygen tanks: Irreversibly inhibits cyclooxygenase via covalent acetylation

5. Two trombones and prostitutes knocked over by cyclone: Decreases synthesis of TXA2 and prostaglandins

6. Fire extinguisher held by screwy man: Is an NSAID

7. Paratrooper making "PTT" sound and mom telling him, "Not Today": No effects on PT or PTT

8. Sub-Zero cold treat/drink stand: Metabolized through zero-order elimination pharmacokinetics

9. "Out of service until new plates arrive" sign next to broken platelets: The effects of aspirin last until new platelets are produced

10. Small asp slithers around broken plates: At low doses, it decreases platelet aggregation (decreases risk of clot formation)

11. Heat lamp: At intermediate doses it can be used to treat fever

12. Guy getting massage: At intermediate doses, it is an analgesic

13. Fireman uses fire extinguisher on heat lamp: Is an anti-inflammatory

14. Hypnotist makes guy flushed with a colorful gem on rope next to man with nightstick: Can prevent flushing caused by gemfibrozil and niacin

15. Kawasaki motorcycle: Used as part of the treatment for Kawasaki disease

16. Footprints or holes left from running: May cause gastric ulcers

17. Runner squishing rodent: Can lead to GI bleeding

18. Couple tramples kidney bean plants: Can lead to acute kidney injury

19. "Asp interstate" sign hit by car crushing kidney plants: Can lead to interstitial nephritis

20. Girl covering ears from loud bell: Can cause tinnitus

21. Cyclone makes guy cough and wheeze: Can cause allergic reactions

22. Ray of sun shines on kid: Can cause Reye syndrome in children treated with aspirin for viral infection

23. Burning kid burns sack on kid and water splashes in face: Reye syndrome can be neurotoxic and lead to cerebral edema

24. Battery vendor lady in pajamas hyperventilating: Can cause respiratory alkalosis (early)

25. Hyperventilating battery bus driver gets out of bus, spewing green acid: Can transition to a mixed metabolic acidosis-respiratory alkalosis (later)

26. Fire hydrant spraying water, causing red balloons to pop: May induce hemolysis in patients with G6PD deficiency

27. Falling power lines causing couple to let go of hands: Overdose may cause uncoupling of the electron transport chain

See Figure 9.11.1 - Pharmacologic Effects on Arachidonic Acid Synthesis (Musculoskeletal Pharmacology, Section 1, Page 223)

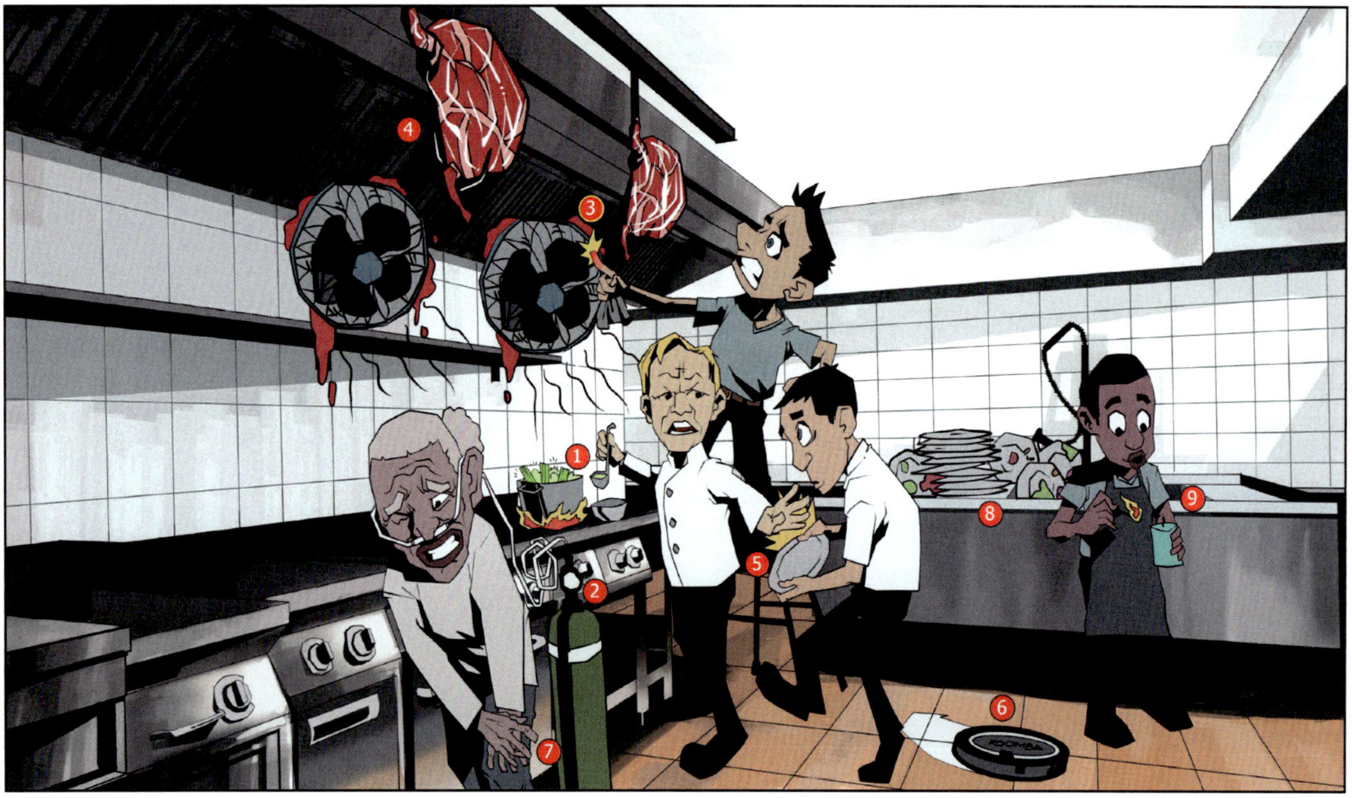

1. Celery soup: Celecoxib

2. Oxygen tank with two restricted cyclone fans used to cool chefs: Reversibly and selectively inhibits the cyclooxygenase isoform 2 (COX-2)

3. Red buildup on cyclone fans and injured red thumb of technician: COX-2 is found in inflammatory cells and the vascular endothelium and mediates inflammation and pain

4. Unused, stomach-shaped bags of meat: Does not have the corrosive effects of other NSAIDs on the gastrointestinal lining (spares COX-1 inhibition)

5. Chef spares plate and instead wants to use bowl for celery soup: Spares platelet function (TXA2 production is dependent of COX-1)

6. Roombas cleaning kitchen: Used to treat rheumatoid arthritis

7. Old chef holding her knee: Used to treat osteoarthritis

8. Dirty, unorganized, stack of plates: Increases the risk of thrombosis

9. Dishwasher man with match: Can cause sulfa allergy

See Figure 9.11.1 - Pharmacologic Effects on Arachidonic Acid Synthesis (Musculoskeletal Pharmacology, Section 1, Page 223)

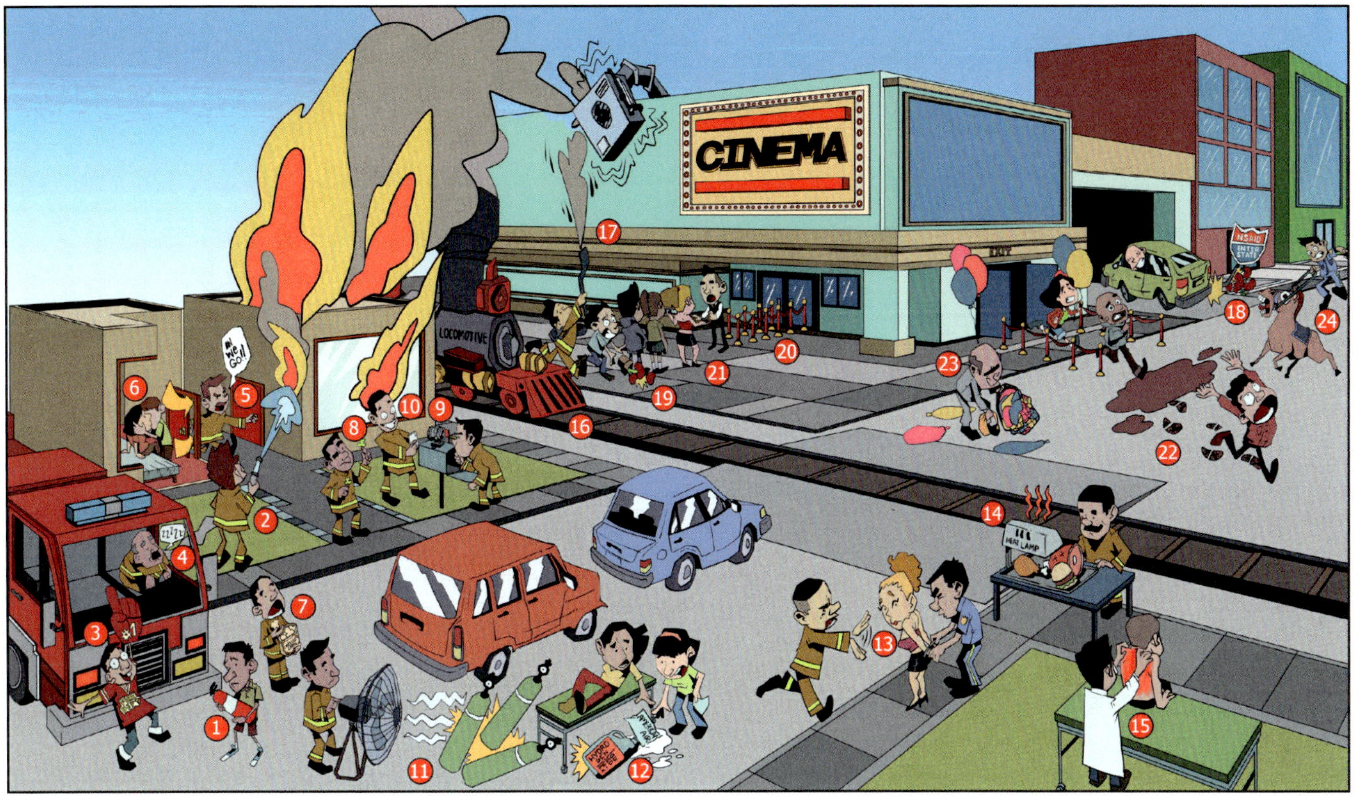

1. Scrawny guy holding fire extinguisher: NSAIDs

2. Fireman spraying water on burning building: Anti-inflammatory

3. Professional fan: Ibuprofen

4. Napping fire chief: Naproxen

5. Team leader shouting, "In we go!": Indomethacin

6. Making out couple behind closed door: Indomethacin is used to close a PDA

7. Firefighter eating kettle corn: Ketorolac

8. Distracted fireman with two four-leaf clovers: Diclofenac

9. Mailbox camera: Meloxicam

10. Pyro fireman taking selfie: Piroxicam

11. Fan blowing little cyclone blowing over three oxygen tanks: Cyclooxygenase (COX) 1 and 2

12. American Airlines (AA) ticket dissolved by peroxide next to oxygen tanks: Cyclooxygenase converts arachidonic acid into cyclic endoperoxides

13. Prostitute getting arrested: Blocks prostaglandin synthesis

14. Heat lamp: Use for fever

15. Paramedic applies ointment to burn victim's back: Use as an analgesic

16. Locomotive quickly passing through city: Increases leukotriene production

17. Spazzing air filtration system next to locomotive: Can cause bronchospasm

18. Guy backing out with car and hits the interstate sign which crushes kidney bean plant: Can cause tubulointerstitial nephritis

19. Firefighter bumping into guy who drops his kidney bean plant in front of cinema: Can cause renal ischemia

20. Afferent ropes pushed tightly together: NSAIDs cause vasoconstriction of the afferent arteriole

21. Prostitute getting blocked near closed off theater ropes: NSAIDs block prostaglandins resulting in vasoconstriction of the afferent arteriole

22. Muddy ulcer shaped footprints: Can cause gastric ulcers

23. Different colored balloons popped and being picked up: Can cause aplastic anemia

24. Mounted police officer bucked off his horse while still holding on reigns: Can cause increased plasma renin

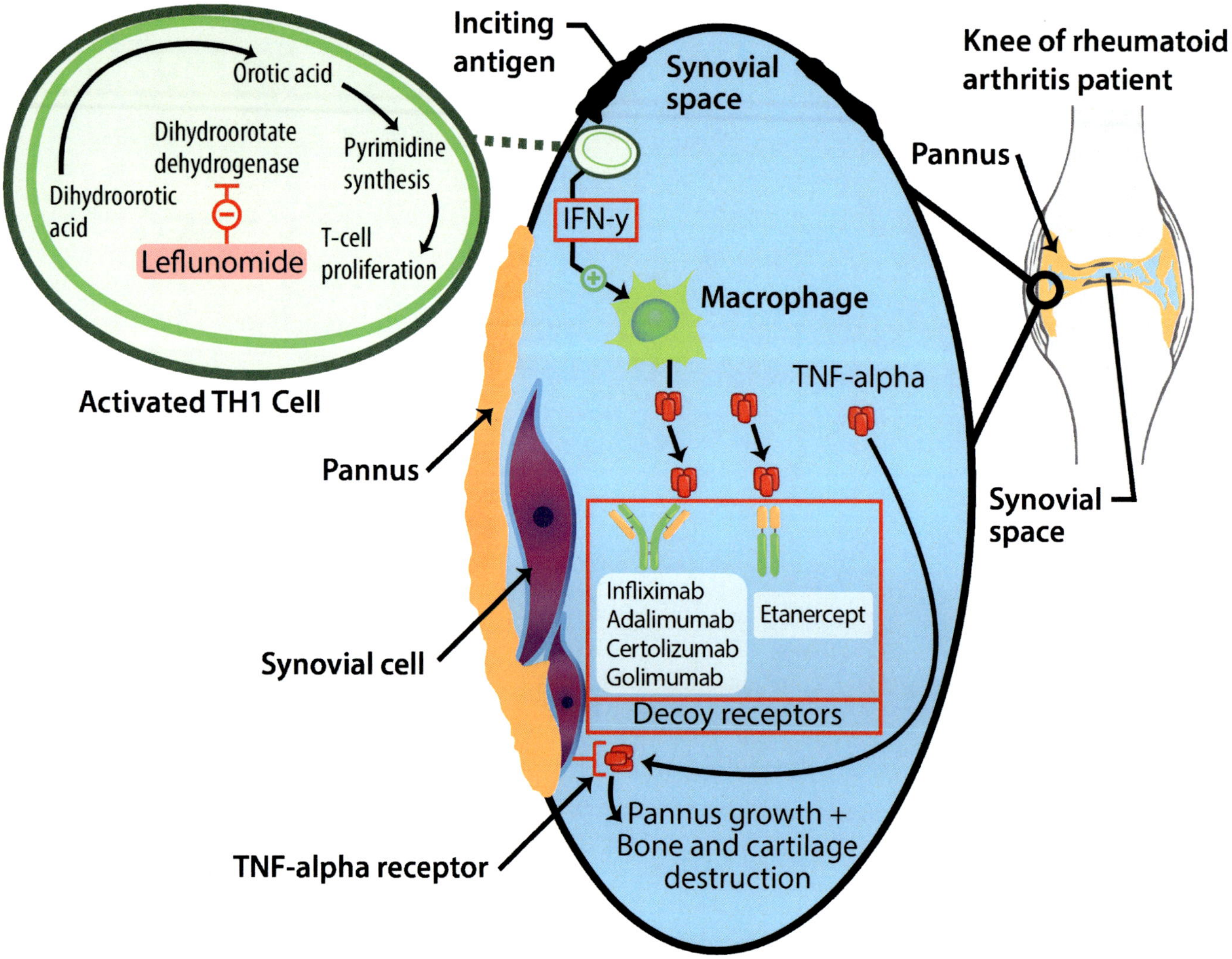

Figure 9.11.2 - TNF Inhibitors and Leflunomide

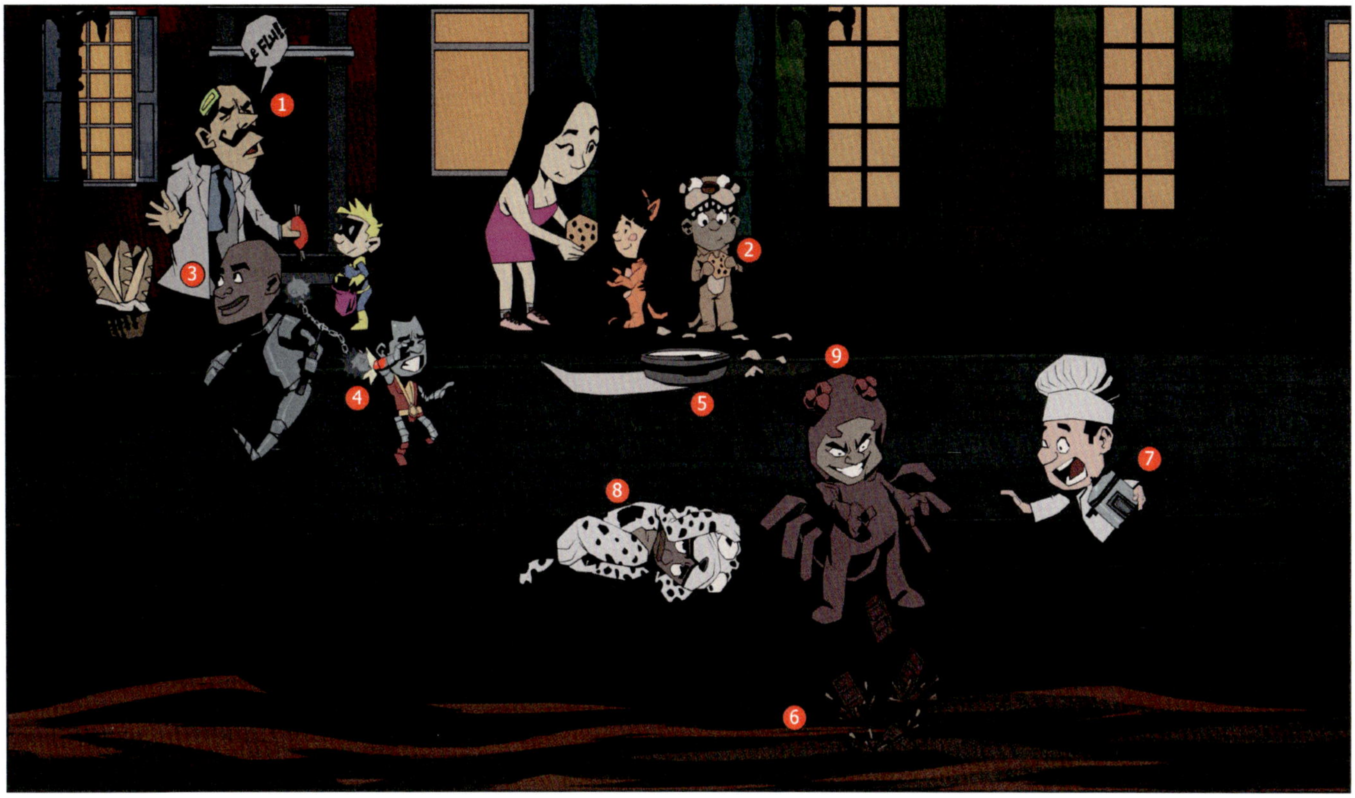

1. "LeFlu!" sneezing French man: Leflunomide

2. Kids immediately eating two hexagon-shaped cookies orally: Reversibly inhibits dihydroorotate dehydrogenase

3. Teenager in knight costume holding a "I" shaped flail being stopped by French man: Suppresses t-cell proliferation

4. "T" shaped flail hits Colossus kid with shiny and scaly armor causing a sore on dog's elbow: Can be used to treat psoriatic arthritis

5. Roomba: Can be used to treat rheumatoid arthritis

6. Bully throwing candy into muddy river: Can cause diarrhea

7. Chef kid with pressure cooker: Can cause hypertension

8. Liver-spotted dalmatian costume kid by river: Can cause hepatotoxicity

9. Tarantula costume: Teratogenic

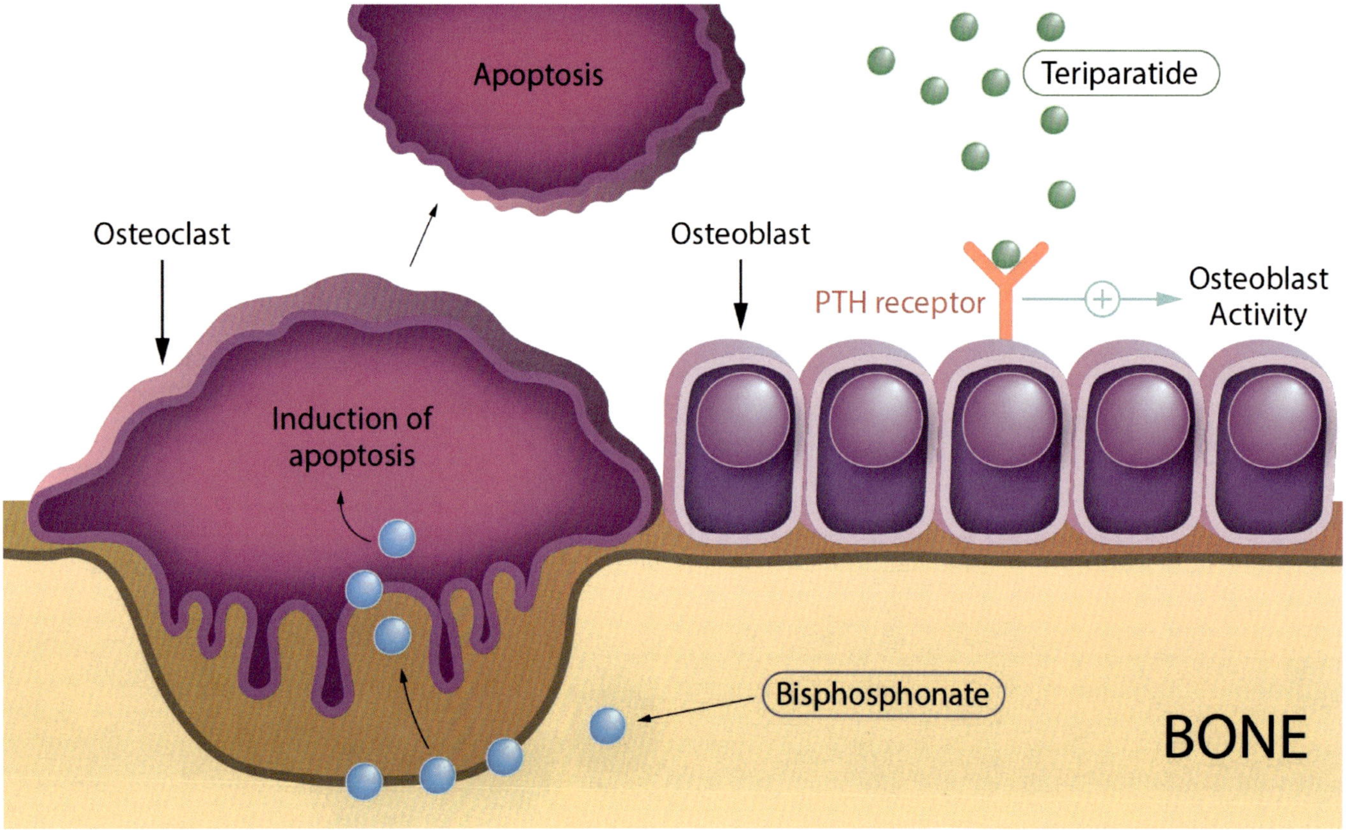

Figure 9.11.3 - Overview of Bisphosphonates and Teriparatide

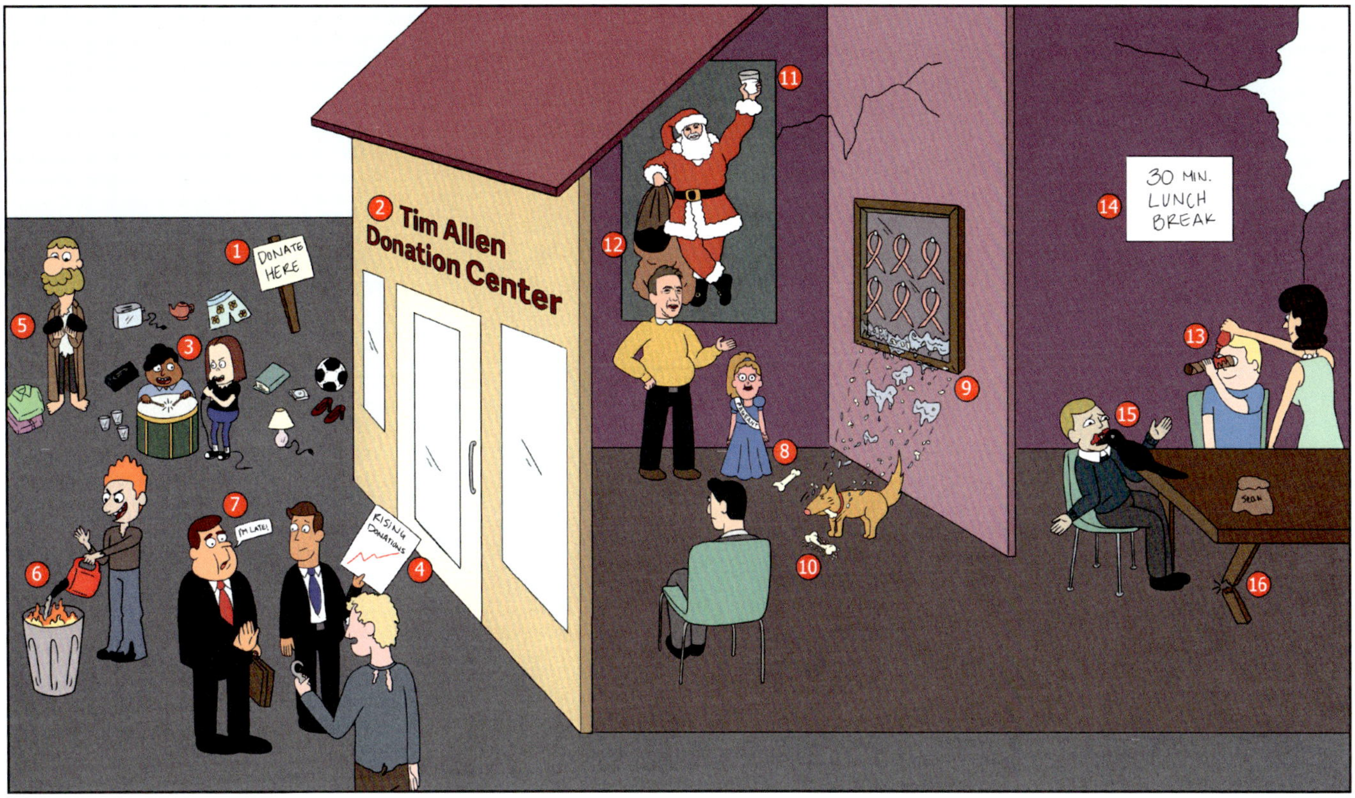

1. "Donate here" sign outside thrift shop: Bisphosphonates all have the suffix, "-dronate"

2. "Tim Allen Donation Center": Alendronate

3. Kids in pretend band with donated items: Ibandronate

4. Rising donations chart: Risedronate

5. Homeless man inspecting soles of donated shoes: Zoledronate

6. Pyro homeless man: Works by acting as pyrophosphate analog

7. Donor refusing to buy clasp because he is late to his meeting: Blocks osteoclast activity

8. Pageant girl with dog bone inside thrift store: Use for Paget disease of the bone

9. Bits of dog bone spread over pink cancer ribbons inside thrift store: Use for metastatic bone disease

10. Chewed dog bone: use for osteoporosis

11. Santa painting with milk held high: Use for hypercalcemia

12. Santa painting holding bag of coal: Use for osteogenesis imperfecta

13. Esophagus shaped paper towel roll with ketchup: Can cause esophagitis

14. "30 min. lunch break" sign: Prevent bisphosphonate-induced esophagitis by remaining upright for 30 minutes after swallowing

15. Crow pecking at worker's jaw: Can cause jaw osteonecrosis

16. Broken table leg: Can cause atypical femoral stress fractures

See Figure 9.11.3 - Overview of Bisphosphonates and Teriparatide (Musculoskeletal Pharmacology, Section 6, Page 231)

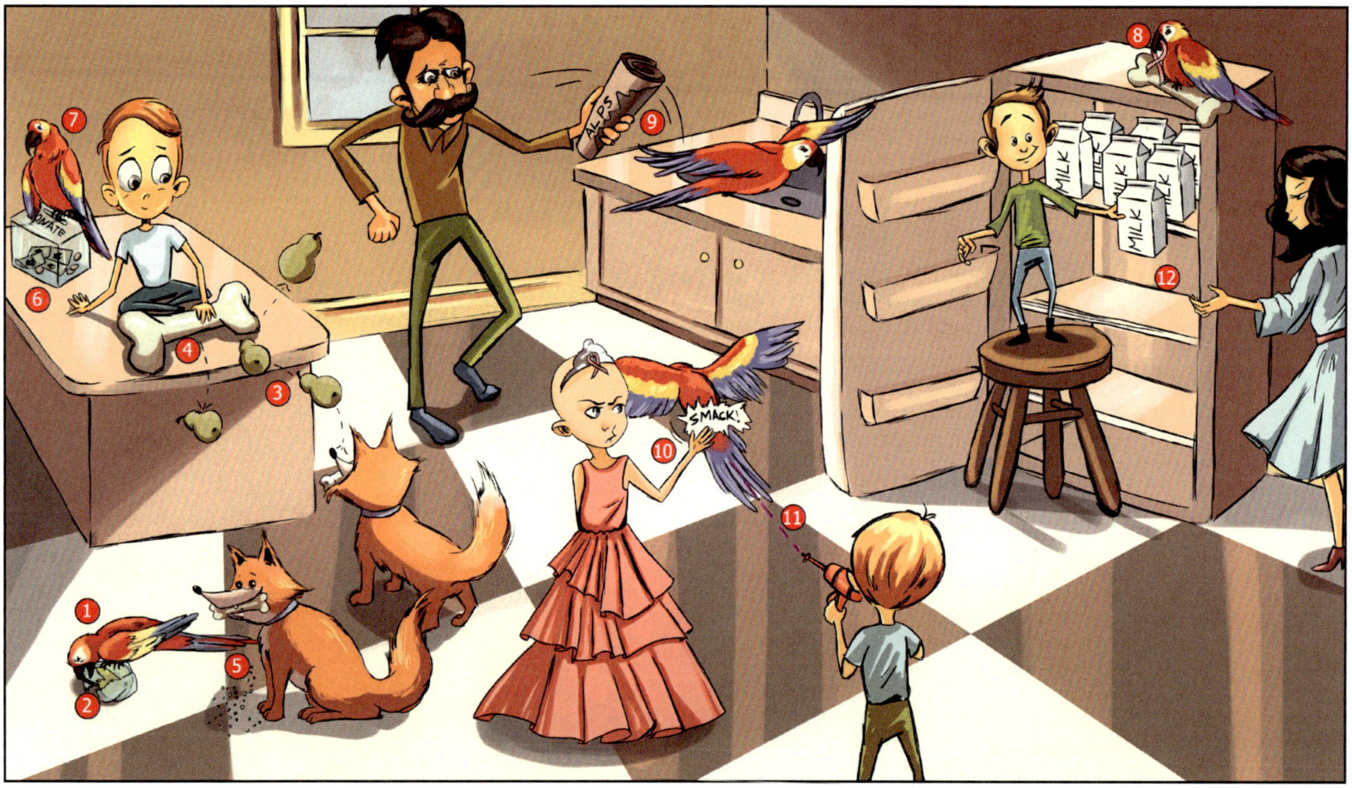

1. Parrot tearing into pear: Teriparatide

2. Wrapped pear that parrot is trying to tear: Recombinant "para"thyroid Hormone analog (PTH)

3. Dog tossing pears trying to hit large bone one by one: Pulsatile administration increases bone growth

4. Kid holding onto bone allowing bone to grow: Bone growth occurs due to osteoblast activity

5. Bone fragments from dog's mouth: Used to treat osteoporosis

6. "Donate" box: All bisphosphonates end with the suffix "-dronate"

7. Parrot perched on donation box near the large bone: Teriparatide is superior to bisphosphonates in terms of increasing bone growth

8. Parrot with bone that has pink cancer ribbon on: Can increase the risk of osteosarcoma

9. Father shooing parrot out of kitchen with ALPS magazine: Avoid using teriparatide in patients with high alkaline phosphatase (ALP) of undetermined origin

10. Girl in pageant dress smacking parrot: Should not be used in patients with Paget disease of the bone or in patients who have had cancer

11. Boy shooting parrot with laser gun: Should not be used in patients who have had radiation therapy

12. Kid handling carton of milk to mother: Can cause hypercalcemia transiently

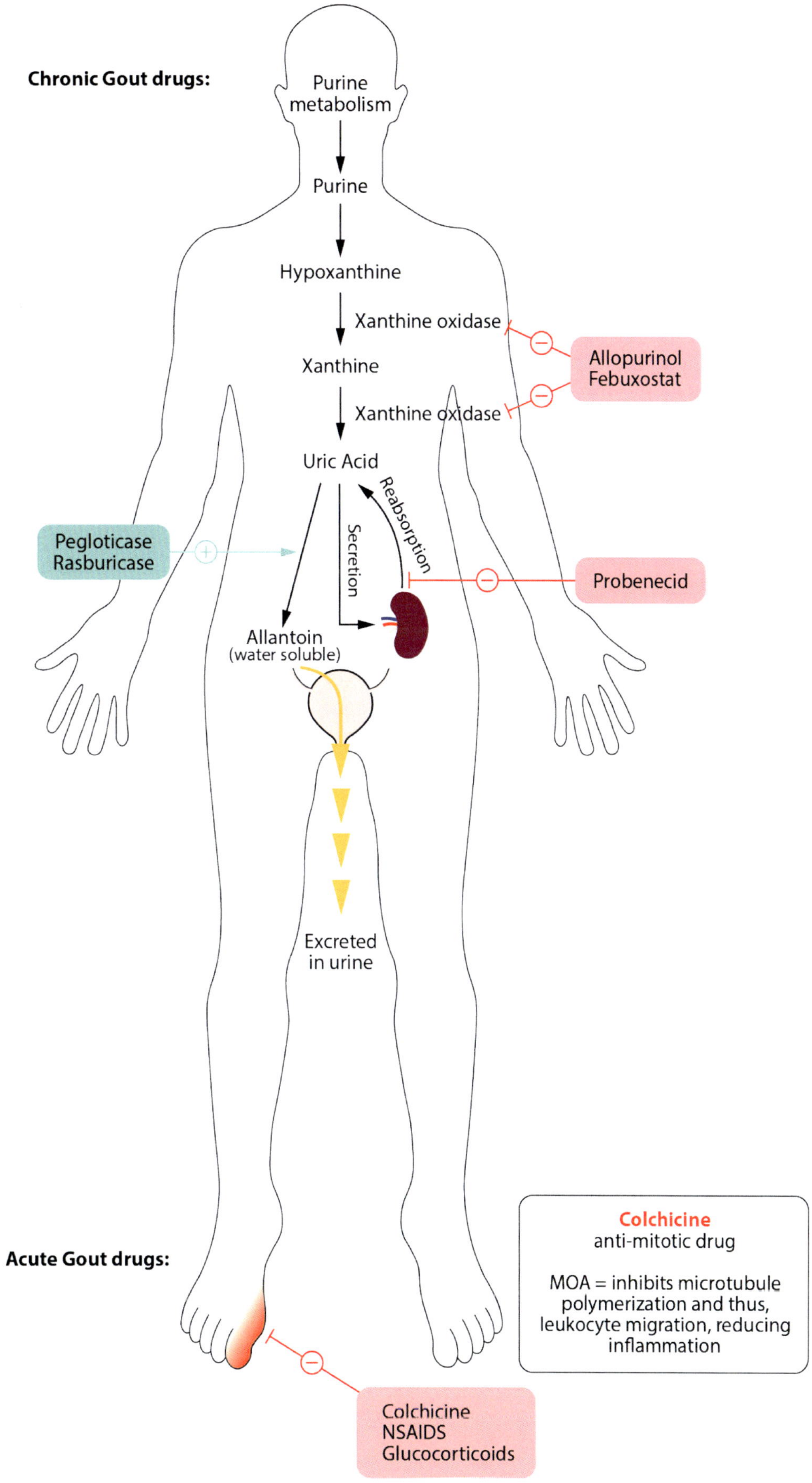

Figure 9.10.10 - Gout and Tumor Lysis Nephropathy Drug Overview

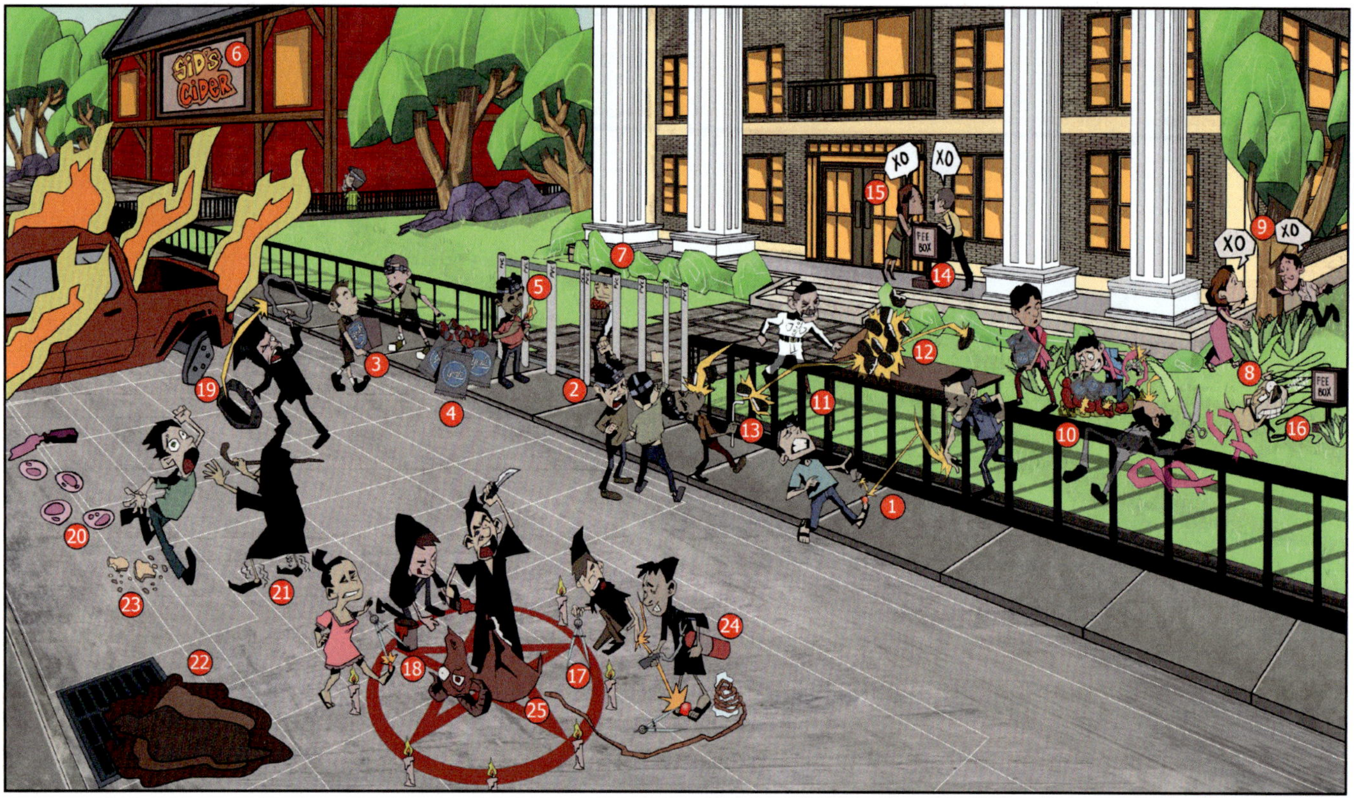

1. Guard preemptively clearing out protest and hits protester's toe, causing it to swell: Preventive therapy for gout (i.e. chronic treatment)

2. Go pro-wearing protesters: Probenecid

3. York peppermint patty delivery man is unable to get through the PVC fence due to protesters: Probenecid prevents uric acid from being reabsorbed in the PCT

4. Kidney shaped stones weighing down York patties: Probenecid can cause precipitation of uric acid calculi

5. Protester lighting match: Probenecid is a sulfa drug

6. "Sid's Cider" sign: Probenecid can be used to prevent cidofovir-related nephrotoxicity

7. PVC fence blocking politician with pennies from reaching street: Probenecid prevents penicillin from being secreted leading to higher serum levels of penicillin

8. Aloe plants on yard: Allopurinol

9. Couple kissing, "XO", separated by aloe plant: Allopurinol blocks xanthine oxidase

10. Guy ripping cancer ribbon while destroying kidney bean plants and dropping York patties near aloe plant: Allopurinol can be used to prevent tumor-lysis nephropathy

11. Peg-leg politician with case: Pegloticase

12. York patties flying off of table by peg-leg politician: Pegloticase is a recombinant uricase that catalyzes uric acid breakdown

13. Guy using allen wrench to break in is hit by York patty: Uric acid is broken down to allantoin which is more water soluble

14. "Fee Box" in yard: Febuxostat

15. Employees blowing kisses, "XO": Febuxostat blocks xanthine oxidase

16. Dog biting his paw while on a leash by other "Fee Box": Allopurinol and febuxostat can be used to treat Lesch-Nyhan syndrome

17. Satanists accidentally stabs other satanist in toe with protractor kept at acute angle: Acute gout treatment

18. Occult scene with injured toe: Colchicine treats acute gout

19. Satanist ripping inner tube of tire: Colchicine stabilizes tubulin which prevents microtubule polymerization

20. Neutrophil shaped footprints: Stabilizing tubulin prevents neutrophil chemotaxis and degranulation

21. Weak cult member in black robe: Colchicine can cause myopathy

22. Sewage flowing out of storm drain: Colchicine can cause diarrhea

23. Granules of bread from dropped sandwich: Colchicine can cause agranulocytosis

24. Cult member with fire extinguisher has injured toe from protractor: NSAIDs treat acute gout

25. Goat's feet bound by glued chords: Glucocorticoids treat acute gout

See Figure 9.11.2 - TNF Inhibitors and Leflunomide (Musculoskeletal Pharmacology, Section 5, Page 229)

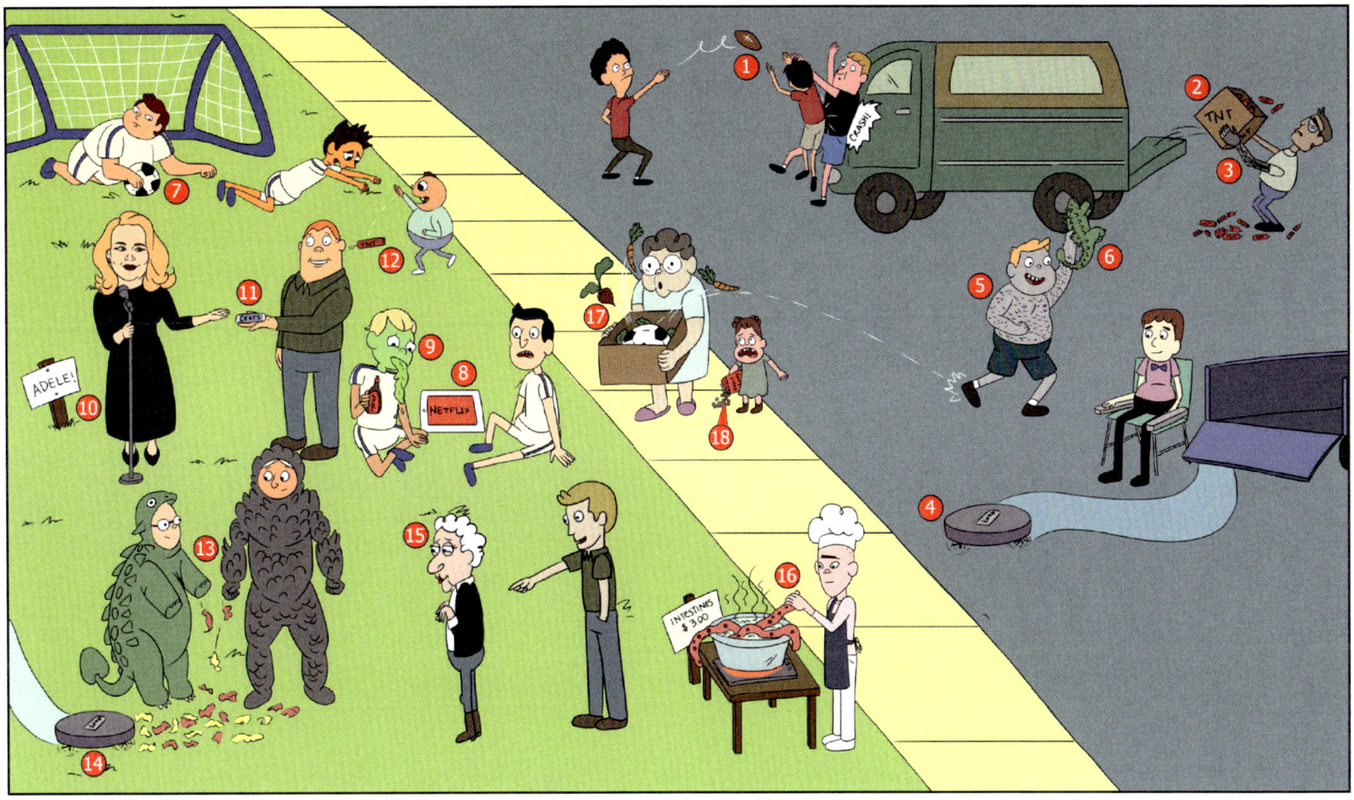

1. Guy intercepting pass: Etanercept

2. Intercepting guy smashes into van knocking out TNT: Etanercept is a TNF-alpha inhibitor

3. Robot arm guy catching TNT box: Etanercept is created through recombinant DNA technology

4. Roomba: Use for rheumatoid arthritis

5. Scale man painted kid: Use for psoriasis

6. Ankylosaurus plush held by scale man painted kid: Use for ankylosing spondylitis

7. Goalie: Golimumab

8. Netflix: Infliximab

9. Guy vomiting holding syrup: Infliximab can cause serum sickness

10. Adele: Adalimumab

11. Certs mints handed to Adele: Certolizumab

12. Player preventing firecracker popping kid between Netflix watching kids, Adele, Certs mints, and goalie: These 4 "mab" drugs (golimumab, infliximab, adalimumab, and certolizumab) work by directly targeting TNF-alpha

13. Scale man and Ankylosaurus mascots: These "mab" drugs can be used for ankylosing spondylitis and psoriasis

14. Roomba cleaning mascot's mess: These "mab" drugs can be used for rheumatoid arthritis

15. Old crone walking on field: These "mab" drugs can be used for Crohn's disease

16. Fried intestines with ulcer-shaped burns: These "mab" drugs can be used for ulcerative colitis

17. Grandma with box of tubers that were knocked out from a soccer ball: All TNF-alpha inhibitors can cause a predisposition to infection, especially TB because TNF-alpha is required to maintain granulomas

18. Fruit loops carried by granddaughter: All TNF-alpha inhibitors can lead to drug-induced SLE

NEUROLOGY PHARMACOLOGY

Section 1 - Epilepsy: Ethosuximide

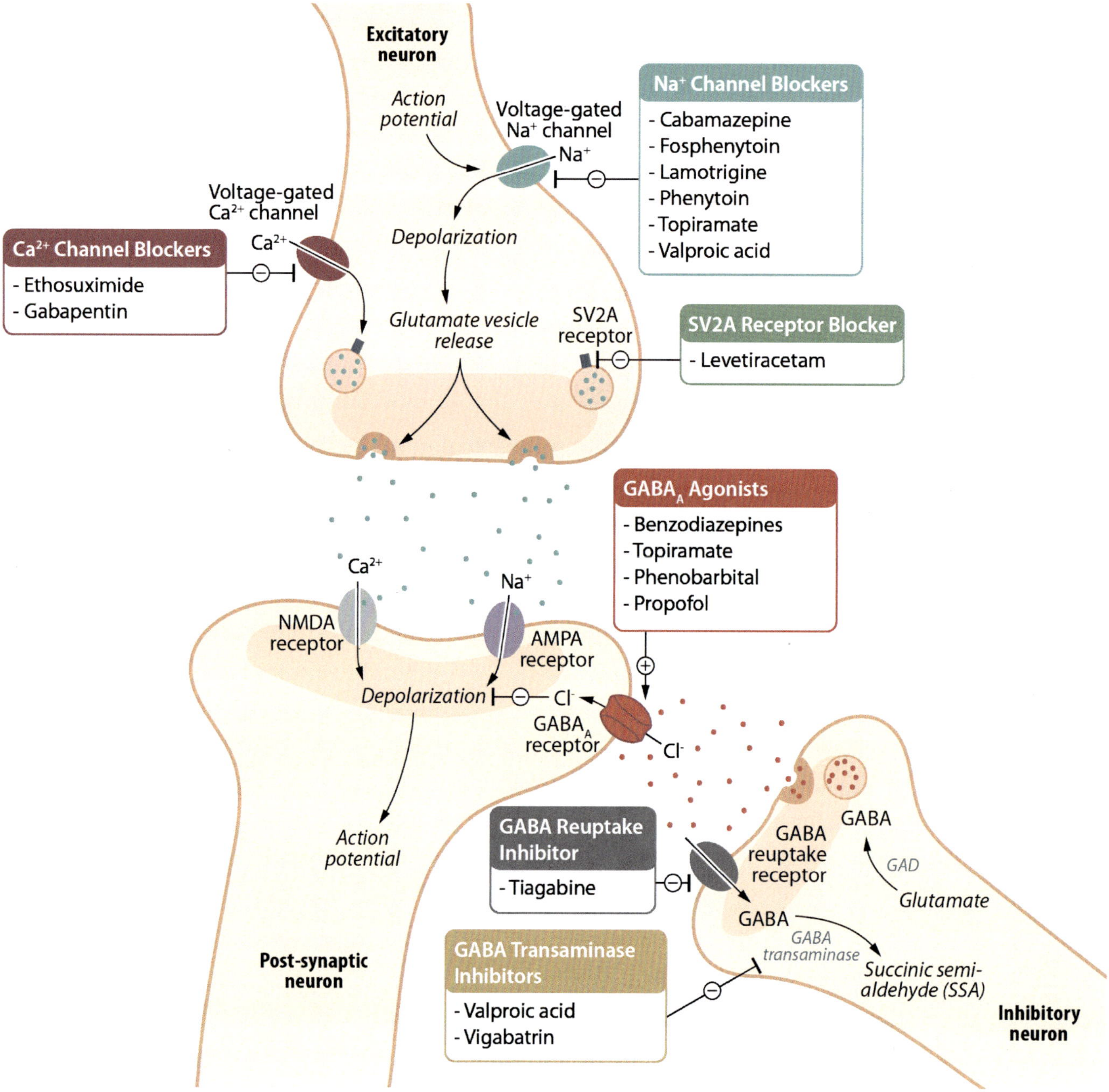

Figure 9.12.1 - Anti-Epileptic Mechanisms

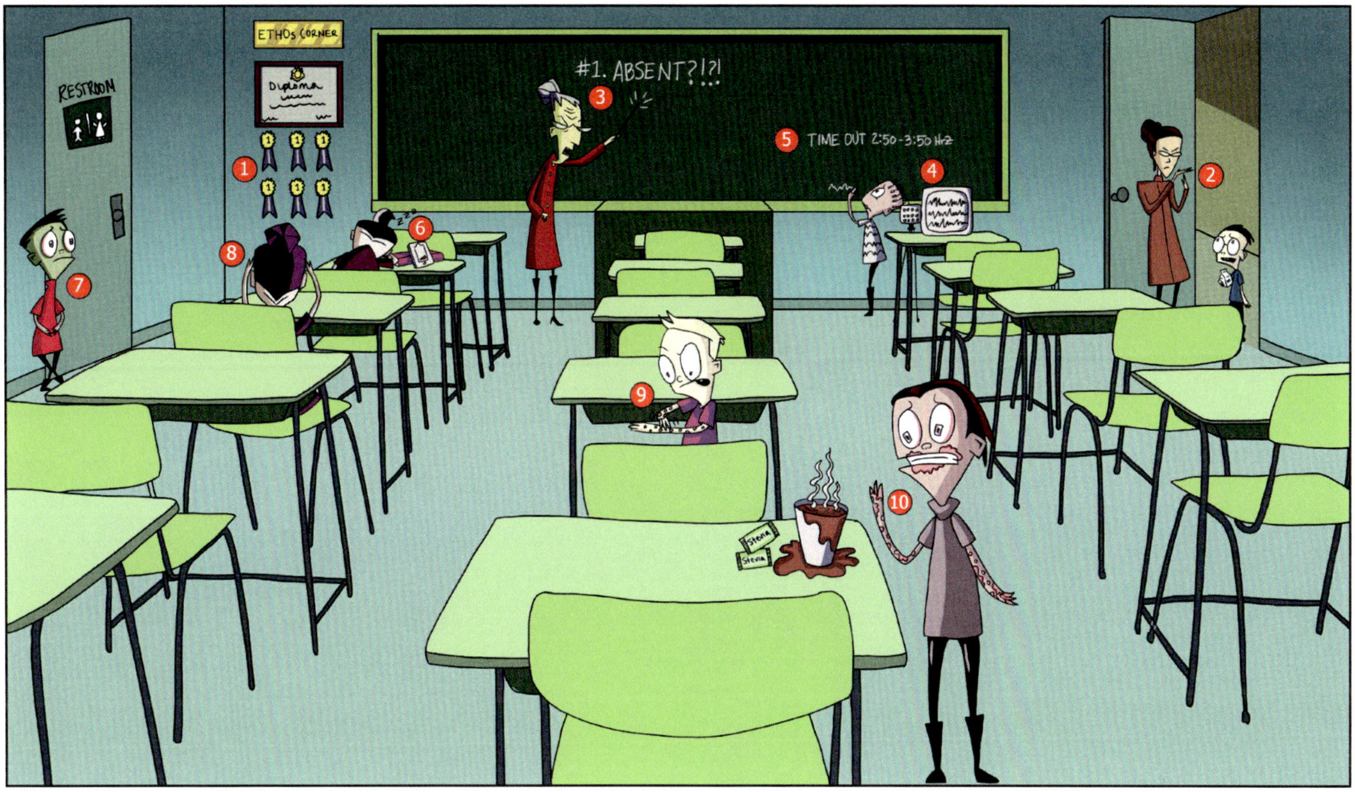

1. Ethos, or the ethical appeal of diplomas: Ethosuximide

2. Teacher aid's T-shaped hands blocking student from bringing milk in classroom: Blocks thalamic voltage-gated T-type Ca^{2+} channels

3. "#1. Absent?!?!" written on board: Use as first line for absence seizures

4. EEG machine with spike and wage patterns next to kid with spike and wave t-shirt: On EEG, absence seizures typically reveal a "spike and wave" pattern

5. "Time out 2:50-3:50 HrZ" on board next to EEG machine: Absence seizures typically have a frequency of 2.5-3.5 Hz

6. Kid passed out with low cell phone battery: Can cause fatigue

7. Distressed kid with green face by bathroom: Can cause GI distress

8. Student holding head in pain: Can cause headache

9. Kid stretching itchy, red bumps: Can cause itching (urticaria)

10. Girl with burnt arms and face from hot chocolate next to stevia packets: Can cause Stevens-Johnson syndrome

See Figure 9.12.1 - Anti-Epileptic Mechanisms (Neurology Pharmacology, Section 1, Page 237)

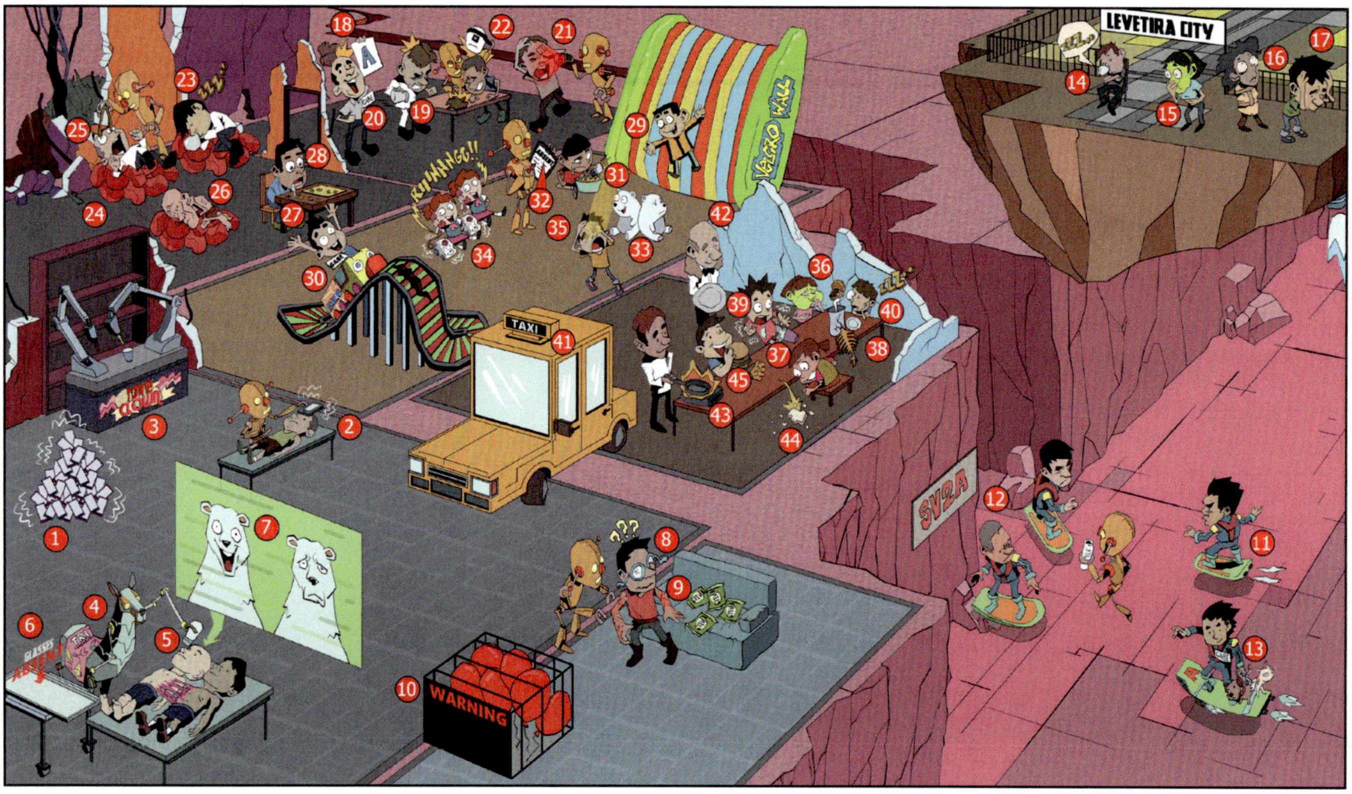

1. Pile of ringing cell phones shaking: Broad-spectrum antiepileptics

2. Ringing cell phone being installed on man's forehead: Use for focal seizures

3. "Tonic Clown" beverage bar: Use for tonic-clonic seizures

4. Robot llama hybrid with trigonometry saddle: Lamotrigine

5. Robot llama surgeon connecting two glued mates together with salt shaker but lid is too tight: Lamotrigine blocks voltage gated Na+ channels and inhibits release of glutamate

6. Tray absent of surgical instruments next to robot llama surgeon: Lamotrigine is used for absence seizures

7. Two polar bears on opposite ends of the emotional spectrum: Lamotrigine is used as a mood stabilizer in bipolar disorder

8. Human's cracked glasses in recovery area: Lamotrigine can cause blurry vision

9. Human's arm red and splotchy near Stevia packets: Lamotrigine can cause Stevens-Johnson syndrome

10. Balloons trapped in a black cage with warning sign on it: Lamotrigine can cause hemophagocytic lymphohistiocytosis (black box warning)

11. Levitating humans on hoverboards: Levetiracetam

12. Humans on hover boards blocking robot with milk from entering narrow pass with "SV2A" sign: Levetiracetam is a SV2A receptor blocker and inhibits voltage gated Ca^{2+} channels

13. "Gabe" cutting glue between glued hybrid pets: Levetiracetam may modulate GABA and glutamate release

14. Sleeping guard on levitating city: Levetiracetam can cause somnolence

15. Nauseous person with green face on levitating city: Levetiracetam can cause nausea

16. Crazy woman on levitating city: Levetiracetam can cause psychiatric symptoms (especially changes in personality)

17. Person holding head in pain on levitating city: Levetiracetam can cause headache

18. Toupee-wearing human slaves: Topiramate

19. Toupee-wearing human slave with blocked salt shaker: Topiramate works by blocking voltage-gated Na+ channels

20. Toupee-wearing health inspector named "Gabe" with his "A" rating: Topiramate allosterically binds to GABA-A receptor and increase GABA

21. Person grabbing head in pain with bright, red light in eyes: Use topiramate for migraine prophylaxis

22. Toupee-wearing slave being hit in head with pressure cooker: Use topiramate for idiopathic intracranial hypertension

23. Toupee-wearing human asleep: Topiramate can cause somnolence

24. Kidney-shaped stones that toupee-wearing human is sleeping on: Topiramate can cause kidney stones

25. Robot pressing tongs into toupee-wearing human's eye: Topiramate can cause glaucoma

26. Skinny human slave on kidney shaped stones: Topiramate can cause weight loss

27. Word game with no found words next to toupee-wearing humans: Topiramate can cause word-finding difficulties

28. Human staring blankly while drooling next to word game: Topiramate can cause cognitive slowing

29. Velcro wall: Valproic acid (valproate)

30. "Gabe" driving the ammo train uphill and being stopped by broken tracks at the top: Valproic acid inhibits GABA transaminase leading to increased GABA

31. Closed salt shaker near velcro wall: Valproic acid inactivates Na+ channels

32. "Absent" on robot's clipboard next to velcro wall: Valproic acid can be used for absence seizures

33. Two stuffed polar bears expressing different emotions next to velcro wall: Valproic acid can be used as a mood stabilizer in patients with bipolar disorder

34. Two clone children with their ringing phones next to velcro wall: Valproic acid can be used myoclonic seizures

35. Kid grabbing head in pain with bright light in his eyes: Valproic acid can be used for migraine prophylaxis

36. Nauseous child slave with green face next to picnic table: Valproic acid can cause GI upset

37. Kid with liver-shaped water stain at picnic table: Valproic acid can cause hepatotoxicity

38. Tarantula on pale, dying potted plant whose roots are spilling out on picnic table: Valproic acid is teratogenic (neural tube defects)

39. Trembling kid at picnic table: Valproic acid can cause tremor

40. Sleeping kid at picnic table: Valproic acid can cause sedation

41. Taxi in room with picnic table: Valproic acid can cause ataxia

42. Bald waiter serving kids at picnic table: Valproic acid can cause alopecia

43. Flaming pan on picnic table: Valproic acid can cause pancreatitis

44. Grain crumbs on the ground near picnic table: Valproic acid can cause agranulocytosis

45. Obese kid eating food at picnic table: Valproic acid can cause weight gain

See Figure 9.12.1 - Anti-Epileptic Mechanisms (Neurology Pharmacology, Section 1, Page 237)

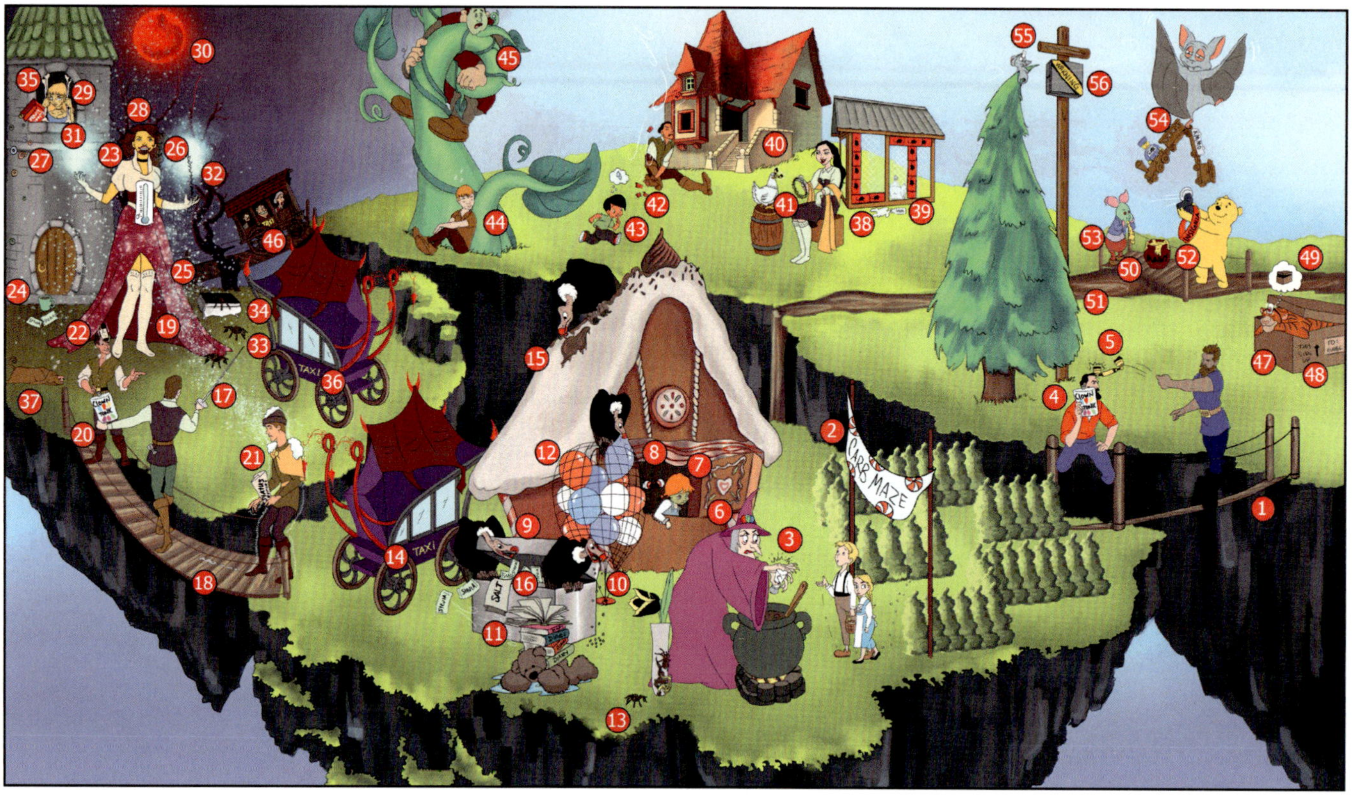

1. Narrow, shaky rope bridges: Narrow-spectrum antiepileptics

2. Hansel and Gretel leaving carb trail in pine maze: Carbamazepine

3. Evil witch's clogged salt shaker: Carbamazepine works by inactivating Na^+ channels

4. Man drinking colorful clown tonic: Use carbamazepine for generalized tonic-clonic seizures

5. Shaking GPS device implanted into the woodsman's forehead: Use carbamazepine for focal seizures

6. Three gems on witch's hat: Use carbamazepine as first line treatment for trigeminal neuralgia

7. Child in house nauseous from being fed candy: Carbamazepine can cause nausea

8. Crossed eyes watching child inside house: Carbamazepine can cause diplopia

9. Vulture opening garbage can that looks like chrome box: Carbamazepine induces cytochrome P-450

10. Vulture dropping white grain crumbs on the ground: Carbamazepine can cause agranulocytosis

11. Empty salt bag and wet teddy bear with swollen limbs under wet stack of diaries being dried by wind: Carbamazepine can cause hyponatremia and edema due to SIADH

12. Vulture popping multi-colored balloons in net: Carbamazepine can cause aplastic anemia

13. Tarantula crawling up tulip plant with exposed roots: Carbamazepine is teratogenic during the first trimester and can cause cleft lip/palate and spina bifida

14. Witch's taxi carriage: Carbamazepine can cause ataxia

15. Vulture pecking at liver-shaped chocolate stain on roof: Carbamazepine can cause hepatotoxicity

16. Stevia packets falling out of chrome box garbage can: Carbamazepine can cause Steven-Johnson syndrome

17. Fencing prince crossing narrow, shaky bridge: Phenytoin

18. Prince's clogged salt shaker: Phenytoin works via inactivation of Na^+ channels

19. Enchantress trying to eliminate the prince with zero degree weather: Phenytoin works via zero order elimination (constant rate of elimination)

20. Fencing prince drinking clown tonic: Use phenytoin as a first line prophylaxis and treatment of tonic-clonic seizures

21. Status report brought to fencing prince by violently shaking messenger: Use phenytoin as a first line prophylaxis and treatment of status epilepticus

22. Shaking GPS device implanted into page's forehead: Use phenytoin for focal seizures

23. Enchantress's prominent gums: Phenytoin can cause gingival hyperplasia

24. Stevia packets next to enchantress's hot chocolate: Phenytoin can cause Steven-Johnson syndrome

25. Enchantress wearing dress with pink sequins: Phenytoin can cause DRESS syndrome

26. Enchantress's facial hair: Phenytoin can cause hirsutism

27. Princess in tower knocking over box of fruit loops: Phenytoin can cause drug-induced lupus

28. Enchantress's yellow/brown skin: Phenytoin can cause yellow brown skin

29. Princess's yellow brown skin: Phenytoin can cause yellow brown skin

30. Blood moon and barren trees: Phenytoin can cause megaloblastic anemia due to folate deficiency

31. Princess trying to break brittle brone-liek bars on her window: Phenytoin can cause osteopenia

32. Enchantress wearing gloves and knee-high socks with barbed wire want: Phenytoin can cause peripheral neuropathy

33. Enchantress's army of tarantulas directed against fencing prince: Phenytoin is teratogenic (can cause fetal hydantoin syndrome)

34. Tarantula army climbing out of open chrome box: Phenytoin can cause induction of cytochrome P-450

35. Princess's spinning eyes: Phenytoin canc ause nystagmus and diplopia (toxicity)

36. Enchantress's taxi carriage: Phenytoin can cause ataxia (toxicity)

37. Sleeping guard dog: Phenytoin can cause sedation (toxicity)

38. Woman grabbing next to chicken pen made of tin: Gabapentin

39. Chickens blocked from getting milk by "T" and "L" shaped gates covered with mouse towels: Gabapentin inhibits voltage-gated calcium channels (T-type and L-type) in neurons of the thalamus

40. Shaking GPS device implanted ito chicken's forehead: Use gabapentin for focal seizure

41. Woman wearing gloves and knee-high socks and holding barbed wire: Use gabapentin for peripheral neuropathy

42. Shingles falling onto husband's foot: Use gabapentin for postherpetic neuralgia

43. Jack's dry mouth and thirstiness while running from giant: Gabapentin can cause dry mouth

44. Sleeping man by beanstalk: Gabapentin can cause somnolence

45. Nauseous giant with green face: Gabapentin canc ause nausea

46. Townspeople arriving in taxi carriage: Gabapentin can cause ataxia

47. Tiger hiding in box: Tiagabine

48. Box marked with up arrow and "TO GABE" label: Tiagabine works by inhibiting GABA reuptake → increased GABA

49. Shaking GPS device implanted into Tigger's forehead: Use tigabine for focal seizures (with or without consciousness impairment)

50. Nauseous Piglet vomiting up honey: Tiagabine can cause nausea and vomiting

51. Bridge crossing muddy river: Tiagabine can cause diarrhea

52. Pooh Bear taking photo with insignia camera and blinding Piglet with camera flash: Tiagabine can cause insomnia

53. Heavy-set Piglet in tight clothing after eating honey: Tiagabine can cause weight changes

54. Vampire bat flying upwards carrying broken toy train loaded with ammo in A formation with conductor named Gabe: Vigabatrin inhibits GABA transaminase → increased GABA

55. Shaking GPS device impaired into baby bat's forehead: Use vigabatrin for refractory focal seizures

56. Vampire bat about to fly into black box warning sign: Vigabatrin can cause irreversible vision loss (black box warning)

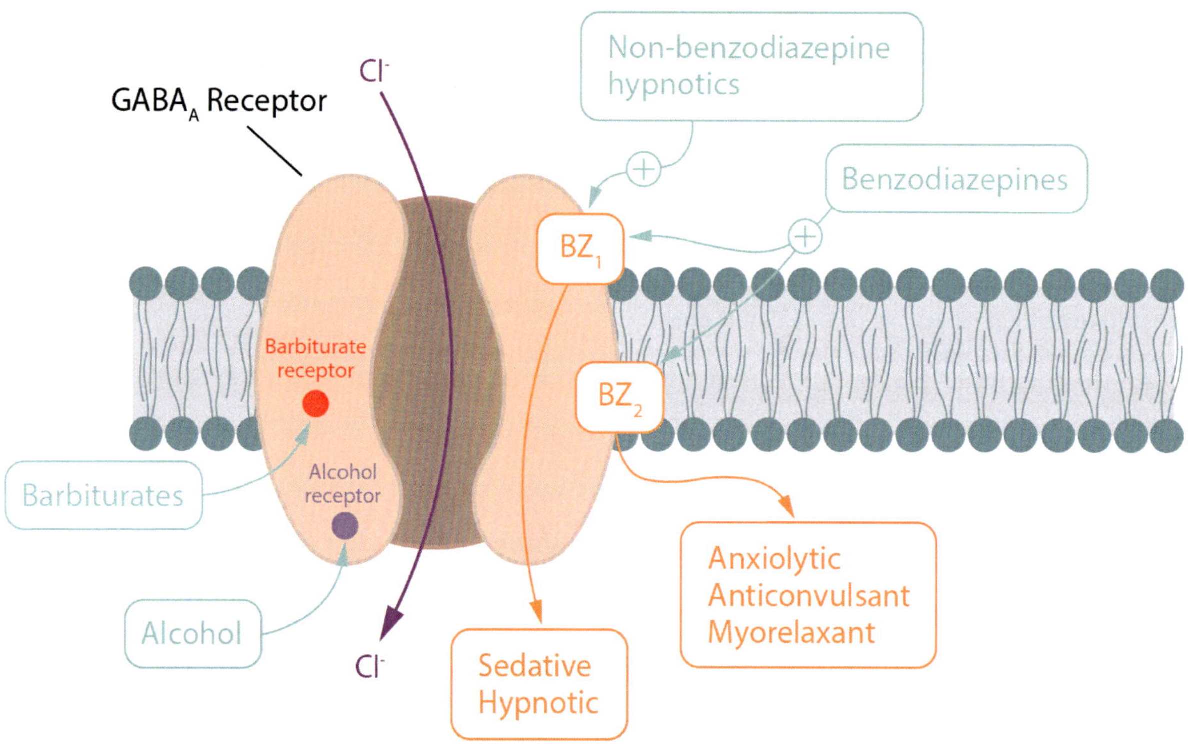

Figure 9.12.2 - Effects of Medications that Act on the GABA-A Receptor

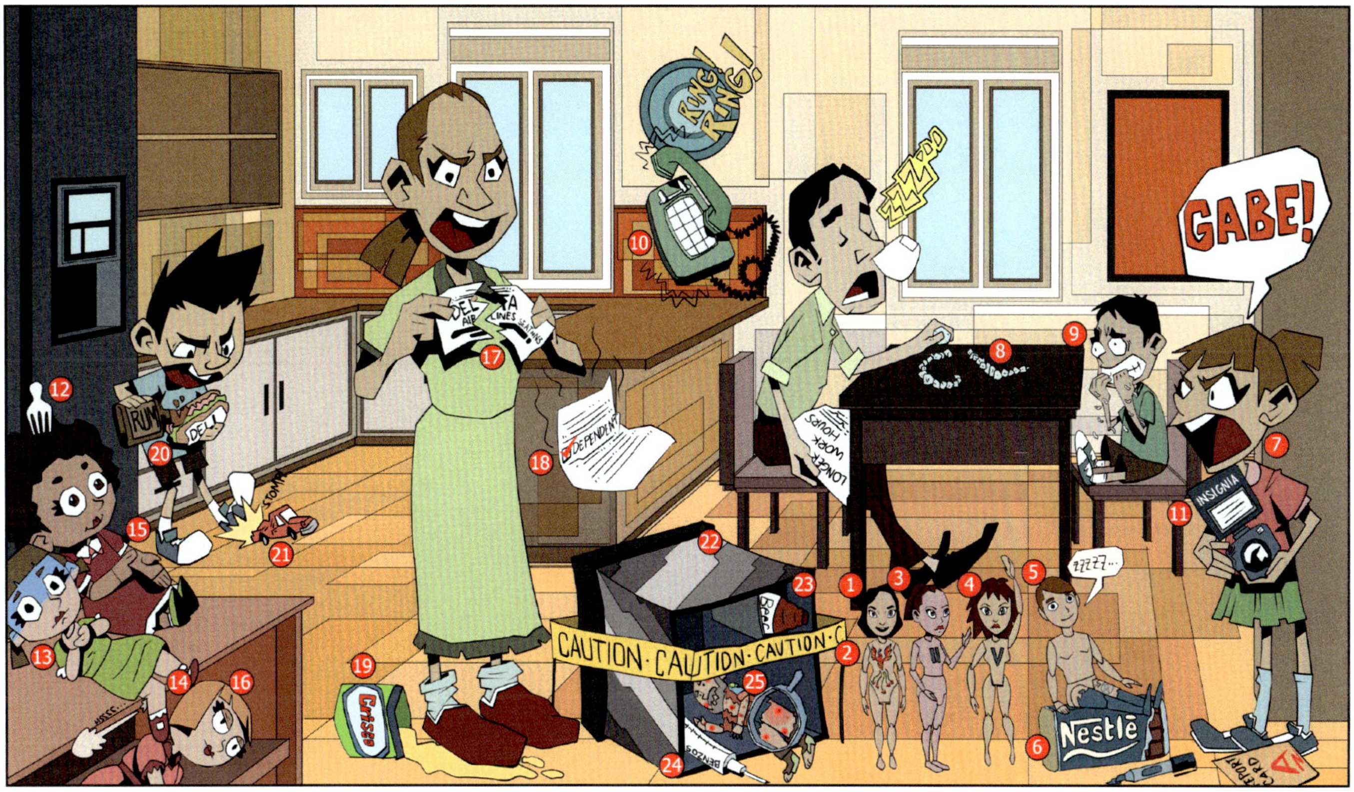

1. Barbies: Barbiturates

2. Barbie painted with phoenix design: Phenobarbital

3. Barbie painted with Roman numeral "II" for second in command: Secobarbital

4. Barbie painted with Roman numeral "V" for fifth in command: Pentobarbital

5. Ken doll with thighs colored with blue pen: Thiopental

6. Ken doll with thighs colored sleeping on Nestle bar: Thiopental can be used to induce anesthesia

7. Girl yelling for her brother Gabe with Gabe's "A" report card on floor: Stimulates the GABAa receptor

8. Father scooping chloride compound pills into "CL" shape with note announcing longer work hours: Results in chloride channels being open for longer

9. Anxious little brother biting nails: Can be used for anxiety

10. Phone ringing off the hook: Can be used for seizures

11. Sister holding insignia camera: Can be used for insomnia

12. Comb stuck in doll's hair: Can cause CNS depression

13. Doll with hands around throat: Can cause respiratory depression

14. Doll with punctured inflatable limbs that are deflating quickly: Can cause hypotension

15. Doll checking radial pulse while resting: Can cause bradycardia

16. Doll with drooping eyelids on lower shelf: Causes a decrease in REM sleep

17. Delta plane tickets being torn in half: Causes a decrease in delta wave (N_3) sleep

18. Tax form with "dependent" box checked: Can cause dependence

19. Puddle of melted Crisco oil soaking into mom's shoes and floor: Has high lipid solubility

20. Gabe pouring rum over deli sandwich: Can cause delirium

21. Gabe stomping on crushed toy car: Life-threatening cardiovascular collapse

22. Open chrome box of Barbies: Induces cytochrome P-450

23. Hidden beer in chrome box marked off with caution tape: Contraindicated with alcohol ingestion

24. Benzos syringe in chrome box marked off with caution tape: Contraindicated with benzodiazepines

25. Poor, imprisoned Barbie doll with burn marks and torn clothes in chrome box marked off with caution tape: Contraindicated in porphyria

See Figure 9.12.2 - Effects of Medications that Act on the GABA-A Receptor (Neurology pharmacology, Section 4, Page 243)

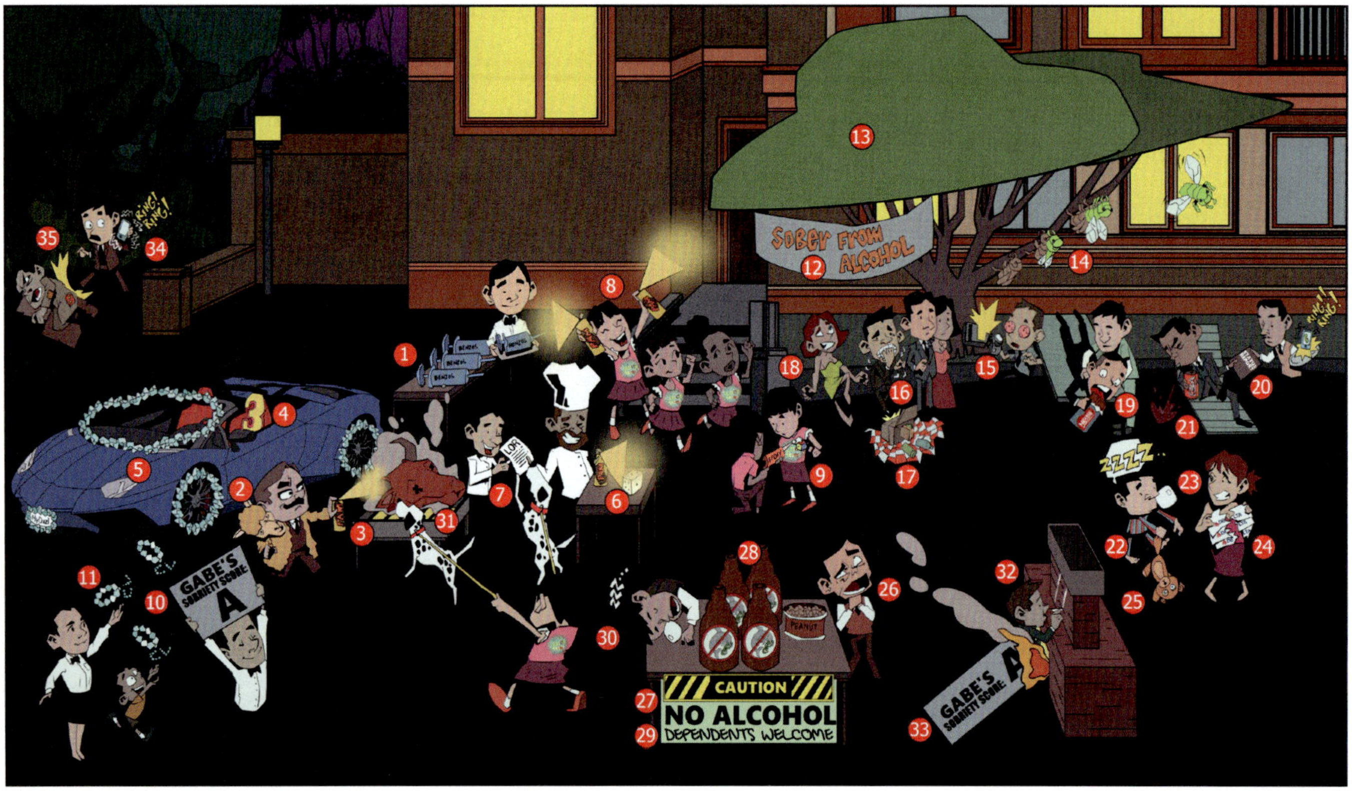

1. Walter handing out blue syringes with benzos: Benzodiazepines

2. Short guest wearing an alpaca coat: Alprazolam

3. Short guest spraying Pam cooking spray on burning ox on grill: Oxazepam

4. Driver seat in short guest's Lamborghini marked with lucky number "3": Triazolam

5. "My Dazl" license plate on short guest's bedazzled car: Midazolam

6. Die on table coated with Pam cooking spray: Diazepam

7. Chef spraying Pam giving Letter of Recommendation (LOR) drenched in Pam to apprentice chef: Lorazepam

8. Dancing team spraying Pam: Temazepam

9. Colored die being glued onto dancer's uniform with an epoxy glue gun: Chlordiazepoxide

10. Sign saying "Gabe's sobriety score: A": Benzodiazepines stimulate GABAa

11. Server tossing "CL" necklaces with chloride crystals to guests near "Gabe's sobriety score: A" sign one at a time: Stimulates GABAa receptors by increasing frequency of the Cl- channel opening

12. "Sober from alcohol" banner: Use detoxification, especially for alcohol withdrawal

13. Acadia tree: Can be used for akathisia

14. Shedding and flying cicadas: Akathisia is a feeling of restlessness and wanting to crawl out of one's skin

15. Photographer with Insignia camera pointing flash at his own face: Use for insomnia (has sedative effects)

16. Anxious guy biting nails: Use for anxiety

17. Trampled and disordered picnic set-up: Use for panic disorder

18. Guest with muscle spasms from dancing too much: Use for muscle spasticity

19. Guest eating Nestle bar while getting a massage: Use as a general anesthetic (has amnestic and muscle relaxant effects)

20. Walter giving ringing phone to guest while giving status report: Use for seizures and status epilepticus

21. Red can of Coke: Use for cocaine intoxication

22. Kid sleepwalking through party: Use for sleepwalking

23. Guest scared by sleepwalking kid: Use for night terrors

24. Scared guest accidentally ripping up 3 Delta airline tickets: Decreased delta wave (N_3) sleep

25. Upside-down teddy bear with fluttering eyes: Decreased REM sleep

26. Guest struggling to breathe after choking: Can cause respiratory depression

27. Big sign with yellow caution tape saying "no alcohol" on table: Contraindicated with alcohol

28. Bottles of root beer on table with caution tape: Contraindicated with 1st generation antihistamines due to sedation

29. "Dependents welcome" sign on table: Can cause dependence

30. Sleeping bartender resting head on table: Can cause sedation

31. Dalmatian sniffing at ox getting sprayed with Pam on grill and second Dalmation pawing at chef holding LOR: Lorazepam, oxazepam and temazepam can be used for those with liver disease who drink a "LOT"

32. Guest kneeling while drawing on chimney flue with chalk: Treat overdoses with flumazenil

33. Burning "Gabe's sobriety score: A" sign in fireplace: Flumazenil is a competitie GABAa receptor antagonist

34. Guy withdrawing from party perimeters with ringing phone: Can precipitate seizures due to acute withdrawal

35. Guy accidentally disturbing sleeping hobo while withdrawing from party: Acute withdrawal can cause sleep disturbances

See Figure 9.12.2 - Effects of Medications that Act on the GABA-A Receptor (Neurology pharmacology, section 4, Page 243)

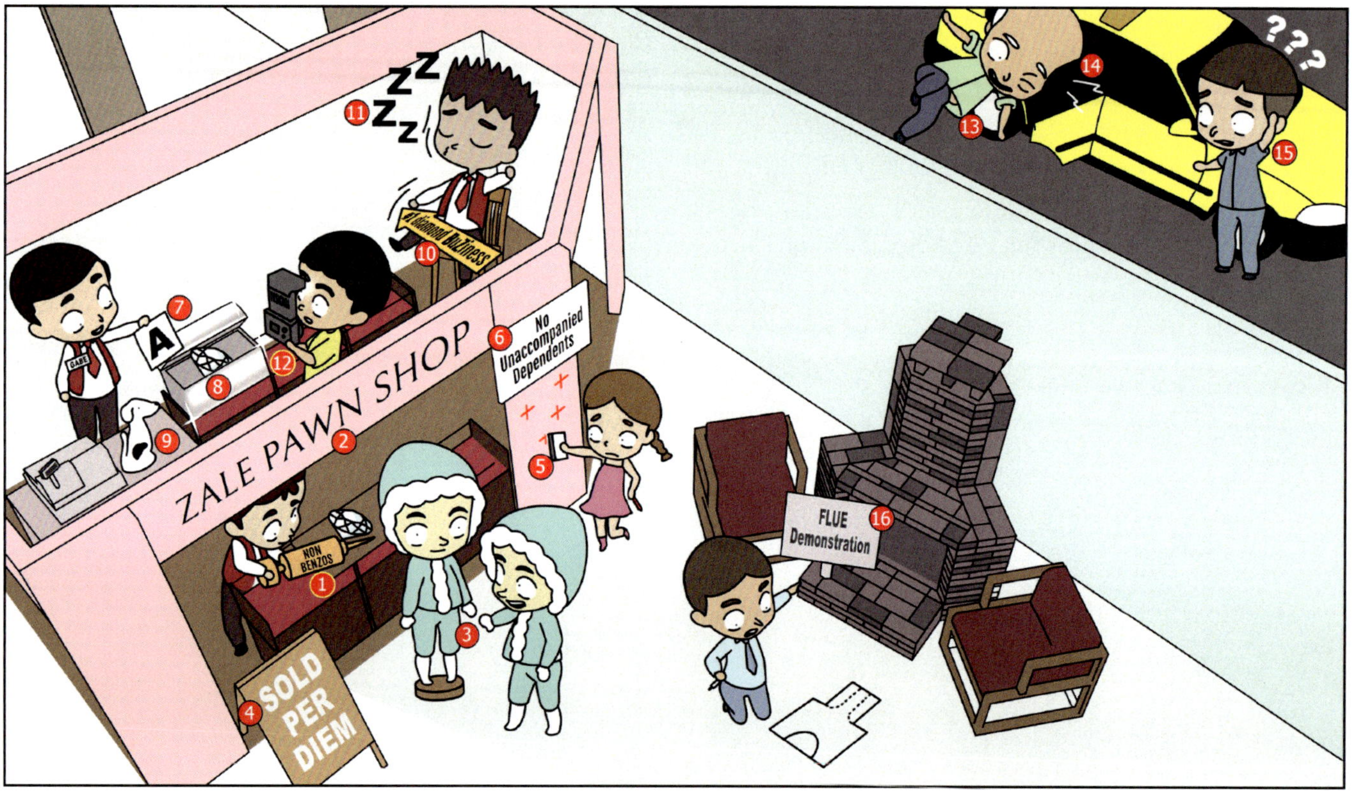

1. "Non-benzos" label on yellow syringe: Non-benzodiazepine hypnotics
2. "Zale Pawn Shop" sign: Zaleplon
3. Eskimo trying to sell wax clone of himself: Eszopiclone
4. "Sold per diem" sign: Zolpidem
5. Girl erasing addition symbols written on wall: Does not cause addiction
6. "No unaccompanied dependents" sign: Low dependence
7. Gabe holding onto letter "A" sign: Binds GABAa receptor
8. Diamond kept inside chrome box: Metabolized by cytochrome P-450
9. Liver-spotted Dalmatian figurine on desk next to chrome box: Metabolism takes place in the liver
10. Employee holding "#1 diamond BuZiness" sign for advertising: Specifically binds to the BZ1 site on the GABAa receptor
11. Guy falling asleep right after sitting down: Rapid onset of action
12. Insignia camera flashing in customer's eyes: Use for insomnia
13. Elderly man falling over while getting out of taxi: Can cause central ataxia
14. Elderly man hitting head on taxi door: Can cause headaches
15. Confused taxi driver not knowing how to help elderly man: Can cause confusion
16. Kneeling salesman demonstrating how chimney flue works on antique fireplace in pawnshop: Treat overdoses with flumazenil

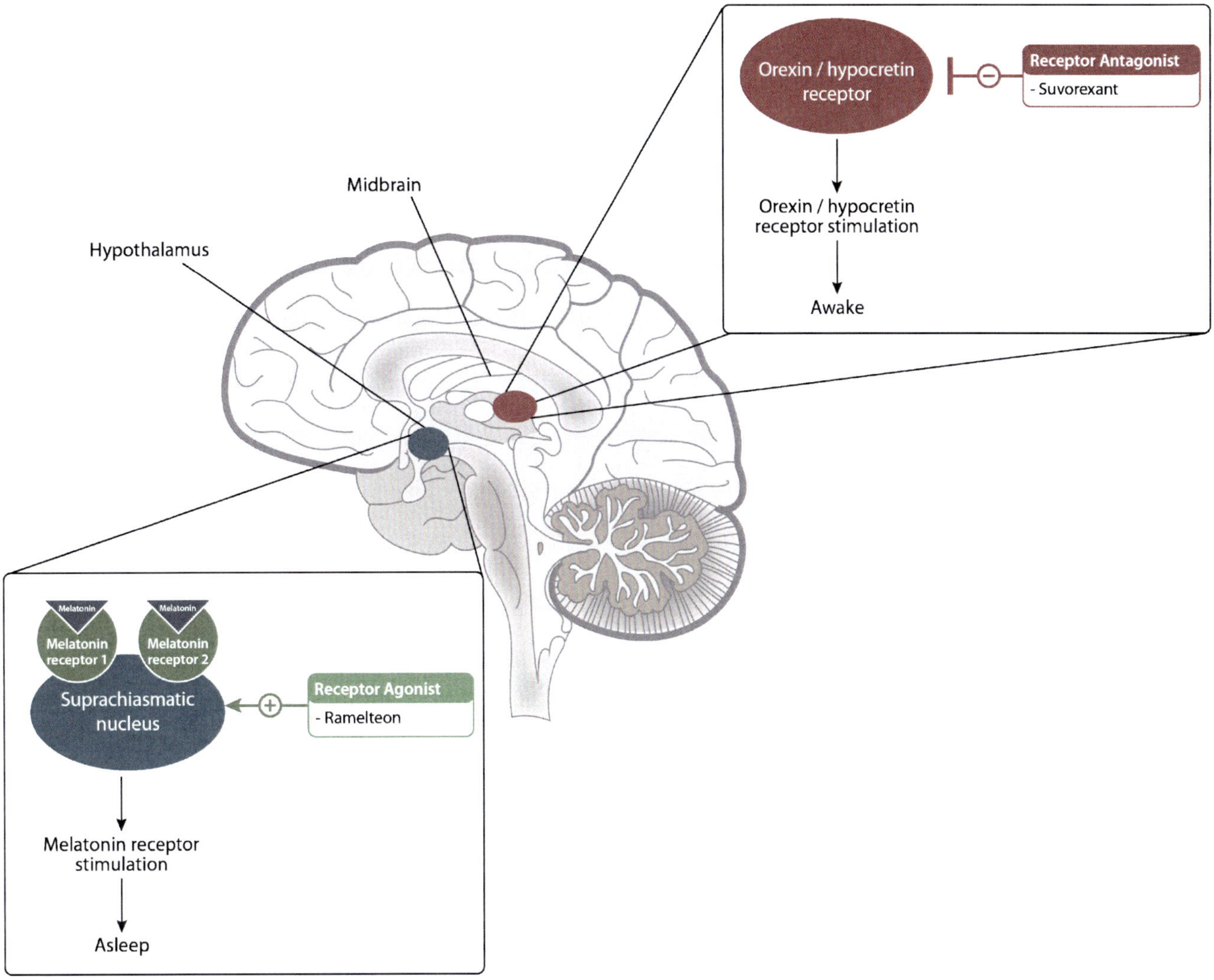

Figure 9.12.3 - Mechanism of Suvorexant and Ramelteon

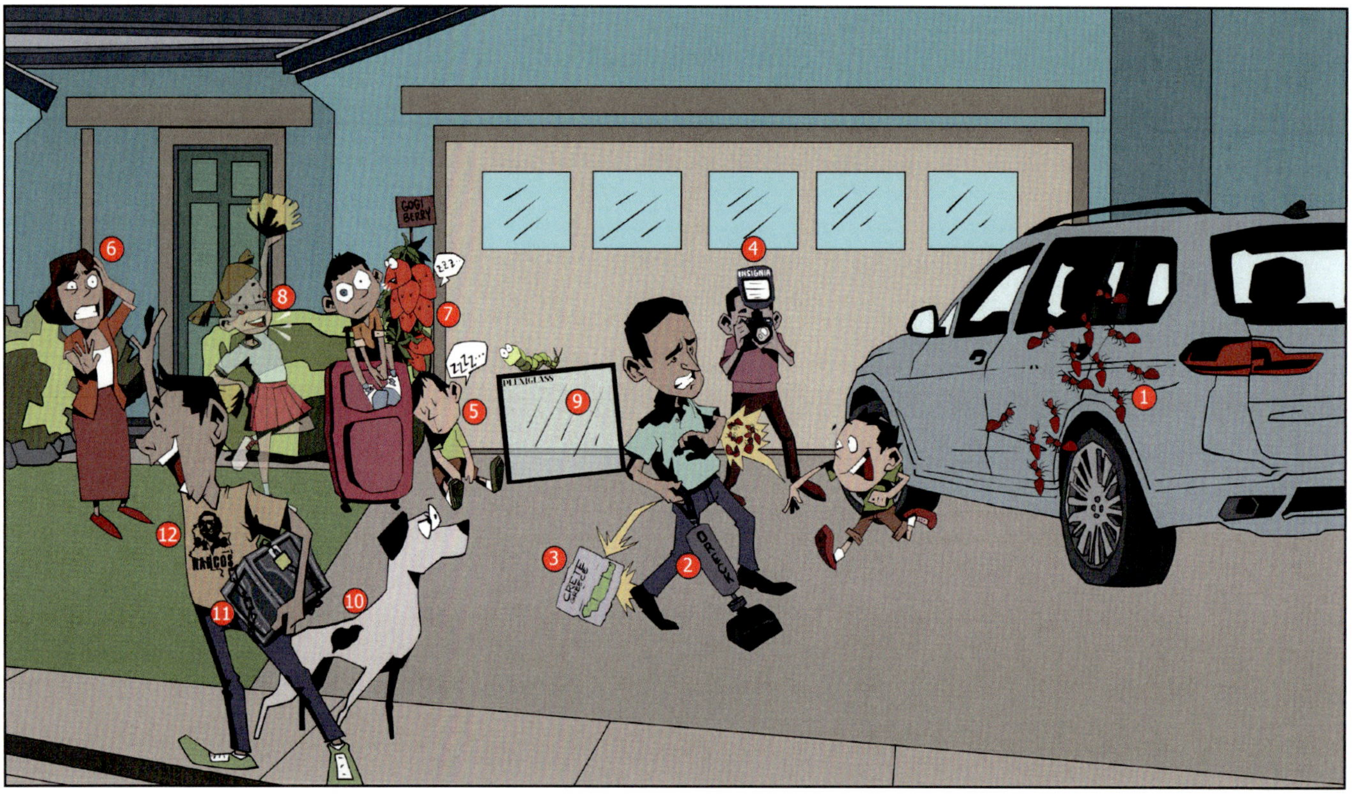

1. SUV covered in ants: Suvorexant

2. Kid picking ants off SUV and throwing them at dat with Oreck vacuum: Orexin receptor antagonist

3. Map of Crete falling out of dad's pocket onto ground near Oreck vacuum: Hypocretin is another name for orexin

4. Brother taking picture with Insignia camera: Use for insomnia

5. Little brother sleeping in front of yard: Can cause sedation

6. Mom holding head in pain: Can cause headaches

7. Brother hallucinating about bench of goji berries taking a nap and talking to him: Can cause hypnagogic hallucinations (auditory hallucinations while falling asleep)

8. Brother hallucinating about peppy cheerleader with pompoms: Can cause hypnopompic hallucinations (auditory hallucinations upon walking)

9. Caterpillar crawling on piece of plexiglass: Can cause cataplexy

10. Liver-spotted dog being taken away by owner: Do not use with liver disease

11. Mother telling neighbor with locked chrome boxes to go away: Do not use in combination with strong CYP3A4 inhibitors

12. Guy being told to go away, wearing Narcos shirt: Do not use in patients with narcolepsy

See Figure 9.12.3 - Mechanism of Suvorexant and Ramelteon (Neurology, Section 7, Page 248)

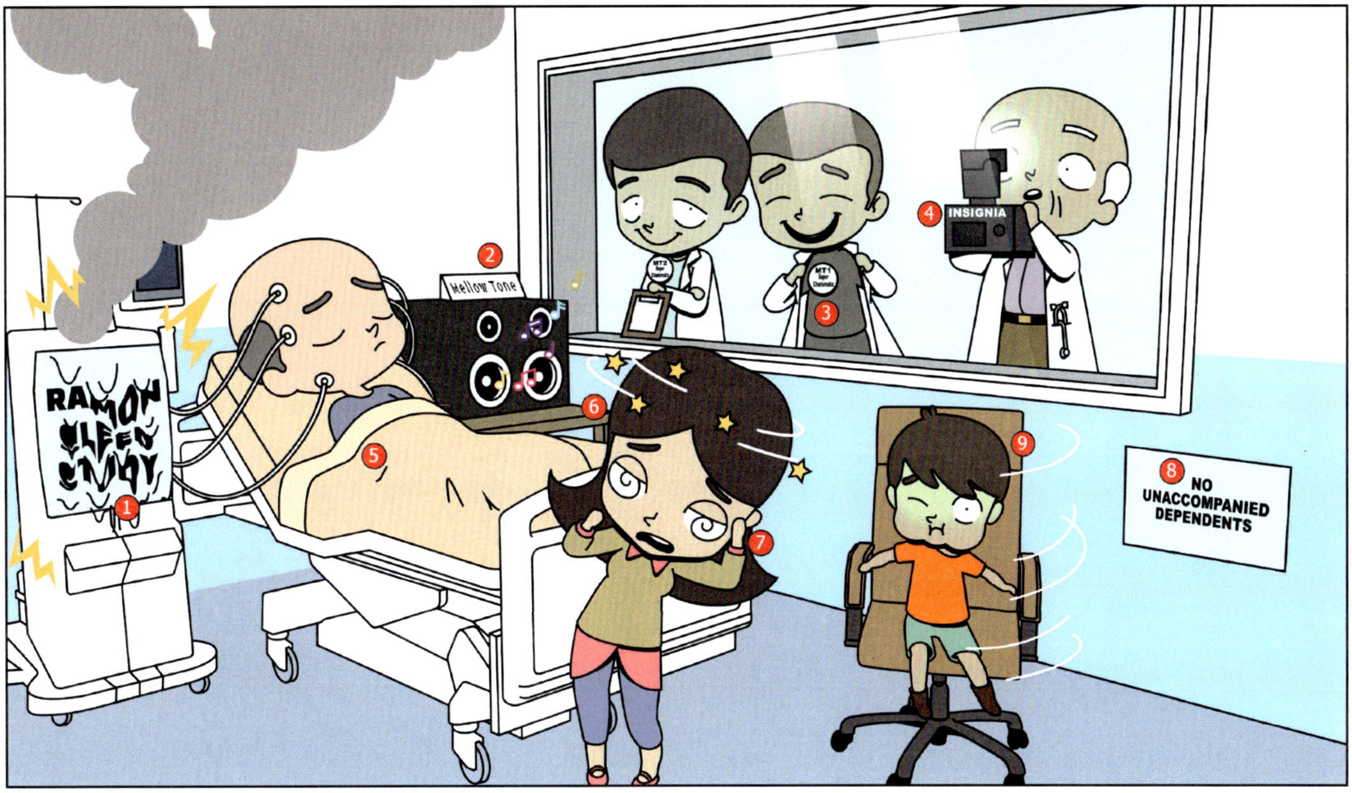

1. Sleep monitor machine with melting "Ramon" label: Ramelteon

2. Speaker playing music with mellow tones: Acts as a melatonin receptor agonist

3. Medical trainees wearing "MT1" and "MT2" stickers that say "super charismatic": Binds MT_1 and MT_2 in the suprachiasmatic nucleus

4. Attending holding Insignia camera with flash going off in his eyes: Use for insomnia

5. Sleeping patient: Can cause fatigue

6. Wife dizzy due to fumes from broken machine: Can cause dizziness

7. Wife holding head in pain due to fumes: Can cause headaches

8. "No unaccompanied dependents" sign in sleep study room: Does not cause dependence

9. Child nauseous from spinning in chair: Can cause nausea and vomiting

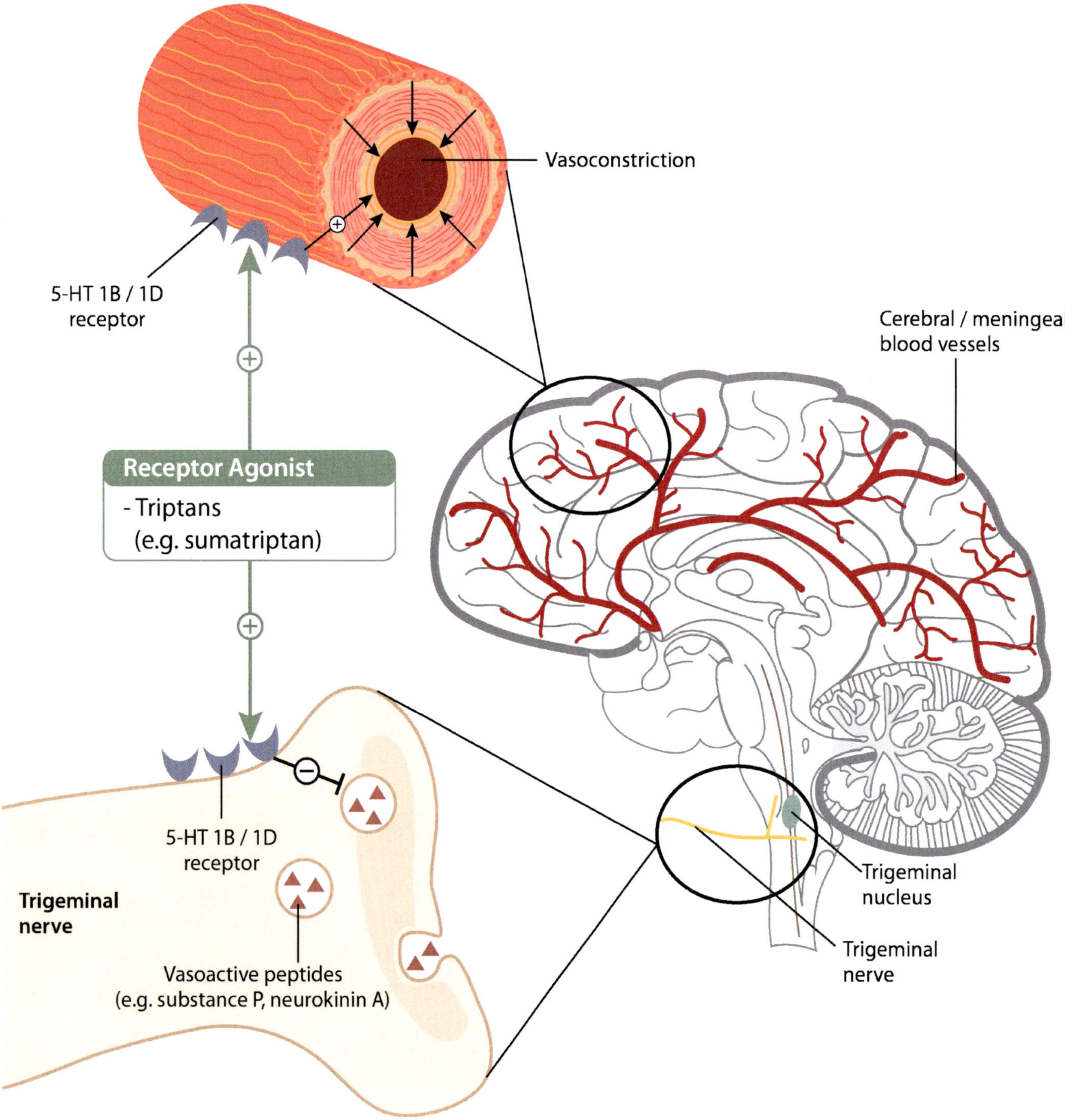

Figure 9.12.4 - Mechanism of Triptans

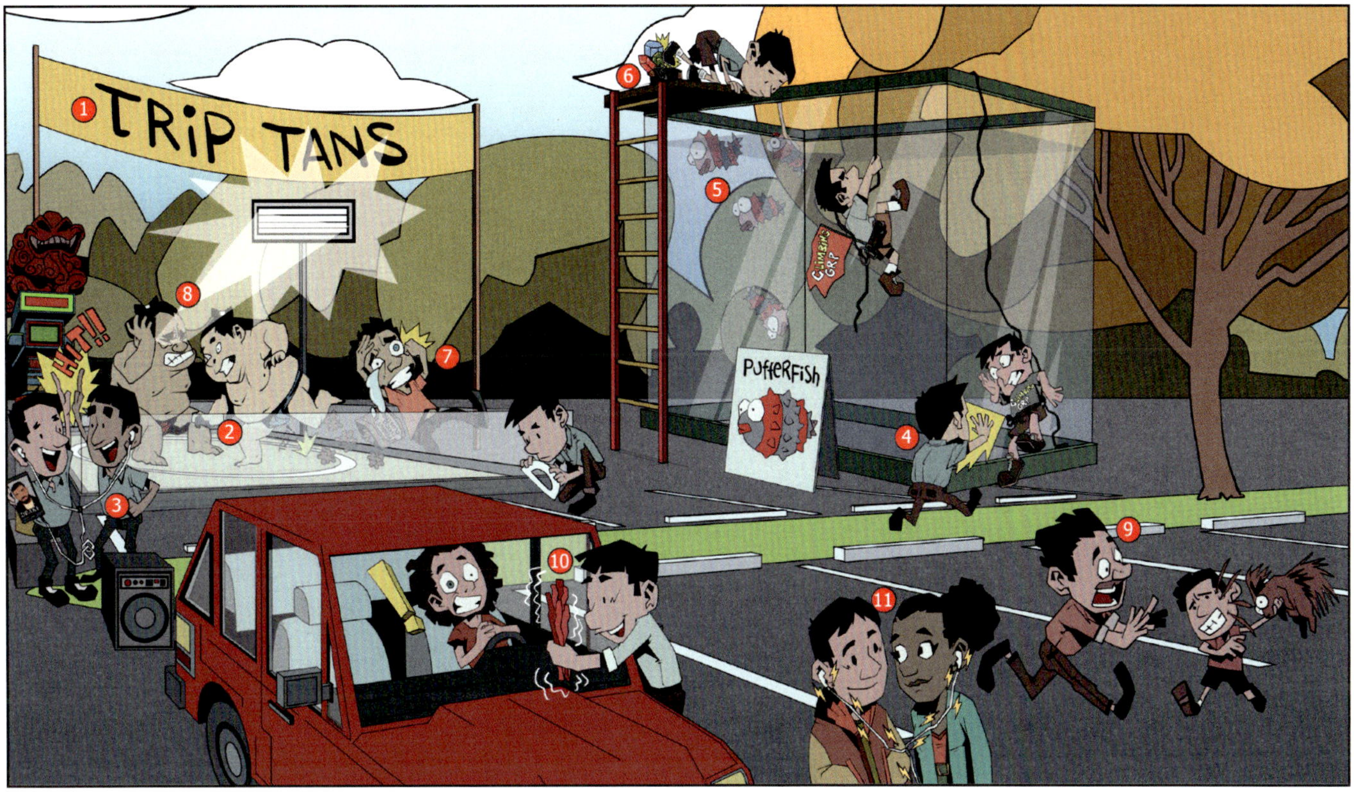

1. "Trip Tans" banner guaranteeing suntans: Triptans

2. Tripping sumo wrestler: Sumatriptan

3. Kids high-fiving while sharing a Drake tune through the same headphones next to bass speaker: 5-HT1B/1D agonist

4. Climbing group member of "Climbing GRP" t-shirt being blocked from climbing fish tank: Sumatriptan blocks the release of calcitonin gene-related peptide (CGRP)

5. Relaxed, constricted puffer fish with red stripes: Works by inducing vasoconstriction

6. Guy stepping on bag with three gems: Inhibits trigeminal nerve activation

7. Guy eating peanut clusters giving himself a headache and event worker holding measurement device at acute angle: Use for acute cluster headache

8. Sumo wrestler blinded by Insignia camera flash holding head in pain: Use for acute migraine

9. Kid covered in porcupine needles: Sumatriptan can cause mild paresthesia

10. Woman grabbing her chest inside car while salesman is shaking red licorice: Sumatriptan can cause coronary artery vasospasm

11. Electric volts from headphones shocking couple sharing a tune: Sumatriptan can cause serotonin syndrome

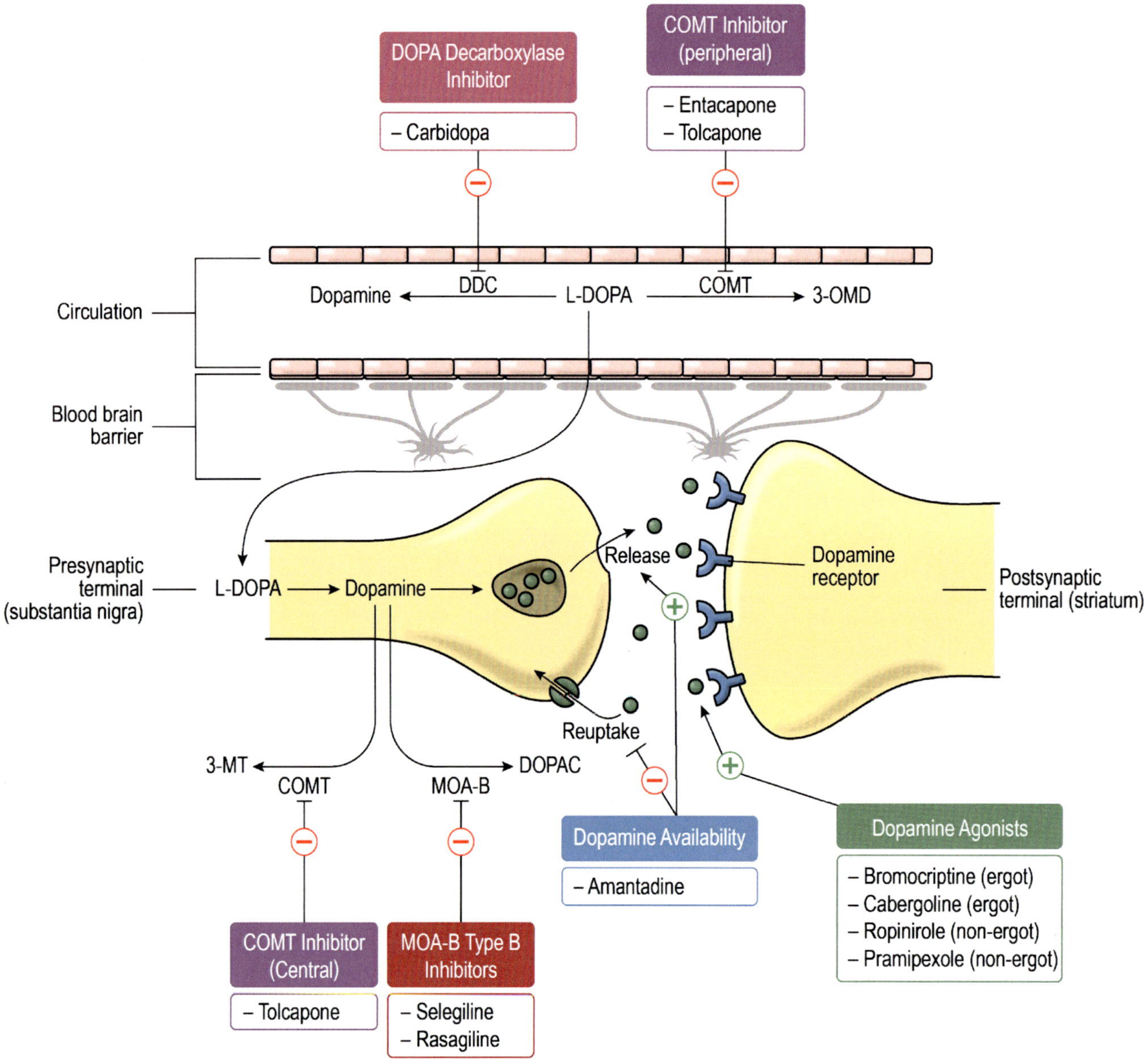

Figure 9.12.5 - Drugs that Interact with Dopamine Pathways

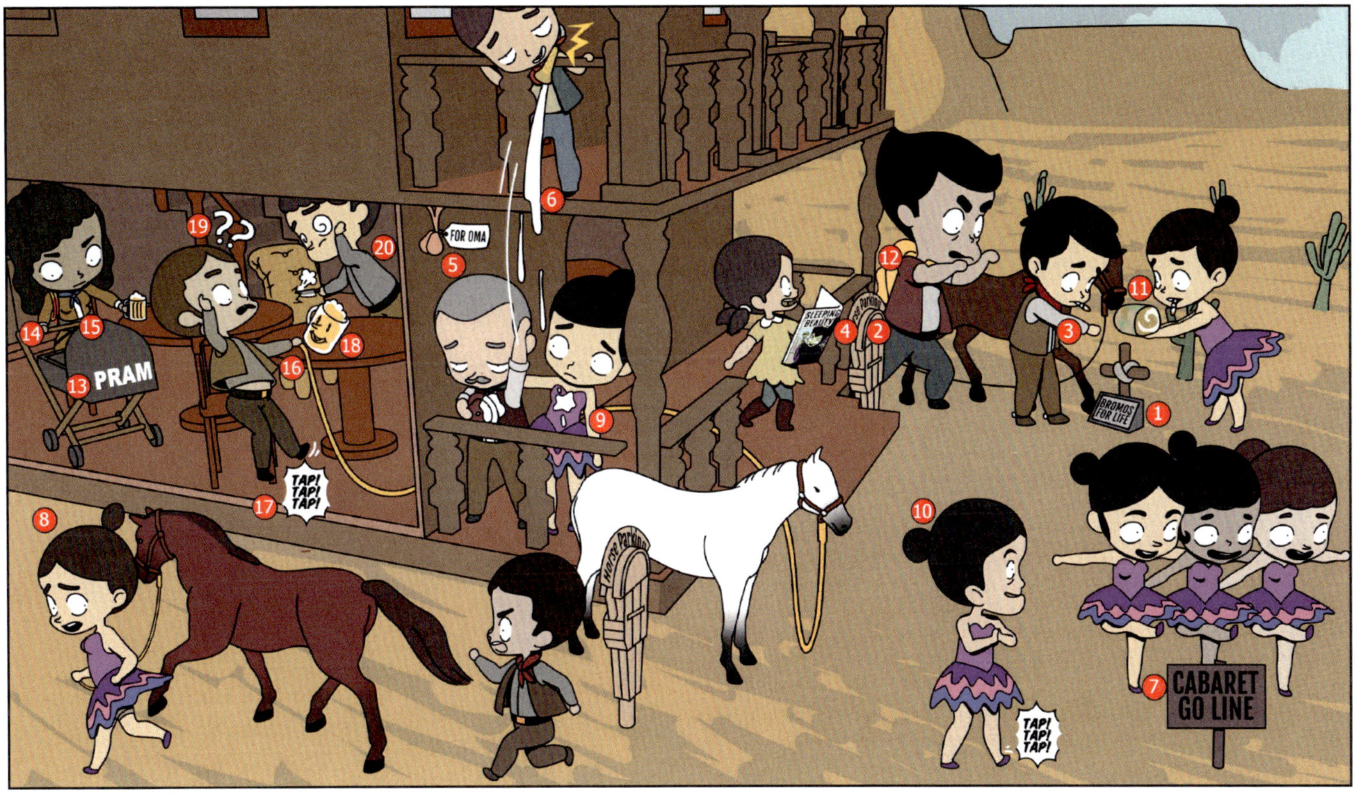

1. Cowboy next to crypt with tombstone reading, "Bromos for life": Bromocriptine

2. Parking meter by tombstone: Use for Parkinson disease

3. Cowboy smoking dope: Dopamine agonist

4. Maleficent with staff of neurological power on comic book cover: Bromocriptine can cause neuroleptic malignant syndrome

5. Two budding pears hanging from ceiling with tag reading, "for Oma": Use bromocriptine for pituitary adenoma

6. Two people on lower floor underneath budding pears who have milk spilt on them: Bromocriptine can be used for prolactinemia and galactorrhea from pituitary adenoma

7. Dancers near "Cabaret Go Line" sign: Cabergoline

8. Manager yelling at dancer who parked her horse out front: Cabergoline is not used for Parkinson disease

9. Cabaret dancer under budding pears with milk on chest: Cabergoline can be used for prolactinoma and galactorrhea from pituitary adenoma

10. Head cabaret dancer tapping her foot restlessly to the rhythm: Cabergoline can be used for restless leg syndrome

11. Cabaret dancer giving mourning cowboy moldy rye bread: Bromocriptine and cabergoline are ergot-derived (fungus that grows on rye)

12. Enormous, rough-faced guy approaching cowboy and dancer: Bromocriptine or cabergoline can be used for acromegaly

13. Mom with "pram" stroller: Pramipexole

14. Rope rolled up in a lasso on mom's shoulder: Ropinirole

15. Bloody rope on shoulder of mom who strangled her husband impulsively: Pramipexole and ropinirole can decrease inhibition and increase impulsivity (adverse effect)

16. Guy sitting next to "pram" stroller holding rope tied to horse near parking meter: Use pramipexole and ropinirole for Parkinson's disease

17. Guy restlessly tapping foot while waiting for beer: Pramipexole and ropinirole can be used for restless leg syndrome

18. Guy hallucinating smiling beer talking to him: Pramipexole and ropinirole can cause hallucinations

19. Guy confused by hallucinations: Pramipexole and ropinirole can cause confusion

20. Guy stabbing inflatable chair in knife fight: pramipexole and ropinirole can cause postural hypotension

See Figure 9.12.5 - Drugs that Interact with Dopamine Pathways (Neurology Pharmacology, Section 10, Page 253)

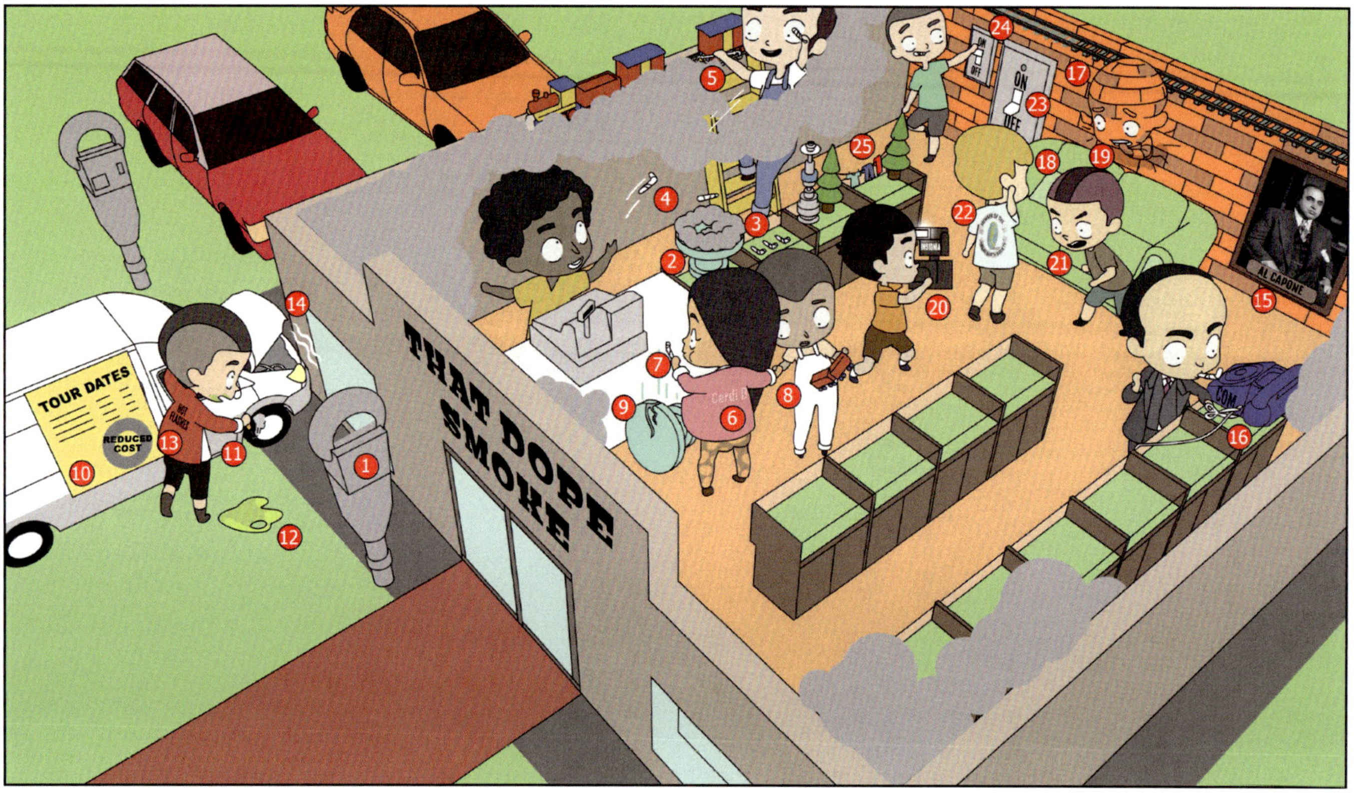

1. Dope shop with parking meter out front: Used for Parkinson disease

2. Dope device with levitating cloud of smoke: Levodopa

3. Display cause holding L-shaped joints next to levitating dope device: Levodopa is an analog of L-DOPA

4. L-shaped joint being tossed upward and breaking through smoke barrier: Levodopa (L-DOPA) can cross the blood brain barrier

5. Worker straightening out of L-shaped joint into linear shape above smoke cloud while pulling model train cars apart: L-DOPA gets converted to dopamine in the CNS by DOPA decarboxylase

6. Cardi B smoking dope: Carbidopa

7. Cardi B eating L-shaped joints next to joint being tossed upwards and levitating: Carbidopa is given with levodopa to increase bioavailability of L-DOPA for the CNS

8. Cardi B preventing worker below smoke clouds from separating model train cars: Carbidopa is a peripheral DOPA decarboxylase inhibitor → increased L-DOPA entering the CNS

9. Levitating dope device being knocked over under the cloud: Decreased peripheral conversation of L-DOPA to dopamine → decreased peripheral adverse effects of levodopa

10. "Reduced Cost" sign listening concerts on Cardi B's tour bus: Carbidopa reduces the peripheral side effects of levodopa

11. Cardi B's drummer accidentally stabbing deflating tire with keys while leaning against van for support: Carbidopa can reduce postural hypotension

12. Fresh puddle of vomit next to drummer: Carbidopa can reduce nausea/vomiting

13. Drummer wearing "Hot Flashes" jacket: Carbidopa can reduce hot flashes

14. Cardi B's tour bus engine rattling: Carbidopa can reduce risk of arrhythmias

15. Al Capone photo on wall of dope shop: Entacapone and tolcapone

16. Owner dressed as Al Capone smoking L-shaped joint while cutting COM telephone: Entacapone and tolcapone inhibit COMT → decreases L-DOPA degradation → increased L-DOPA levels

17. Kid hallucinating after smoking joint given to him by owner: Entacapone and tolcapone can cause hallucinations

18. Kid confused by hallucinations: Entacapone and tolcapone can cause confusion

19. Hallucinating kid biting nails nervously: Entacapone and tolcapone can cause anxiety

20. Insignia camera flash going off in photographer's eyes: Entacapone and tolcapone can cause insomnia

21. Angry, irritable guy going to confront photographer: Entacapone and tolcapone can cause agitation

22. Hallucinating kid wearing "Flat Earth Society" shirt: Entacapone and tolcapone can cause delusion

23. On-off switch in back of store: As disease progresses, patients taking levodopa can experience an "on-off" phenomenon (large motor fluctuations independent of levodopa dosing interval)

24. Guy smoking tiny L-shaped joint and flipping smaller switch on "on" position: Reducing dose helps alleviate these "on-off" effects

25. Strange, smokable display of two pine trees with clothesline strung between them: If reducing isn't possible, atypical antipsychotics (e.g. clozapine) may be helpful in reducing adverse effects

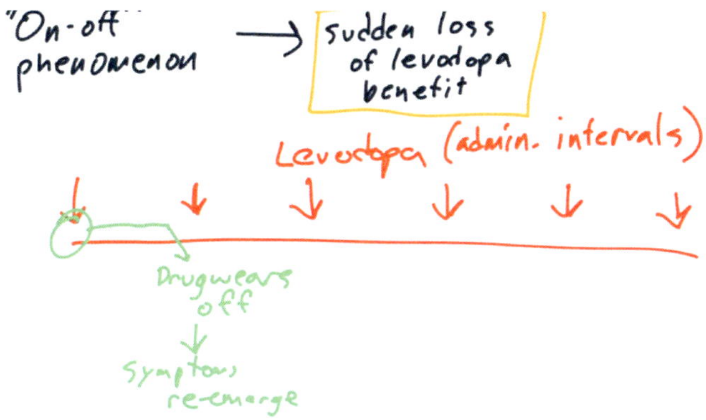

See Figure 9.12.5 - Drugs that Interact with Dopamine Pathways (Neurology Pharmacology, Section 10, Page 253)

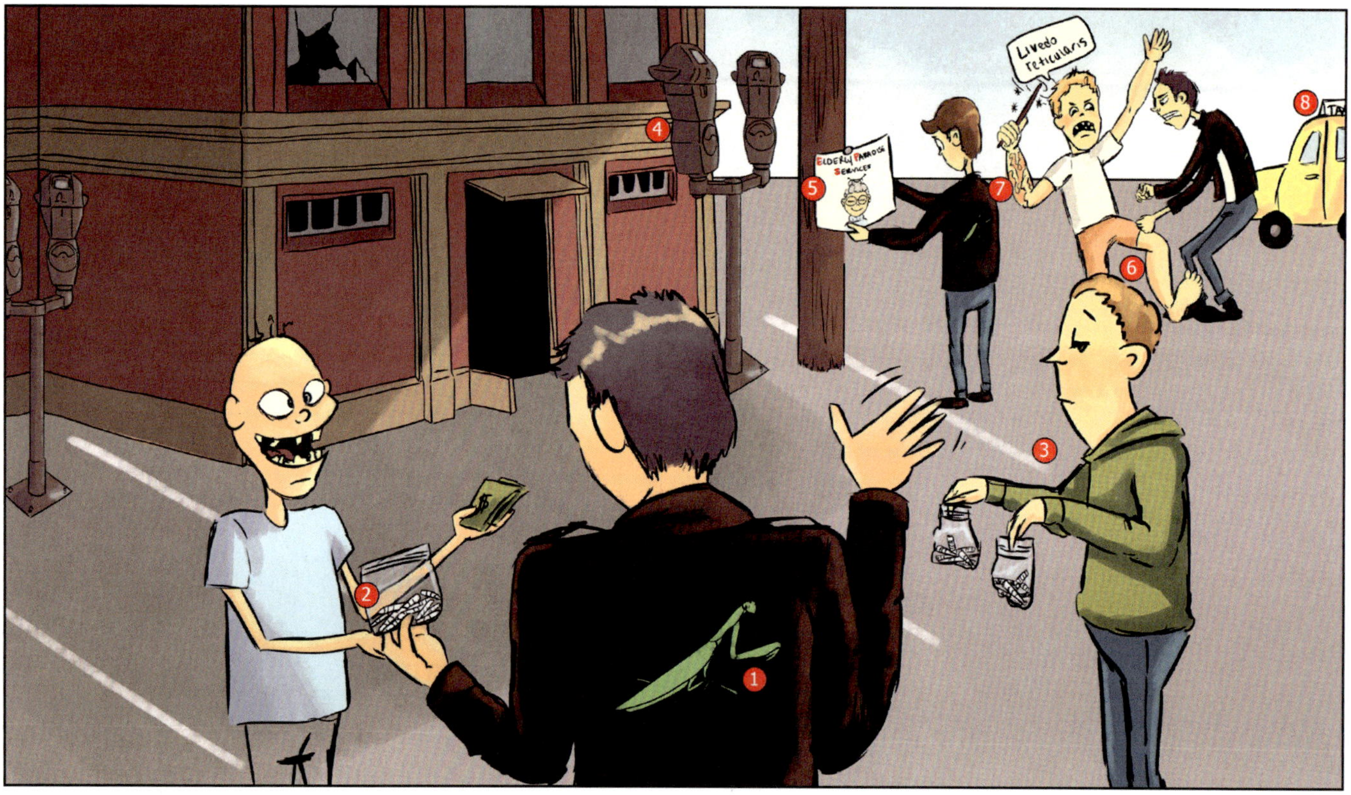

1. Dealer with praying mantis gang symbol on jacket: Amantadine

2. Dealer holding bag of dope: Dopamine

3. Dealer selling dope to one guy while refusing to take it back from the other: Increases dopamine release and decreases dopamine reuptake

4. Parking meters: Used to treat Parkinson's disease

5. Dealer's son in praying mantis jacket hanging up EPS ad to adverse his "Elder Paradise Service": Used to treat extrapyramidal symptoms

6. Headlight reflecting off mobster's eyes: Cataracts

7. Junkie's mottled and discolored arm holding wand: Can cause livedo reticularis

8. Taxi gang members arrived are waiting in background: Can cause ataxia

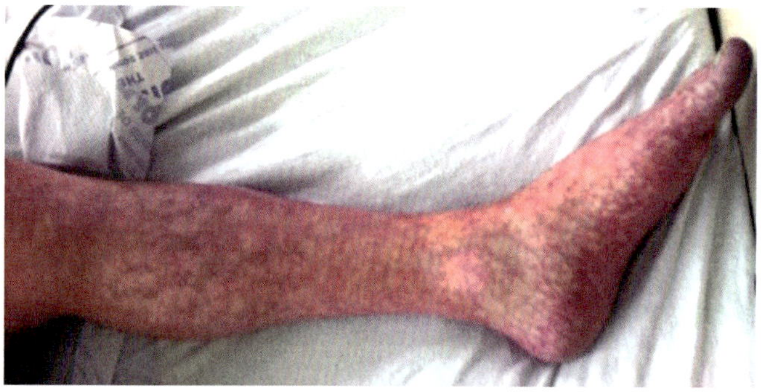

Photo Credit: Natsupawat T et al via Wiki CC SA 3.0

Figure 9.12.6 - Livedo Reticularis

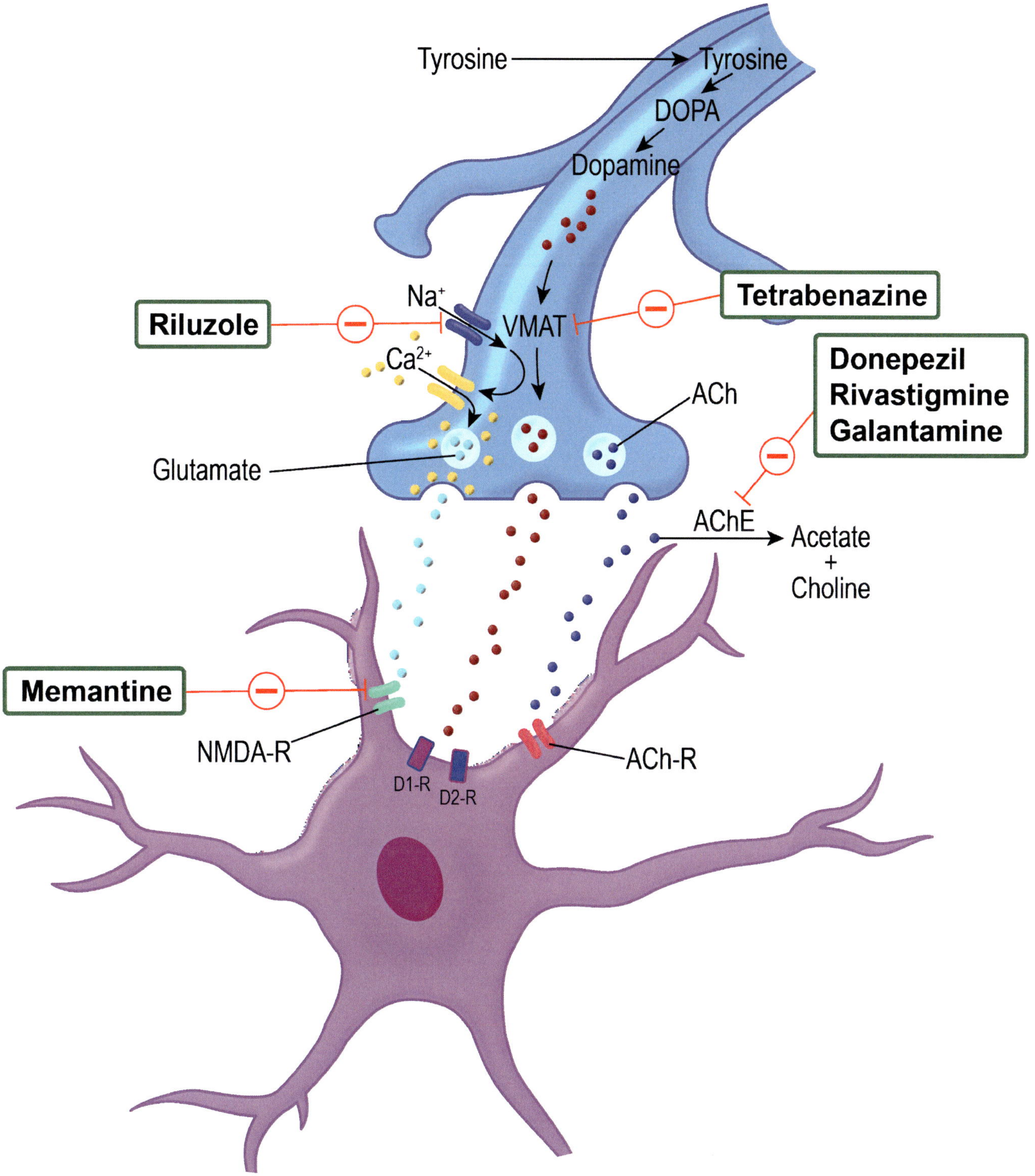

Figure 9.12.7 - Riluzole, Tetrabenazine, Memantine, and AChE Inhibitors Used for Dementia

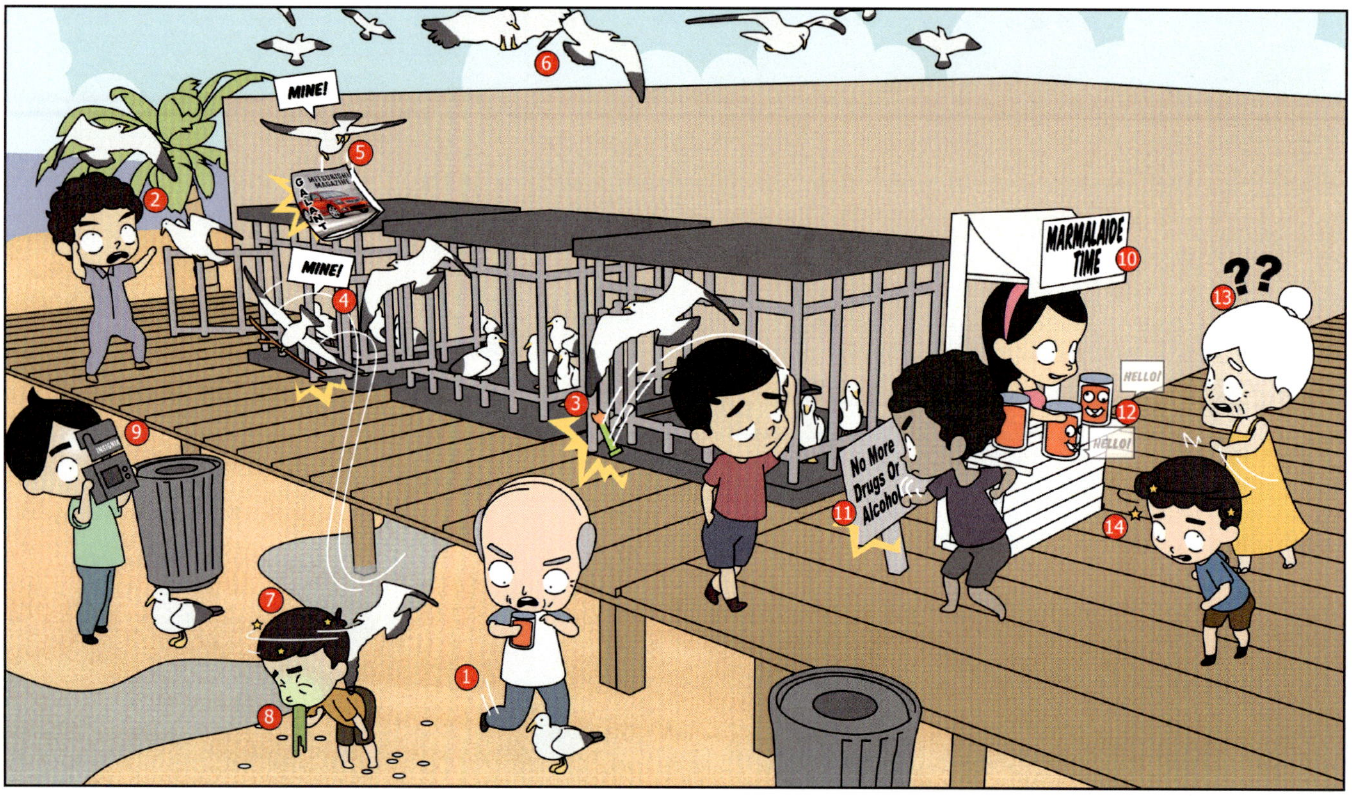

1. Older man scolding inanimate object: Used for moderate to advanced Alzeimer's dementia

2. A man trying to capture seagulls in cage to help reduce the seagull population: Acetylcholinesterase (AChE) normally reduces acetylcholine levels

3. Man tossing finished ("done") Pez dispenser over shoulder and accidentally releasing seagulls: donepezil block AChE

4. Seagull with stick flying over river while shouting "mine" hitting cage and opening door: Rivastigmine blocks AChE

5. Seagull saying "mine" and carrying magazine with Mitsubishi Galant on cover: Galantamine block AChE

6. Seagulls escaping from all 3 cages: All 3 of these drugs increase acetylcholine levels

7. Seagull making kid dizzy: Can cause dizziness

8. Kid vomiting: Can cause nausea

9. Tourist with Insignia camera flash going off in his face: Can cause insomnia

10. Girl running "Marmalade Time" marmalade stand: Memantine

11. Kid punching "no more drugs or alcohol" sign on pier in frustration: Memantine is an NMDA receptor antagonist

12. Hallucinating old lady: Memantine can cause hallucinations

13. Old lady confused by hallucinations: Memantine can cause confusion

14. Old lady hitting kid and making him dizzy: Memantine can cause dizziness

See Figure 9.12.7 - Riluzole, Tetrabenazine, Memantine, and AChE Inhibitors used for Dementia (Neurology Pharmacology, Section 13, Page 258)

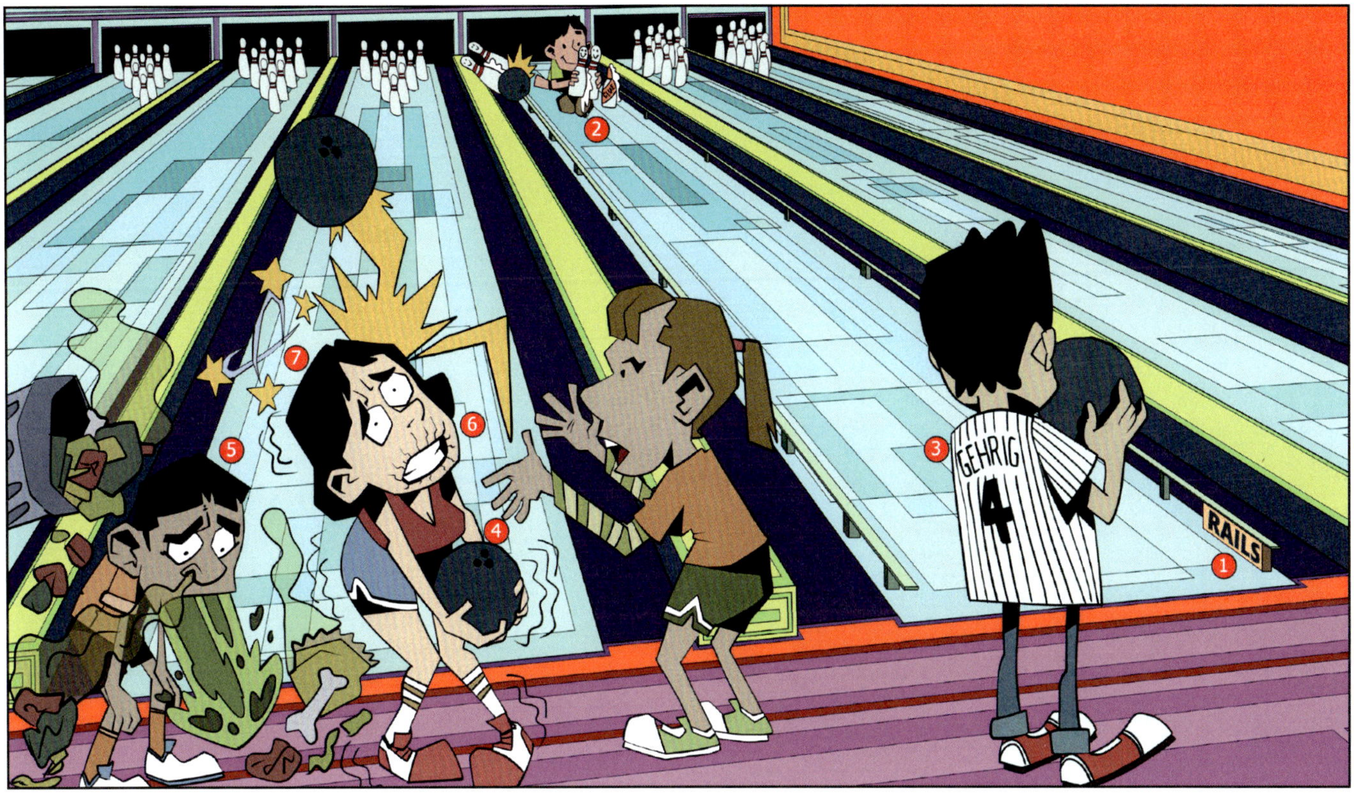

1. Bumper rails at bowling alley: Riluzole

2. Kid gluing bowling pins together in pairs and ball knocking one pair into the gutter, where they get blocked from being reset at the end of the lane: Neuroprotective and blocks glutamine neurotransmission in CNS

3. Teenager wearing Lou Gehrig jersey: Used for ALS (Lou Gehrig's disease)

4. Girl struggling to hold heavy bowling ball: Can cause weakness

5. Vomiting guy disgusted by overflowing garbage: Can cause nausea and vomiting

6. Weak girl with dry mouth and severely chapped lips: Can cause dry mouth

7. Dizzy, weak girl being hit in the head with bowling ball: Can cause dizziness

See Figure 9.12.7 - Riluzole, Tetrabenazine, Memantine, and AChE Inhibitors used for Dementia (Neurology Pharmacology, Section 13, Page 258)

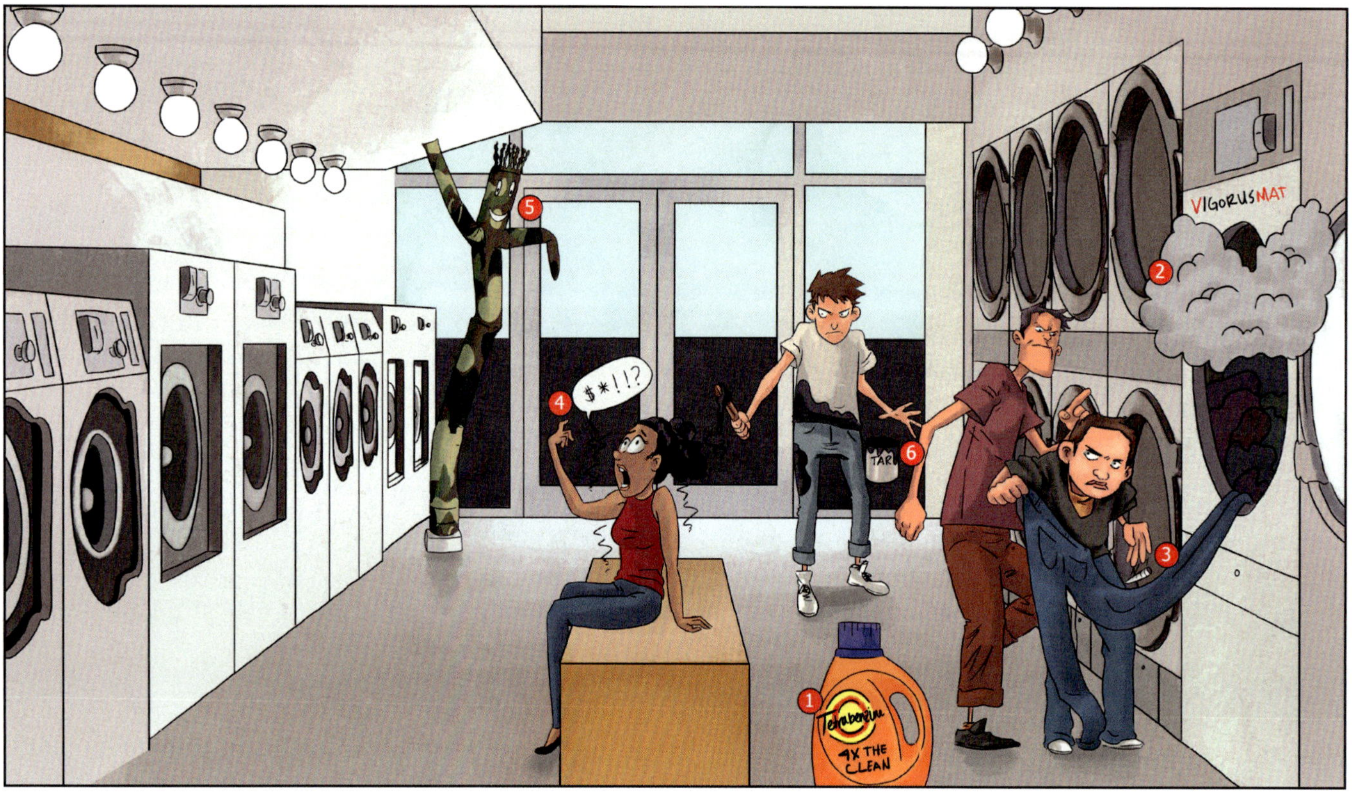

1. Tetrabenazine laundry detergent: Tetrabenazine

2. Malfunctioning "Vigorous MAT" laundry machine with smoke billowing out: Inhibits vesicular monoamine transporter (VMAT)

3. Kid taking out clothes and throwing dope ruined by laundry machine on the ground: Decreased dopamine release

4. Lady with Tourette syndrome exhibiting tics: Used for intractable and distressing tics in Tourette syndrome

5. Camouflage promotional airman dancing: Used for Huntington's chorea

6. Frustrated worker covered in tar holding tar-covered applicator stick: Used for tardive dyskinesia

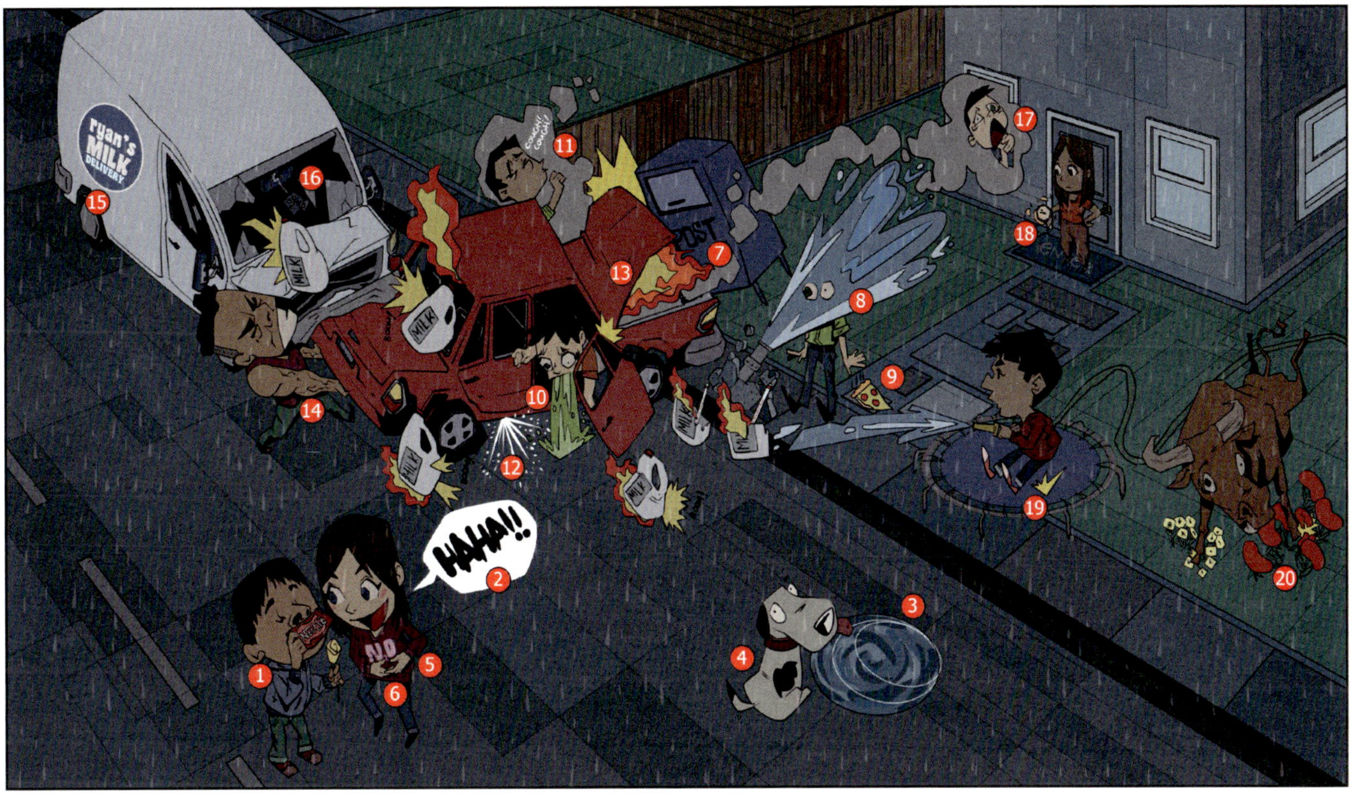

1. Kid inhaling the smell of Nestle candy bar: Inhaled anesthetics

2. Kid sniffing candy bar picking a flower in the rain for his girlfriend: Most inhaled anesthetic drug names end with the suffix, "-flurane"

3. Rain ripples that look like halos in water puddle: Halothane

4. Liver-spotted dog sitting next to puddle: Halothane is hepatotoxic

5. Girl wearing a sweater saying, "N2" laughing: Nitrous oxide (N_2O)

6. Girl laughing and holding belly: Can cause bowel distention

7. Postal box marked "post" being smashed by swerving car: Inhaled anesthetics enhance inhibitory postsynaptic channel activity

8. Bystander blasted in face by water from ruptured water line: Causes increased cerebral flow

9. Bystander dropping his food after getting sprayed in head: Causes decreased cerebral metabolic demand

10. Passenger climbing out of crashed car and vomiting: Can cause vomiting and nausea

11. Passenger coughing from car smoke: Can cause coughing

12. Car scraping along ground due to blown out ("depressed") tires and creating sparks: May cause cardiac depression

13. Car fire spreading to milk jugs with thermometers in them: Can cause malignant hyperthermia via excessive calcium from sarcoplasmic reticulum

14. Guy dragging burning car away with contracted muscles: Malignant hyperthermia causes severe muscle contractions

15. Van marked "Ryan's Milk Delivery" crashing and causing milk jugs to fly everywhere and explode: Mutations in the ryanodine receptor results in increased calcium release from the sarcoplasmic reticulum

16. Dominos hanging from rearview mirror of crashed car: Malignant hyperthermia is an autosomal dominant condition

17. Guy inside house, choking from smoke due to crashed cars: Inhaled anesthetics can cause respiratory depression

18. Mother standing on "enter" mat holding shaking alarm clock indicating time for dinner: Enflurane can cause seizures

19. Teenager jumping on trampoline and using hose to put out fire: Malignant hyperthermia is treated with dantrolene

20. Ox trampling wild kidney bean plants and flowers in the rain: Methoxyflurane is nephrotoxic

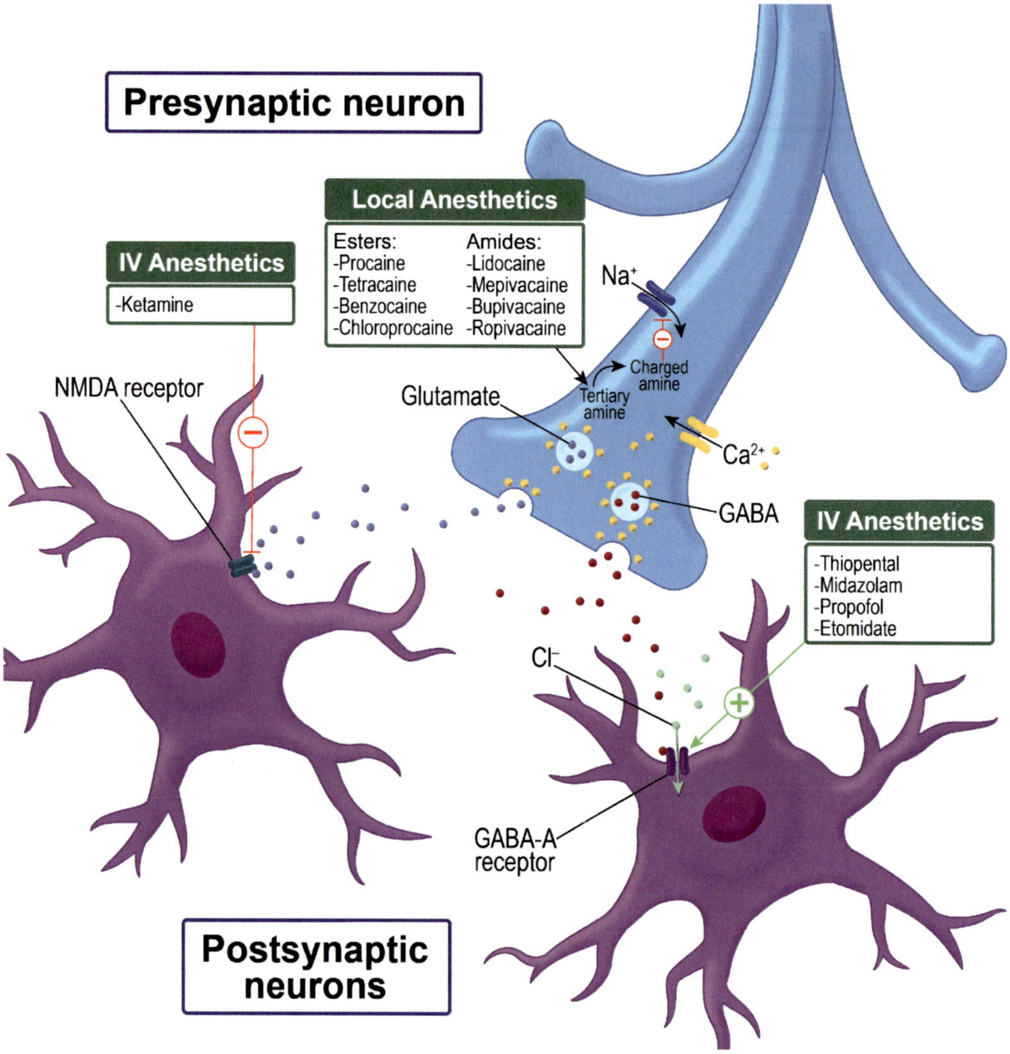

Figure 9.12.8 - Mechanism of Local and IV Anesthetics

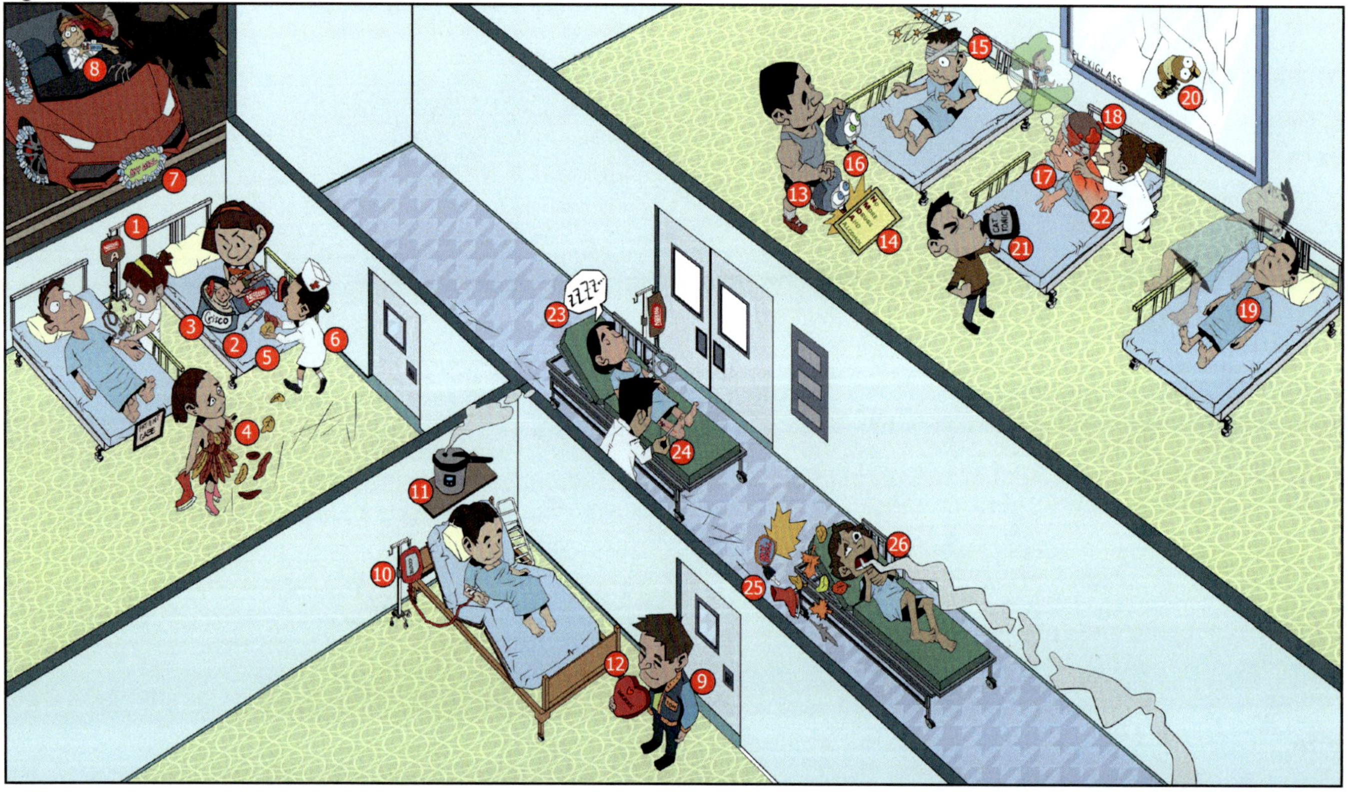

1. Nurse treating patient named Gabe with IV bolus filled with Grade "A" Nestle chocolate: IV anesthetics work by stimulating GABA-A receptors (except ketamine)

2. Gabe's little sister drawing pentagrams on Ken doll's thighs with a pen: Thiopental

3. Sister dumping Ken doll with decorated thighs and Nestle bar into Crisco oil: Thiopental has high lipid solubility

4. Gabe's pro skater mom wearing fall-themed costume with leaves falling off: Propofol

5. Sister mixing fall leaves into the Crisco: Propofol has high lipid solubility

6. ICU nurse: Propofol is common in ICU setting in which patients need prolonged sedation

7. Surgeon injecting himself with blue benzos syringe before getting out of car with "My Dazi" license plate: Midazolam

8. Dementor sucking memories out of the front of "My Dazl" surgeon's head: Midazolam can cause anterograde amnesia

9. Tom Cruise visiting inpatient girlfriend for hospital date: Etomidate

10. Tom's date getting blood transfusion due to her unstable condition while lying on unstable hospital bed: Etomidate is used for patients with hemodynamic instability

11. Gently depressurizing pressure cooker releasing steam above Tom's date's head: Etomidate decreases ICP

12. Tom giving unopened heart-shaped chocolate box to girlfriend: Etomidate has little to no effect on the cardiovascular system

13. Physical therapy trainer demonstrating how to use kettlebell: Ketamine

14. Trainer knocking over "No More Drugs and Alcohol" sign with kettlebell: Ketamine is an NMDA receptor antagonist

15. Disoriented patient with bandaged head waking up in a daze: Ketamine can cause disorientation upon emergence from sedation

16. Disoriented patient hallucinating that kettlebells are talking to him: Ketamine can cause hallucinations upon emergence from sedation

17. Patient waking up from vivid dream: Ketamine can cause vivid dreams upon emergence from sedation

18. Patient with blood-soaked bandages on head: Ketamine increases cerebral blood flow

19. Patient having an out-of-body experiences while asleep: Ketamine can cause dissociative amnesia

20. Caterpillar on plexiglass observation window: Can cause a state similar to that of cataplexy

21. Friend bringing patient "Cat Tonic" moonshine: Can cause a state similar to that of catatonia

22. Nurse rubbing patients red and sore back to ease patient's pain: Use for analgesia

23. Patient being put to sleep with Nestle chocolate IV: Used for anesthesia induction

24. Patient being stitched up quickly while sedated: Used for short surgical procedures

25. Pro skater's fallen leaves are dropped skate by ""My Dazl" keychain next to hospital bed's deflating tire: Midazolam and propofol can cause low blood pressure

26. Patient choking on visitor's cigarette smoke: Midazolam and propofol can cause respiratory depression

See Figure 9.12.8 - Mechanism of Local and IV Anesthetics (Neurology Pharmacology, Section 17, Page 263)

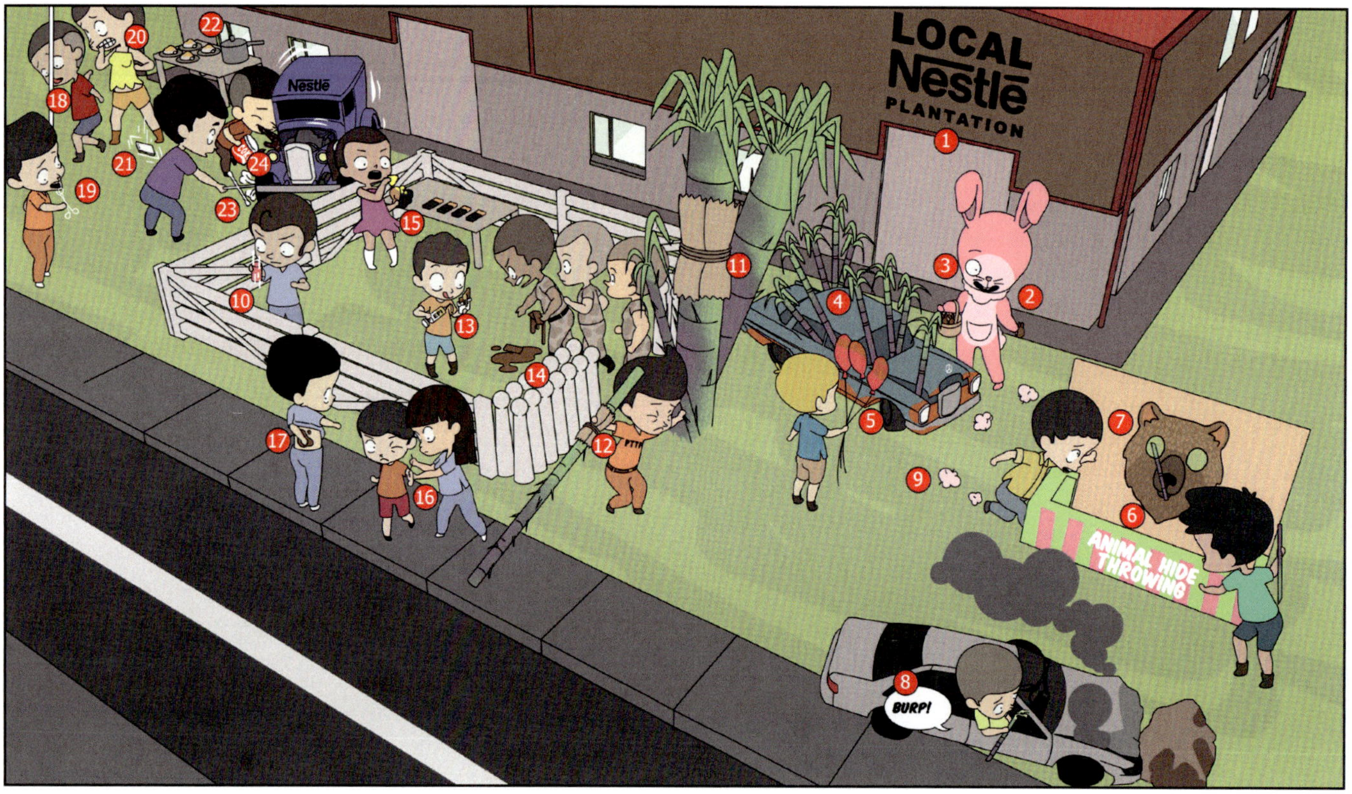

1. Local Nestle plantation: Local anesthetics

2. Easter Bunny handing out samples to visitors: Esters

3. One-eyed Easter Bunny costume: All esters have only one "i" in their names (e.g. procaine, tetracaine, benzocaine, chloroprocaine)

4. Antique Benz car outside with sugar canes growing through it: Benzocaine

5. Rusty antique Benz with sugar canes turning balloons brown after rubbing against them: Benzocaine can cause methemoglobinemia

6. Kid aiming at bear's eyes in carnival game: Amides

7. "Aim for the 2 eyes" carnival game: Amides have two "i"s in their names (e.g. lidocaine, mepivacaine, bupivacaine, ropivacaine)

8. Drunk guy burping with chewing on sugarcane after crashing his car: Bupivacaine can cause severe cardiovascular toxicity

9. Kid allergic to bunnies running away from Easter Bunny and leaning on "aim for the 2 eyes" stand: If allergic to esters, give amides

10. Guy inside fence holding blocked salt shaker: Block Na^+ channels by binding to specific receptors on the inner portion of the channel

11. Worker pulling up sugar cane sticks from small to large and pulling up ones wrapped in cloth first: Nerves are blocked in this order: Small-diameter myelinated → small-diameter unmyelinated → large myelinated → large unmyelinated

12. Worker pulling up sugar cane sticks wearing "PTTP" shirt: Sensations are lost in this order: Pain, temperature, touch, pressure (PTTP)

13. Kid injecting himself with enhanced Nestle chocolate-filled Epipen: Can be given with epinephrine to enhance local anesthetic effects

14. Head Marine in group of three getting angry at melted chocolate and blocking other Marines from entering area with bilayer fence: Local anesthetics are tertiary amines that enter the membrane unchanged → become charged → bind to ion channels to block them

15. Girl pouring vinegar onto battery-shaped Nestle bars, causing them to swell and be unable to fit into her mouth: In acidic tissues, alkaline anesthetics are charged and cannot penetrate the membrane effectively

16. Kid outside fence area getting stitches: Used for minor surgical procedures

17. Guy rubbing nestle chocolate along his spine: Use for spinal anesthesia

18. Kid licking metal flagpole after assuming it was edible: Can cause a metallic taste

19. Guy numb from dentist's anesthetics with dentist's forceps still on lips: Can cause perioral numbness

20. Nervous mom biting nails after son licks flagpole: Can cause anxiety

21. Nervous mom dropping ringing phone: Can progress to seizures

22. Pressure cooker making food for visitors: Can cause hypertension

23. Deflating tire on Nestle car: Can cause hypotension

24. Guy spraying Coke out of his nose onto shaking Nestle car's engine: Can cause arrhythmia

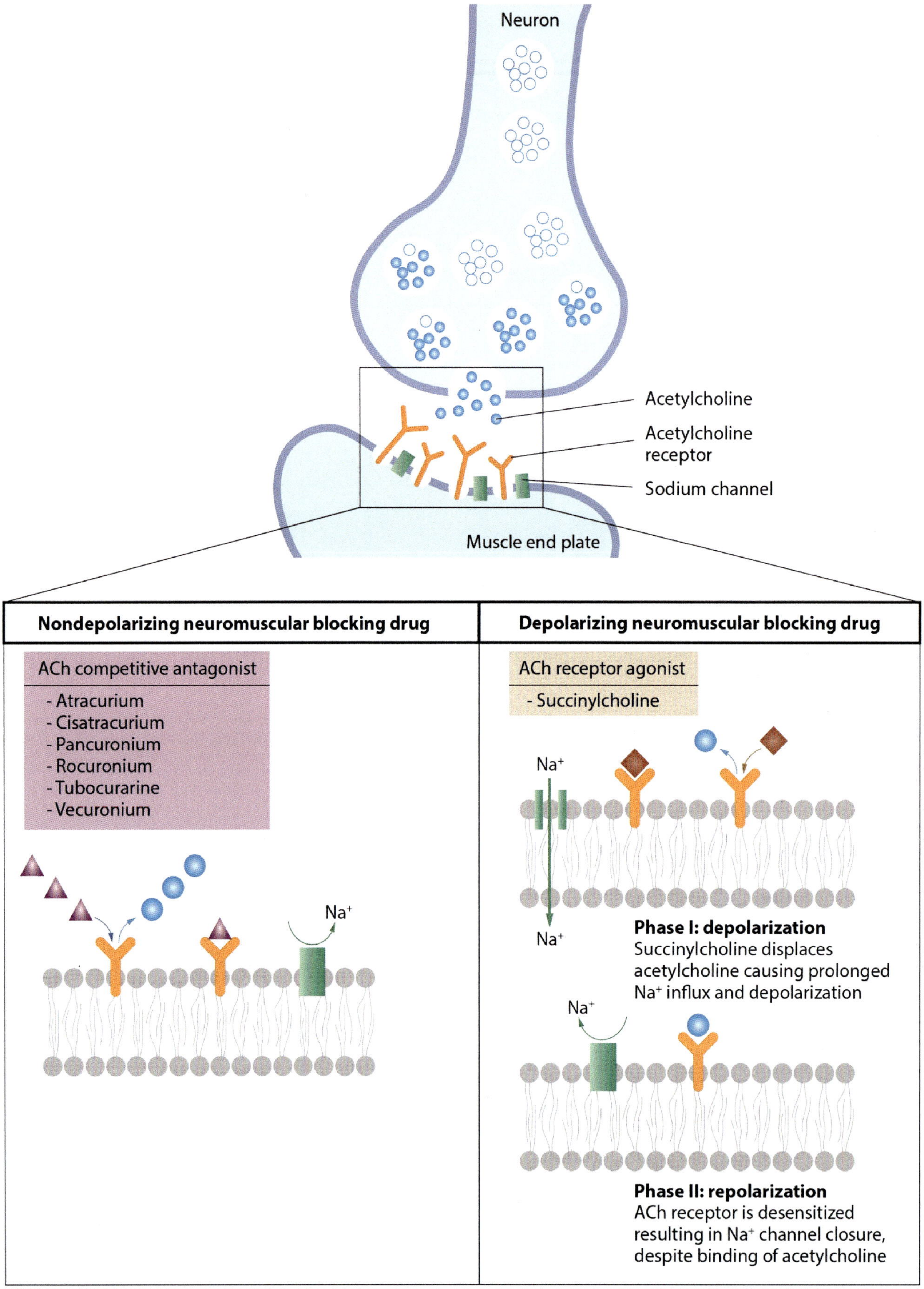

Figure 9.12.9 - Neuromuscular Blocking Drugs

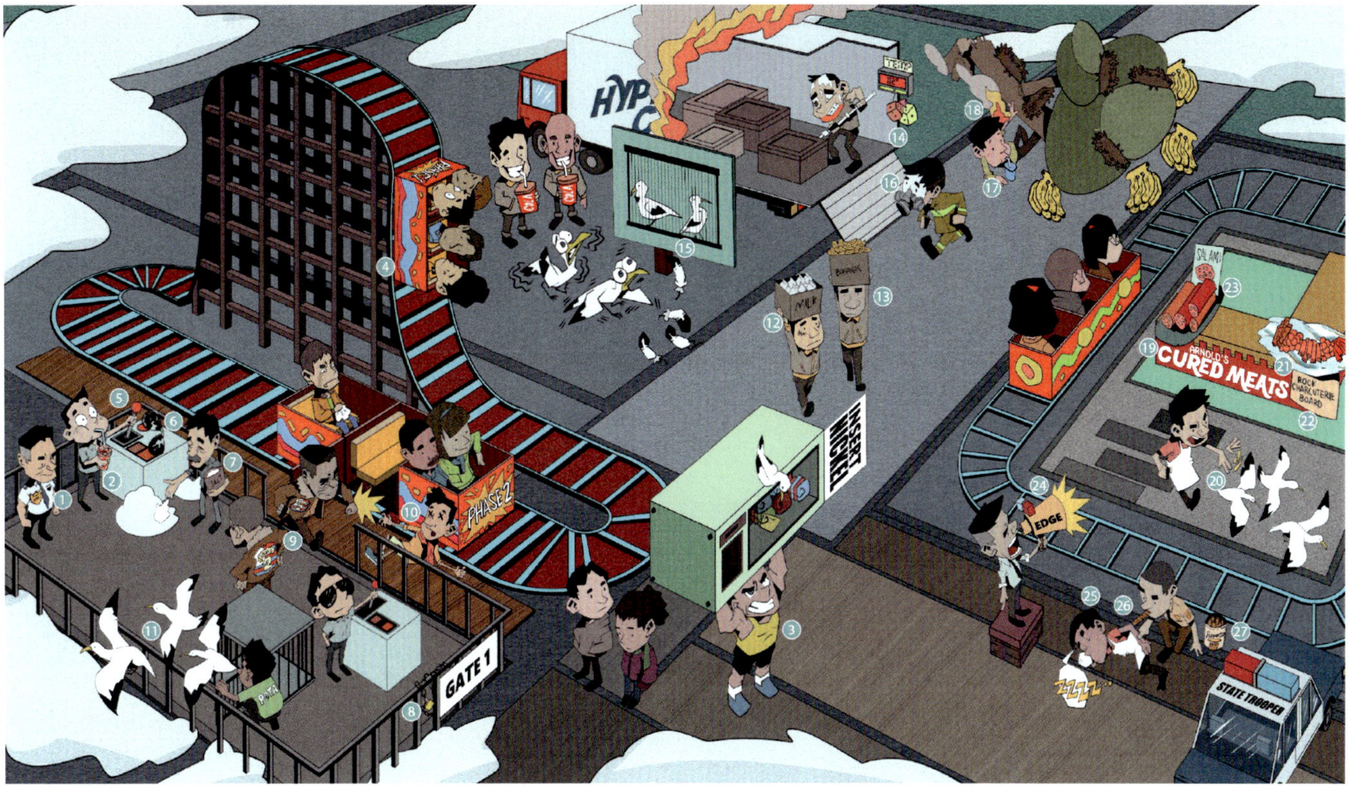

1. Blocked off and guarded control panel section of roller coaster in amusement park: Neuromuscular blocking drugs

2. Roller coaster operator sucking in cola drink through straw: Succinylcholine

3. Strong guy lifting up "insert nickel" vending machine with seagull perched on it: Succinylcholine is a strong nicotinic acetylcholine receptor agonist

4. Roller coaster stopped and sustained in mid-climb position: Sustains depolarization at neuromuscular end plate

5. Roller coaster operator with fully extended arm: Prevents muscle contraction

6. Broken pair of polarized sunglasses on control panel right on top of joystick: Succinylcholine sustains depolarization of the neuromuscular end plate → prevents muscle contraction

7. Park worker scattering big bag of deicing salt inside gated section: Na^+ channels around the plate becoming inactivated and are unable to reopen

8. Irreversible lock and chain on control panel area gate marked "gate 1": No antidote for Phase I of the succinylcholine blockade aka the prolonged depolarization phase

9. Two policemen next to second operator with fully extended arm and unbroken polarized sunglasses: Phase II occurs when repolarization takes place but the receptors are still desensitized

10. Officer with "squad 2" jacket punches kid and knocks him out: Leads to flaccid paralysis

11. Officer with "squad 2" jacket distracted while PETA activist releases seagulls: Cholinesterase inhibitors can reverse Phase II of blockade

12. Truck worker holding box of milk above head: Succinylcholine may cause hypercalcemia

13. Truck worker carrying box of bananas high above head: Succinylcholine may cause hyperkalemia

14. Worker inside hot truck holding lead pipe with ripped sleeve exposing rigid muscle: Succinylcholine may cause malignant hyperthermia

15. Seagulls paralyzed with fear in front of picture of seagulls in cage while two workers watch and suck cola through straws: Patients with pseudocholinesterase deficiency experience decreased succinylcholine breakdown → prolonged paralysis

16. Firefighter wearing CPAP-like mask: Prolonged apnea

17. Falling tree with several seagull nests and bunches of bananas crushing burned visitor: Certain pathologic states → upregulation of muscle nicotinic ACh receptors → acute hyperkalemia after succinylcholine administration

18. Falling tree crushing the burned visitor: In patients with crush injuries, burn injuries, myopathies, denerving injuries or disease (e.g. quadriplegia and Guillain-Barre syndrome) → upregulation of muscle nicotinic ACh receptor and/or rhabdomyolysis → release of large amounts of potassium when succinylcholine is administered

19. "Cured Meats" stand: Non-depolarizing neuromuscular junction drugs

20. Seagulls competing for food and blocked by cured meats worker: Non-depolarizing blocking agents are competitive ACh antagonists

21. Tray of cured meats: Atracurium

22. Cured meats served on fancy rock charcuterie board: Rocuronium

23. Tee cured meat stand with salami: Tubocurarine

24. Health inspector with EDGE megaphone and neon lights kicking out cured meat stand: Reverse nondepolarizing neuromuscular junction drugs using acetylcholinesterase (AChE) inhibitors: Neostigmine and edrophonium

25. Worker asleep on ground: AChE inhibitors may cause bradycardia

26. State trooper checking sleeping guy's pulse: Atropine can be given to reverse bradycardia caused by AChE inhibitors

27. State trooper with Pirouette cookie in mouth like cigar: Glycopyrrolate can be given to reverse bradycardia caused by AChE inhibitors

See Figure 9.2.4 - Tizanidine and Baclofen Mechanism (Autonomics in Pharmacology, Section III, Page 31)

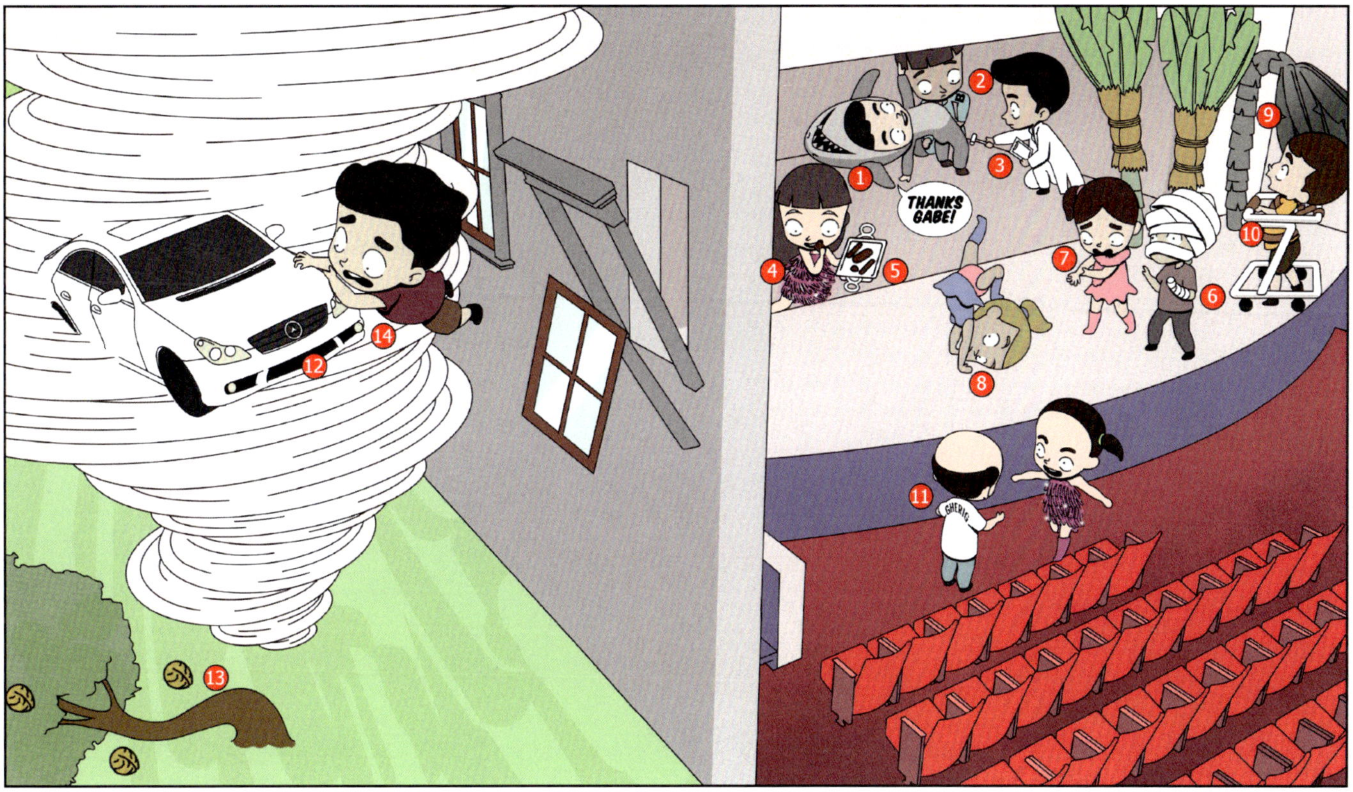

1. Actor in shark costume bending backwards to get low with back fin: Baclofen

2. Actor's boss Gabe trying to fix shark guy's injured back: Baclofen acts as an agonist at the GABAb receptor in the spinal cord

3. Shark guy has no response to reflex hammer: Baclofen decreased excitability of the spinal reflexes

4. Dancer wearing tinsel-covered dress: Tizanidine

5. Tinsel dress dancer gorging herself with treats from tray with 2 alpha-shaped handles: Tizanidine is a centrally acting α_2 agonist

6. Lady's burned head wrapped in bandages: Tizanidine or baclofen can be used as monotherapy for the treatment of spastically caused by spinal cord or brain disease

7. Dancer with muscle spasm: Tizanidine or baclofen can be used for muscle spasticity

8. Dancer distorting her body during performances: Tizanidine or baclofen can be used for dystonia

9. Palm tree wilting and dying after being unwrapped: Tizanidine or baclofen can be used for multiple sclerosis

10. Kid with cerebral palsy on stage: Tizanidine or baclofen can be used for cerebral palsy

11. Dancer off stage running to hug dad wearing Lou Gehrig jersey: Tizanidine can be used for amyotrophic lateral sclerosis (ALS)

12. Cyclone sucking up Mercedes Benz: Cyclobenzaprine

13. Topped over, "relaxed" walnut tree after cyclone: Cyclobenzaprine acts within the brainstem to relax muscles

14. Man grabbing onto Mercedes Benz while holding right arm with his left to check for pain: Cyclobenzaprine relieves pain and muscle spasticity

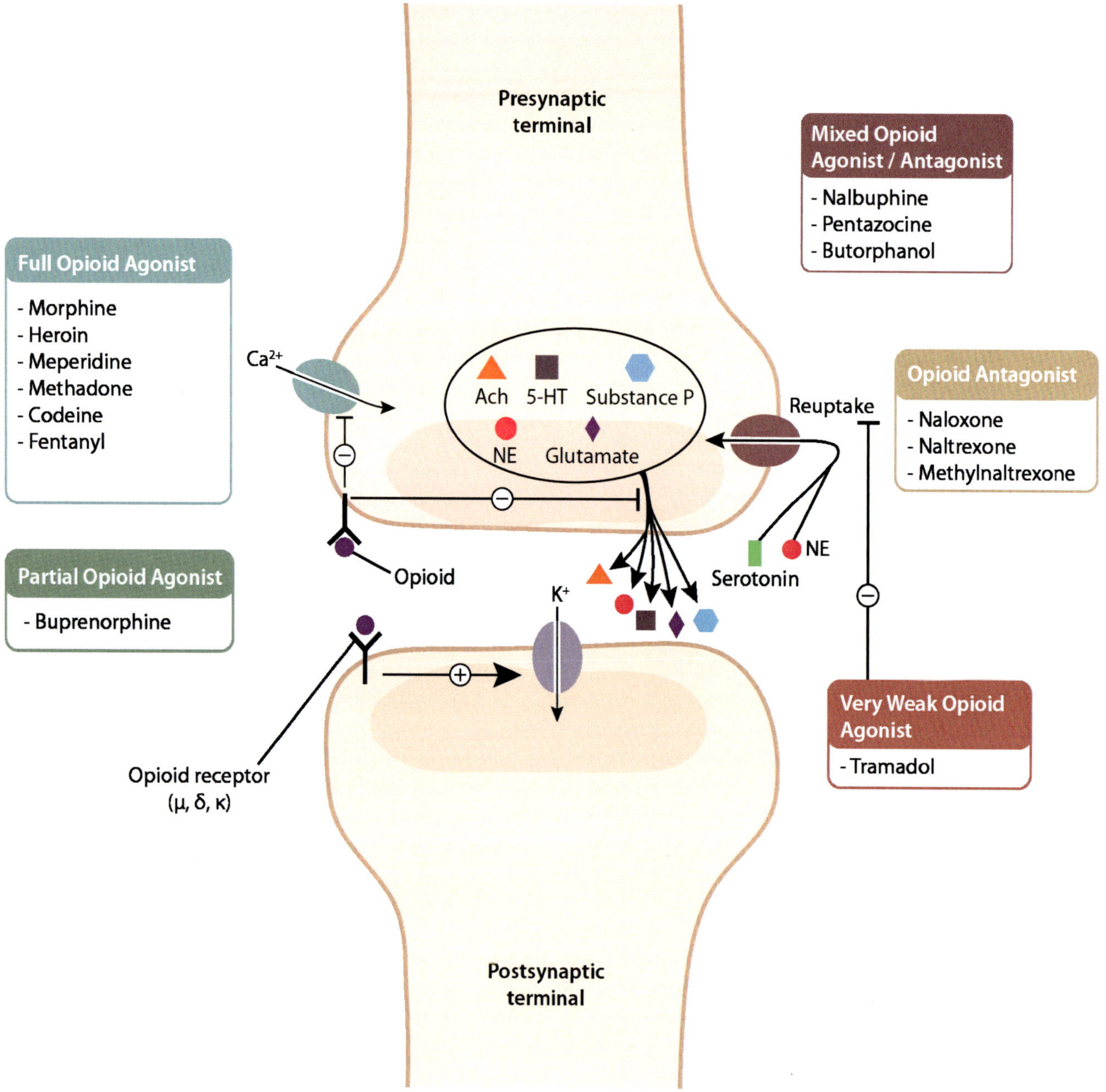

Figure 9.12.10 - Pharmacologic Effects on Opioid Receptors

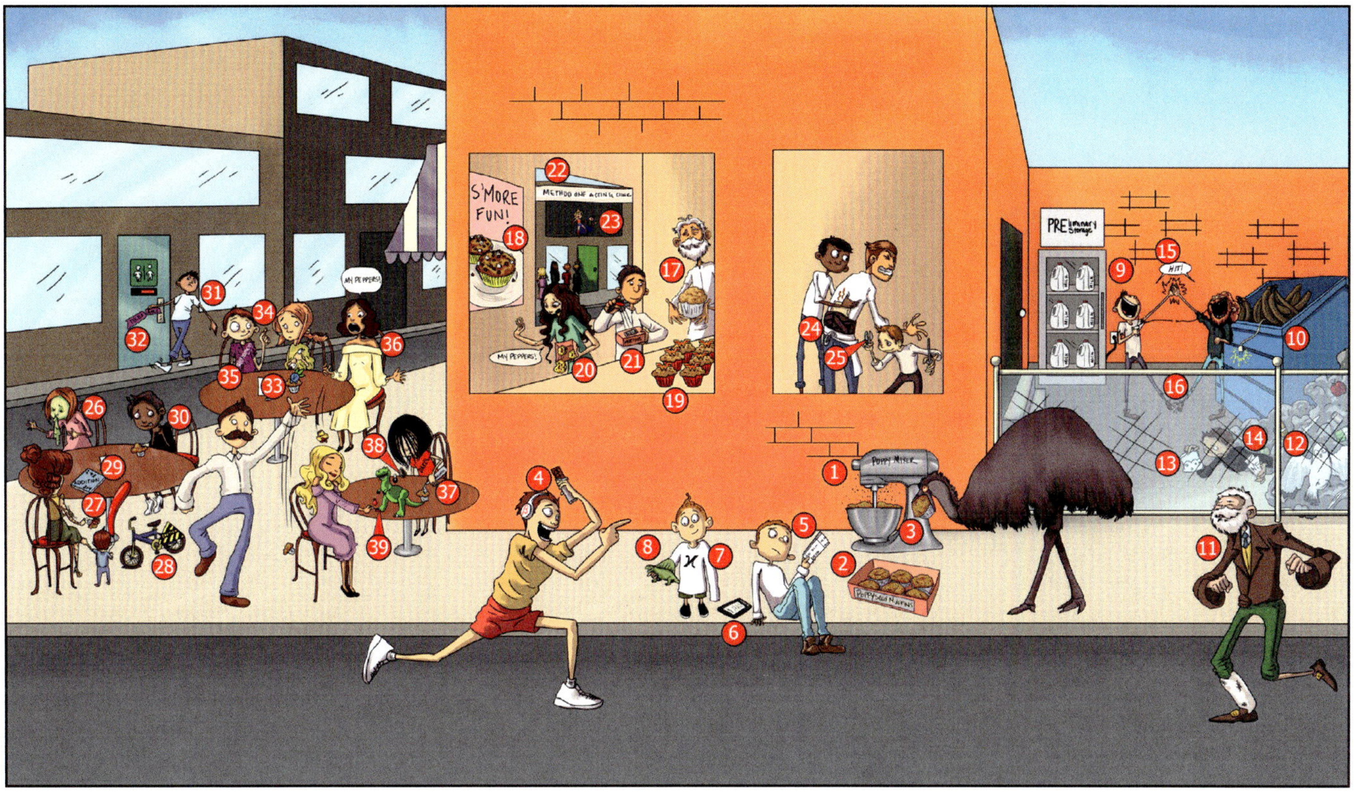

1. Electric mixer mixing poppy seed muffins: Opioid analgesics

2. Box of poppy seed muffins on street: Agonist at opioid receptors

3. Emu eating poppy seed muffin: μ receptor (mu receptor)

4. Runner wearing Beats headphones (marked with beta sign) and holding chocolate while chasing emu: β-endorphin binds to mu receptors

5. Student holding Delta airline ticket: δ receptor (delta receptor)

6. Student with tickets has e-reader Kindle: Enkephalin binds to delta receptors

7. Student's little brother wearing kappa fraternity shirt: ϰ receptor (kappa receptor)

8. Kid in kappa shirt holding dinosaur toy with fin on back: Dynorphin binds to kappa receptors

9. Closed, plugged-in fridge of milk behind bakery: receptor stimulation will close presynaptic Ca^{2+} channels

10. Open dumpster full of bananas and unplugged cables: Receptor stimulation will also open the postsynaptic K^{+} channels (hyperpolarized)

11. Old man with leg in cast who is not in pain skipping around: Decreased transmission of pain

12. Seagull trapped under garbage: Inhibits release of ACh

13. Kid holding bag of pea-like substance trapped under garbage: Inhibits release of substance P

14. Map marked "NE" in trapped kid's hand: Inhibits release of NE

15. Guys sharing a tune and high-fiving, causing headphone cord to break: Inhibits release of 5-HT

16. Mates glued together and using broken headphone cord: Inhibits release of glutamate

17. Big poppy seed muffin full of seeds: Full opioid agonists

18. Ad for "s'more fun" muffins: Morphine

19. Wonder Woman-themed muffins: Heroin

20. Customer saying "my peppers!" as she drops her pepper muffins: Meperidine

21. Barcode on muffin box: Codeine

22. Method One acting school: Methadone

23. Actor preventing heroine from falling out of Method One school window: Methadone is used for maintenance programs for heroin addicts

24. Baker with persistent back pain even after heat pack and massage: Use opioids for moderate to severe pain or refactor pain

25. Lung-shaped paring knife that is dripping wet: Use for acute pulmonary edema

26. Vomiting customer sitting outside: Opioids can cause nausea and vomiting

27. Itching customer with muffin decorated with flower and son holding long red balloon: Opioids can cause pruritus *mu-opioid stimulation causes histamine release leading to vasodilation and itching)

28. Deflating wheel on bike marked with "caution" sign: Use cautiously in patients with hypotension

29. Son's addition math book on table: Addiction possible

30. Person struggling to breathe after choking on muffin: Can cause respiratory depression

31. Person taking time in bathroom: Can cause constipation (mu opioid stimulation shows gut motility)

32. Impatient person ripping tolerance sign off bathroom door: No tolerance is developed against constipation (i.e. constipation persists even when tolerance has developed in other ways)

33. Girl shaking while struggling to squeeze out icing from piping bag onto muffin decorated with Oddi Pokemon: Sphincter of Oddi spasm → increased pressure in common bile duct → biliary colic (possible, but very rare)

34. Boy holding pin up to his eye: Can cause miosis

35. Boy holding pin wearing tattered t-shirt that says, "tolerance": No tolerance is developed against miosis (i.e. miosis persists even when tolerance has developed in other ways)

36. Lady with wide eyes and dilated pupils yelling "my peppers!" after dropping her muffin: Opposite of most opioids, meperidine causes mydriasis

37. GIrl with hair covering eyes wearing "D.A.R.E." shirt: Additive CNS depression with other drugs

38. Girl with hair covering eyes painting nails: Toxicity (CNS depression) treated with naloxone

39. Girl painting T-rex toy's nails and not realizing that someone dropped poppy seed muffin on her head: relapse prevented with naltrexone once detoxified

See Figure 9.12.10 - Pharmacologic Effects on Opioid Receptors (Psychiatric Pharmacology, Section 21, Page 271)

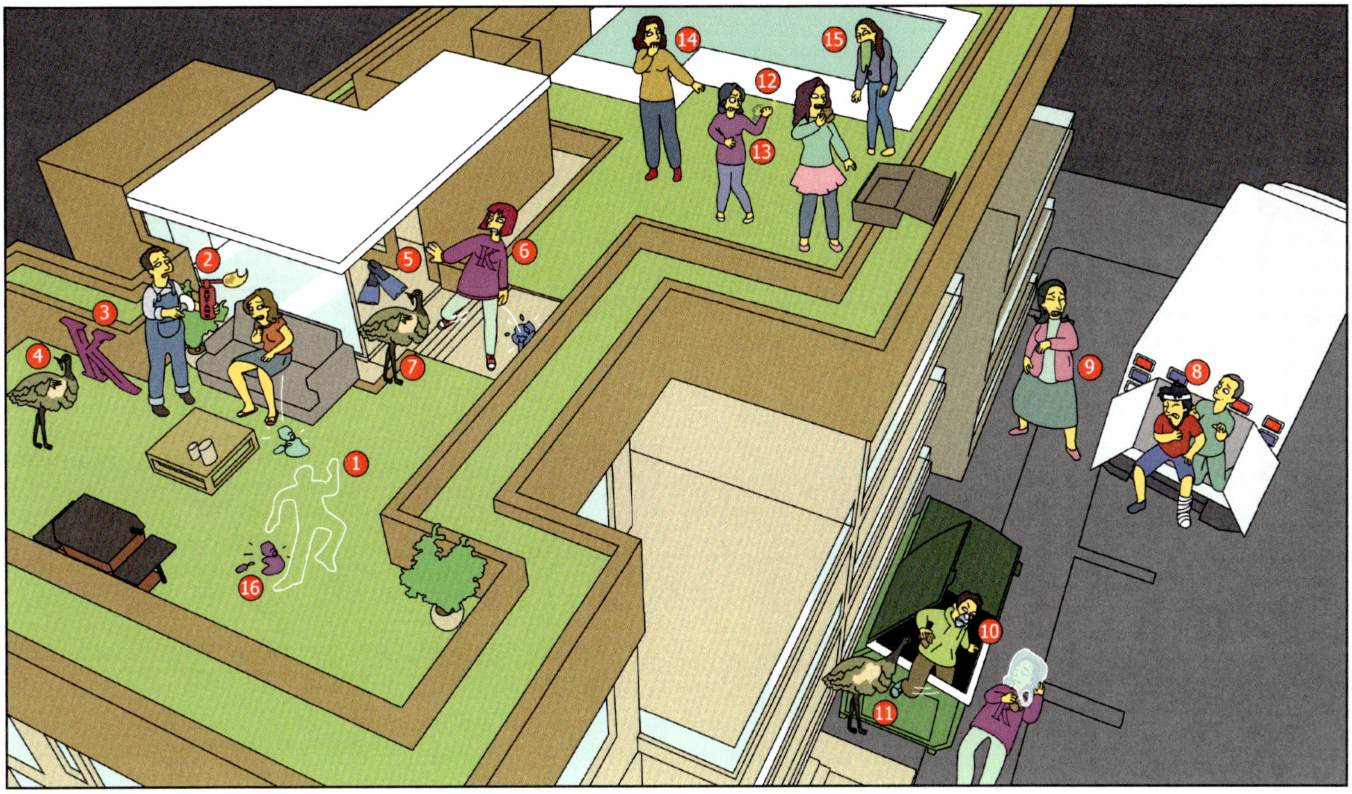

1. Penthouse crime scene: Pentazocine

2. Butane flame to keep traumatized witness warm: Butorphanol

3. Upright K for kappa on fraternity penthouse hear butane flame: Pentazocine and butorphanol are full agonists at kappa opioid receptors

4. Partially feathered emu with bald patches near K: Pentazocine and butorphanol are partial agonists at mu opioid receptors

5. Sorority girl with blue nails and blue flipper fins: Nalbuphine

6. Upright K sweatshirt on girl with blue nails: Nalbuphine is a full kappa agonist

7. Blue nail girl blocking path of partially feathered emu: Nalbuphine is a partial mu antagonist

8. Victim in pain near ambulance not being helped by massage: Pentazocine, butorphanol, and nalbuphine can be used for moderate to severe pain

9. Pregnant lady in pain near ambulance: Pentazocine, butorphanol, and nalbuphine can be used for labor and delivery pain

10. Criminal wearing oxygen mask hiding while holding half a poppy seed muffin inside dumpster next to suffocated girl holding full poppy seed muffin: Cause less respiratory depression than full opioid agonists

11. Partially feathered emu withdrawing after being kicked by criminal: In a patient with opioid use disorder, administering a mixed agonist/antagonist can precipitate immediate withdrawal

12. Angry girl in penthouse shaking fist at other girl eating last poppy seed muffin: Withdrawal includes irritability and anger

13. Angry girl holding stomach from hunger: Abdominal pain with withdrawal

14. Anxious girl biting nails as last muffin is taken: Withdrawal includes anxiety

15. Vomiting girl: Withdrawal includes nausea and vomiting

16. Spilled bottles of nail polish scattered around penthouse near nail girl, butane flame, and crime scene: Nalbuphine, butorphanol, and pentazocine not easily reversed with naloxone

See Figure 9.12.10 - Pharmacologic Effects on Opioid Receptors (Psychiatric Pharmacology, Section 21, Page 271)

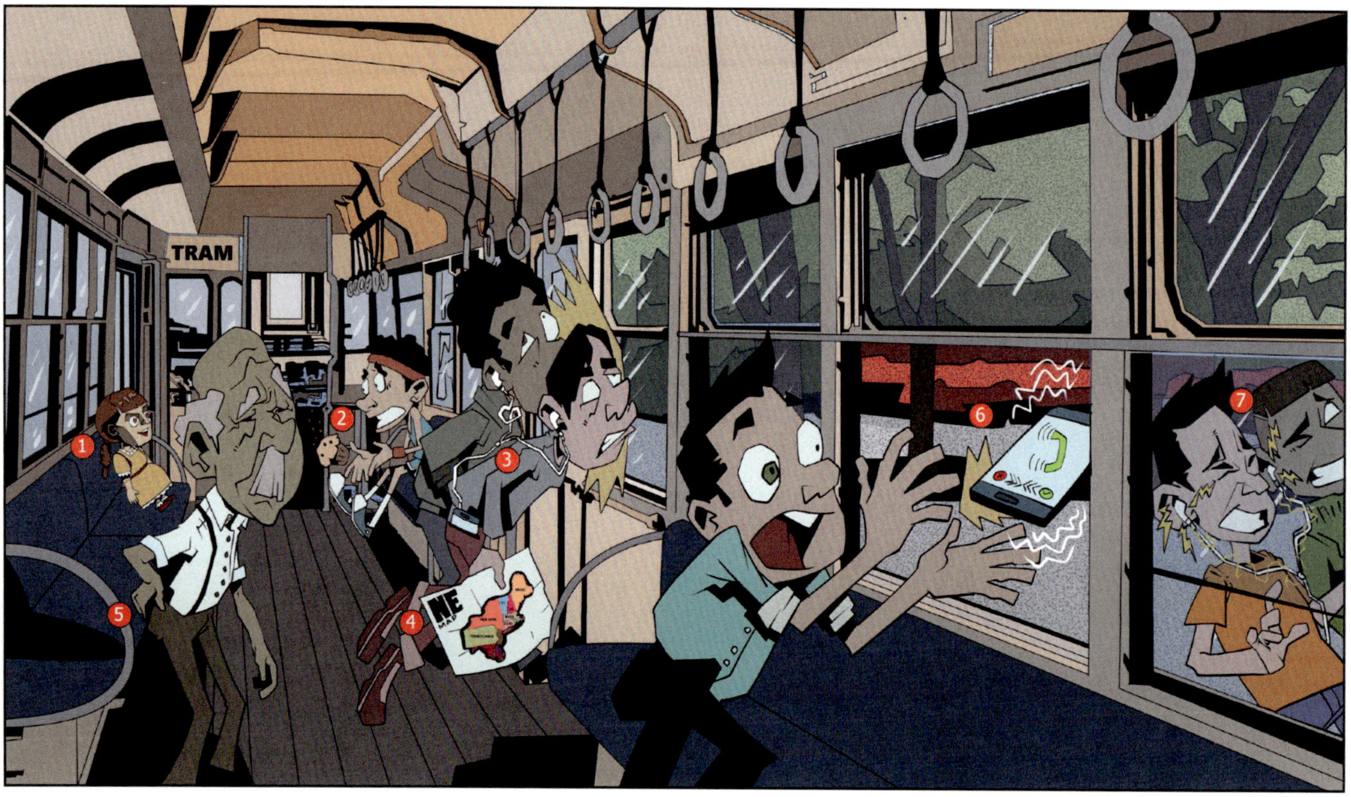

1. Doll on tram: Tramadol

2. Weak guy dropping poppy seed muffin on floor: Weak opioid agonist

3. Two guys slamming into doors while sharing a tune: Inhibits reuptake of serotonin

4. Guy holding map of New England marked "NE": Inhibitors reuptake of norepinephrine (NE)

5. Old man holding back in pain while preparing to sit: Use for chronic pain

6. Phone vibrating and falling out of tram window: Can cause seizures

7. Guys sharing a tune while being shocked by electrical short caused by passing tram: Can cause serotonin syndrome

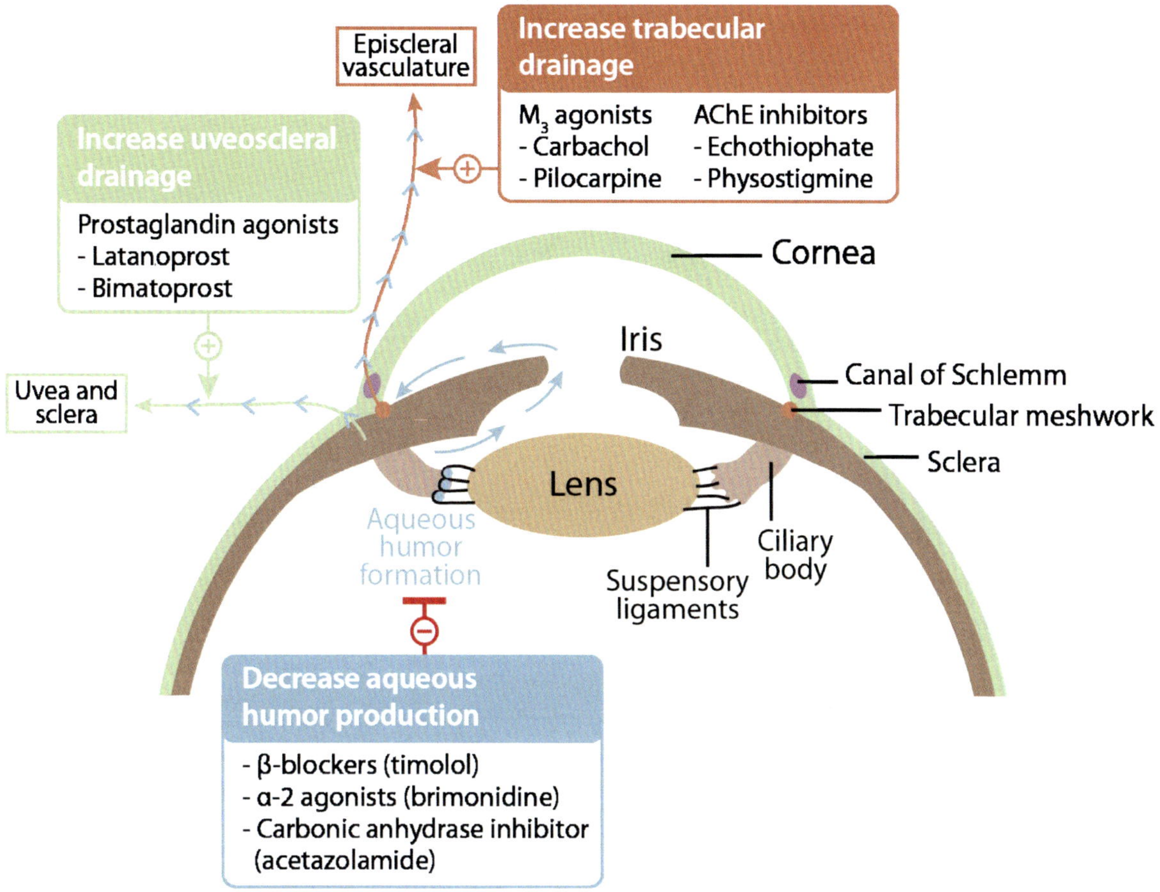

Figure 9.12.11 - Glaucoma Drugs

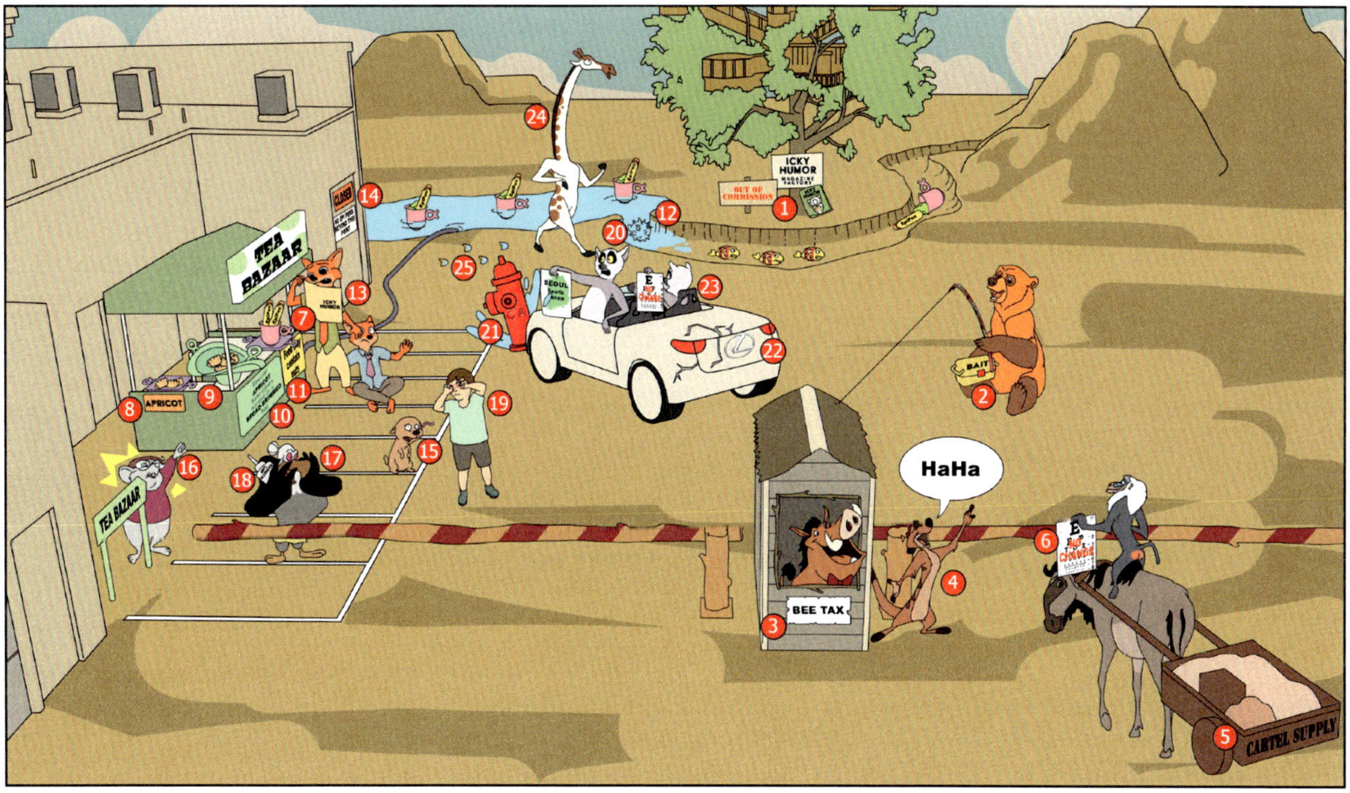

1. Icky Humor Magazine factory out of commission: Decreased aqueous humor synthesis

2. Snagged fishing pole with boat attached to bait tackle box, preventing bear from going through toll booth: Beta blockers

3. "Bee Tax" sign on toll booth to bee nature reserve: Betaxolol

4. Timone laughing out loud (LOL) at stuck fishing pole: Timolol

5. Cartel supply cart trying to get through gate: Careolol

6. Cartel driver holding up "no visual changes" document: No pupillary or vision changes

7. Tea cup with one alpha-shaped handle and tray with two alpha-shaped handles: Alpha agonists

8. Apricot bear claws on alpha dessert tray: Apraclonidine (α_2)

9. Fancy wide-brimmed hat dessert tray with two alpha-shaped handles: Brimonidine (α_2)

10. Lack of water after river is used up by dessert stand prevents production of Icky Humor Magazine: Decreases aqueous humor synthesis (apraclonidine, brimonidine)

11. Epipens provided inside alpha 1 teacup and on alpha 2 dessert tray: Epinephrine activates α_1 and α_2 receptors

12. Dessert stand sending Epipens to three deflated, constricted pufferfish in dried-up river: Epinephrine can also decrease aqueous humor synthesis via α_1 vasoconstriction

13. Vendor's large, dilated pupils from shock while reading Icky Humor Magazine: Epinephrine can cause mydriasis because of its α_1 agonism

14. Wide-eyed vendor covering and accidentally squeezing friend's eye near closed door with "no Epipens buoyed this point" sign: Do not use epinephrine in closed-angle glaucoma cause mydriasis can increase intraocular pressure

15. Prairie dog with worm in eye: Can cause foreign body sensation (feels like sand in the eyes)

16. Mouse with broken glasses after bumping into tea shop/dessert stand sign: Can cause blurry vision

17. Eagle with red, irritated eyes from sand: Can cause ocular hyperemia

18. Eagle sneezing with irritated, watery eyes and using anti-allergy eye drops: Can cause ocular allergic reactions

19. Guy rubbing itchy eyes with sand in them: Can cause ocular pruritus

20. Lemur in Lexus with Seul, South Korea map: Acetazolamide

21. Lexus crashing into fire hydrant: Inhibits carbonic anhydrase

22. Cracked back of Lexus: Decreased CSF production in choroid plexus

23. Lemur holding document with eye exam that says, "no change": No pupillary or vision changers

24. Tall male (man) giraffe walking near river: Mannitol

25. Tall man's footprints pulling in water by creating depressions next to river: Mannitol diuresis can decrease CSF volume

See Figure 9.12.11 - Glaucoma Drugs (Neurology Pharmacology, Section 24, Page 276)

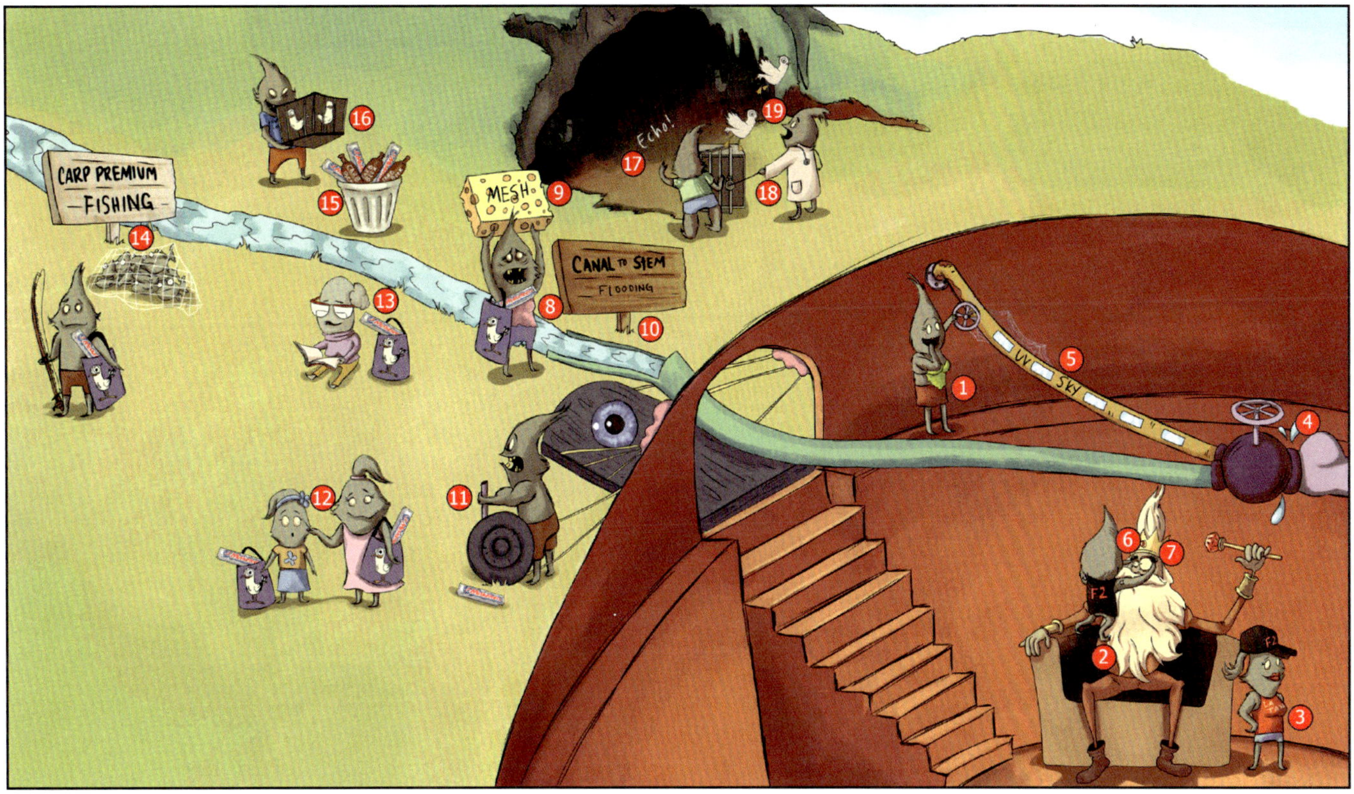

1. Two prostitutes next to gnome king: Prostaglandins

2. Prostitute with F2 shirt, two alpha tattoos and blue toenail polish putting false eyelashes on king: Bimatoprost is a PGF2α analog

3. Prostitute with LA fan shirt and F2 hat: Latanoprost is a PgF2α analog

4. Prostitute opening valve that allows liquid from clogged over-pressurized pipe to flow into smaller yellow pipe: Increased aqueous humor outflow through uveoscleral pathway

5. Prostitute opening valve into yellow backup pipe with "UV sky" label: Increased aqueous humor outflow through uveoscleral pathway

6. Prostitute applying false lashes on king: Eyelash growth (may be intentional)

7. Dark glue on king's eyes to help eyelashes stick: Darkens color of iris (browning)

8. Worker gnome with seagull purse containing 3 Musketeers bar: Cholinominmetics (M_3)

9. Worker gnome holding up sponge marked "mesh" and removing it from canal to allow water flow: Cholinomimetics increase aqueous outflow by opening the trabecular meshwork

10. Sign marked "canal to stem flooding" near worker gnome: By opening the trabecular meshwork, more aqueous can flow through canal of Schlemm

11. Worker gnome with 3 Musketeers bar contracting muscles to lower drawbridge with eye painted on by decreasing tension in ropes attached to drawbridge: M_2 stimulation → ciliary muscle contraction

12. Mother holding pin to daughter's eye to fix headband while both carry seagull purses with 3 Musketeers bars: All cholinomimetics can cause miosis (contraction of pupillary "iris" sphincter muscles)

13. Elderly gnome wearing hyperfocusing bifocal glasses with seagull purse and 3 Musketeers bar: Can cause cyclospasm

14. Fisherman with seagull bag and 3 Musketeers bar next to pile of carp and "carp premium fishing" sign: Pilocarpine (direct M3 stimulation)

15. Garbage can full of carb-rich alcohol and 3 Musketeers bars: Carbachol (direct M_3 stimulation)

16. No carb-rich alcohol inside cage full of seagulls: Carbachol is a "carbon copy" of acetylcholine (but resistant to AChE)

17. Gnome with thick thighs calling into cave with seagull cages and hearing echo back: Echothiophate (indirect M_3 stinumation)

18. Gnome physician with stick freeing caged seagulls: Physostigmine (indirect M_3 stimulation)

19. Physician and gnome with thick thighs releasing caged seagulls, which fly up into sky: Echothiophate and physostigmine block AChE → M_3 stimulation

PSYCHIATRIC PHARMACOLOGY

Section 1 - Serotonin Syndrome

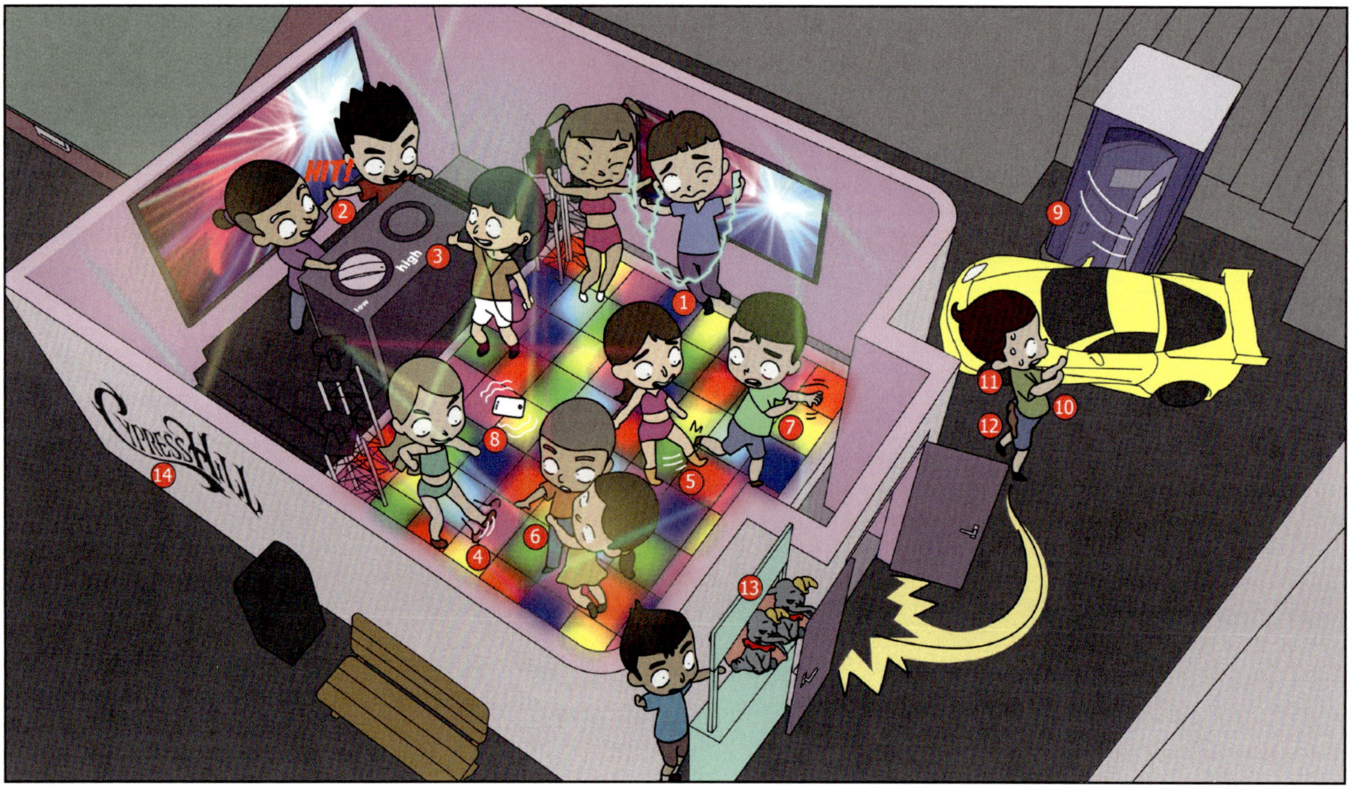

1. Couple sharing a tune through headphones and get shocked at a club: Serotonin syndrome

2. Two DJs give each other a high five and make "Hit!" sound: The scientific name for serotonin is 5-HIT

3. DJs turn up the sound from low to high: Caused by any drug that increases 5-HT (serotonin)

4. Girl moving her foot so fast in blurs: Clonus

5. Girl's knee being kicked which caused her to kick outward like a reflex hammer: Hyperreflexia

6. Rigid uncomfortable man dancing with girlfriend: Hypertonia

7. Guy shaking from embarrassment from kicking girl's knee: Tremors

8. Phone shaking and ringing on floor: Seizures

9. Bathroom automatic door malfunctioning: Autonomic instability

10. Sweating and burning drugged person next to bathroom: Hyperthermia

11. Drugged guy with large beads of sweat next to bathroom: Diaphoresis

12. Guy trying to make it to the bathroom but is blocked by car and poops his pants: Diarrhea

13. Plush elephants that look wasted outside of club: Altered mental status

14. "Cypress Hill" band graphic on wall outside of club: Treat with cyproheptadine ($5\text{-}HT_2$ receptor agonist)

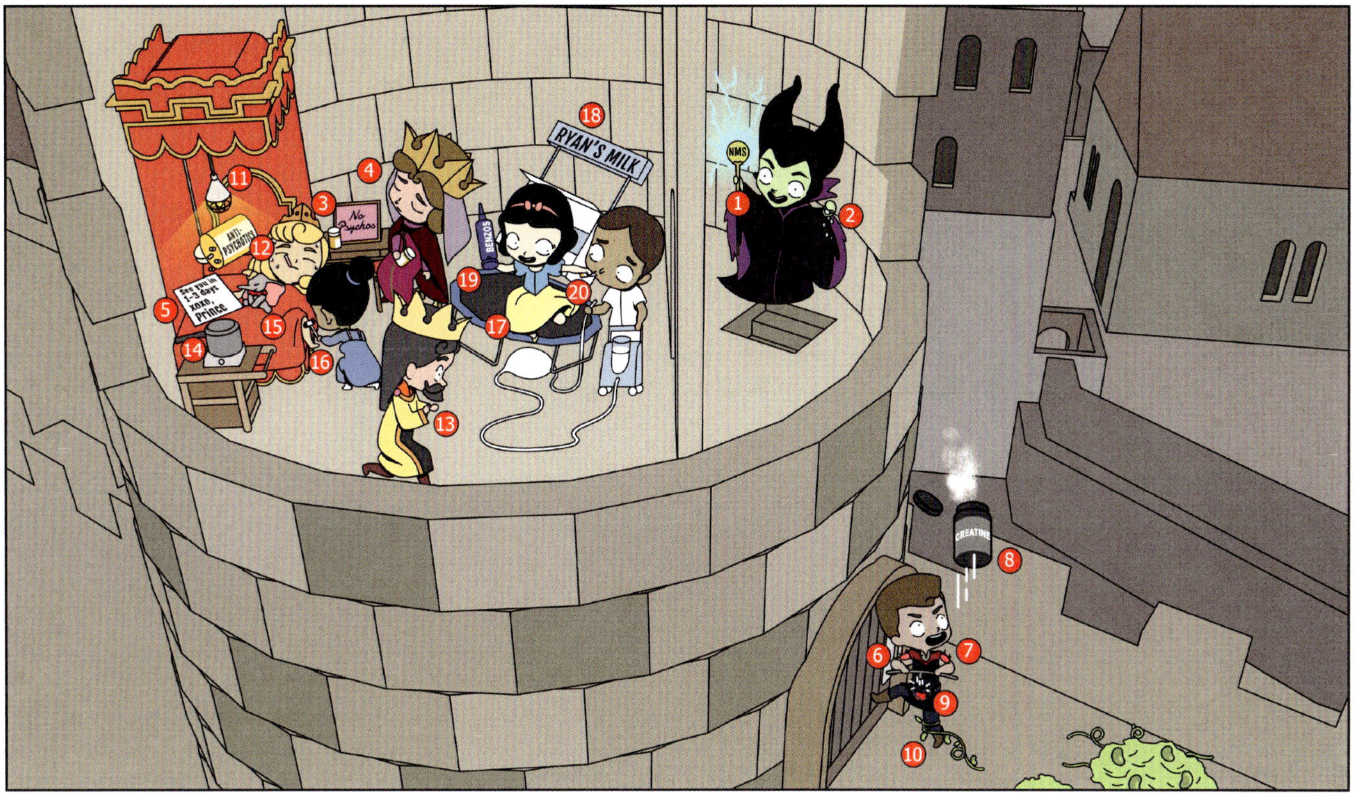

1. Maleficent with "NMS" staff: Neuroleptic malignant syndrome (NMS)

2. Maleficent crushing dope in hand: Although the exact mechanism is uncertain, the prevailing theory about the cause of NMS symptoms is dopamine antagonism

3. Cursive "No Psychos" sign next to antipsychotics pill bottle around ill Sleeping Beauty: NMS typically occurs after using antipsychotics (typical and atypical)

4. Sleeping Beauty's mom asleep next to Sleeping Beauty: Need to have a genetic predisposition to develop NMS

5. "See you in 1-3 days" note from Prince Phillip: Onset is 1-3 days after taking antipsychotics

6. Prince being unable to bend rigid pipe: Can cause muscle rigidity

7. Prince's ruptured arm muscles: Muscle rigidity leads to rhabdomyolysis (muscle breakdown)

8. Creatine bottle kicked in the air by prince: Skeletal muscles release creatine kinase (CK) into the blood when breaking down → serum CK

9. Red jelly on prince's crotch: Skeletal muscles also release myoglobin which readily enters the urine (myoglobinuria) and often gives the urine a red or brown tint

10. Kidney bean vine wrapped around prince's leg from trampled kidney bean plant: Myoglobinuria can lead to renal failure

11. Heat lamp next to sleeping beauty: NMS can cause hyperthermia

12. Heat lamp causes Sleeping Beauty to sweat: NMS can cause diaphoresis

13. Kind checking his radial pulse while running around: NMS can cause tachycardia

14. Pressure cooker next to Sleeping Beauty: NMS can cause hypertension

15. Stuffed drunk elephant: NMS can cause encephalopathy

16. Nurse hitting knee with reflex hammer but left with no reaction: NMS can cause hyporeflexia

17. Trampoline in room: Treat with dantrolene

18. Snow white on trampoline, knocking over milk stand which kinks the milk pumping hose: Dantrolene prevents release of Ca^{2+} from sarcoplasmic reticulum with skeletal muscle

19. Blue benzos syringe in Snow White's hand: Consider treatment with benzodiazepines

20. Snow White shoving dope in man's mouth: Consider treatment with dopamine agonists

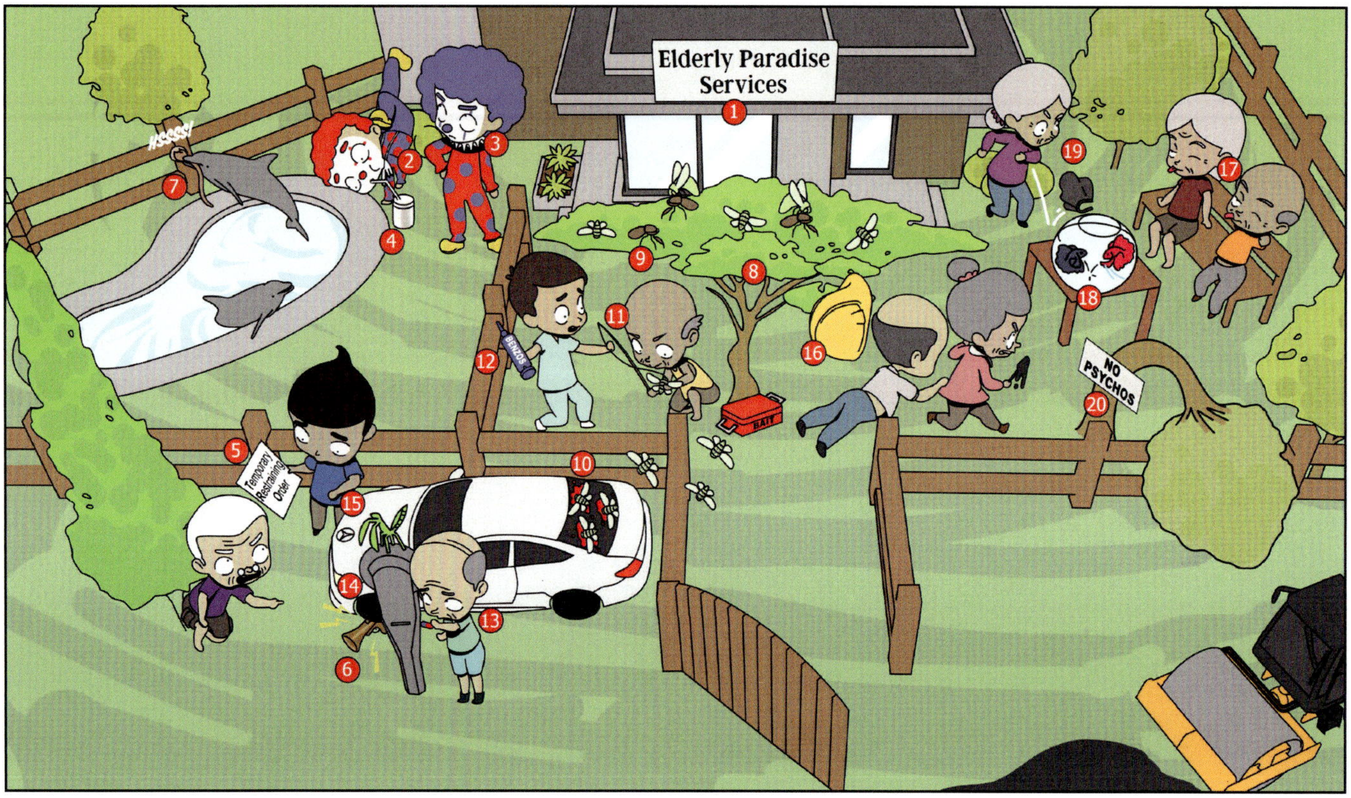

1. "Elderly Paradise Services" sign: Extrapyramidal symptoms (EPS)

2. Contortionist clown next to nursing home: Extrapyramidal symptoms include acute dystonia

3. Annoyed clown rolling eyes: Acute dystonia includes muscle spasm and stiffness and oculogyric crisis (prolonged, involuntary upward gaze)

4. Contortionist clown drinking through straw: Acute dystonia can lead to laryngospasm and require intubation

5. Man next to mercedes benz with "Temporary Restraining Order" next to pine tree: Can treat acute dystonia with benztropine

6. Benz crushing M1 musket: Benztropine is an M_1 antagonist

7. Dolphin holding hissing snake by dystonic clowns: Can treat acute dystonia with diphenhydramine

8. Acadia tree in courtyard: Late EPS include akathisia

9. Cicadas molding skins on acadia tree: Akathisia is a feeling of restlessness and wanting to crawl out of one's skin

10. Smashed cicadas on back of mercedes benz: Can treat akathisia with benztropine

11. Old man not able to put acadia tree cicadas in two handled bait box as bait: Can treat akathisia with beta blockers

12. Blue "Benzos" syringe held by staff member: Can treat akathisia with benzodiazepines

13. Old man using pills as parking meter coins: Late PES include drug-induced parkinsonism

14. Parking meter guy near benz: Drug-induced parkinsonism can be treated with benztropine

15. Praying mantis on parking meter near old man: Drug-induced parkinsonism can be treated with amantadine

16. Contractor diving on woman who stole his tar-mixing stick: Very late EPS symptoms include tardive dyskinesia

17. Old couple with mocking facial expressions: Tardive dyskinesia can include orofacial chorea

18. Due leading to dead gray tetra fish bouncing in fish bowl: Can treat tardive dyskinesia with deutetrabenazine

19. Old woman throwing veil and veil bouncing: Can treat tardive dyskinesia with valbenazine

20. "No psychos" sign nailed to atypical tree: Can treat tardive dyskinesia with atypical antipsychotics

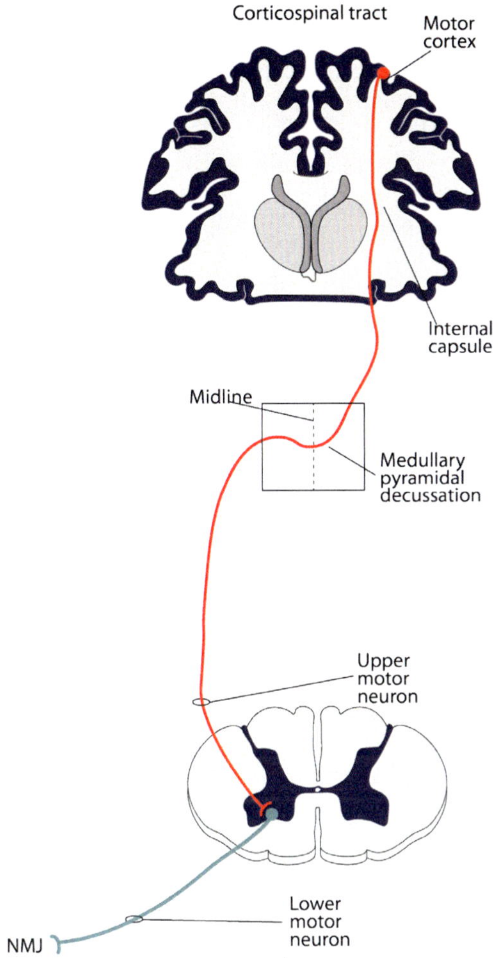

Figure 9.13.1 - Corticospinal Tract

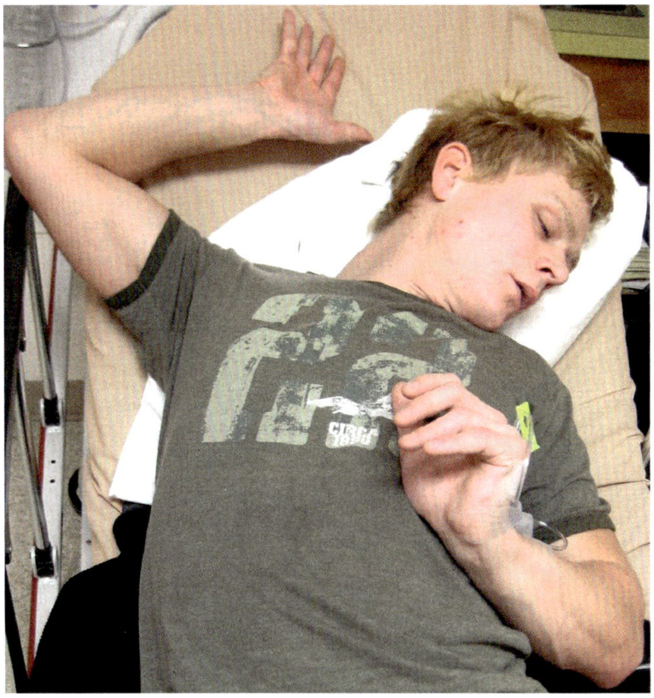
Photo Credit: James Heilman, MD / CC BY-SA (https://creativecommons.org/licenses/by-sa/3.0)

Figure 9.13.3 - Acute Dystonia

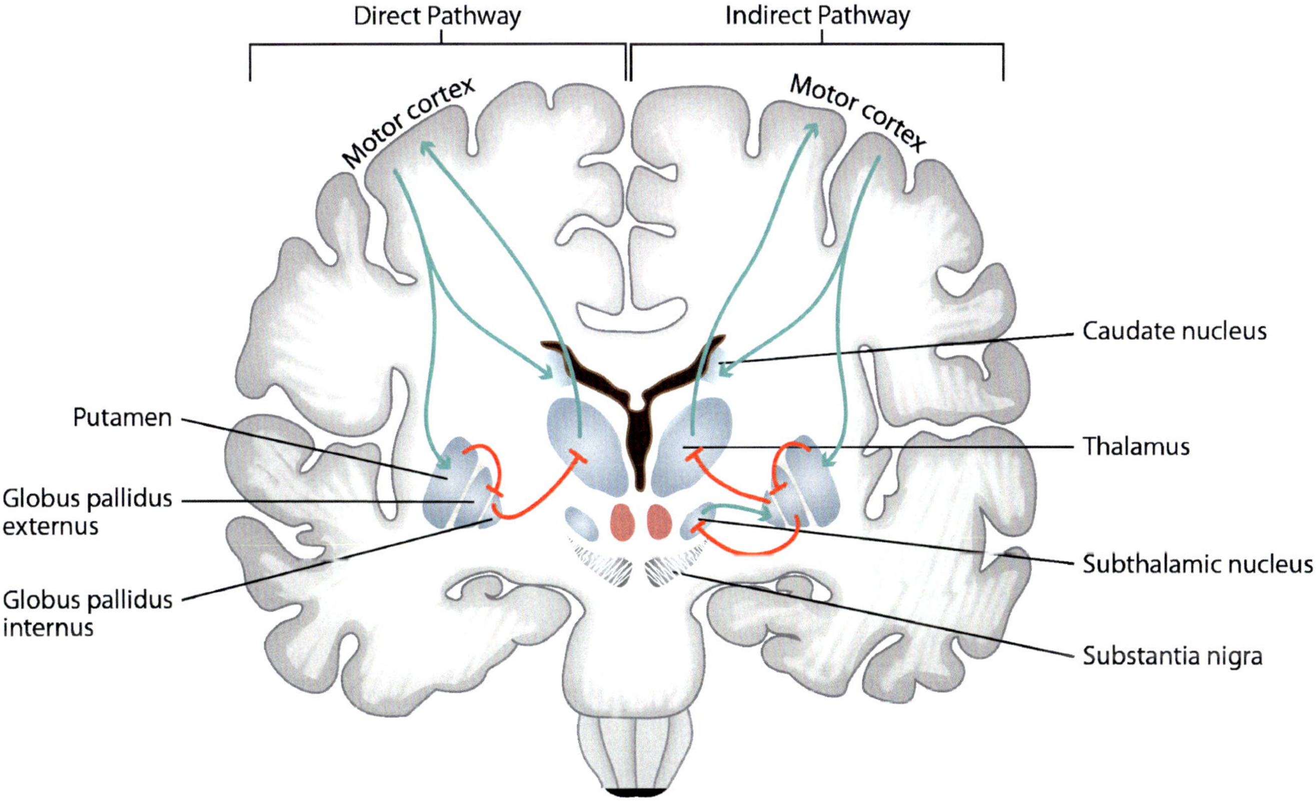

Figure 9.13.2 - Pyramidal and Extrapyramidal Systems

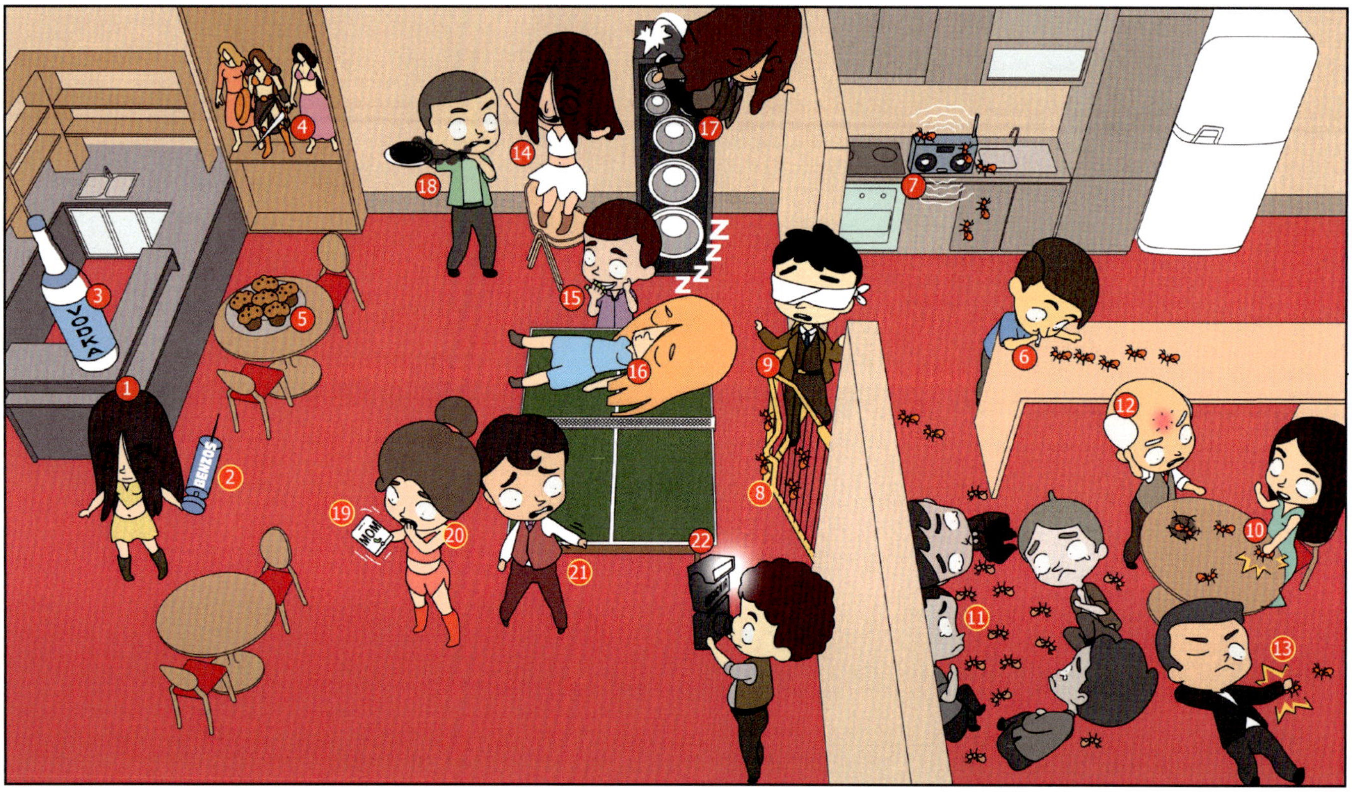

1. Woman with long, droopy hair over face: CNS depressants

2. Blue "Benzos" syringe held by woman: Benzodiazepines

3. Vodka on bar shelf: Alcohol

4. Barbarian barbies on display: Barbiturates

5. Poppy seed muffins on table: Opioids

6. Man snorting ants in kitchen: Inhalants

7. Broken boombox in kitchen with ants: Inhalant intoxication can cause slurred speech

8. Ant-covered doggy gate: Inhalant intoxication can cause disturbed gait

9. Man with blindfold running into gate: Inhalant intoxication can cause disorientation

10. Angry woman crushing ant in room next to kitchen: Inhalant withdrawal can cause irritability

11. Four guys laying in fetal position with dead ants: Inhalant withdrawal can cause dysphoria

12. Man smashing ants with head and holding his head: Inhalant withdrawal can cause headaches

13. Loner unable to sleep and smashing ants: Inhalant withdrawal can cause sleep disturbances

14. Woman with droopy hair dancing on chair and smiling: Intoxication can cause mood elevation

15. Man who isn't biting his nails because of thimbles: Intoxication can cause decreased anxiety

16. Woman sleeping on ping pong table: Intoxication can cause sedation

17. Man with droopy hair belly flopping onto floor with no regard of his well being: Intoxication can cause behavioral disinhibition

18. Man choking on burnt pizza smoke: Intoxication can cause respiratory depression

19. Woman's hair withdrawn to bun and her phone shaking: Withdrawal can cause seizures

20. Woman with phone biting nails: Withdrawal can cause anxiety

21. Man's shaking arm near ping pong table: Withdrawal can cause tremor

22. Man with Insignia brand camera flashing himself in eyes: Withdrawal can cause insomnia

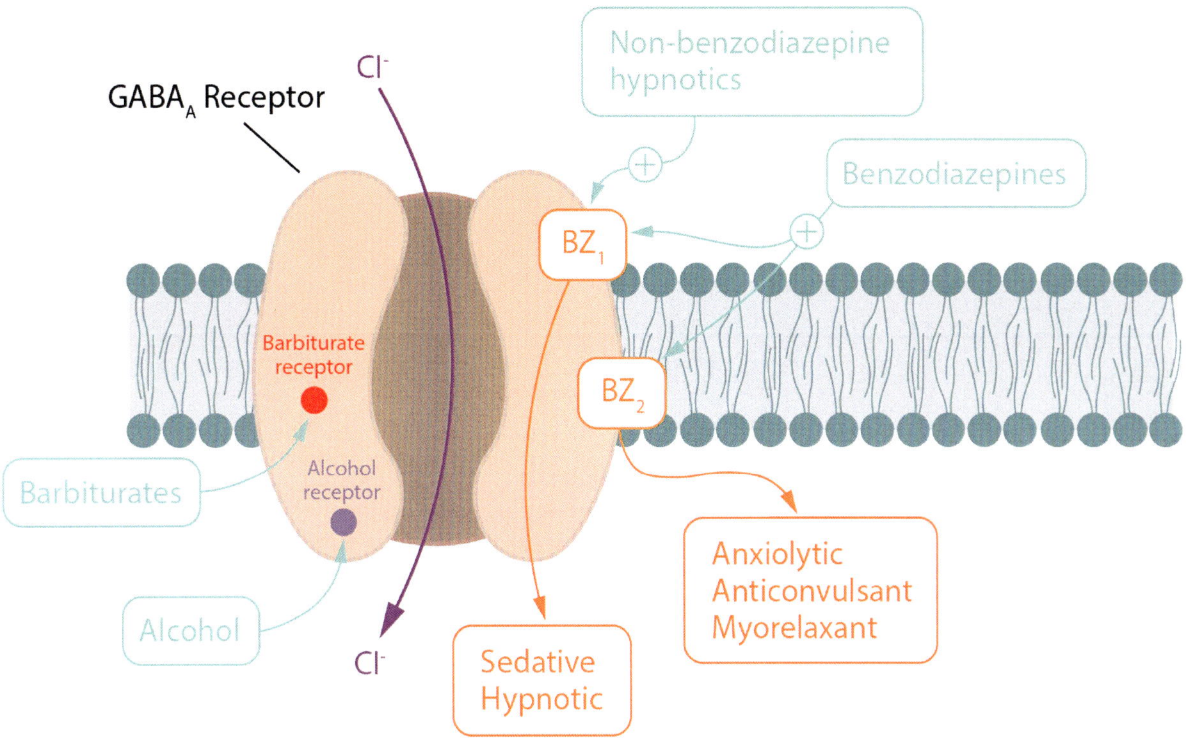

Figure 9.13.4 - Effects of Medications that Act on the GABA-A Receptor

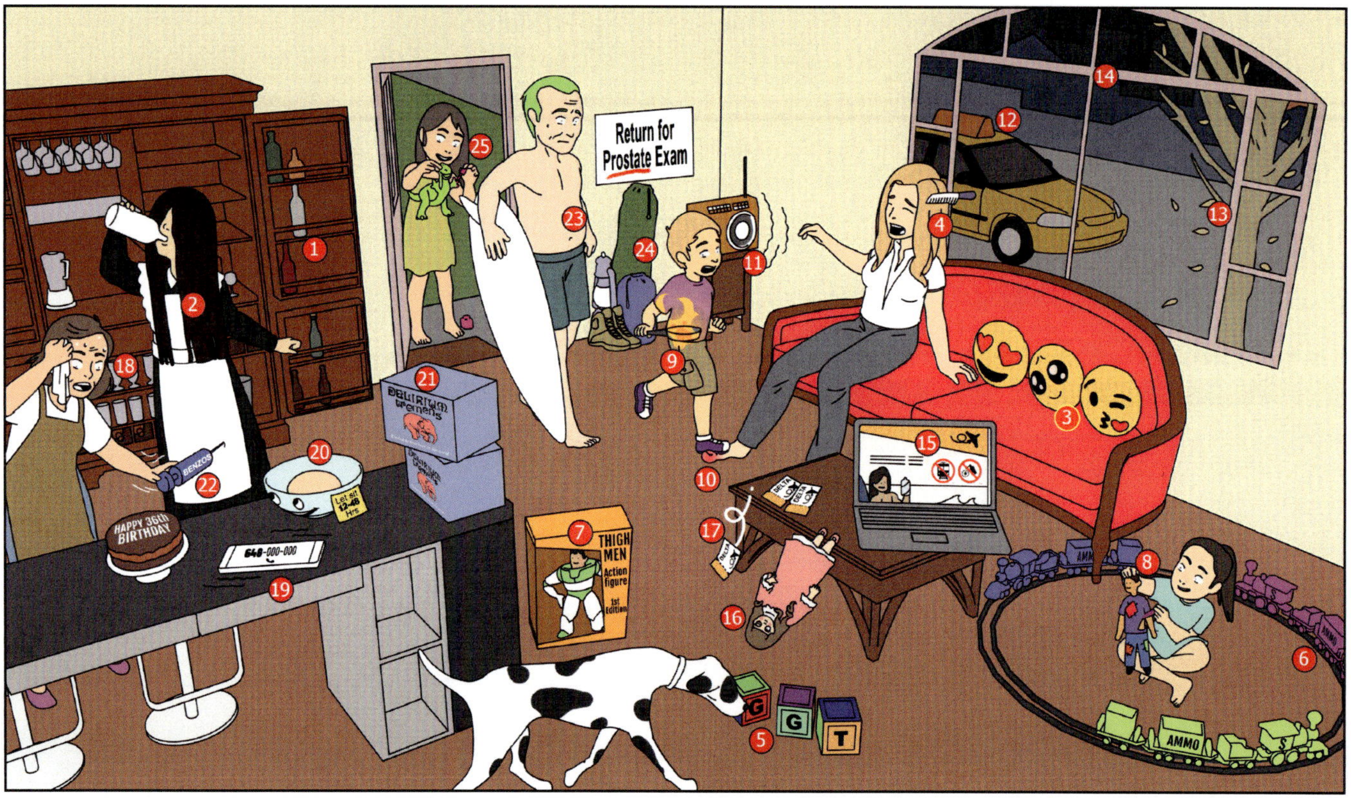

1. Liquor cabinet in living room: Alcohol

2. Maid with long hair covering her face: CNS depressant

3. Emoji pillows on velvet couch: Can cause emotional lability

4. Comb stuck in passed out woman's hair: Can cause coma

5. Liver-spotted dog smelling blocks that spell "GGT": Serum GGT (gamma-glutamyltransferase) is a sensitive indicator of alcohol use

6. Two "S" ammo trains to one "L" ammo train: AST > ALT 2 : 1

7. "Thigh men" first edition action figure on ground: Can cause a thiamine (B_1) deficiency

8. Girl exacerbating doll's torn clothes: Alcohol can exacerbate porphyria

9. Boy with flaming pans: Can cause acute and chronic pancreatitis

10. Boy steps on mom's big toe: Can precipitate gout

11. Radio with broken speaker next to boy: Can cause slurred speech

12. Taxi outside: Can cause ataxia

13. Tree with little foliage: Causes a folate deficiency

14. Blacked out section of city: Can cause blackouts

15. "No metro" and "no grease" hair dye advertisement on laptop with di-ad surfer: Avoid with metronidazole and griseofulvin due to the risk of a disulfiram-like reaction

16. Doll with fluttering eyes falling off table: Can cause decreased REM sleep

17. Three Delta airplane tickets on table with one falling on floor: Can cause decreased delta wave sleep (N_3)

18. Nervous mom trying to finish "Happy 36th Birthday" cake: Withdrawal can cause tremors, insomnia, diaphoresis, agitation, GI upset: 3-36 hrs

19. Ringing phone with "648" number: Withdrawal seizures: 6-48 hrs

20. Post-it note that reads, "Let sit 12-48 hours" on talking bowl: Hallucinations (usually auditory): 12-48 hours

21. Two forty-eight packs of delirium tremens beer: Delirium tremens 48-96 hrs

22. Blue "Benzos" syringe held by nervous mom: Benzodiazepines are used for alcohol withdrawal

23. Surfer with dyed hair: Treat alcoholism with disulfiram

24. Camping gear near "Return for Prostate Exam" note: Treat alcoholism with acamprosate

25. T-rex getting nails painted: Treat alcoholism with naltrexone

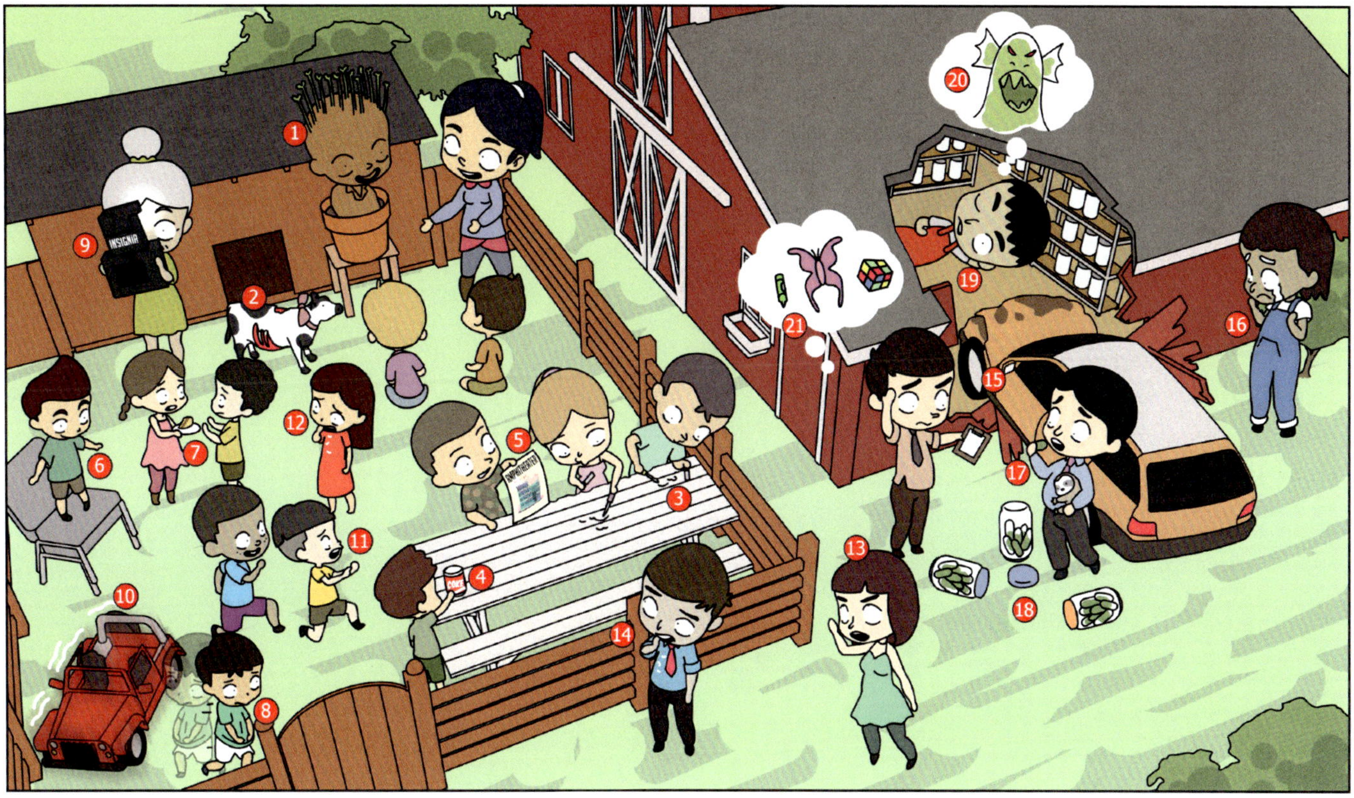

1. Chia pet with hair sticking up: CNS stimulants

2. Rotting calf fiend: Caffeine

3. Teens digging deep nicks into wooden table: Nicotine

4. Can of coke on table: Cocaine

5. Free concert at local amphitheater for marines: Amphetamines

6. Proud kid standing on stack of chairs: Intoxication can cause mood elevation

7. Kid rejecting lunch from sweet girl: Intoxication can cause decreased appetite

8. Nervous pacing kid tugging on his shirt: Intoxication can cause psychomotor agitation

9. Principal flashing eyes with Insignia brand camera: Intoxication can cause insomnia

10. Shaking toy car: Intoxication can cause cardiac arrhythmias

11. Kid checking his radial pulse while running away from bully: Intoxication can cause tachycardia

12. Girl anxiously biting fingernails: Intoxication can cause anxiety

13. Irritated mom outside of fence: Withdrawal can cause irritability

14. Dad outside of fence, biting nails: Withdrawal can cause anxiety

15. Crashed car at nearby farm: Withdrawal can cause post-use crash

16. Sad farmer crying at crashed car: Withdrawal can cause depression

17. Dad with stuffed sloth outside of fence: Withdrawal can cause lethargy

18. Dad eating pickles outside of fence: Withdrawal can cause increased appetite

19. Irritated man who was woken up inside of nearby barn: Withdrawal can cause sleep disturbances

20. Lazy farmhand's nightmare: Withdrawal can cause vivid nightmares

21. Man distracted by thoughts outside of fence: Withdrawal can cause difficulty concentrating

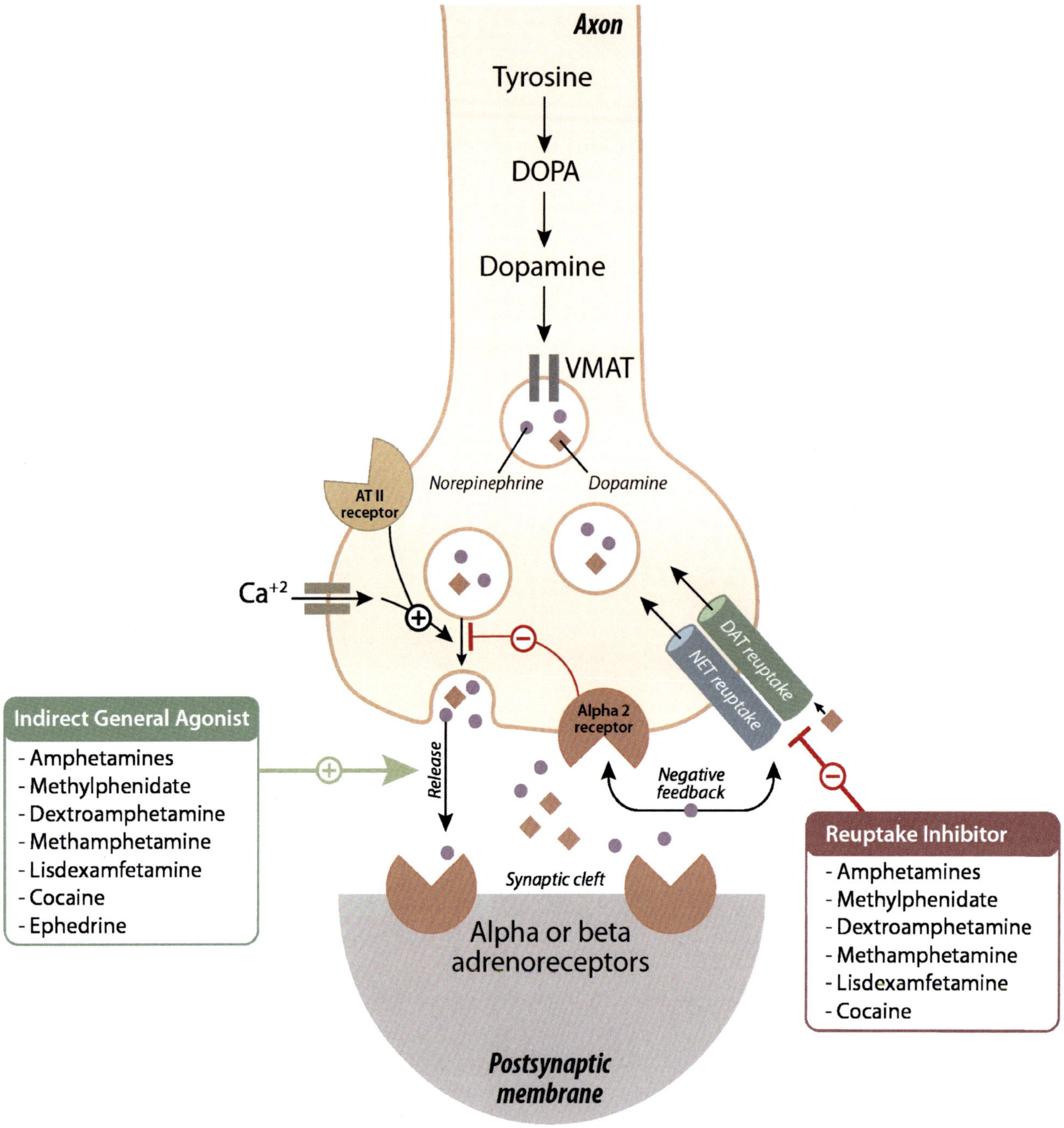

Figure 9.13.5 - Effects of Stimulants on Adrenergic Neurotransmitters

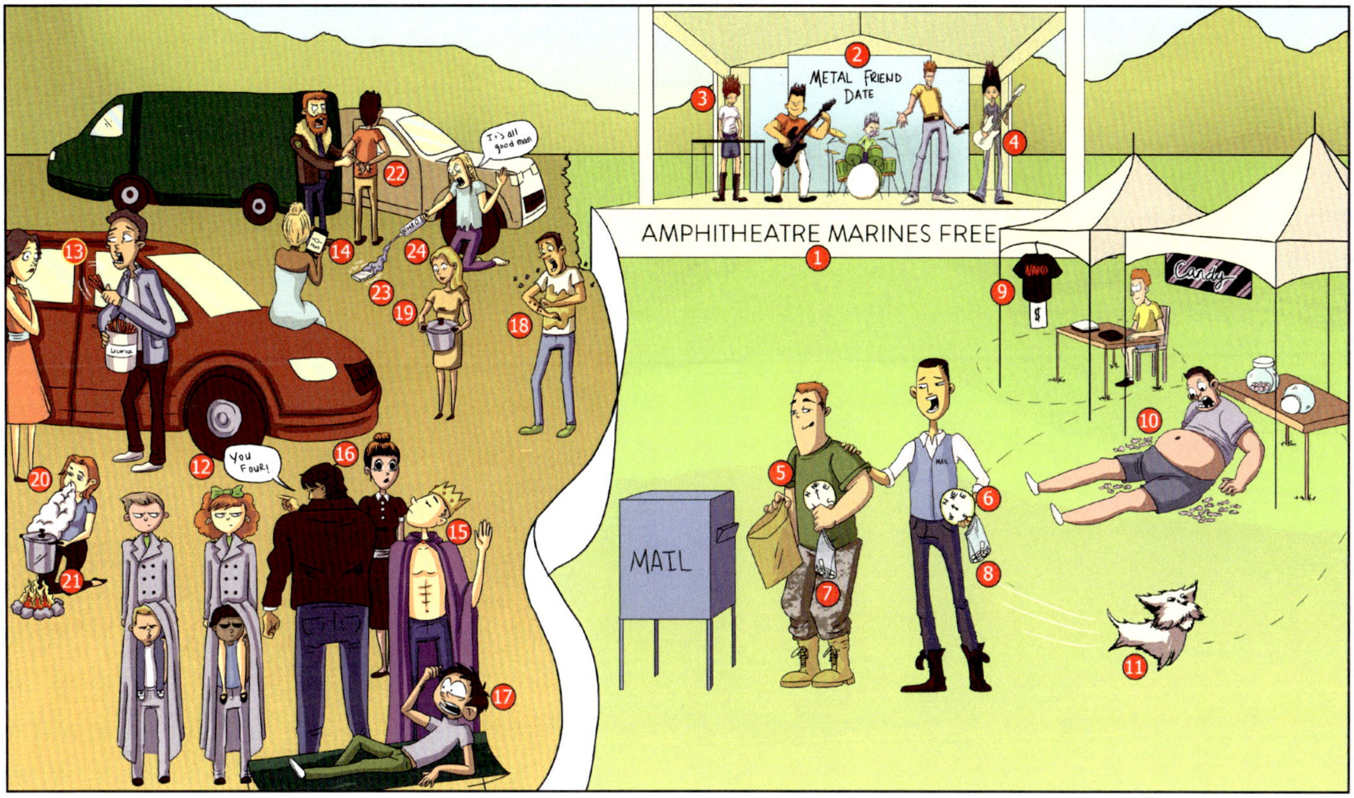

1. Amphitheater: Amphetamines

2. "Metal Friend Date" rock band performing: Methylphenidate

3. Band member's hair sticking up: CNS stimulants

4. Scrawny base guitarist: Weak base

5. Mailman stopping marine from mailing compass that only points to "NE": Works by inhibiting reuptake of NE

6. Mailman making his compass only point "NE": Works by stimulating the release of NE

7. Mailman stopping marine from mailing dope: Works by inhibiting dopamine reuptake

8. Mailman pulling out more dope: Works by stimulating dopamine release

9. "Narcos" shirt for sale: Used for narcolepsy

10. Fat man who binged on candy: Used to treat binge-eating disorder

11. Small, yappy dog running around: Used to treat ADHD

12. Bouncer saying, "You four" outside of concert: Can cause euphoria

13. Woman grabbing her chest while guy tries to sell her shaken up red licorice from car: Can cause coronary vasospasms

14. Woman taking panoramic picture: Can cause paranoia

15. Man with king crown and robe with nose in air outside of concert: Can cause grandiosity

16. Woman with wide, dilated pupils aimed at crowned man: Can cause pupillary dilation

17. Bouncer laying on cot awake focusing on hair on his air: Can cause prolonged wakefulness and attention

18. Man who spilled food on himself and scratching himself to get rid of bugs: Can cause skin excoriation with methamphetamine

19. Pressure cooker held by woman outside of concert: Can cause hypertension

20. Woman inhaling steam from pressure cooker outside of concert: Can cause pulmonary arterial hypertension

21. Woman heating up pressure cooker over fire: Can cause fever

22. Man getting arrested outside of concert: Can cause cardiac arrest

23. Phone vibrating on ground: Can cause seizures

24. Agitated man squirting blue benzo liquid over vibrating phone: Treat the seizures and agitation with benzodiazepines

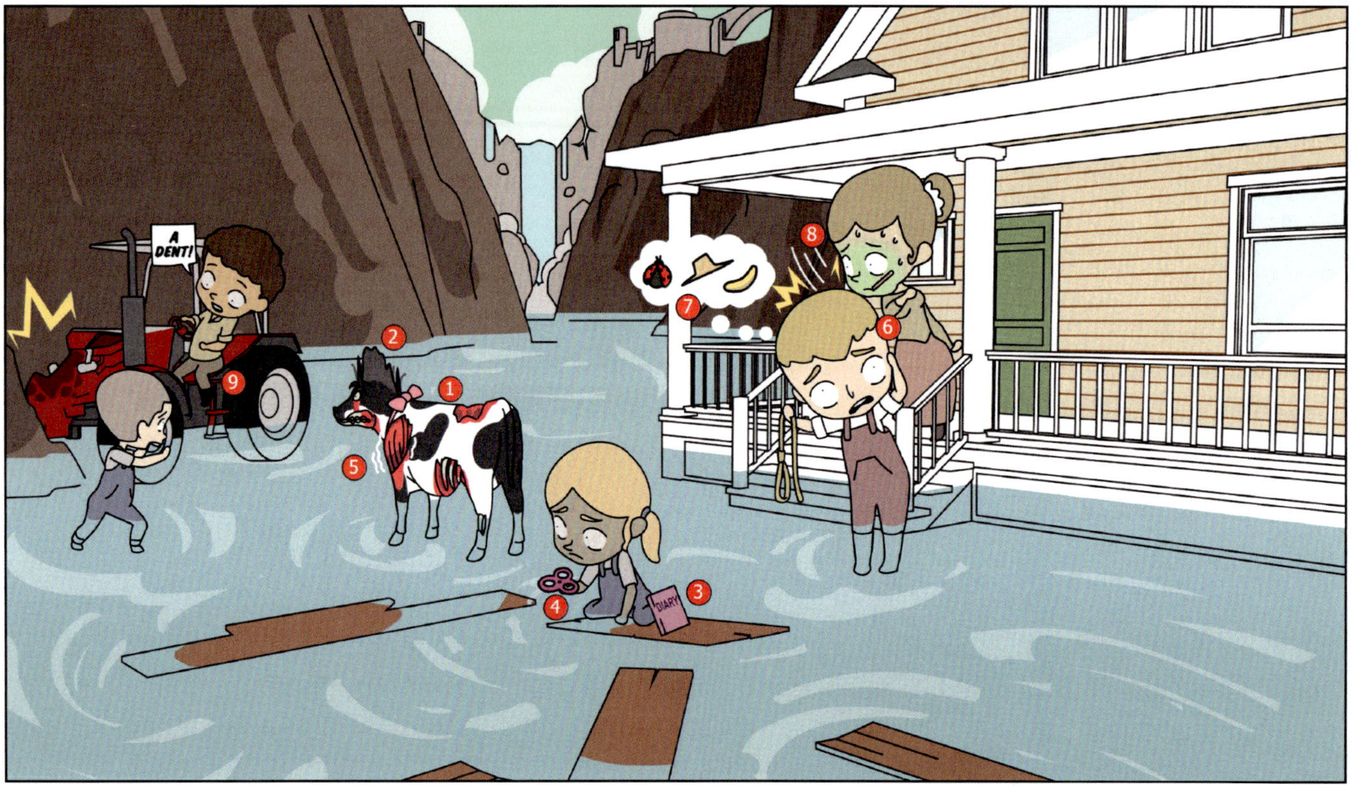

1. Decaying and fiendish-looking calf ravaging ranch: Caffeine

2. Calf with wide eyes and straight hair sticking up: CNS stimulant

3. Girl floating on wooden board with her diary from flood: Increased diuresis

4. Fidget spinner held by ranch girl: Can cause restlessness

5. Calf fiend's muscle twitching: Can cause muscle twitching

6. Rancer holding head from being hit from wife: Withdrawal can cause headache

7. Rancer daydreaming of random items after hit: Withdrawal can cause difficulty concentrating

8. Rancher's wife with green face and sweat droplets from seeing calf: Withdrawal can cause flu-like symptoms

9. Ranch hand saying, "A dent!" with crashed tractor and other ranch hand directing him away: Caffeine is an adenosine receptor antagonist

See Figure 9.13.5 - Effects of Stimulants on Adrenergic Neurotransmitters (Psychiatric Pharmacology, Section 7, Page 287)

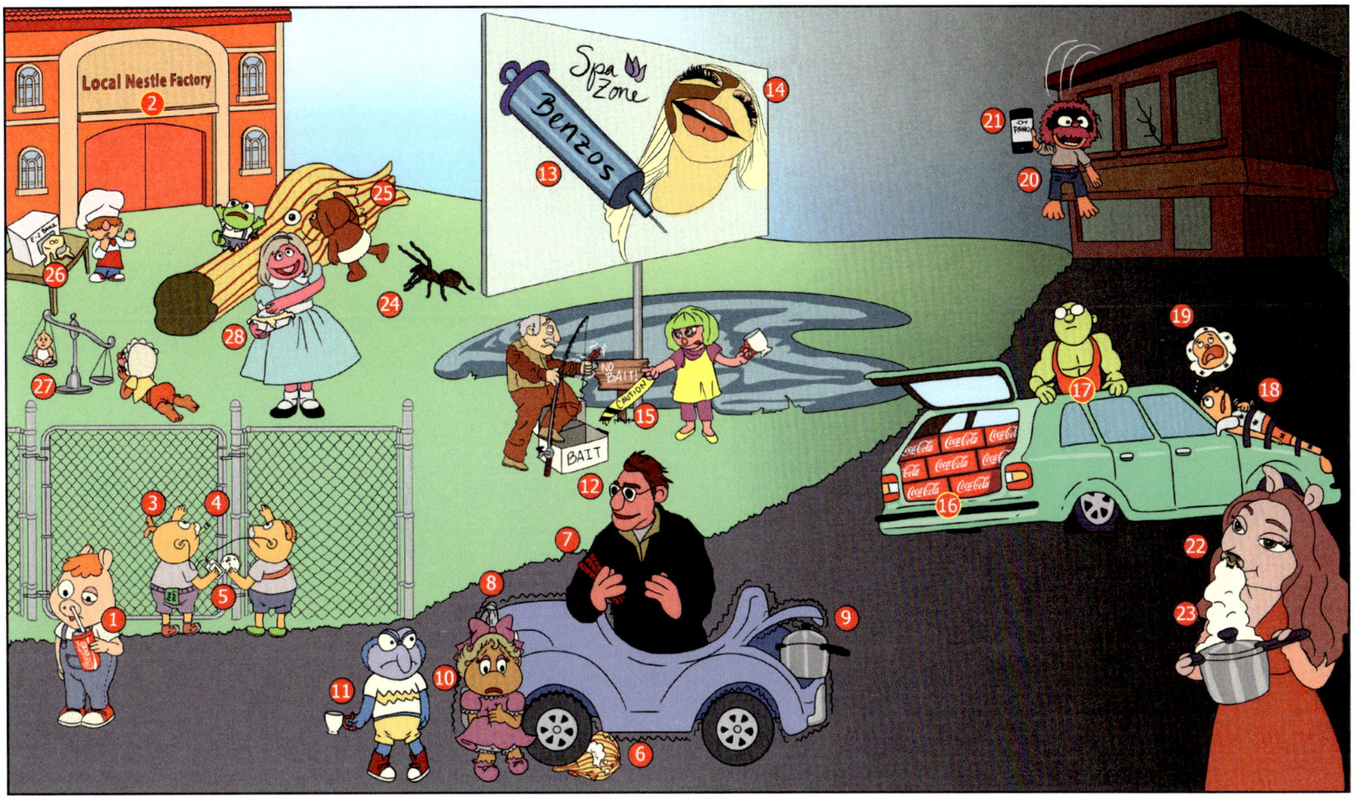

1. Kid snorting coke through straw: Cocaine

2. Local Nestle factory: Can be used for local anesthesia

3. Baby muppets sharing a tune unable to open gate: Cocaine works by inhibiting reuptake of serotonin

4. Rolled dollar bill representing dope in baby muppet's mouth: Inhibits reuptake of dopamine

5. Compass that points "NE" in baby muppets hand: Inhibits reuptake of norepinephrine (NE)

6. Ran over red-striped puffer fish: Causes vasoconstriction (alpha 1 stimulation)

7. Creepy man shaking red licorice in car: Can cause coronary vasospasm

8. Shaking car: Can cause arrhythmia

9. Pressure cooker in trunk of car: Can cause hypertension

10. Muppet girl grabbing chest in shock: Can cause vasospasm → myocardial ischemia → angina

11. Teacup with alpha shaped handle held by angry muppet friend: α-1 activation

12. Muppet man's dilated pupils: Pupil dilation (α-1)

13. Blue "Benzos" syringe advertisement: Treat with benzodiazepines

14. Mud mask on half of model's face on advertisement: Phentolamine for cocaine-induced hypertension

15. Fisherman with red licorice, bait and tackle box next to "No bait" sign near upset woman holding teacup with alpha-shaped handle: Caution when giving β-blockers if cocaine intoxication is suspected (can lead to unopposed α-1 activation → extreme hypertension, coronary vasospasm)

16. Car weighed down with coke cans: Dilated cardiomyopathy

17. Muscular muppet getting out of car: Myocarditis

18. Man arrested on the car: Cardiac arrest (sudden death)

19. Man arrested hallucinating about spiders: Hallucinations, including tactile hallucinations (aka, cocaine crawlies)

20. Muppet jumping from building smiling: Intoxication characterized by impaired judgment and disinhibition

21. Panoramic picture held by crazy muppet: Paranoia

22. Muppet with necrotic nose from nose ring: Chronic use → vasoconstriction and ischemic necrosis → perforated nasal septum

23. Muppet with necrotic nose inhaling pressure cooker steam: Pulmonary hypertension

24. Tarantula near squished pufferfish bounce house: Teratogenicity due to vasoconstriction

25. Muppet tearing through bounce house: Can cause placental abruption

26. Kid pulling cake out of oven prematurely: Can cause preterm birth

27. Light toy baby on scale: Can cause low birth weight

28. Mom preventing bread from rising: Intrauterine growth restriction

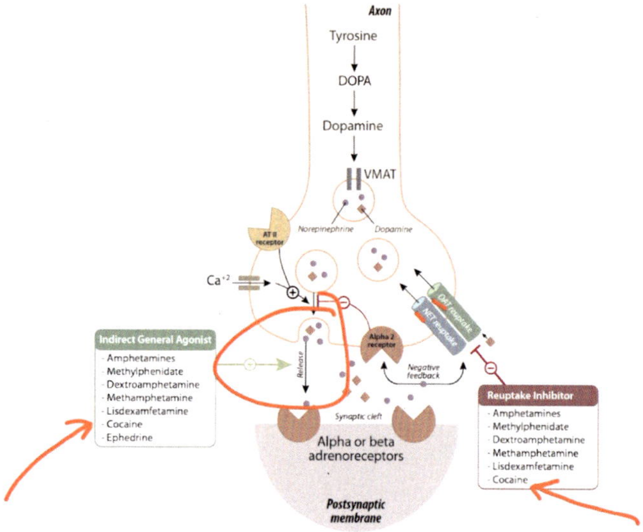

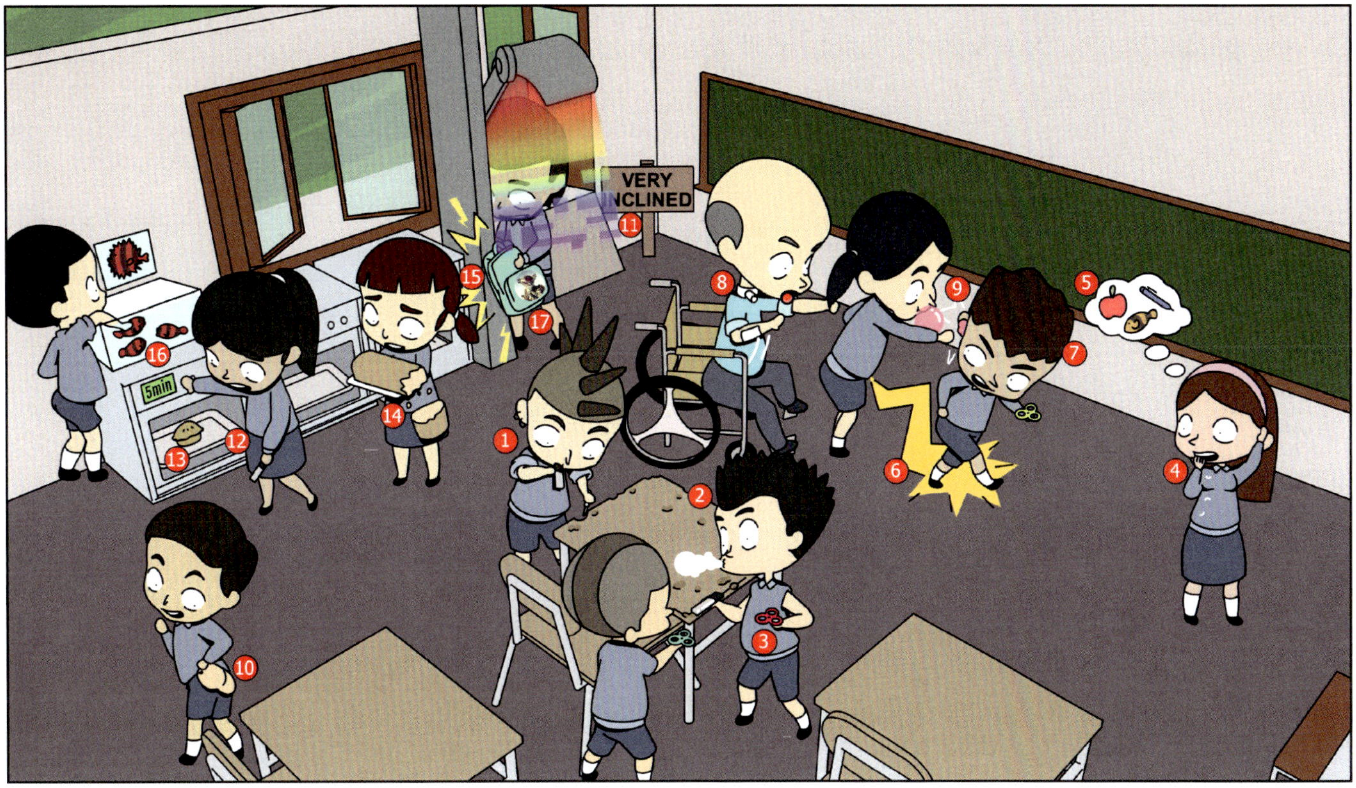

1. Teen carving nicks into desk: Nicotine

2. Wide eyes girl with hair standing straight up: CNS stimulant

3. Fidget spinners: Intoxication can cause restlessness

4. Girl biting nails anxiously away from other teens: Withdrawal can cause anxiety

5. Girl distracted by thoughts: Withdrawal can cause difficulty concentrating

6. Teen pacing around with fidget spinner: Intoxication can cause restlessness

7. Irritated teen with pacing teen: Withdrawal can cause irritability

8. Teacher eating nicotine lozenge and wearing a nicotine patch: Nicotine replacement therapy can take the form of lozenges and patches

9. Teacher trying to stop girl from sticking gum in kids ear: Nicotine replacement therapy can take the form of gum

10. Teen with fake butt prop who doesn't vape: Bupropion can also be taken to help the patient quit

11. "Very Inclined" ramp to enter classroom: Varenicline can also be taken to help the patient quit

12. Teen pulling muffin out to early: Nicotine can cause preterm labor

13. Single muffin baked instead of batch: Nicotine can cause low birth weight

14. Small pan not allowing bread to grow perfectly and piece falling off: Nicotine can cause intrauterine growth restriction

15. Teen being blocked by malfunctioning forcefield: Nicotine can cause placental problems

16. Shriveled up puffer fish with red stripes: Fetal harm results largely from placental vasoconstriction from nicotine

17. Sid the sloth backpack nicotine can cause SIDS

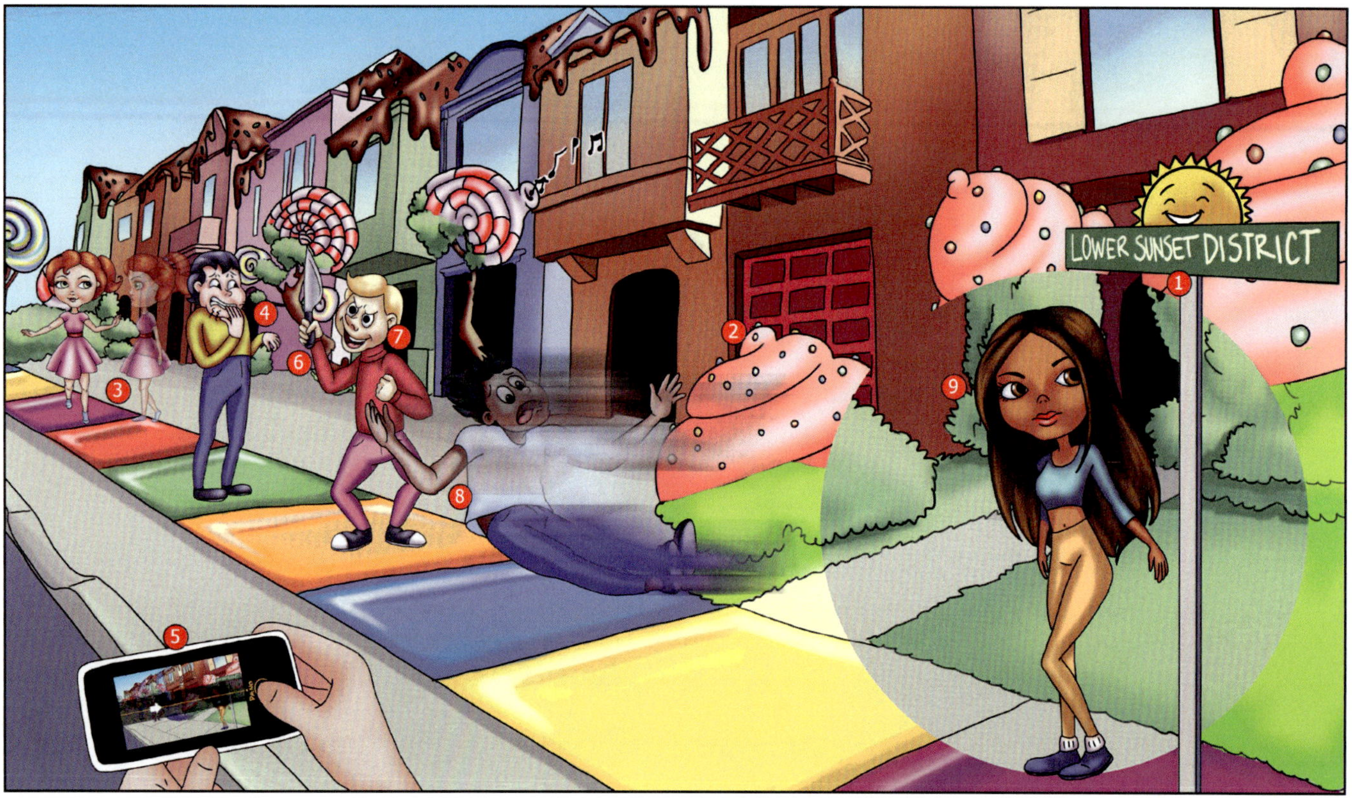

1. "Lower Sunset District" street sign: Lysergic acid diethylamide (LSD)

2. Candy shrubbery, rooftops, and trees throughout street: Can cause perceptual distortion

3. Kid skipping down street while having out of body experience: Can cause depersonalization

4. Man biting fingernails on colorful sidewalk: Can cause anxiety

5. Panorama photo being taken from phone: Can cause Paranoia

6. Psychotic man brandishing kitchen knife: Can cause psychosis

7. Dilation in psychotic man's eyes: Can increase pupil size

8. Man getting thrown backward by unseen force: Can cause flashbacks

9. Girl that seems normal in her own sphere: Diminished response over time (tachyphylaxis)

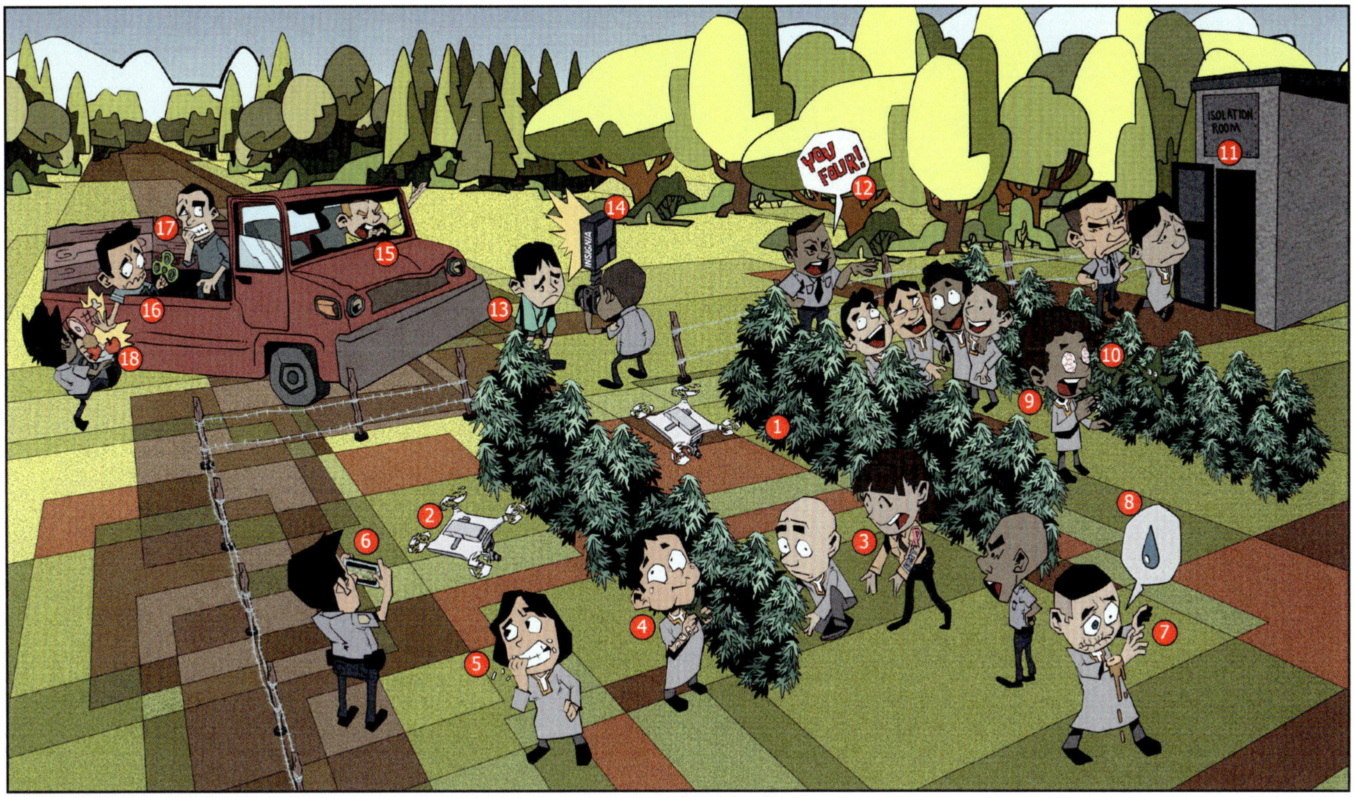

1. Marijuana plants: Marijuana (THC)

2. Drones hovering over marijuana farm: Dronabinol is the pharmaceutical form

3. Anti-medic supervisor yelling at EMT helping cancer patient: Can be used as an antiemetic in chemotherapy

4. Field worker eating marijuana leaves while being watched by drone: Can increase appetite

5. Worker biting fingernails anxiously: Can cause anxiety

6. Panoramic picture on worker's phone: Can cause paranoid delusions

7. Watch slowly melting off man's wrist: Can cause a perception of slowed time

8. Man with dry and cracked mouth after eating leaves and daydreaming about water: Can cause dry mouth

9. Man with bloodshot eyes about to eat a thorn: Can cause impaired judgment

10. Hallucinating man with bloodshot eyes: Can cause hallucination and conjunctival injection

11. Man put in "Isolation Chamber": Can cause social withdrawal

12. Supervisor pointing and saying, "You four!": Can cause euphoria

13. Man being rejected to enter compound: Withdrawal can cause depression

14. Supervisor taking picture of sad man with Insignia brand camera: Withdrawal can cause insomnia

15. Irritable driver outside of compound: Withdrawal can cause irritability

16. Restless kid with fidget spinner on back of truck: Withdrawal can cause restlessness

17. Man biting fingernails on back of truck: Withdrawal can cause anxiety

18. Guy refusing the food: Withdrawal can cause decreased appetite

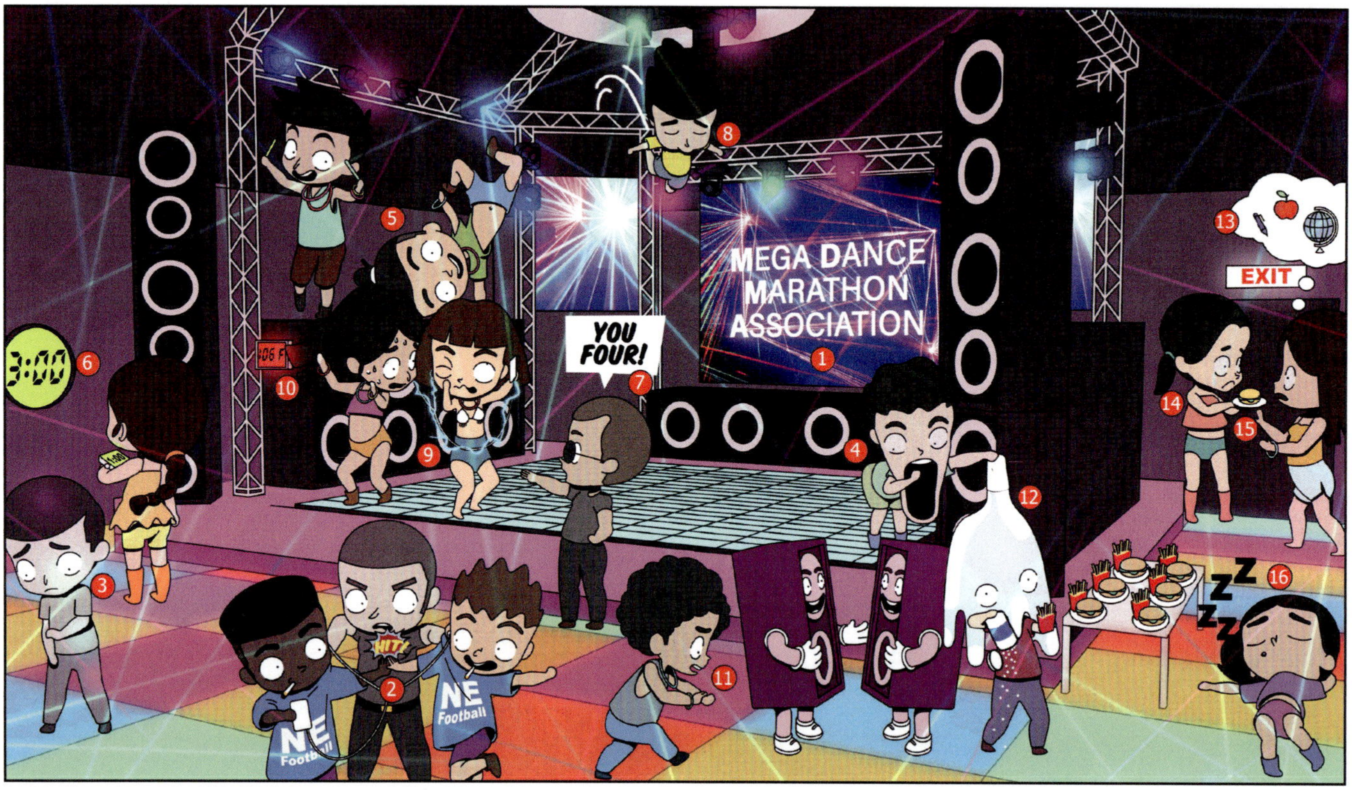

1. "Mega Dance Marathon Association" banner: MDMA is also known as ecstasy

2. Bouncer throwing NE football players sharing a tune bumping fists, "Hit!" out of club: Potent 5-HT, dopamine and NE reuptake inhibitor

3. Regular looking kid who isn't excited surrounded by dull colors: Tachyphylaxis occurs with MDMA

4. Hallucinating raver watching taking speakers: Hallucinogenic stimulant

5. Ravers climbing on stage equipment: Can cause hyperactivity

6. Clocks confusing raver with different times: Can cause distorted perception of time and senses

7. Bouncer shouts, "You four!": Causes euphoria

8. Man driving recklessly off of stage trusses: Causes disinhibition

9. Women being shocked while sharing a tune: Can cause life-threatening serotonin syndrome

10. Woman sweating with white and cold fingers in 106F degrees: Can cause life-threatening hyperthermia

11. Raver pacing while checking radial pulse: Can cause life-threatening sinus tachycardia

12. Raver's head overwhelmed with fluid from salt shaker and drink from hallucinating raver: Can cause life-threatening hyponatremia, which can lead to cerebral edema

13. Raver who is leaving with distracted: Withdrawal can cause difficulty concentrating

14. Sad woman offering hamburger: Withdrawal can cause depression

15. Raver leaving with distracting thought rejecting food: Withdrawal can cause loss of appetite

16. Raver asleep on ground: Withdrawal can cause fatigue

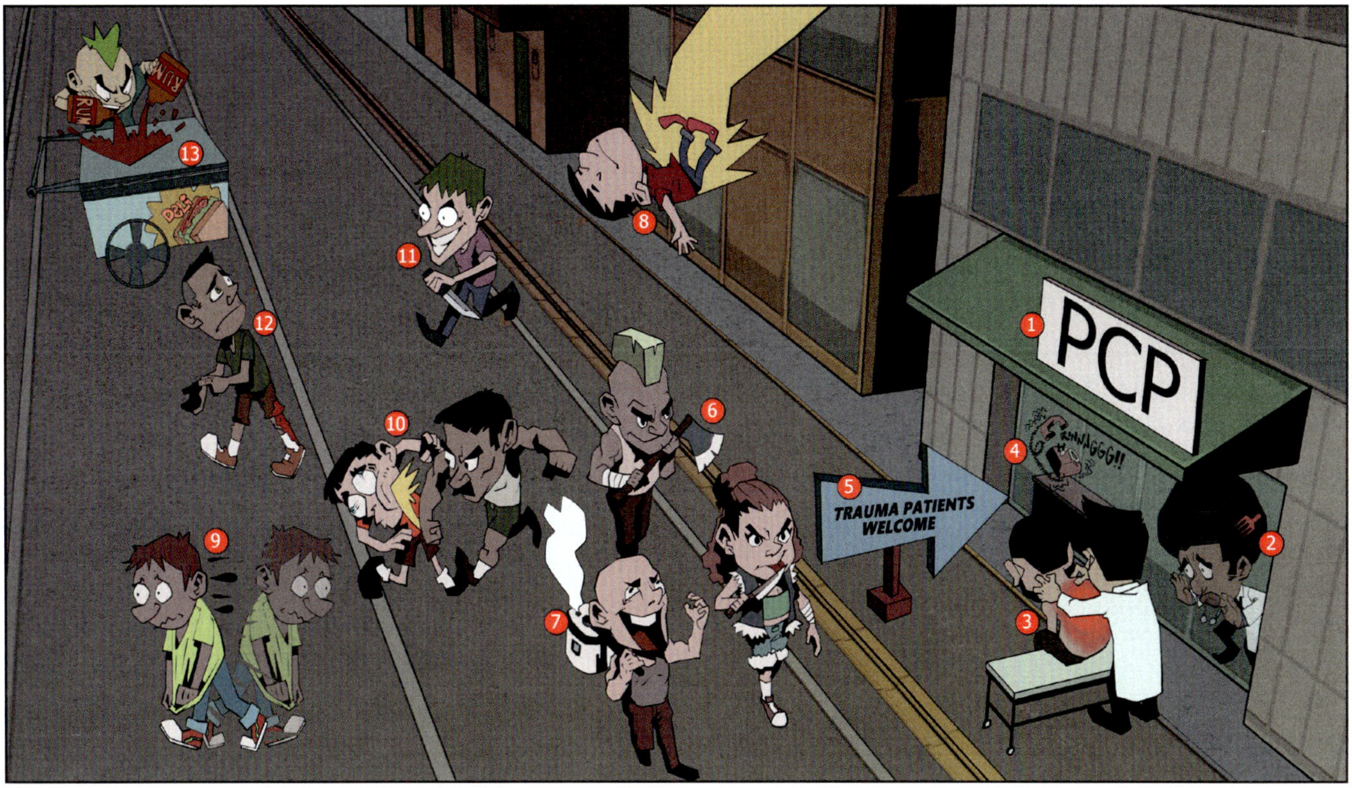

1. Primary care physician (PCP) office: Phencyclidine (PCP)

2. Doctor with comb in his afro: Can cause a coma

3. PA rubbing man's shoulders to alleviate his pain: Acts as an analgesic

4. Phone ringing, "Ringgg!!": Can cause seizures

5. "Trauma patients welcome" sign in front of office: Most common complications is trauma

6. Mad Max characters walking: Can cause violence

7. Pressure cooker held by one of violent characters: Can cause hypertension

8. High man jumping off of roof: Causes people to be impulse and disinhibited

9. Man pacing and picking at his shirt in street: Can cause pacing and purposeless movements (psychomotor agitation)

10. Man's eyes bouncing in different directions after being punched in the face: Can cause vertical and horizontal nystagmus

11. Man with psychotic grin with knife: Can cause psychosis

12. Man checking pulse while trying to run away from psycho: Can cause tachycardia

13. Man pouring rum over deli cart: Can cause delirium

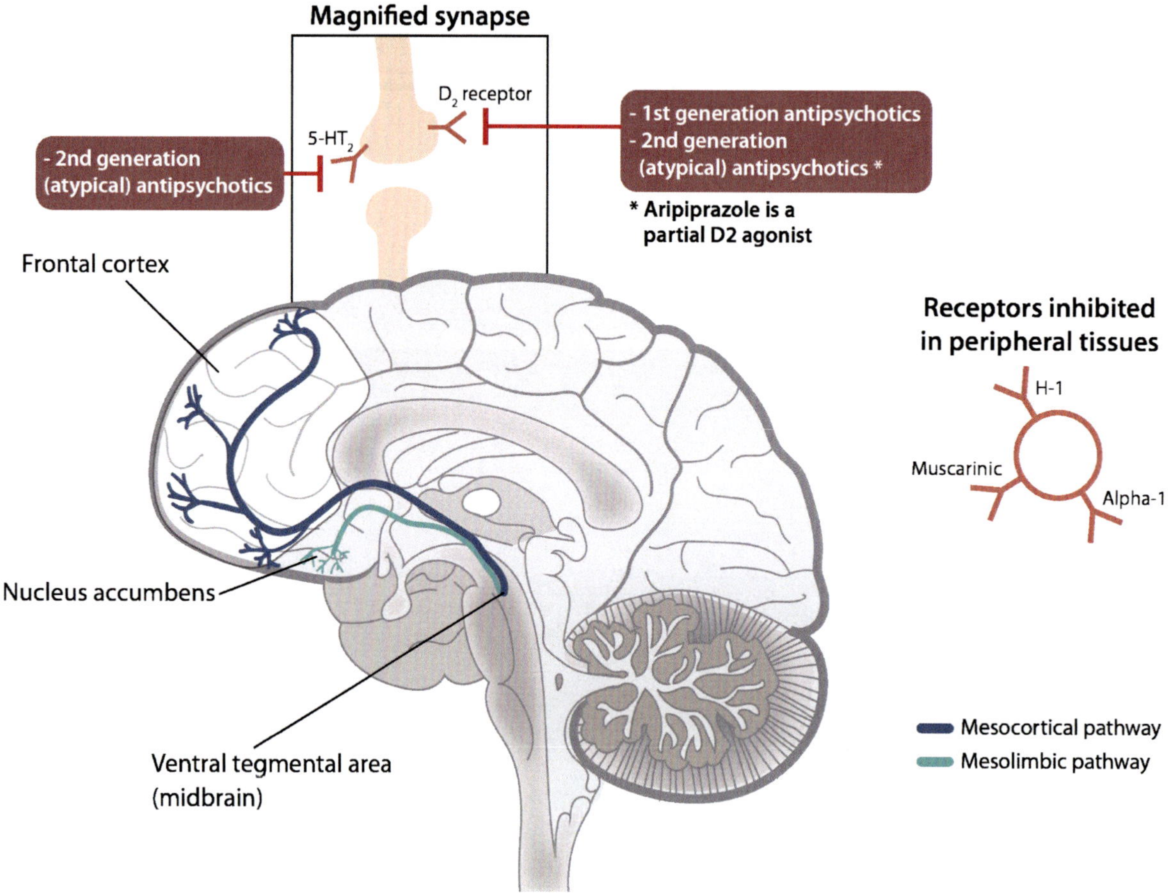

Figure 9.13.6 - Antipsychotic Mechanisms

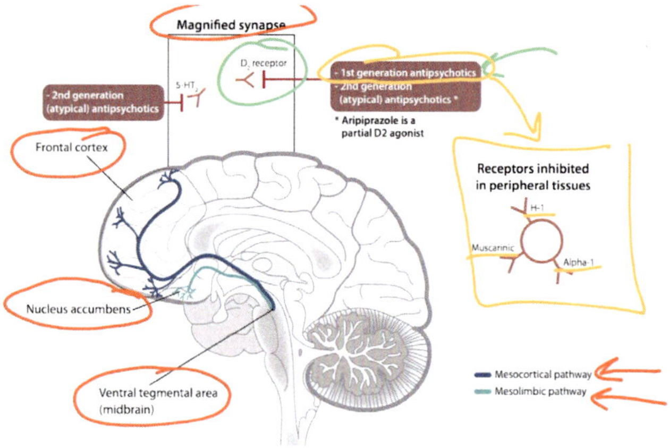

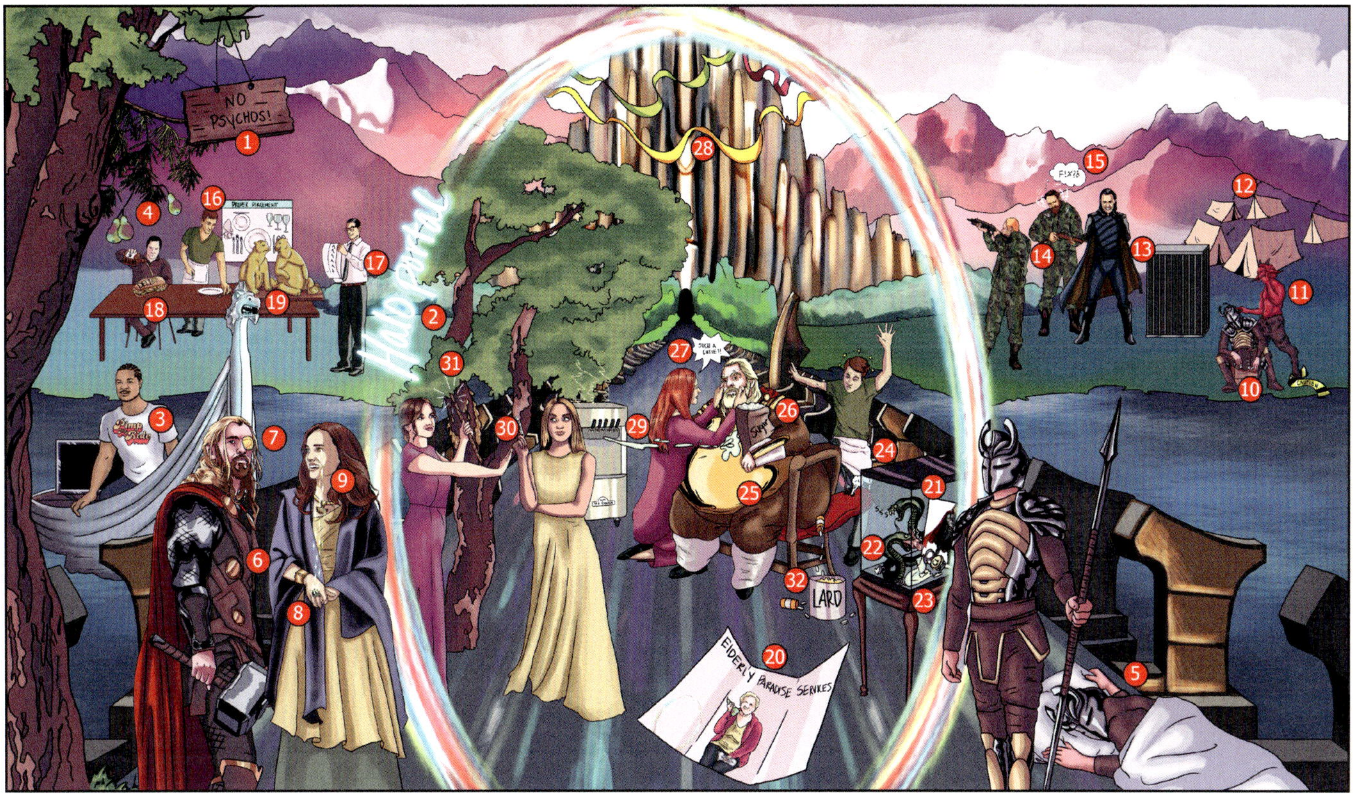

1. "No psychos!" sign: First generation (typical) antipsychotics

2. "Halo Portal" in front of kingdom: Haloperidol

3. Xzibit with "Pimp my Ride" shirt in chrome boat: Pimozide

4. Three pears in pine tree: Trifluoperazine

5. Guard fluffing his pillow while resting: Fluphenazine

6. "Thior" hero: Thioridazine

7. Thior with yellow eyepatch: Thioridazine causes retinal deposits

8. Cute lover "CL" ring worn by Jane: Chlorpromazine

9. Part of the CL ring flew into Jane's eyes: Chlorpromazine causes corneal deposits

10. Warrior with two rolled dopes being blocked: Works by blocking the D2 receptor

11. Demon shouting next to warrior stepping on caution tape: Used cautiously for dementia

12. Lots of tents: Increases cAMP

13. Psychotic man: Used for psychosis

14. Asgardian hunters: Used for Huntington's disease

15. Involuntary twitching and cursing hunter: Use for Tourette syndrome

16. Diagram of obsessive plating chart next to meticulous server: Used to treat obsessive compulsive disorder (OCD)

17. Server's note with only positive sections: Use for 1° positive symptoms in schizophrenia

18. Man pouring rum on deli sandwich: Used to treat delirium

19. Two bears made of bronze on table: Used for bipolar disorder

20. "Elderly Paradise Services", EPS flier inside halo portal: Haloperidol, trifluoperazine and fluphenazine are the most potent and come with the highest risk for EPS

21. Kind Odin's wife's ring is guarded by hissing snake and picture of Thior: Chlorpromazine and thioridazine have an increased risk for antihistamine effects (e.g. sedation)

22. Hot cooked hare: Chlorpromazine and thioridazine have an increased risk for anticholinergic effects (hot, dry, urinary retention)

23. Snake breaking alpha handle teacup near ring and Thior picture: Chlorpromazine and thioridazine have an increased risk for α-blockade

24. Deflating cushing caused by startled server: α-blockade can cause postural hypotension

25. King Odin's large belly: All can cause weight gain

26. King Odin in chair while eating sugar: All can cause hyperglycemia

27. Woman stretching King Odin's cheeks while saying, "Such a cutie!": All can cause QT prolongation

28. Twisted party streamers decorating kingdom: All can cause torsades de pointes

29. Melted milk ice cream splattered on King Odin's chest and dripping down: All can cause hyperprolactinemia and galactorrhea

30. Woman refusing tampon: All can cause oligomenorrhea and/or amenorrhea

31. Ratty-looking sap coming out of tree: All can cause dyslipidemia

32. Tub of lard next to King Odin: All lipid soluble → long half life due to storage in body fat

See Figure 9.13.6 - Antipsychotic Mechanisms (Psychiatric Pharmacology, Section 15, Page 297)

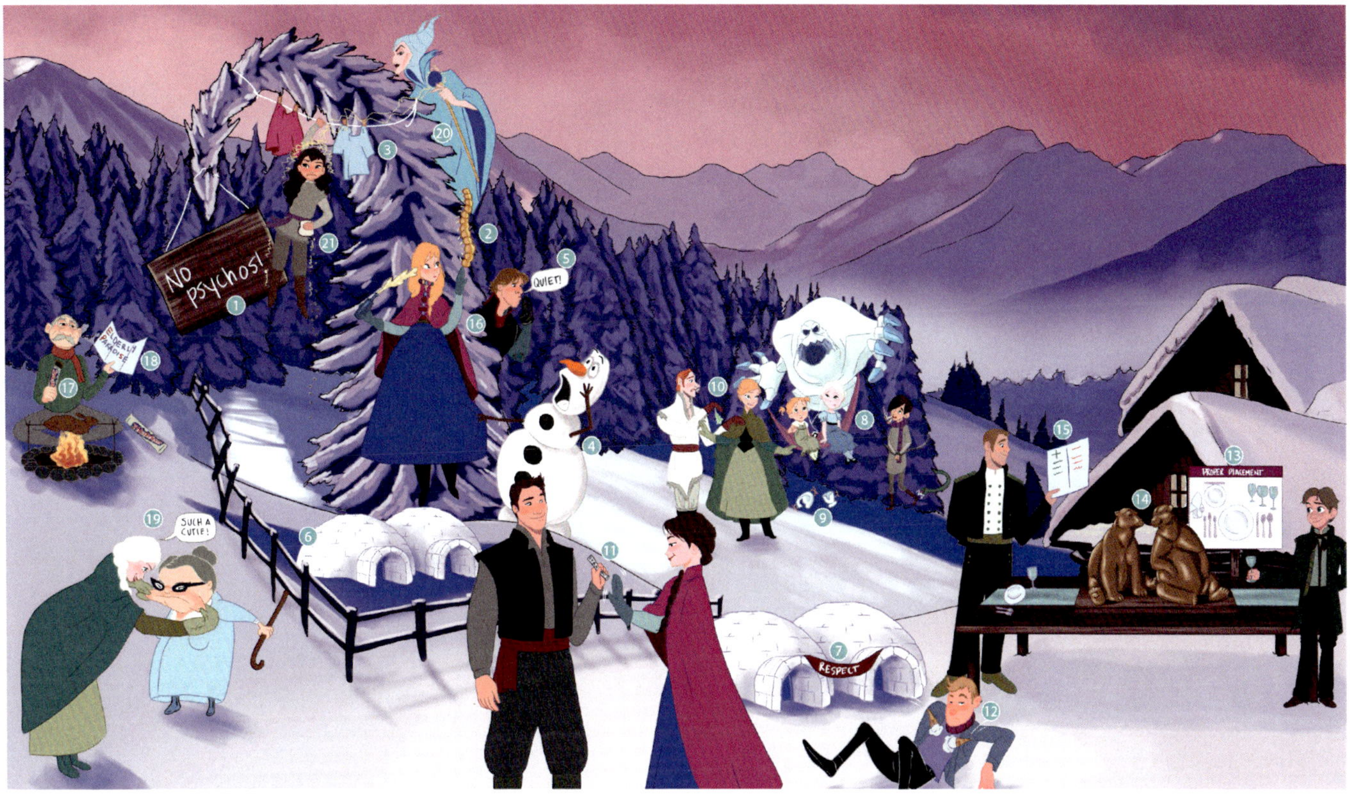

1. "No psychos!" sign on atypically pine tree: Atypical antipsychotics

2. Centipede climbing atypical pine tree: Asenapine

3. Clothesline on atypical pine tree: Clozapine

4. Olof like character at base of pine tree: Olanzapine

5. Kristoff quieting Olof from behind pine tree: Quetiapine

6. Pair of snow domes: Many end with the suffix, "-paridone"

7. Pair of snow domes with "Respect" banner: Risperidone

8. Two kids sharing a tune on two point hammock being blocked from plugging in headphones next to two dopes smoking kid: The mechanism for most drugs in this class is not fully understood, but most are serotonin ($5\text{-}HT_2$) receptor and D_2 receptor blockers

9. Single hissing snake with broken teacup with alpha handle and plate with two alpha handles: Antagonizes H1, α-1 and α-2 receptors

10. Man smoking two dopes who has a pine sol air freshener partially rubbing one shoulder: Aripiprazole works as a partial D_2 agonist

11. Woman refusing feminine hygiene product from boyfriend next to "Respect" banner: Risperidone can cause oligomenorrhea or amenorrhea

12. Man with two ice cream cones on chest: Risperidone can cause gynecomastia and galactorrhea

13. Obsessive waiter arranging plates with chart: Can be used to treat OCD

14. Two polar bear statues, one sad and one happy: Can be used for bipolar disorders

15. Server's note with positives and negatives: Used to treat positive and negative symptoms and schizophrenia

16. Pregnant Anna touching centipede on pine tree near clothesline, quieting man, and Olof while using hot oil: Asenapine, clozapine, quetiapine, olanzapine, cause weight gain, diabetes, and hyperlipidemia

17. Old man eating a 3 Musketeer bar while roasting a hare: Can cause antimuscarinic (anticholinergic effects)

18. Enderly Paradise Services flier next to campfire: 1st Gen. (typical) are more likely to produce EPS and antimuscarinic symptoms compared to 2nd gen. (atypical) antipsychotics

19. Woman pinching mom's cheeks saying, "Such a cutie!": All can cause QT prolongation

20. Maleficent zapping someone on the head: All can cause neuroleptic malignant syndrome (NMS)

21. Kid hanging onto clothesline and whole-grain bread while having a seizure: Clozapine can cause agranulocytosis and seizures

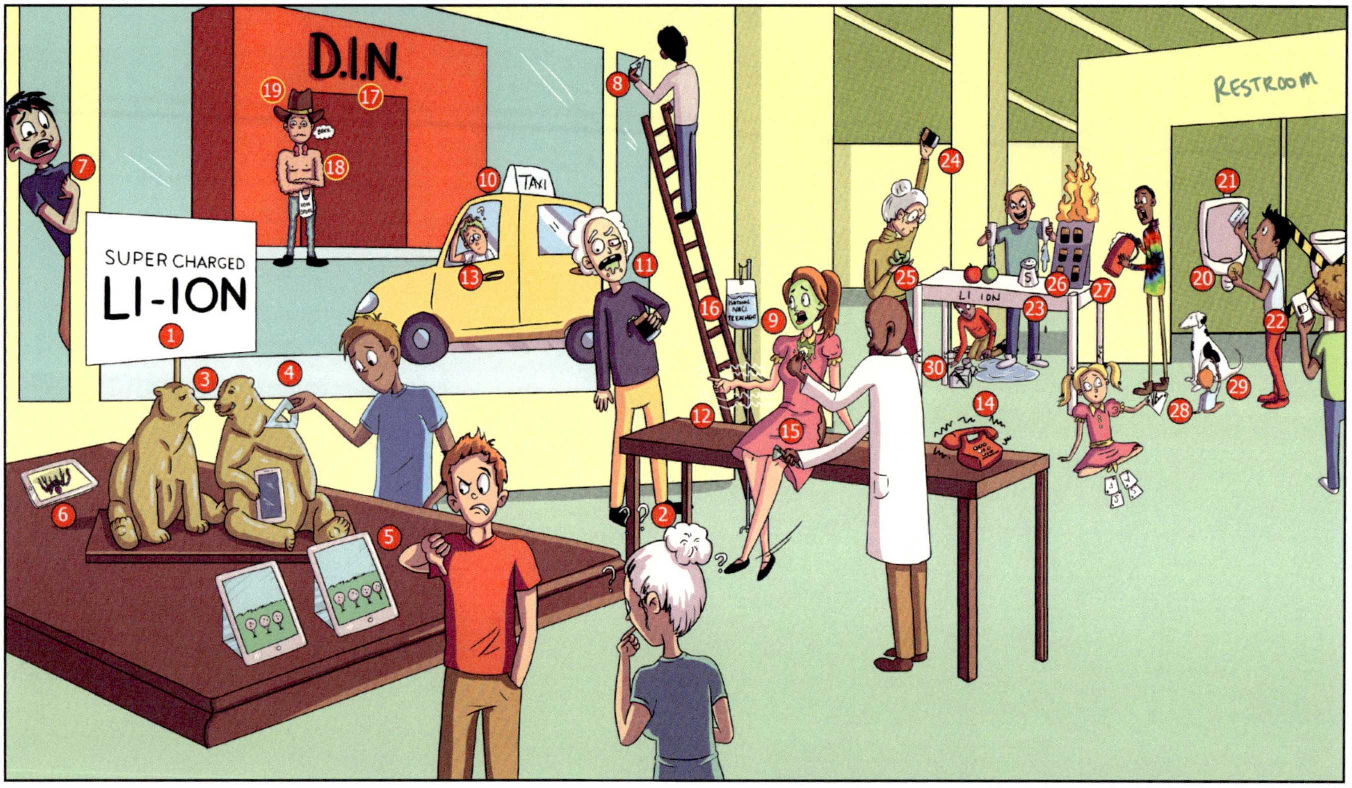

1. "Super charged Li-ion" sign: Lithium

2. Confused customer questioning the mechanism on table: Unclear mechanism

3. Two polar bear statues, one sad and one happy: Use for bipolar disorder

4. Acute angled protractor on happy bear: Use for acute manic episodes

5. Customer giving a thumbs-down to screens with three and four golf balls respectively: Lithium is a goitrogen and inhibits T_3 and T_4 release from the thyroid

6. Tarantula on phone: Teratogenic

7. Narrow window man is hiding behind: Narrow therapeutic window

8. Construction worker measuring angle of window with acute protractor: Acute toxicities

9. Nauseous woman with green face: Acute toxicity can cause GI distress (nausea, vomiting, and diarrhea)

10. Taxi outside of store: Acute toxicity can cause ataxia

11. Man's slurred and garbled speech: Acute toxicity can cause slurred speech

12. Sick nauseous woman's trembling hands: Acute toxicity can cause tremors

13. Confused taxi driver: Acute toxicity can cause confusion

14. Ringing phone in store: Acute toxicity can cause seizures

15. Nauseous woman's hyperreflexic knee: Acute toxicity can cause hyperreflexia

16. IV bag of saline: Treat toxicity with aggressive isotonic NaCl

17. "D.I.N." restaurant outside: Chronic toxicity can lead to nephrogenic diabetes insipidus

18. Shirtless man with "Ion store" bag and untied bowtie shivering: Chronic toxicity can cause hypothyroidism

19. Cowboy hat worn by shirtless man: Neurologic symptoms in chronic toxicity is very similar to those of acute

20. Open urinal: Excreted by the kidneys

21. Man with bun and credit card next to urinal: Monitor levels of BUN/Cr (renal function tests)

22. Customer monitoring lithium phone's battery: Closely monitor serum lithium levels

23. PVC snack tables with salt shaker on top: Lithium is reabsorbed in the PCT through Na+ channels

24. Elderly woman eating kidney beans and raising hand near "Li-ion" table: Kidney damaged can increase lithium toxicity

25. Elderly woman: Elderly patient have increased risk of lithium toxicity

26. Kid depleting water bottles near table: Volume depletion can also increase the chance of lithium toxicity

27. Scrawny firefighter in tie-dye shirt unable to put out li-ion battery fire: Drugs that decrease renal clearance will increase serum lithium levels (e.g. thiazides, NSAIDs)

28. Ripped ace card under firefighter's foot: Drugs that decrease renal clearance will increase serum lithium levels (e.g. ACE inhibitors)

29. Kid poking liver-shaped dog with stick: Cirrhosis can also increase toxicity

30. Broken pump under table: Heart failure can also increase chance for lithium toxicity

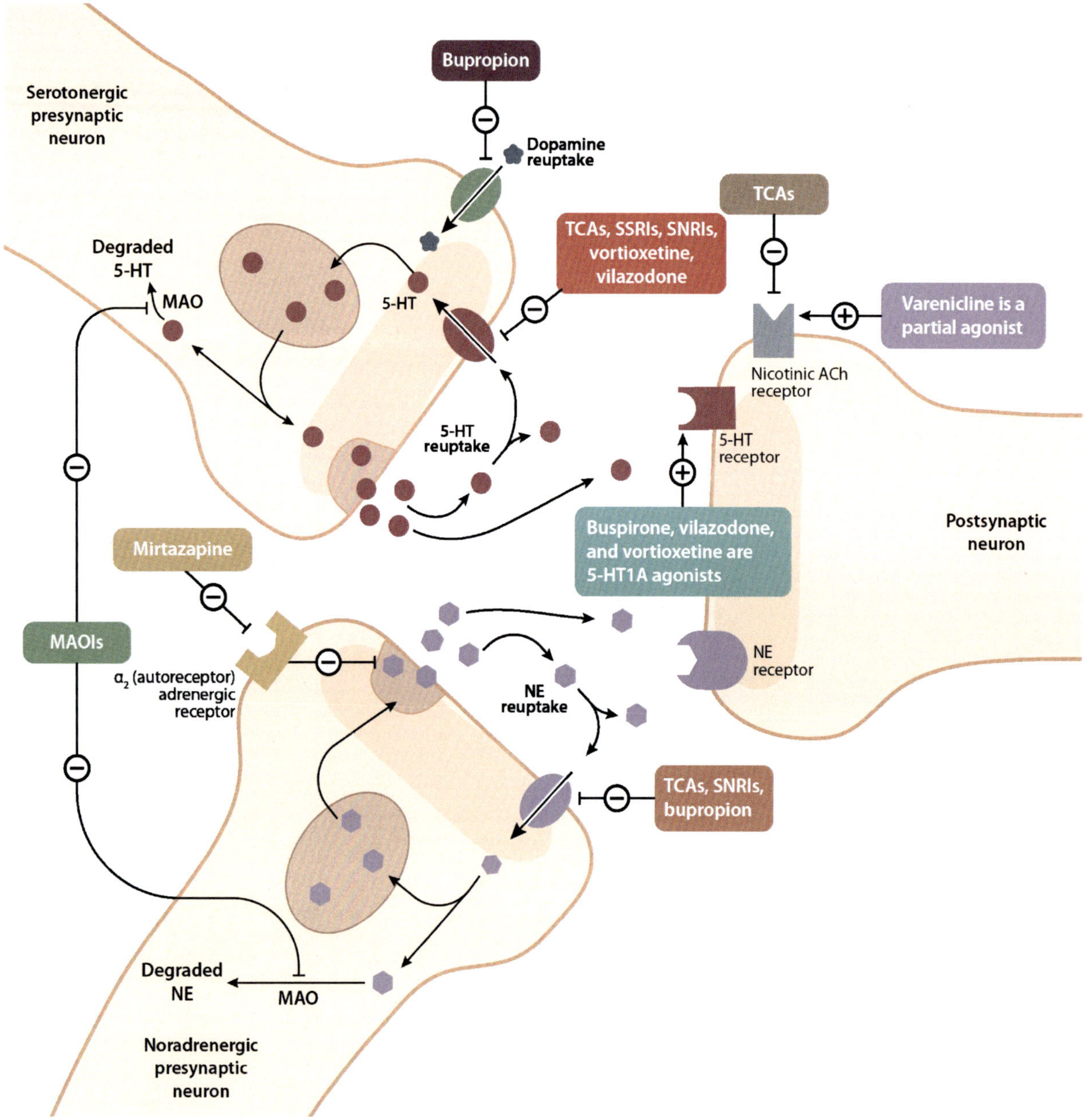

Figure 9.13.7 - Antidepressant Effects on Neurotransmission

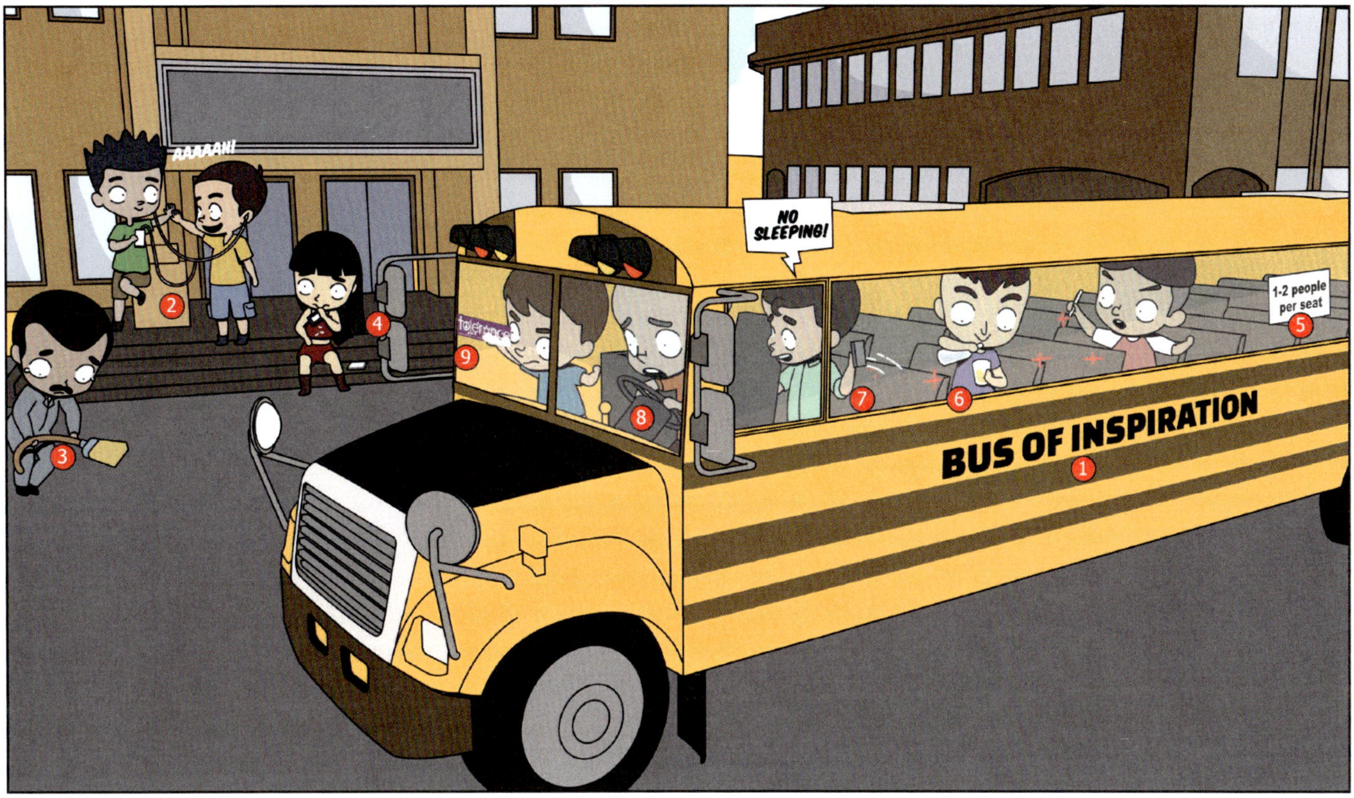

1. "Bus of Inspiration" parked outside prestige school: Buspirone

2. Kids saying, "Ahhh" while high-fiving and sharing a tune: Mechanism: 5-HT_{1a} agonist

3. Sad man holding atypically-shaped broom: Atypical antidepressant

4. Girl anxious about boyfriend with two phones: Can be used as a 2nd line treatment for generalized anxiety disorder (GAD)

5. "1-2 people per seat" sign on school bus: Takes 1-2 weeks to take effect

6. Student pouring alcohol into cup of cooking oil on school bus: Does not interact with alcohol

7. Addition symbols being erased from school bus windows: Does not cause addiction

8. Bus driver rudely woken up: Does not cause sedation

9. Tolerance sticker being scrapped off windshield: Does not cause tolerance

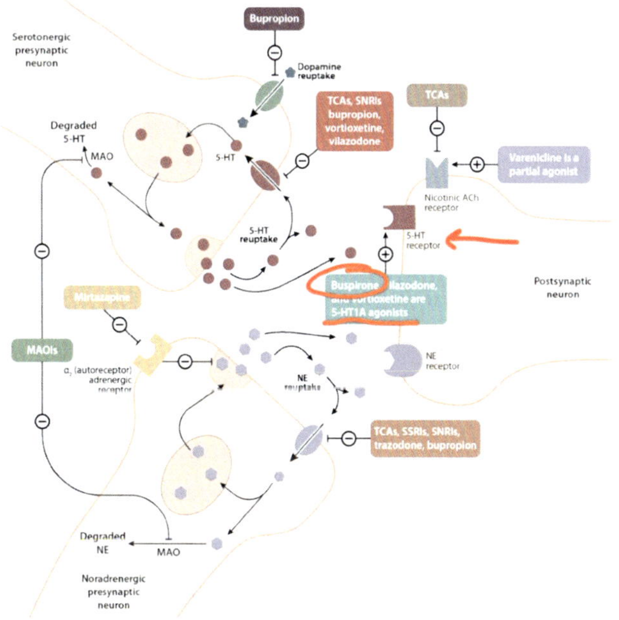

See Figure 9.13.7 - Antidepressant Effects on Neurotransmission (Psychology, Section 18, Page 303)

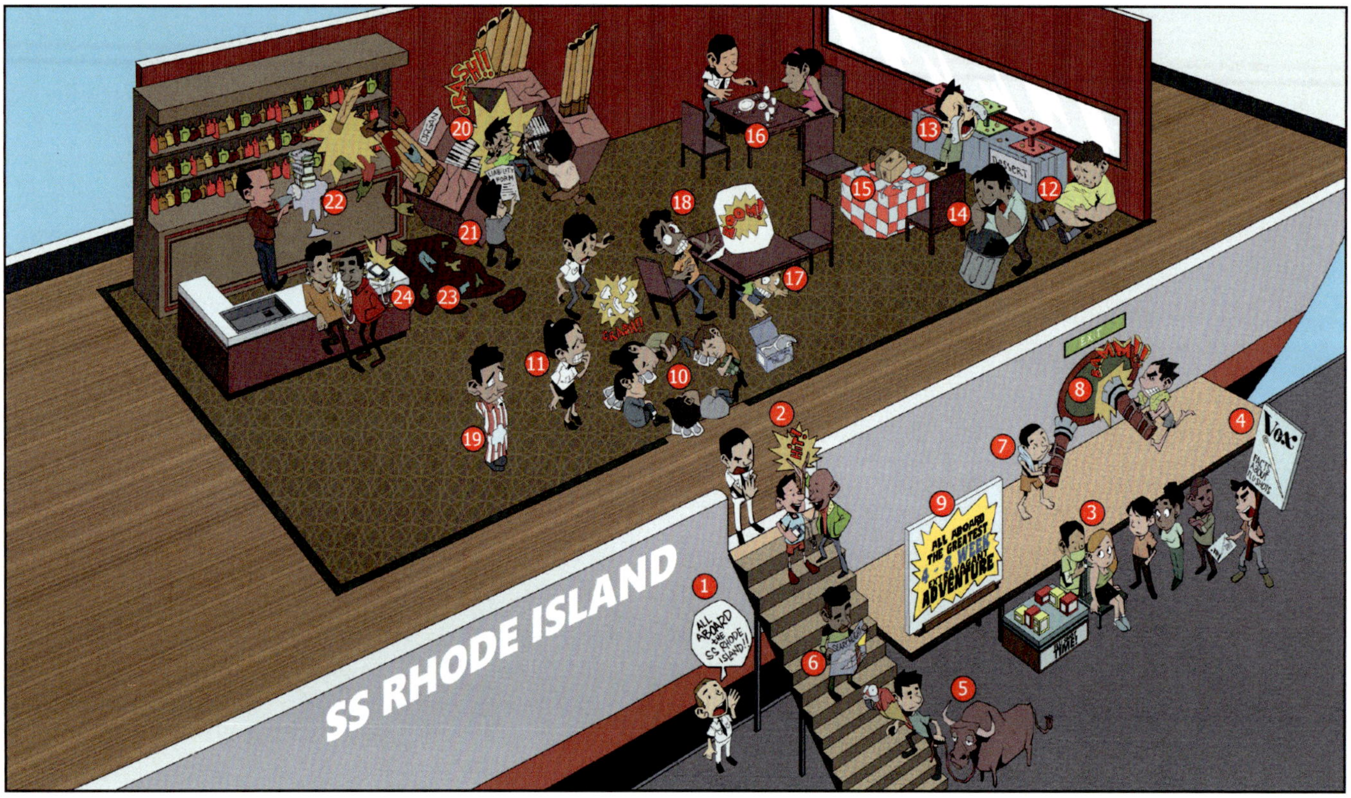

1. "SS Rhode Island" cruise ship: SSRI

2. Cruise worker inhibiting guests to share a tune while high-fiving: Inhibits 5-HT reuptake

3. Flu shot station outside of ship: Fluoxetine

4. Vox logo poster with "Facts about flu shots" written at bottom: Fluvoxamine

5. Parrot and ox with passenger: Paroxetine

6. Searchlight publication: Sertraline

7. Men ramming boat with towels covering ram: Citalopram

8. Men trying to break into the emergency exit door with towel covering ram: Escitalopram

9. "All aboard the greatest 4-6 weeks of extravagant adventure" sign: Takes about 4-8 weeks to have effect

10. Four men who are homesick laying on menstrual pads: Use for premenstrual dysphoric disorder

11. Waiter biting fingernails anxiously: Use for GAD

12. Overweight man near dessert buffet: Use for binge eating disorder

13. Crying passenger next to dessert table: Use for depression

14. Guest vomiting into trash can: Use for bulimia nervosa

15. Picnic-themed table left in chaotic state: Use for panic disorder

16. Obsessive waiter cleaning disordered table: Used to treat obsessive compulsive disorder

17. Anxious man hiding under table: Use for social anxiety disorder

18. Traumatized marine hearing "Boom!" from nearby broken plates: Use for PTSD

19. White frosting over man's crotch while he is in pajamas: Use to treat premature ejaculation

20. Destroyed organ, "Crash!": Can cause anorgasmia

21. Man refusing to sign liability form: Can cause decreased libido

22. Bartender drying wet diaries with blow dryer: Can cause SIADH

23. Chocolate syrup puddle: Can cause GI distress

24. Men sharing a tune with sparks coming out of phone: Can cause serotonin syndrome

See Figure 9.13.7 - Antidepressant Effects on Neurotransmission (Psychology, Section 18, Page 303)

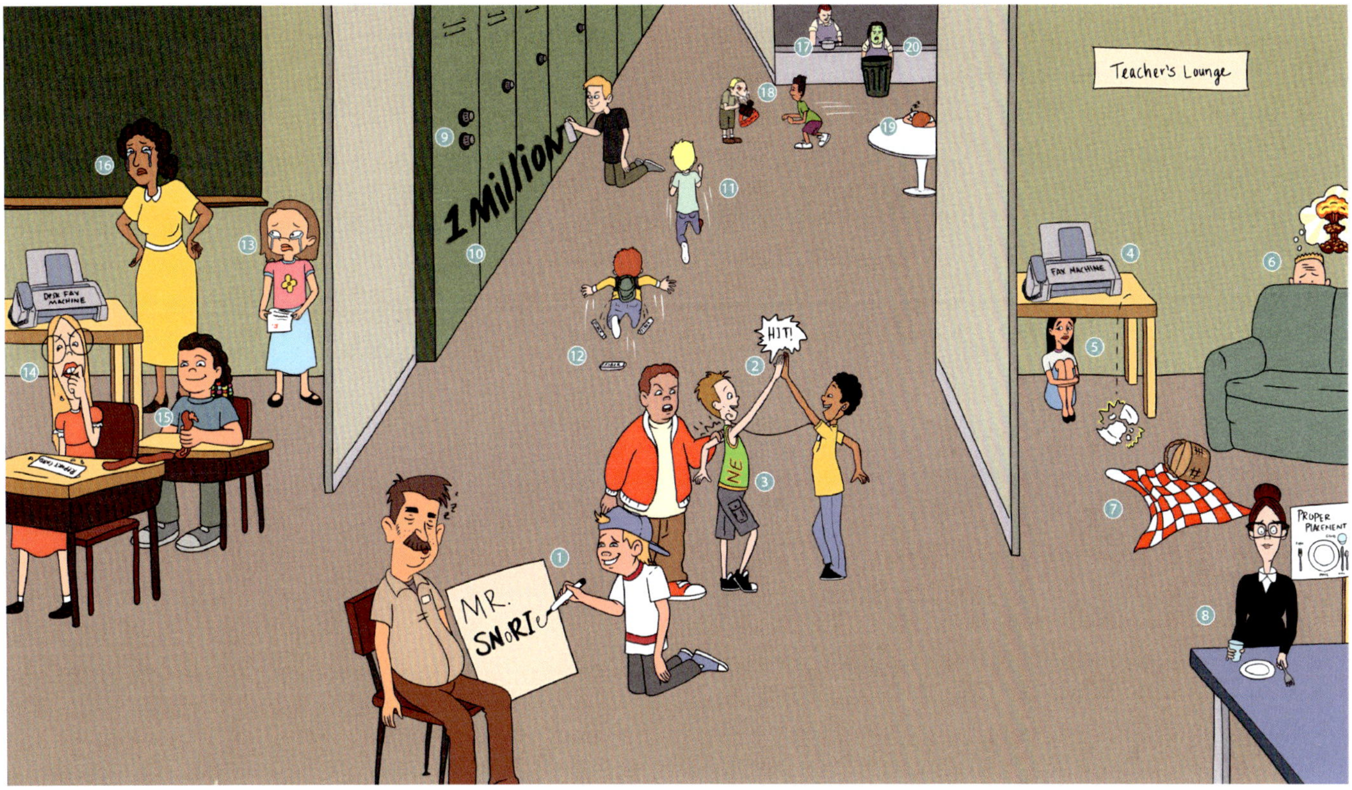

1. "Mr. Snorti" sign to mock teacher: SNRI (serotonin and norepinephrine reuptake inhibitors)

2. Kids sharing a tune while high-fiving and kids in red shirt shoving them: 5-HT (serotonin) reuptake is inhibited

3. "Ne" shirt worn by high-fiving kid: NE reuptake is also inhibited

4. Fax machine: Venlafaxine

5. New teacher hiding under table avoiding kids: Venlafaxine can treat social anxiety disorder

6. Ex-military teacher hiding behind couch while having flashback: Venlafaxine can treat PTSD

7. Picnic basket near fax machine: Venlafaxine can treat panic disorder

8. Obsessive teacher perfecting utensils on table: Venlafaxine can treat OCD

9. Locker with "dual" locks in hallway: Duloxetine

10. "1 Million" spray paint prank on lockers: Milnacipran

11. Students leaving million spray paint scene: Levomilnacipran

12. Kid leaving million scene dropping fiber bars: Use duloxetine, milnacipran, and levomilnacipran for fibromyalgia

13. Student crying in classroom: Use SNRIs for depression

14. Student biting fingernails anxiously: Use SNRIs for generalized anxiety disorder (GAD)

15. Student with dyed beads squeezing sausage links: Use SRNIs for diabetic neuropathy

16. Depressed teacher's desk fax machine: Desvenlafaxine is primarily used for depression

17. Pressure cooker in cafeteria: SRNIs can increase blood pressure

18. Hall monitor flashes himself with Insignia brand camera while trying to take a picture of student checking pulse while running: SNRIs can cause stimulant effects (e.g. tachycardia and insomnia)

19. Kid sleeping on lunch table: SNRIs can cause sedation

20. Nauseous green faced lunch lady: SRNIs can cause nausea

See Figure 9.13.7 - Antidepressant Effects on Neurotransmission (Psychology, Section 18, Page 305)

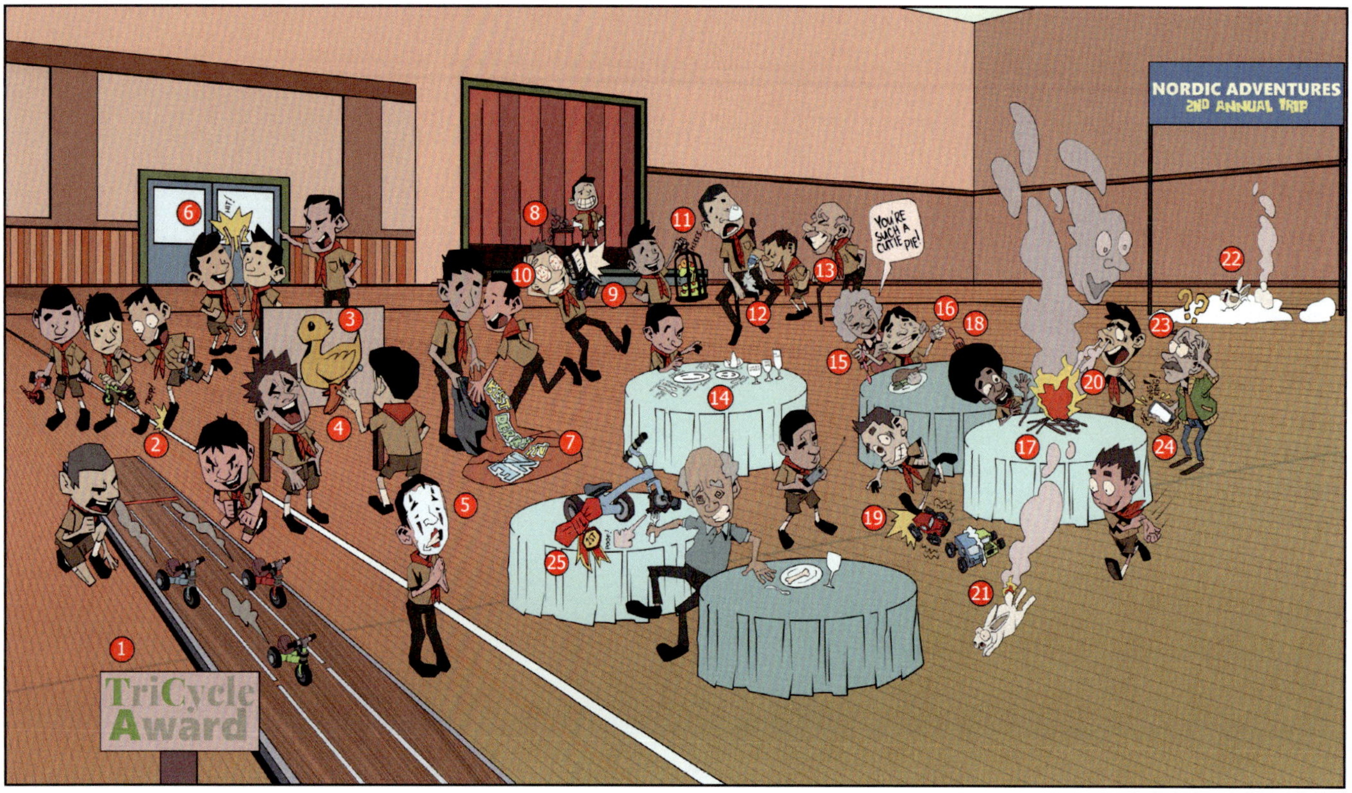

1. "TriCycle Award" sign: Tricyclic antidepressants (TCAs)

2. Tripping scout leaning on his friend: Amitriptyline

3. Pin the bill on the duck game: Doxepin

4. Kid pins bill on duck's crotch and friend mocking him: Amoxapine

5. Praying mime scout: "ipramine" drugs (e.g. imipramine, desipramine, clomipramine)

6. Scouts sharing a turn with high-fiving while leader scolding them and kicking them out: 5-HT reuptake inhibitor

7. "NE" on banner being taken down: NE reuptake inhibitor

8. Scout wearing gloves he used to handle sausages on stage: TCAs are used for peripheral neuropathy

9. Leader flashes himself with Insignia brand camera: Use for insomnia

10. Leader who flashes himself holding his head: Use for migraine prophylaxis

11. Single hissing snake in cage next to sleeping scout leader: H_1 blocker

12. Scout pouring water on sleeping leader's crotch: Used to treat sleep enuresis

13. Old leader with cane holding his sore back: Use for chronic pain management

14. Obsessive scout plating table: Used to treat obsessive compulsive disorder

15. Grandma stretching cheeks of scout who was decorating with twisted streamers: All TCAs can cause QT prolongation leading to torsades de pointes

16. Scout with unused salt shaker: Arrhythmias are due to sodium channel inhibition

17. Fire on top of table: Can cause hyperpyrexia

18. Scout with comb in afro: Can cause coma

19. Two glued cars not rattling next to rattling RC car: $NaHOC_3$ is used to prevent arrhythmias

20. Leader inhaled smoke from fire and can't breathe: Can cause respiratory depression

21. Scout checking his pulse and chasing hare that is on fire: Can cause anticholinergic effects

22. Cooled off rabbit sitting in snow under "Nordic Adventure" banner: Nortriptyline has fewer anticholinergic side effects

23. Confused old man hallucinating: Can cause confusion and hallucinations, especially in the elderly

24. Old man's phone is ringing: Can cause seizures

25. Old man puncturing tire of prized tricycle while rapid change of posture: Can cause postural hypotension

See Figure 9.13.7 - Antidepressant Effects on Neurotransmission (Psychology, Section 18, Page 303)

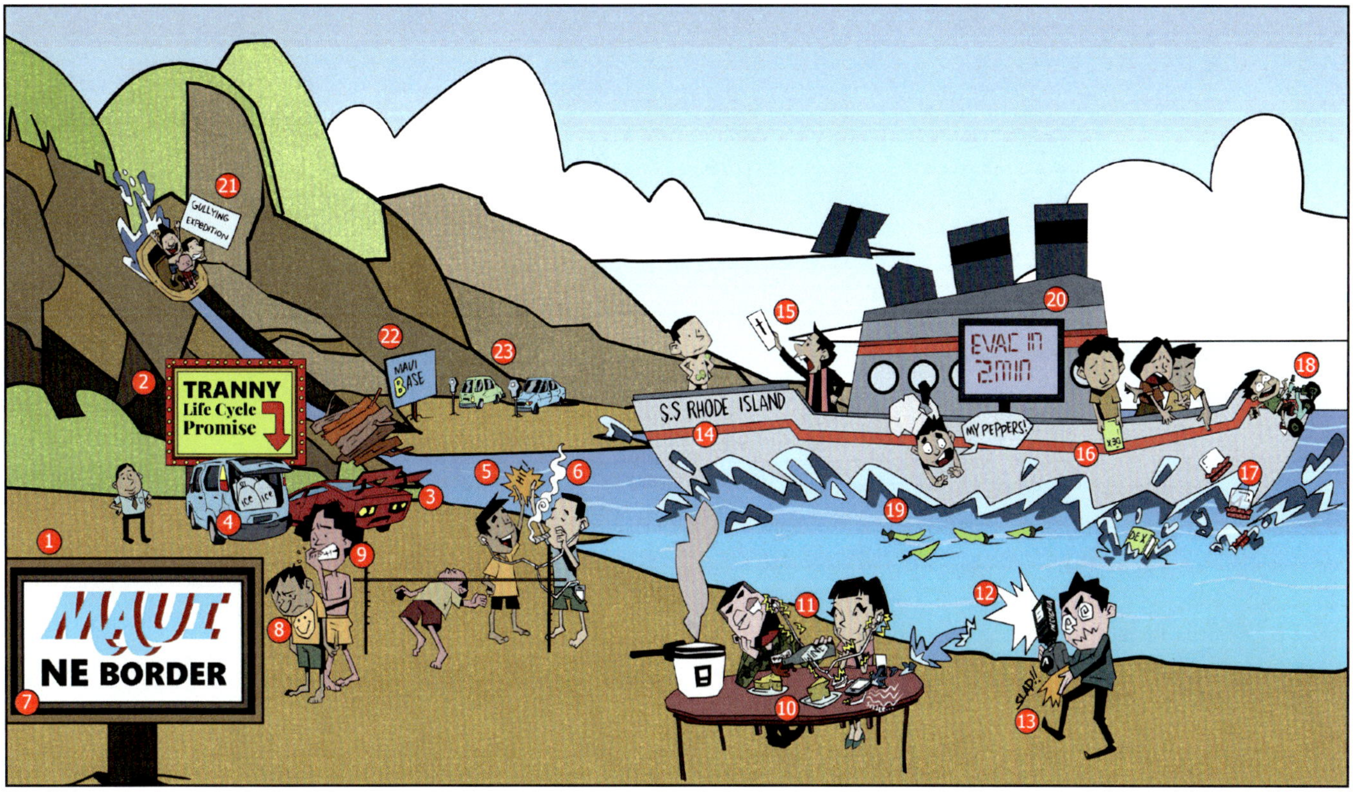

1. "Maui NE Border" sign on beach: MAO inhibitors

2. "Tranny Life Cycle Promise" sign on beach: Tranylcypromine

3. Z-shaped fender on Ferrari: Phenelzine

4. Old box shaped car with bags of ice: Isocarboxazid

5. Men sharing a tune high-fiving each other: Increased levels of 5-HT

6. High-fiving man smoking dope: Increased levels of dopamine

7. NE on "Maui Border" sign: Increased levels of NE

8. Atypically depressed man with smiley face shirt: Used for atypical depression (depression with emotional reactivity)

9. Man biting fingernails anxiously: Used to treat anxiety

10. Tired marine who recently got home with precursor of cheese and wine next to pressure cooker: Increased risk of hypertensive crisis with tyramine containing foods (e.g. wine and cheese)

11. Marine with girlfriend sharing a tune with a shock in headphones: Can cause serotonin syndrome

12. Man with flashing Insignia brand camera: Can cause insomnia

13. Photographer hitting the camera: Can cause agitation

14. SS Rhode Island ship falling apart: Contraindicated with SSRIs

15. St. John on a forbidden boat shouting at man with warts: Contraindicated with St. John's Wort

16. Man throwing "Dex" phone books off of ship: Contraindicated with dextromethorphan

17. Linen lids getting tossed off of ship: Contraindicated with linezolid

18. Kid on tricycle falling off of ship: Contraindicated with TCAs

19. Man diving down for his peppers saying, "My peppers!": Contraindicate with meperidine

20. "Evac in 2 Min" sign on ship: Wait 2 weeks after stopping MAOIs to start serotonergic drugs or stop dietary restrictions

21. Runoff rafting with "Gullying expedition" sign: Selegiline and rasagiline

22. "Maui Base" sign at end of raft: Selegiline and rasagiline selectively inhibit MAO-B

23. Parking meters near base gulley: Selegiline and rasagiline are used mainly for Parkinson's

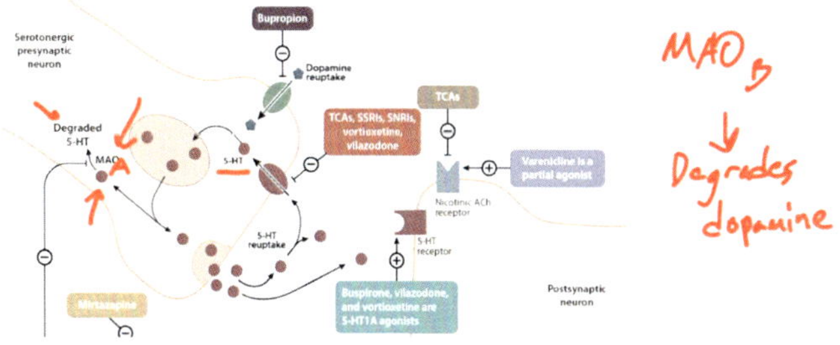

See Figure 9.13.7 - Antidepressant Effects on Neurotransmission (Psychology, Section 18, Page 303)

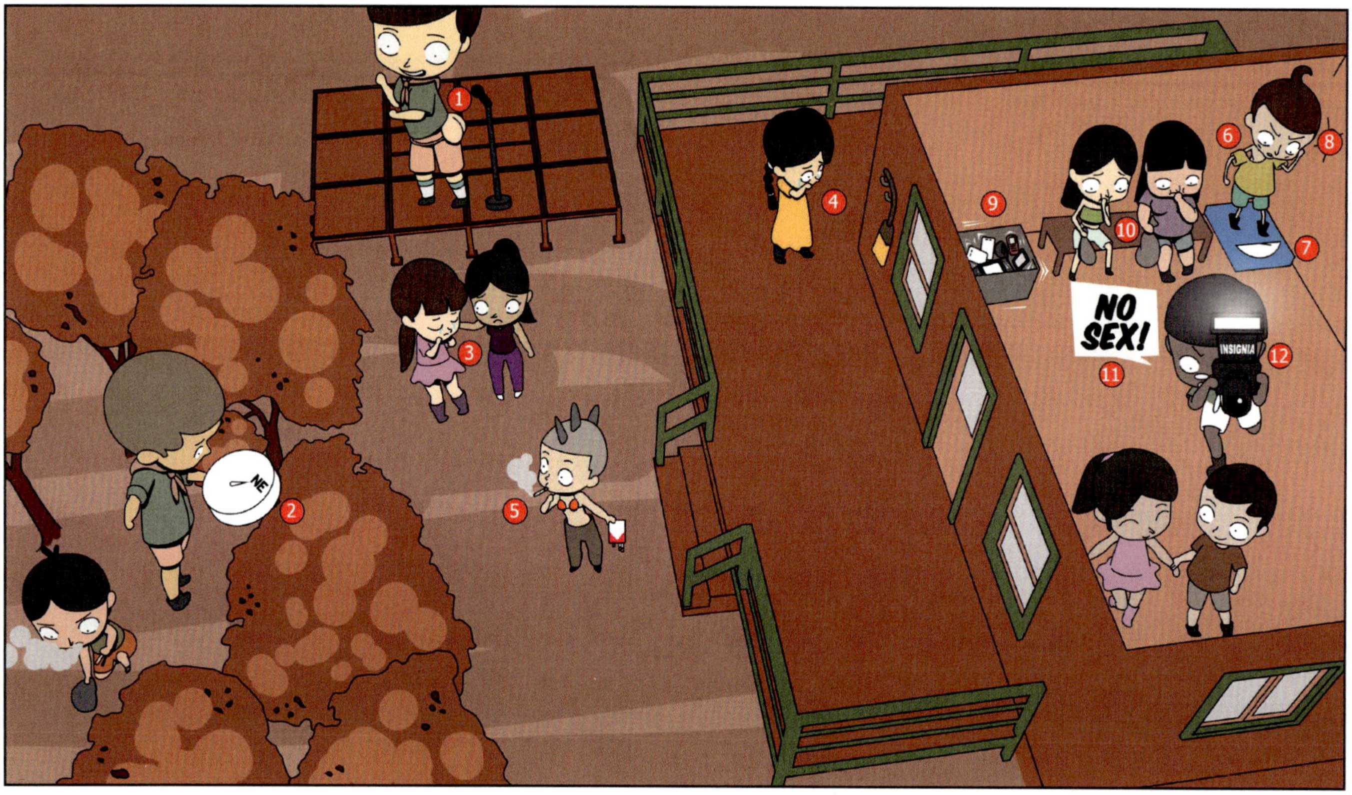

1. Camp counselor with bum prop: Bupropion

2. Counselor with compass pointing NE and a teen smoking dope outside of camp lost: Works as norepinephrine and dopamine reuptake inhibitor (NDRI)

3. Crying teenager next to counselor with bum prop: Used to treat depression

4. Depressed teen looking at atypical shape broom: Considered an atypical antidepressant

5. Teen with mohawk smoking cigarette: Used to treat smoking

6. Wild, constantly moving teen inside lodge: Can cause stimulant effects

7. Wild teen on scale inside lodge: Can cause weight loss

8. Teen holding head inside lodge: Can cause headaches

9. Box of ringing cell phones inside lodge: Can cause seizures

10. Very skinny and obese teens holding bags inside lodge: Seizures are more likely when the patient is anorexic or bulimic

11. Teen couple holding hands while counselor says, "No Sex" inside lodge: No sexual side effects

12. Counselor with Insignia brand camera flashing teen couple: Can cause insomnia

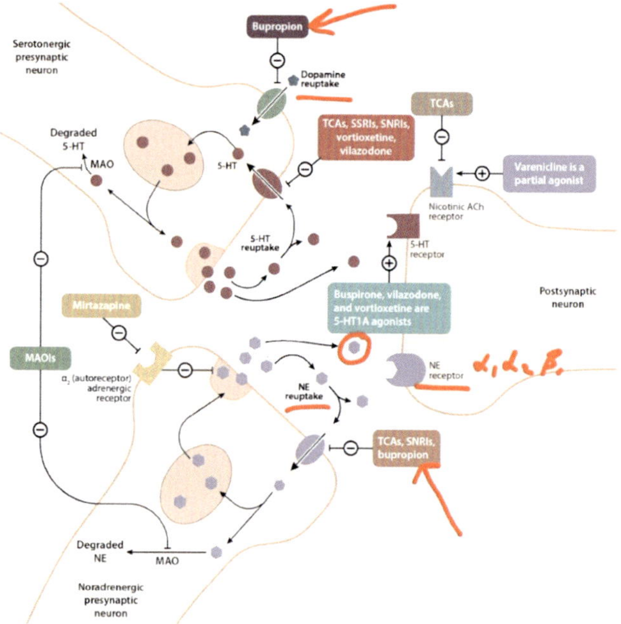

See Figure 9.13.7 - Antidepressant Effects on Neurotransmission (Psychology, Section 18, Page 303)

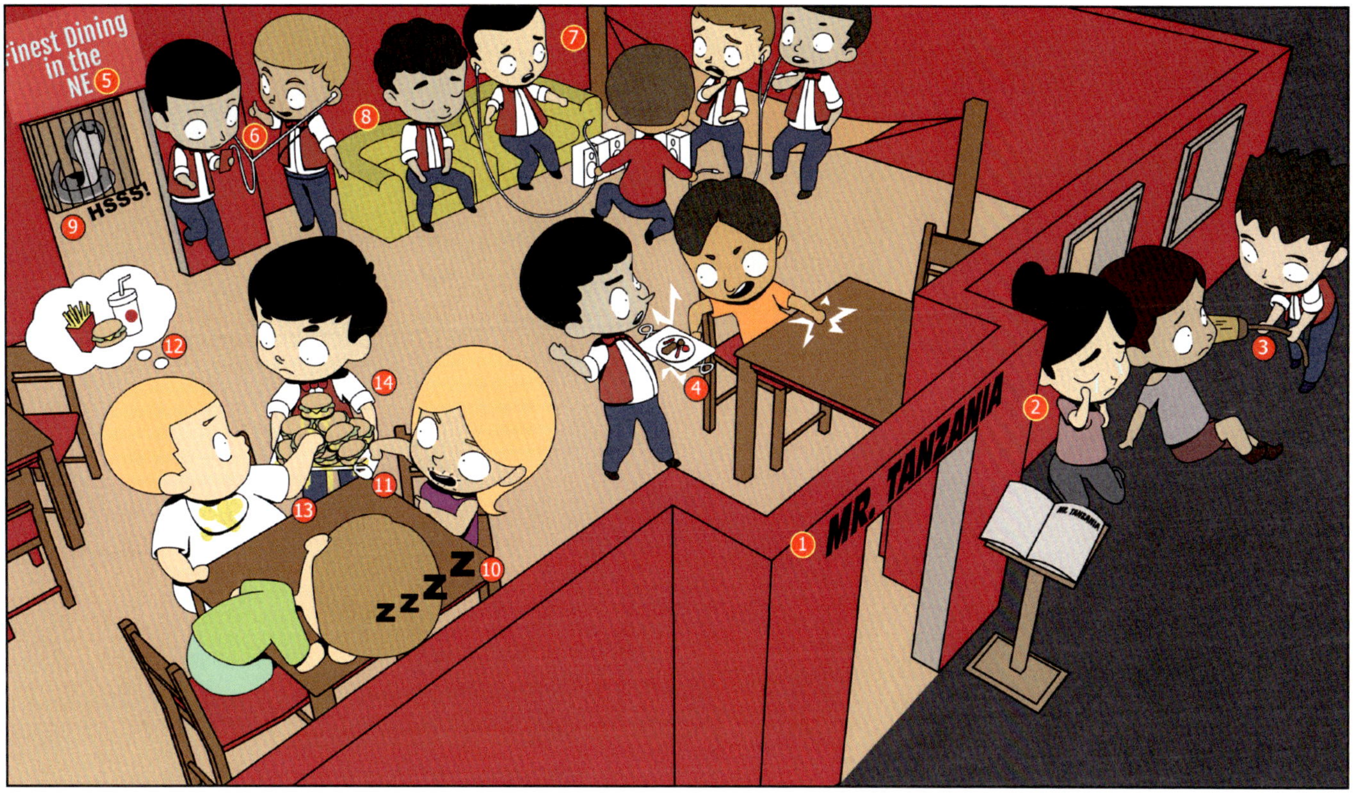

1. "Mr. Tanzania" sign on restaurant: Mirtazapine

2. Homeless sad couple outside of restaurant: Used to treat depression

3. Employee handing over atypical broom to homeless sad couple: Atypical antidepressant

4. Customer pushing tray away with two alpha handles: Alpha-2 antagonist

5. "Finest Dining in the NE" sign inside restaurant: Increased release of norepinephrine (NE)

6. Employees sharing a tuen and one asking to turn music up: increases serotonin

7. Waiters sharing a tune in a hammock hung by two poles while manager smacks and unplugs headphones: 5-HT_2 receptor antagonist

8. Waiters on a "3"-shaped couch sharing a tune while manager smacks and unplugs headphones: 5-HT_3 receptor antagonist

9. Single hissing snake cage in kitchen: Histamine-1 antagonist

10. Customer sleeping on table: Can cause sedation

11. Customer's wife pouring over empty glass: Can cause dehydration

12. Kid daydreaming of food: Can increase appetite

13. Obese kid daydreaming of food: Can cause eight gain

14. Waiter with hamburgers: Can increase cholesterol

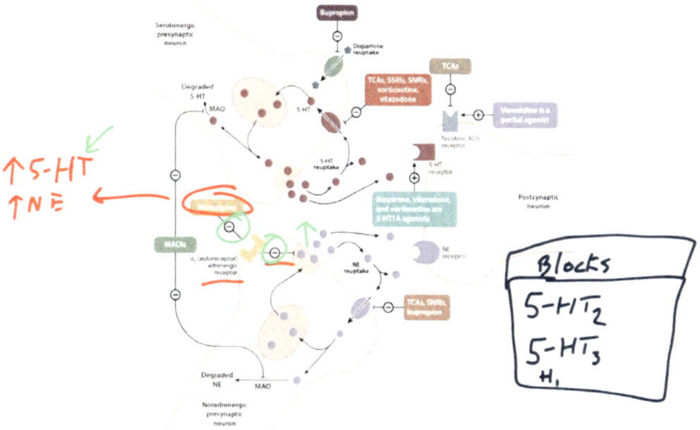

See Figure 9.13.7 - Antidepressant Effects on Neurotransmission (Psychology, Section 18, Page 305)

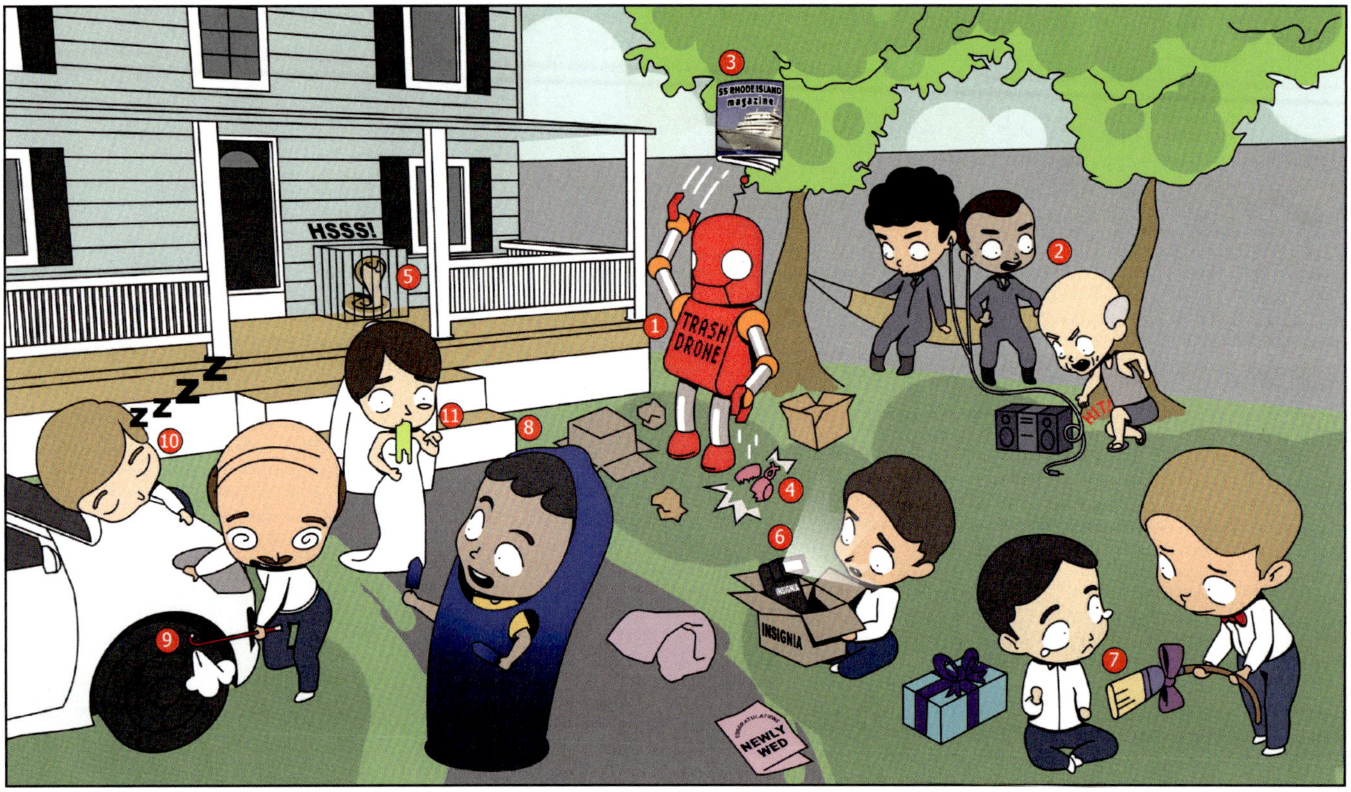

1. "Trash Drone" robot: Trazodone

2. Movers sharing a tune on a hammock hung at two points with man hitting the jack with five fingers: $5\text{-}HT_2$ blocker

3. Picture of the SS Rhode Island thrown up instead of away: Acts as a weak SSRI

4. "Trash Drone" robot breaking alpha-handled tea cup: Blocks alpha-1 activity

5. Single hissing snake in cage: Blocks H-1 activity

6. Boy getting flashed by Insignia brand camera: Primary use is for insomnia treatment

7. Man giving atypical broom to depressed kid: Secondary Use as an atypical antidepressant

8. Dark colored popsicle salesman: Can cause priapism

9. Older man standing up quickly as he deflate a tire: Can cause postural hypotension

10. Son-in-law sleeping on car: Can cause sedation

11. Vomiting bride: Can cause nausea and vomiting

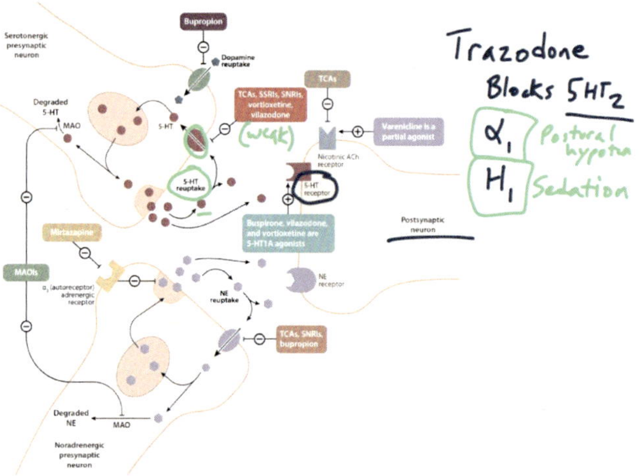

See Figure 9.13.7 - Antidepressant Effects on Neurotransmission (Psychology, Section 18, Page 302)

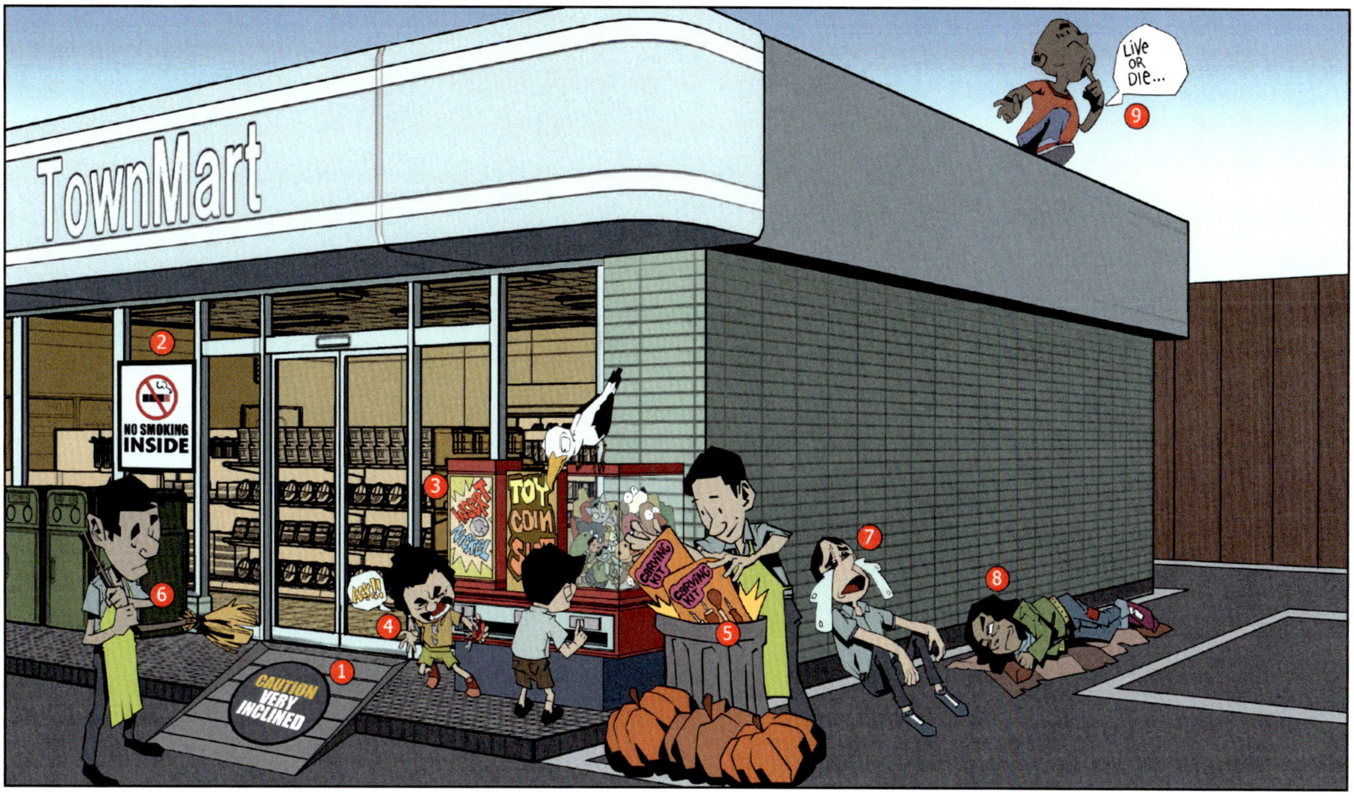

1. “Caution: Very Inclined” stamp on ramp: Varenicline

2. “No Smoking Inside” sign on front doors: Use to help with smoking cessation

3. Kid inserting part of nickel into machine with seagull on top of it: Partial agonist of nicotinic ACh receptors

4. Kid choking on cigarette next to nickel: Prevents nicotine from producing a reward response

5. Worder throwing away carving kits: Decreased nicotine cravings

6. Sad shop worker holding atypical broomstick: Atypical antidepressant

7. Man crying on side of store: Can cause depressed mood

8. Homeless man who can’ sleep on side of store: Can cause sleep disturbances

9. Man on the roof of store contemplating suicide, “Live or die..”: Can cause suicidal ideation

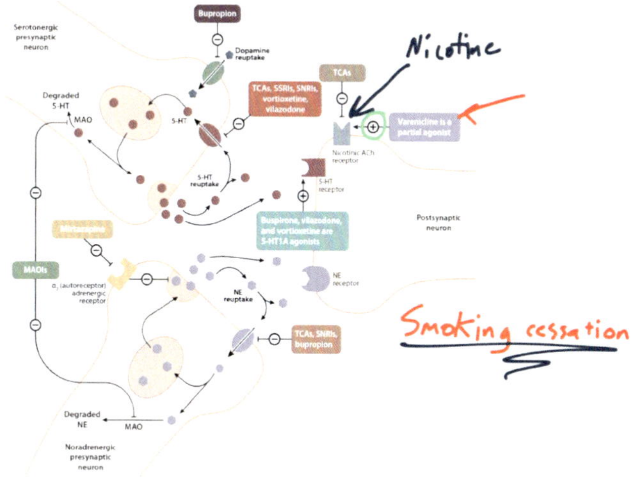

See Figure 9.13.7 - Antidepressant Effects on Neurotransmission (Psychology, Section 18, Page 302)

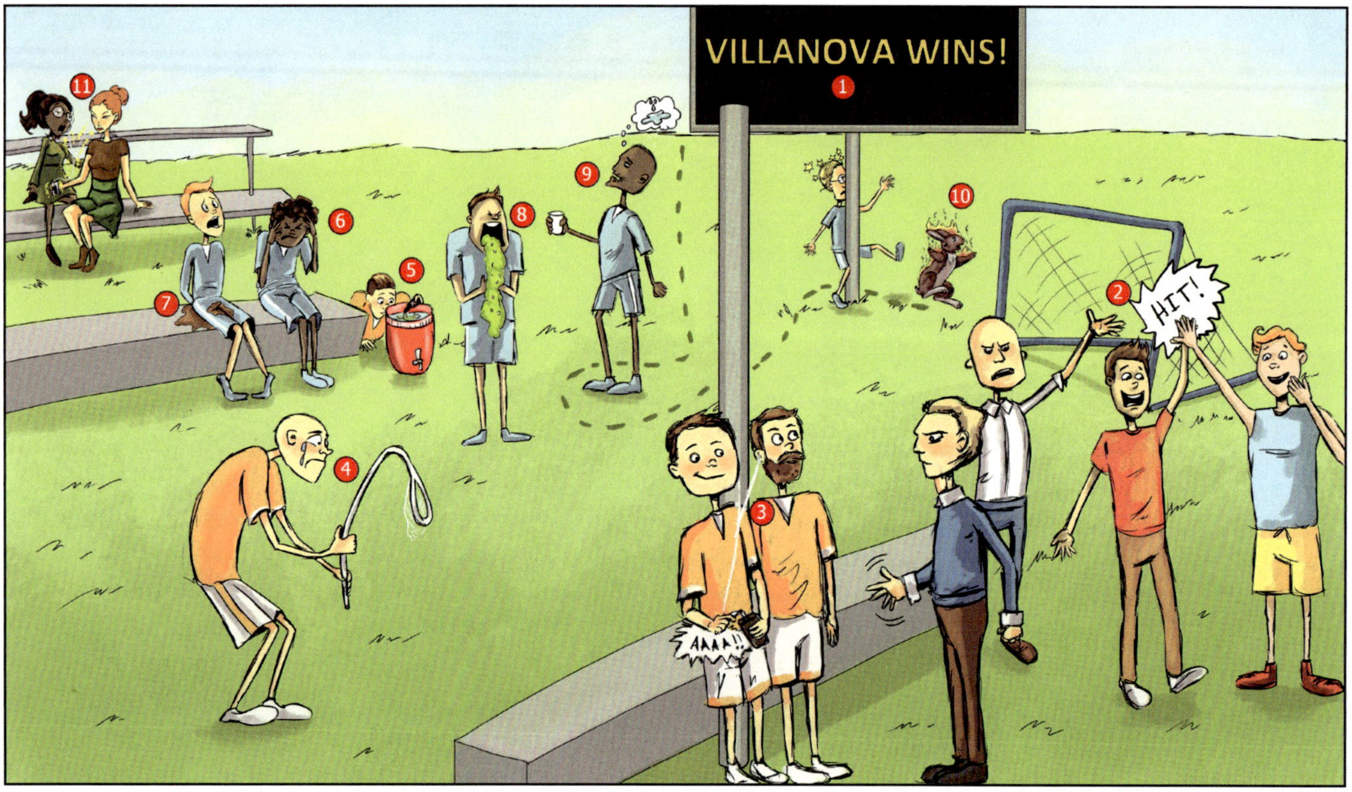

1. "Villanova Wins!" university sign: Vilazodone

2. Coach angry at other team high-fiving and trying to stop them: Inhibits 5-HT reuptake

3. Two players sharing a tune and plug partially into MP3 player playing, "Aaa!!": 5-HT_{1a} partial agonist

4. Sad player with atypical lacrosse stick: Atypical antidepressant

5. Player poisoning Gatorade cooler: Side effects

6. Player holding head in pain: Can cause headaches

7. Player covered in diarrhea on bench: Can cause diarrhea

8. Player vomiting near poisoned Gatorade: Can cause nausea

9. Thirsty player thinking about water: Can cause dry mouth

10. Player who is dizzy trying to catch burning hare: Can cause anticholinergic side effects such as blurry vision and dizziness

11. Women getting shocked by headphones while sharing a tune: Serotonin syndrome

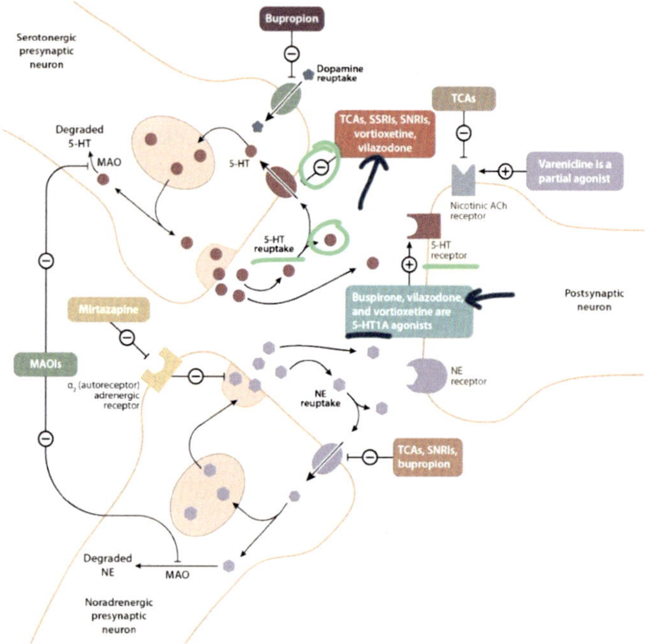

See Figure 9.13.7 - Antidepressant Effects on Neurotransmission (Psychology, Section 18, Page 302)

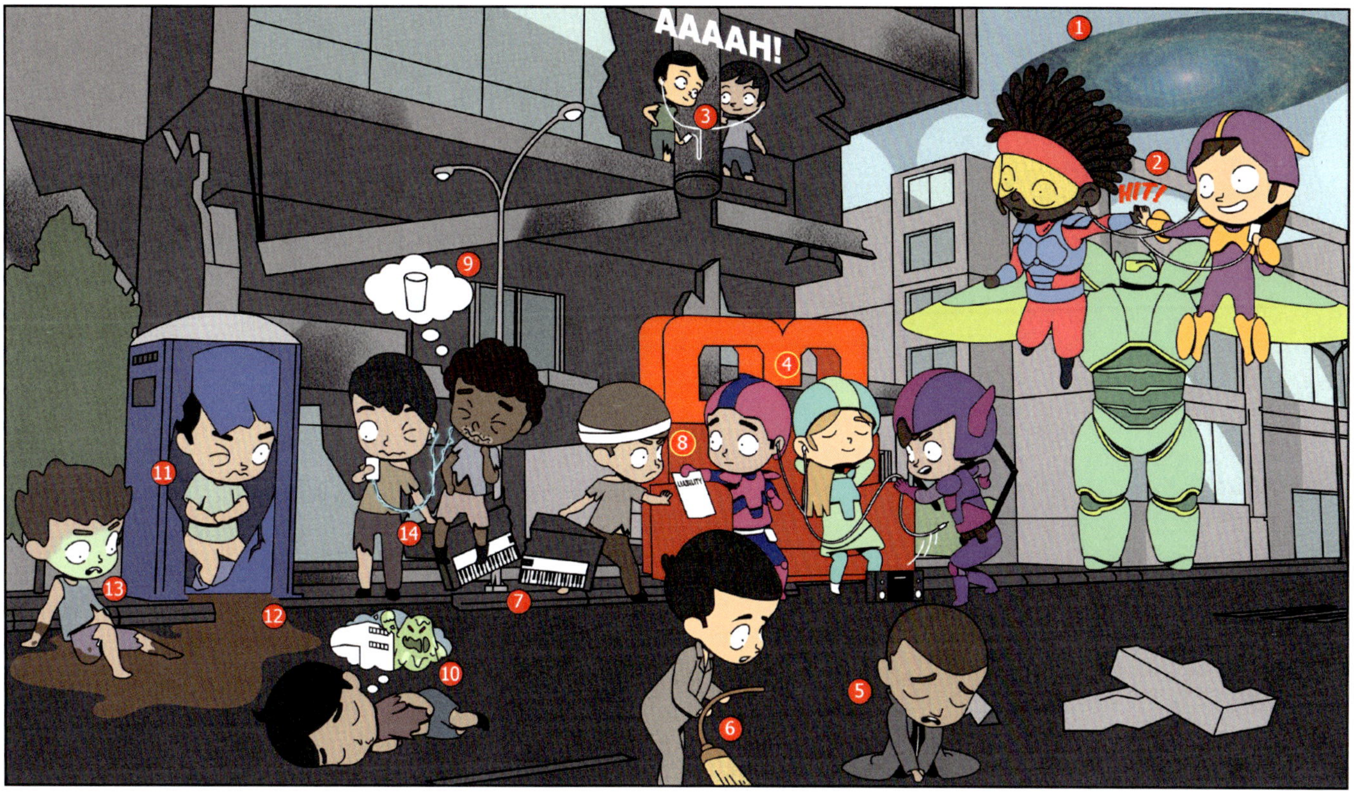

1. Vortex team traveling from vortex: Vortioxetine

2. Big hero yelling at team members while they share a tune and high-fiving each other: Inhibits 5-HT reuptake

3. Two men sharing a screaming, "Ahhh!!!" tune by a single pillar: Antagonizes 5-HT₁ₐ receptor

4. Superheroes sitting on a "3"-shaped couch sharing a tune with another five finger hitting the headphone jack: 5-HT₃ receptor antagonist

5. Depressed supervillain on ground: Use for major depressive disorder (MDD)

6. Atypical broom held by janitor: Atypical antidepressant

7. Broken organ: Can cause anorgasmia

8. Man refusing to sign the liability form: Can cause decreased libido

9. Dehydrated, thirsty man thinking of water: Can cause xerostomia

10. Sleeping man on street with weird dreams: Can cause abnormal dreams

11. Constipated man: Can cause constipation

12. Diarrhea in street: Can cause diarrhea

13. Nauseas man with green face: Can cause nausea

14. Man sharing a tune being shocked by headphones: Can cause serotonin syndrome

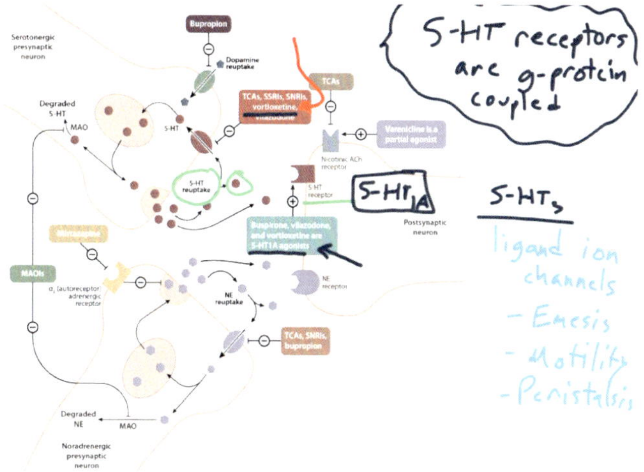

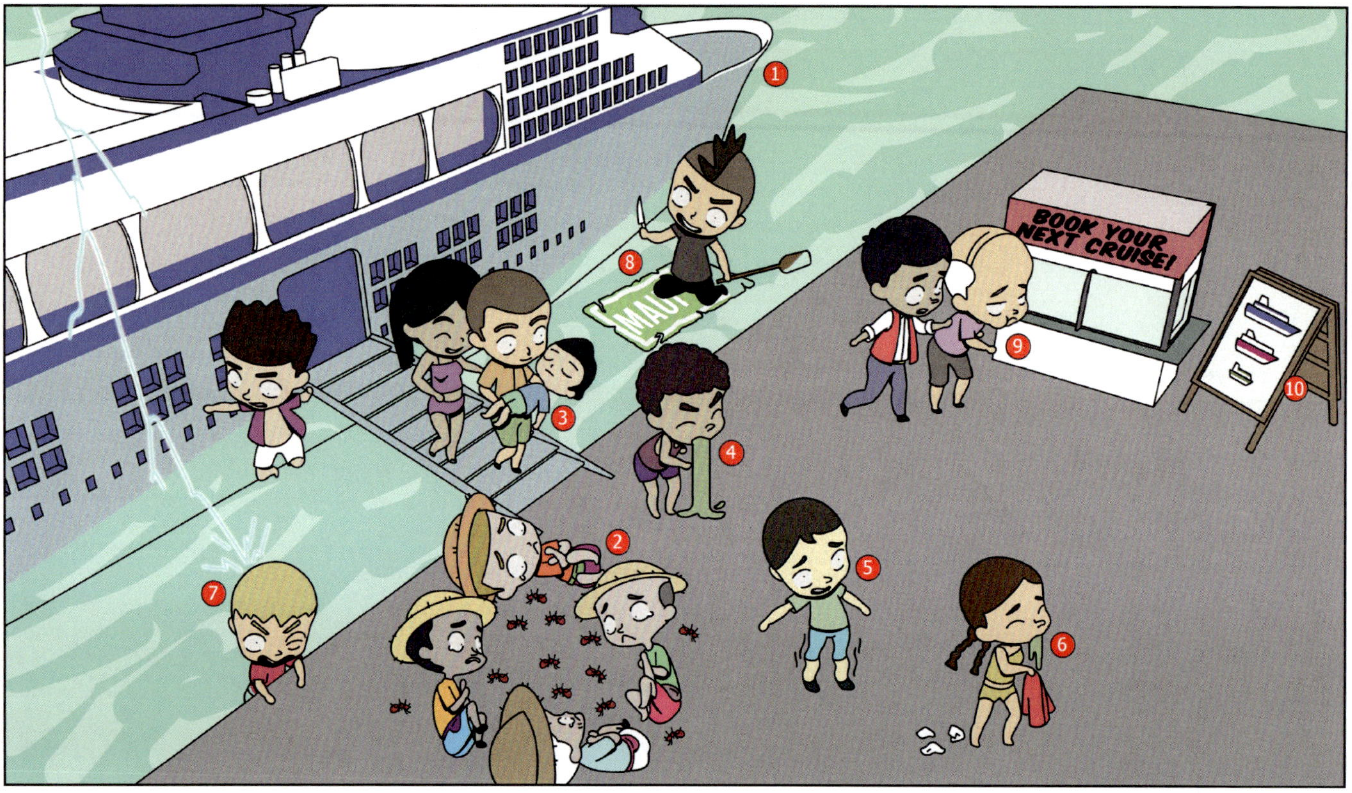

1. Cruise ship ending its trip: Antidepressant discontinuation syndrome

2. Dysphoric passengers in fetal position surrounded by ants: Dysphoria

3. Sleeping boy: Can cause fatigue

4. Vomiting passenger on dock: Can cause GI distress

5. Wobbly passenger on dock: Can cause difficulties with balancing

6. Vomiting passenger with trail tissues behind her and seater: Can cause flu-like symptoms

7. Man leaving cruise ship then being struck by lightning: Sensory disturbances and irritability are more common with abrupt SSRI discontinuation

8. Psycho on "Maui" sign boat: Abrupt MAOI reduction may cause psychosis

9. Depressed old man signing up for another cruise: Treat antidepressant discontinuation by restarting or increasing the antidepressant dose

10. Arranged cruise ship sign showing ships from largest to smallest: Discontinue antidepressants after a gradual taper

Figure 9.12.10 - Pharmacologic Effects on Opioid Receptors (Neurology Pharmacology, Section 18, Page 302)

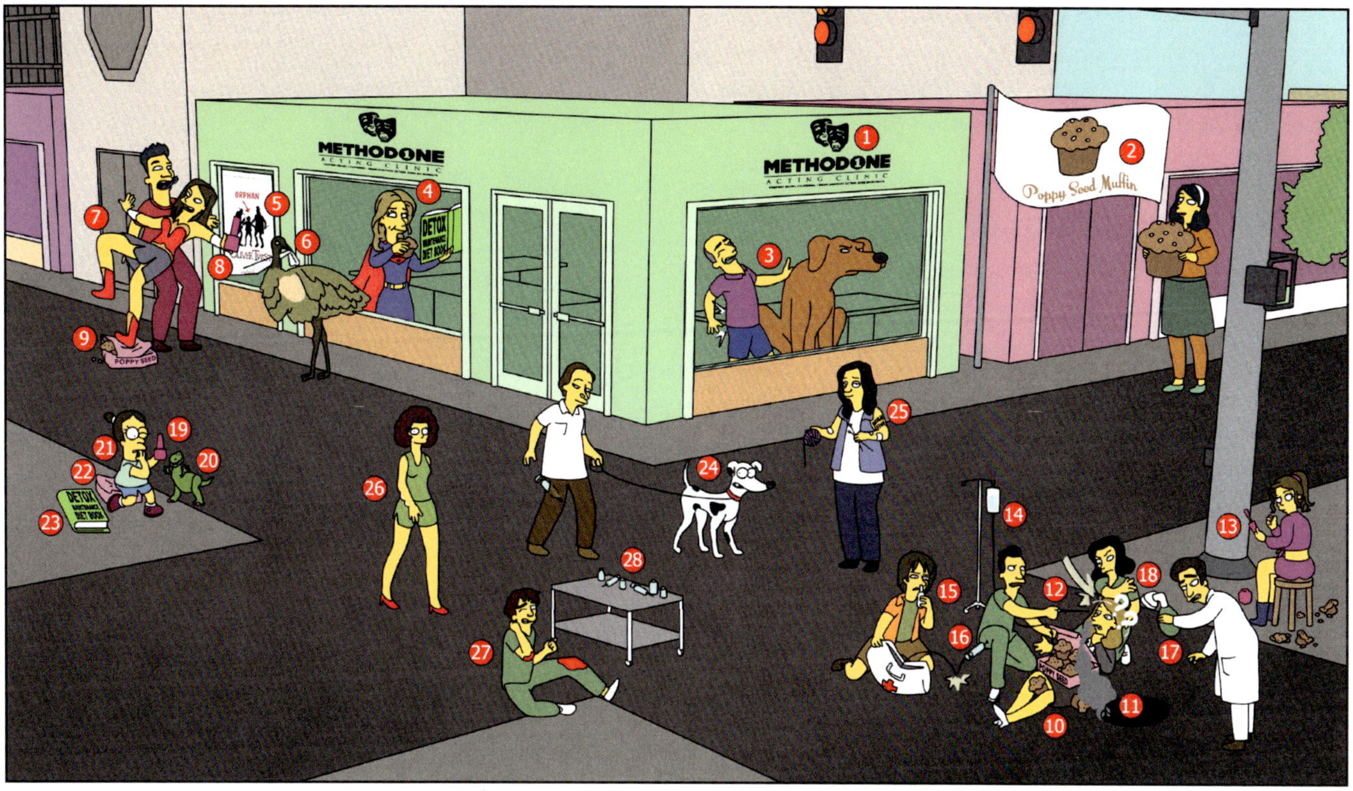

1. "Method One" acting clinic: Methadone

2. Big and full poppyseed muffin flag next to clinic: Methadone is long–acting opiate (full agent)

3. Man in pain pushing a large and stubborn dog: Methadone is used for refractory pain

4. Heroine actress reading her detox maintenance book while nibbling on muffin: Methadone is a long-lasting oral opiate used for heroin detox or long-term maintenance therapy

5. Actor with blue pen in his mouth, studying orphan poster: Buprenorphine is taken in a sublingual form

6. Partially-feathered emu tugging at orphan poster: Buprenorphine is a partial agonist at mu opioid receptors

7. Man with blue pen catching heroine woman falling: Buprenorphine is used to prevent relapse for heroin addicts

8. Heroine actress holding nail polish: Buprenorphine is formulated with naloxone

9. Heroine crushing poppy seed muffin box: Naloxone is a full opioid antagonist

10. Confused woman eating poppy seed muffins sitting in road: Acute opioid overdose

11. Confused woman with poppyseed muffins struggling to breathe because of weid gas: Acute opioid overdose can also cause respiratory depression

12. Nurse holding pin close to confused girl's eyes: Acute opioid overdose also causes miosis

13. Self-absorbed girl painting her nails; Use naloxone for acute overdose

14. IV next to nurse for confused woman: Ideally, naloxone is administered via the IV route

15. Man spraying nasal spray up his nose: outside hospital setting naloxone can be taken as a nasal spray

16. Needle injecting nurse's thigh: Naloxone can be administered via an IM injection

17. Doctor holding ventilation bag mask near confused poppyseed girl: Carefully monitor respiration and provide bag mask ventilation until naloxone kicks in and reverses respiratory depression

18. Nurse elevating woman's head and smacking her awake: Naloxone is intended to reverse CNS depression

19. Girl painting nails on T-Rex toy: Naltrexone

20. Toy T-rex has long fingernails: Naltrexone is long acting

21. Girl sucking on her thumb: Naltrexone is taken orally

22. Girl is sitting and crushing muffin box: Naltrexone is an opioid antagonist

23. Detox maintenance diet book next to nail painting girl: Naltrexone is used after detoxification to help maintain sobriety

24. IV drug user walking liver-spotted dalmatian in middle of street: Intravenous drug users at increased risk for hepatitis

25. Man with knitting needles, band aids, and high-five tattoo in middle of street: Intravenous drug users at increased risk for HIV

26. Woman walking passed drug deal with infected wounds on arms: Intravenous drug users at increased risk for abscesses

27. Dirty and bacteria-infected wounds: Intravenous drug users at increased risk for bacteremia

28. Cart with drugs and needles only on the right side of cart: Intravenous drug users at increased risk for right-sided endocarditis

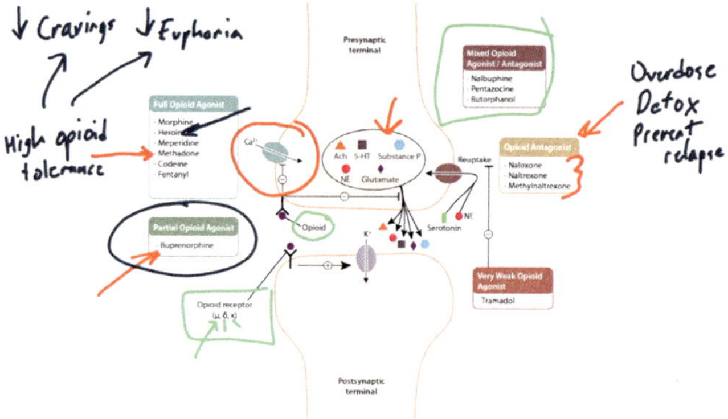

RENAL PHARMACOLOGY

Section 1 - Mannitol

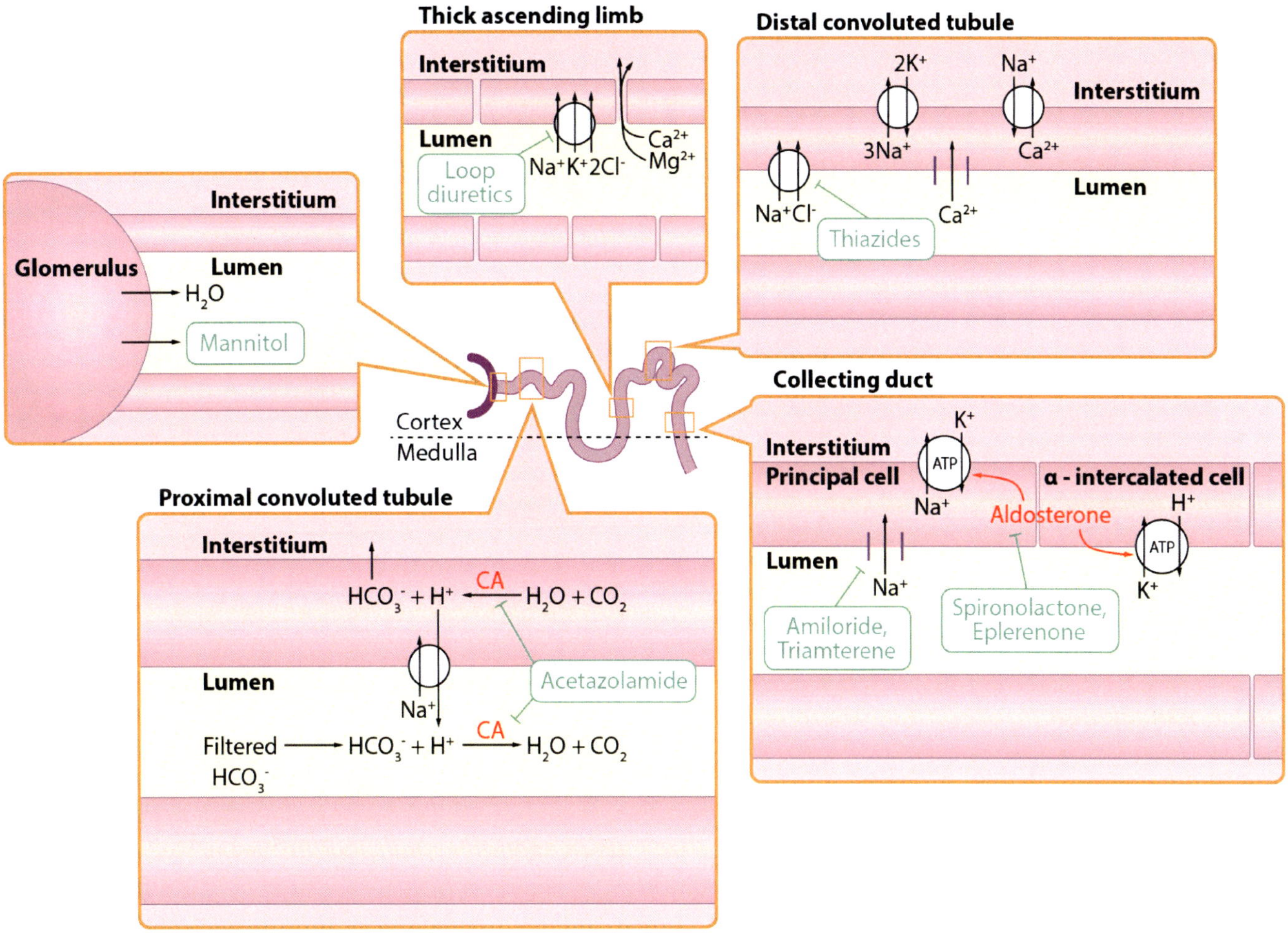

Figure 9.14.1 - Renal Pharmacology Overview

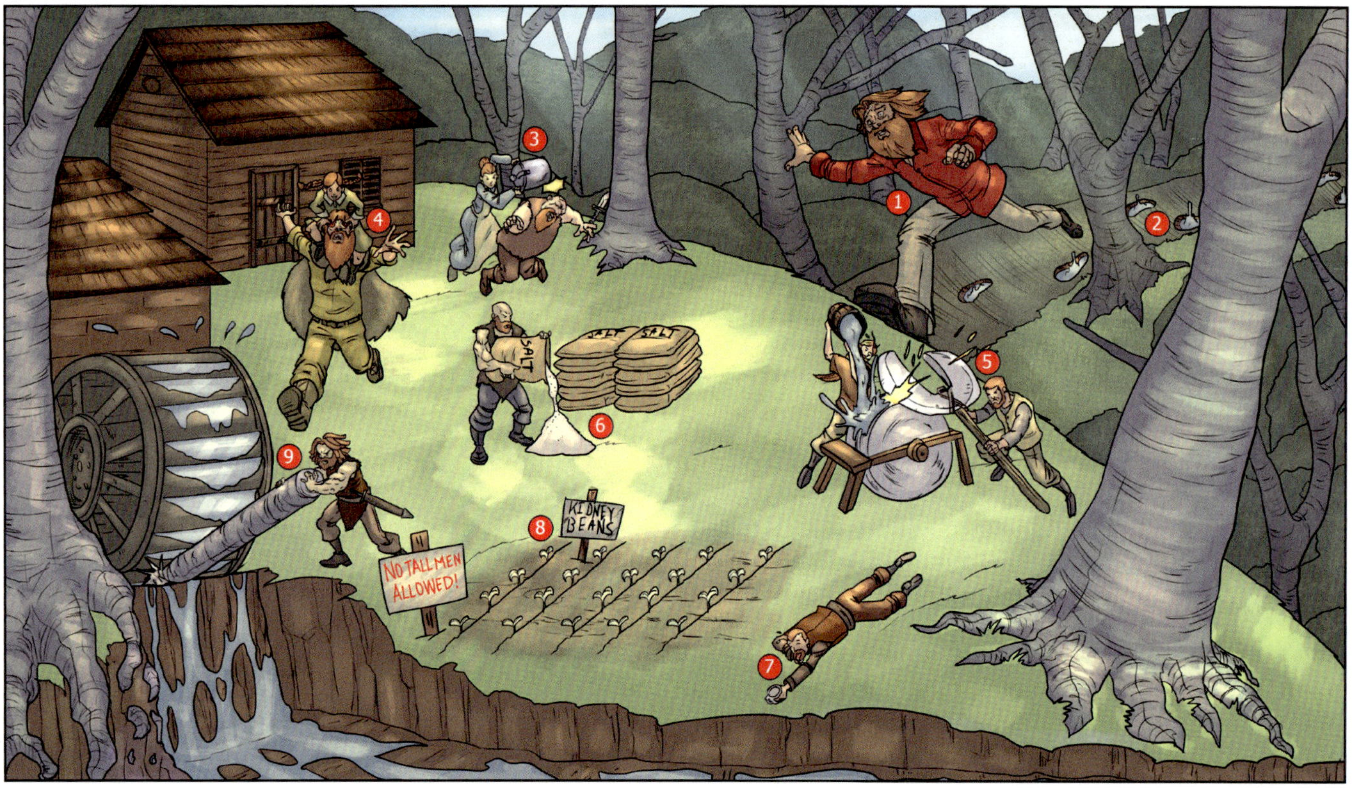

1. Tall man: Mannitol

2. Water in footprints left by tall man: Acts as an osmotic diuretic

3. Woman hitting viking over the head with a pressure cooker: Used to treat intracranial hypertension

4. Eyeballs being pressed on: used to treat intraocular pressure

5. Lung shaped ax being sharpened with water: Can cause pulmonary edema

6. Bags of salt, one being poured out: Can cause high or low sodium

7. Thirsty man next to empty stream: Cna cause dehydration

8. Dried out kidney plants next to "No Tall Men Allowed" sign: Contraindicated in renal failure

10. Jammed water pump next to "No Tall Men Allowed" sign: Contraindicated in heart failure

See Figure 9.14.1 - Renal Pharmacology Overview (Renal Pharmacology, Section 1, Page 318)

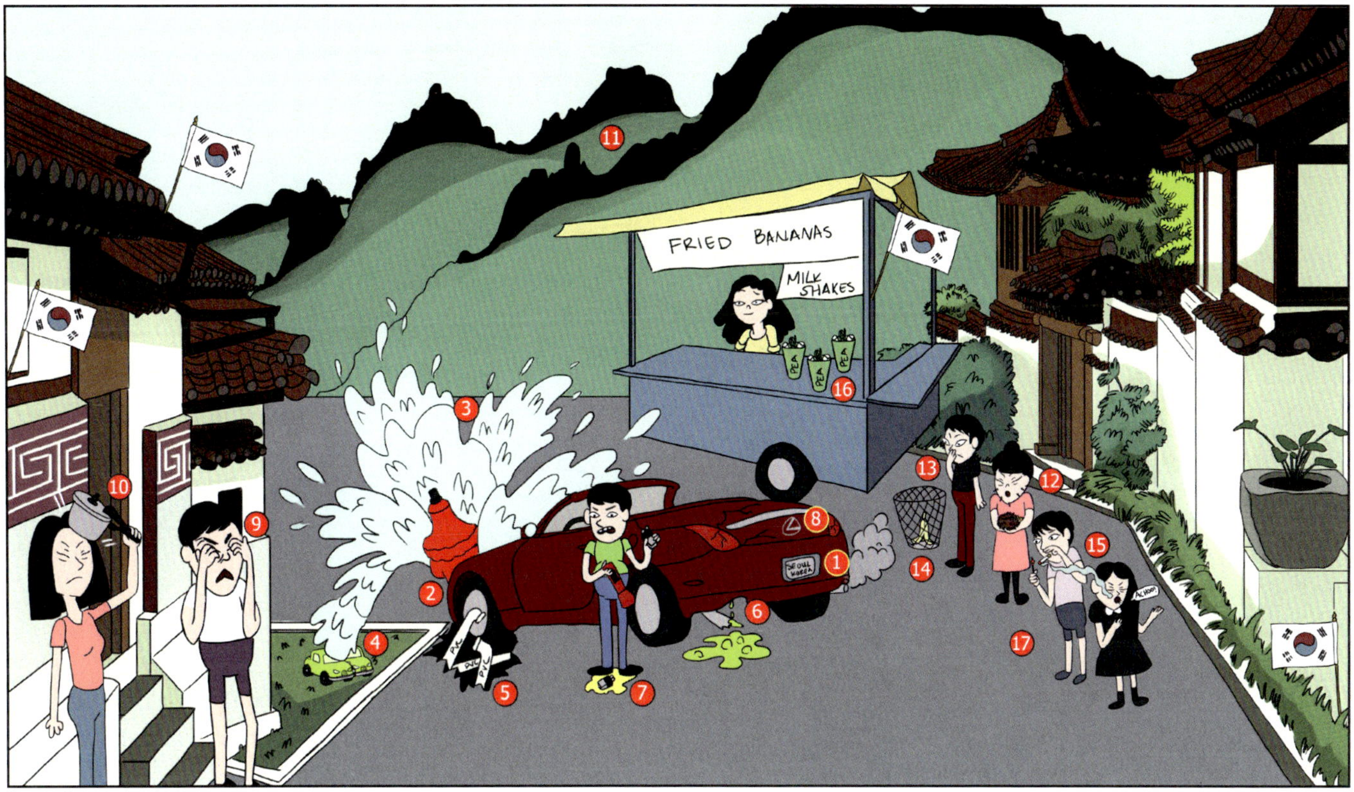

1. Korean flag, roof, and license plate in Seoul, Korea: Acetazolamide

2. Car crashing into a fire hydrant: Is a carbonic anhydrase inhibitor

3. Water gushing from a fire hydrant: Increases urinary volume

4. Two toy cars glued together getting splashed with water: Causes self-limited sodium bicarbonate diuresis

5. PVC pipes: Predominantly affects the proximal convoluted tubule (PCT)

6. Leaking battery acid: Induces a metabolic acidosis

7. Alkaline battery in yellow liquid: Alkalinizes urine

8. Lexus symbol on back of the car: Decreases CSF production in the choroid plexus

9. Man pressing on his eyes: Used to treat glaucoma

10. Woman hitting herself in the head with a pressure cooker: Can be used for idiopathic intracranial hypertension

11. Blackened top of the mountains: Used to treat altitude sickness

12. Woman's face poked by porcupine quills: May cause paresthesias

13. Stinky aroma coming from car: May cause ammonia toxicity

14. Banana peel in the trash can: Can cause hypokalemia

15. Match lighting a cigarette, causing a girl to sneeze: May cause sulfa allergy

16. Pea shakes with chunks of ice cream: Promotes calcium phosphate stone formation

17. Acid leaking from car and the normally spaced banana stand line: Causes a normal anion gap metabolic acidosis

See Figure 9.14.1 - Renal Pharmacology Overview (Renal Pharmacology, Section 1, Page 318)

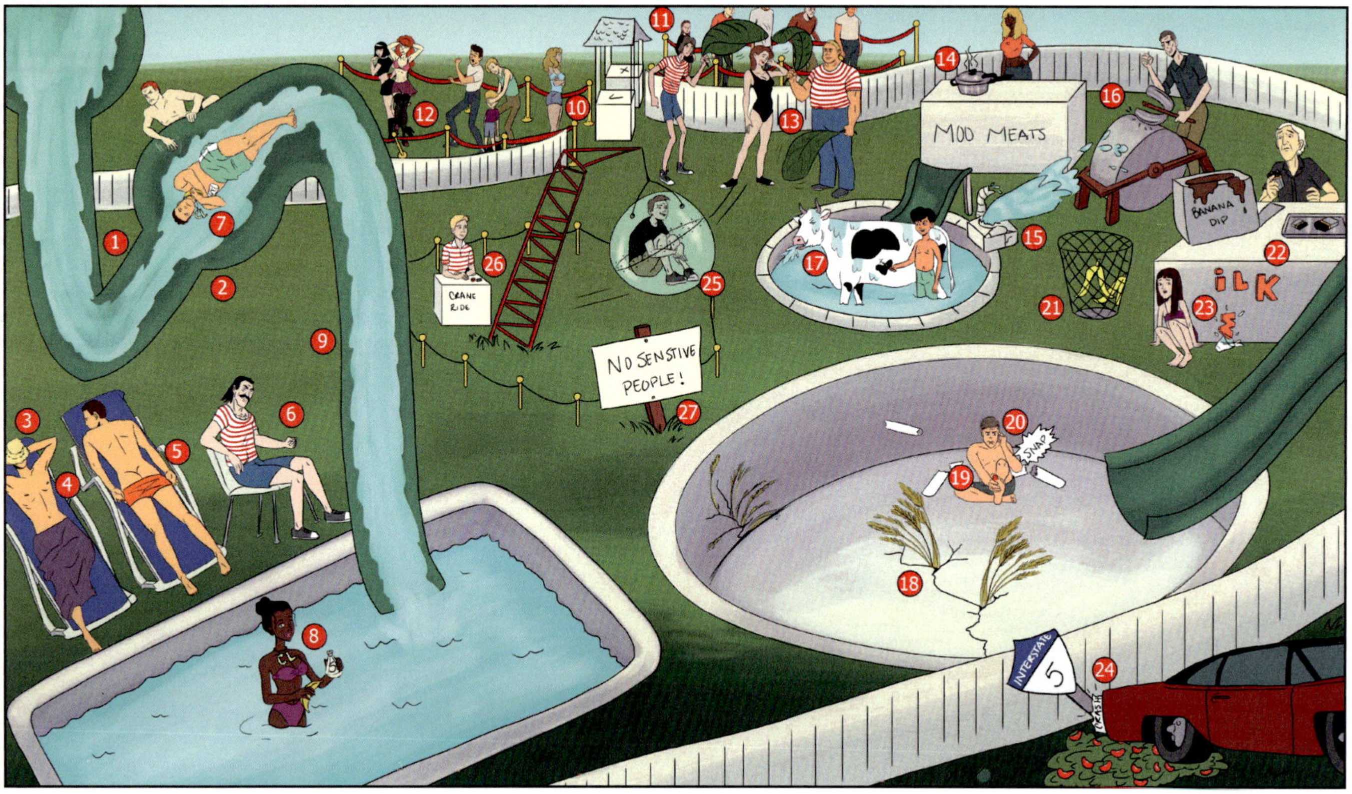

1. Looped water slide: Loop diuretics

2. Thick, ascending portion of waterslide: Loop diuretics work at the thick ascending limb of the Loop of Henle

3. Fur hat on sunbather: Furosemide

4. Sunbather's exposed torso: Torsemide

5. Sunbather tanning his bum: Bumetanide

6. Lifeguard lighting a match: Made of sulfonamides

7. Waterslide goer clutching salt, banana, and wearing "CL" necklace from lifeguard: Loop diuretics block sodium/potassium/chloride pumps (NKCC) on the ascending limb of the Loop of Henle

8. Swimmer in the pool with salt, banana, and "CL" necklace: Sodium, potassium, and chloride are excreted in the urine

9. Splash-free slide: Decreased sodium and chloride in medullary interstitium → decreased osmotic power out of the descending limb → more water remains in the filtrate → increased excretion of water

10. Entrance line marked by red velvet rope: Afferent arteriole

11. Exit line marked by red velvet rope: Efferent arteriole

12. Prostitutes causing park-goers to expand red velvet ropes: Loop diuretics stimulate prostoglandin release which act to dilate the afferent arteriole → increased filtration and excretion

13. Palm frond fans: Use for nephrotic syndrome

14. Pressure cooker on food stand: Use for hypertension

15. Broken pool pump: Use for heart failure

16. Man sharpening his lung-shaped ax and water splashing on whetstone: Use for pulmonary edema

17. Liver-spotted cow spitting out water from being poked by little stick: Use for edema and ascites from liver cirrhosis

18. Dried out pool: Can cause dehydration

19. Swimmer hurting his big toe by landing on PVC pipe: Can cause gout (hyperuricemia)

20. "SNAP!" noise hurting swimmer's ear: Can cause ototoxicity

21. Banana peels in trash can: Can cause hypokalemia

22. Batteries leaking acid on metal plate: Can cause metabolic alkalosis

23. Letter "M" falling on glass of milk in front of milk stand: Can increase calcium and magnesium excretion at the Loop of Henle

24. Car smashing interstate sign and kidney bean plants: Can cause acute interstitial nephritis

25. Crane ride: Ethacrynic acid

26. Lifeguard without matches at crane ride: Ethacrynic acid is not a sulfonamide

27. Sign reading "NO SENSITIVE PEOPLE!": Ethacrynic acid doesn't sulfonamide-related hypersensitivity

See Figure 9.14.1 - Renal Pharmacology Overview (Renal Pharmacology, Section 1, Page 303)

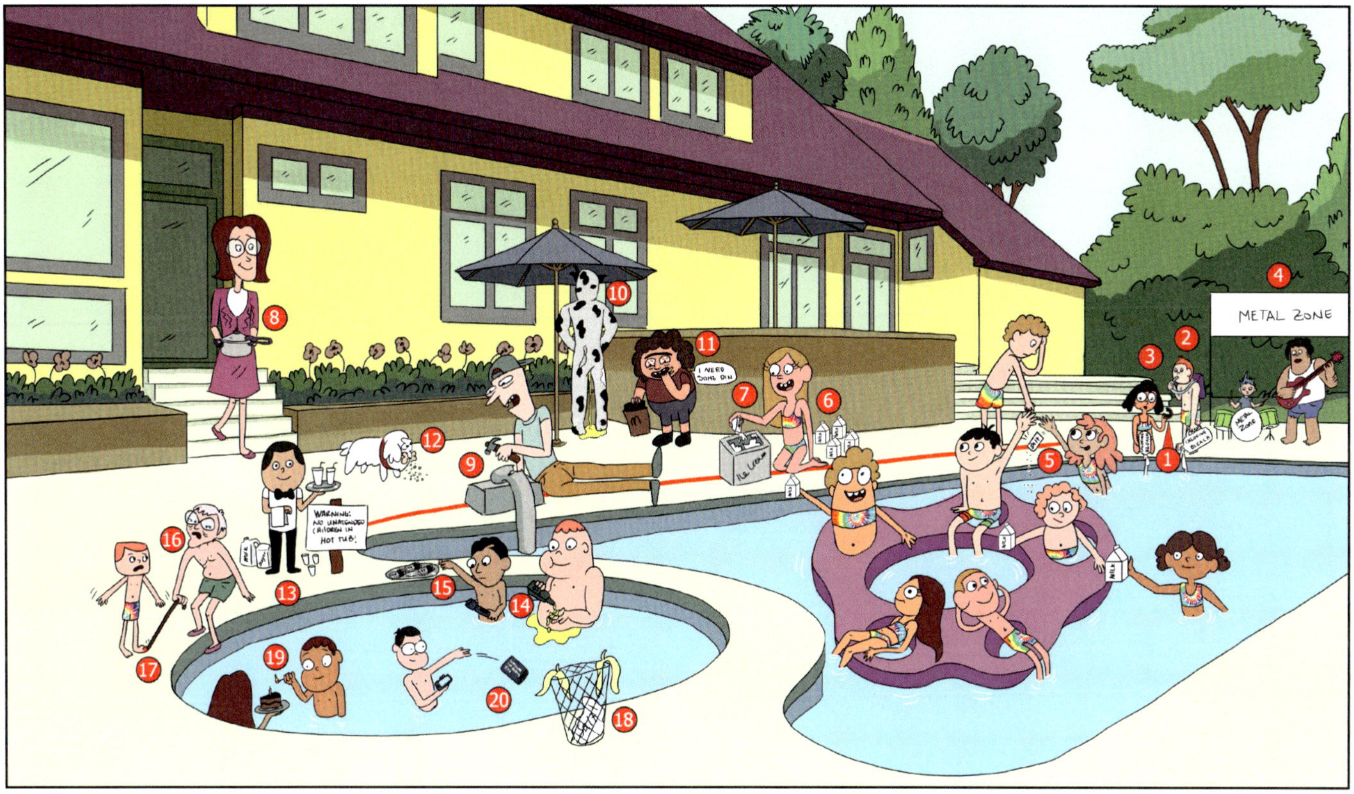

1. Tie-dye shorts: Thiazide diuretics

2. Tie-dyed kid staying hydrated while chlorinating the pool: Hydrochlorothiazide

3. Girl eating donut while chlorinating the pool: Chlorthalidone

4. Banner reading, "metal zone" above rock metal band: Metolazone

5. Salt being blocked from convoluted tube and being spilled in pool: Inhibits NaCl reabsorption in the early DCT

6. Milk being passed outside of the pool to red line: Increases calcium reabsorption

7. Chunks of ice cream: used to treat calcium kidney stones

8. Pressure cooker in mother's hands: Used to treat hypertension

9. Broken pool pump: used to treat heart failure

10. Brother dressed as a cow, urinating: Used to treat idiopathic hypercalciuria

11. Boy saing, "I need some DIN!": Used to treat diabetes insipidus (nephrogenic) or DIN

12. Dog chewing bone into pieces: Used to treat osteoporosis

13. Cups of milk and sugar next to warning sign: May cause hyperglycemia and hypercalcemia

14. Oil on chubby kid's hands in hot tub: May cause hyperlipidemia

15. Alkaline batteries on a metal tray next to hot tub: May cause a metabolic acidosis

16. Frail old man crawling into hot tub: May cause muscle weakness

17. Boy with hurt toe: May cause hyperuricemia which can cause gout

18. Empty bag of salt banana peels in the trash can: Can cause hypokalemia and hyponatremia

19. Match used to light birthday cake: May cause sulfa allergy

20. Throwing away a lithium battery in trash can: Thiazide diuretics affect the clearance of lithium

See Figure 9.14.1 - Renal Pharmacology Overview (Renal Pharmacology, Section 1, Page 303)

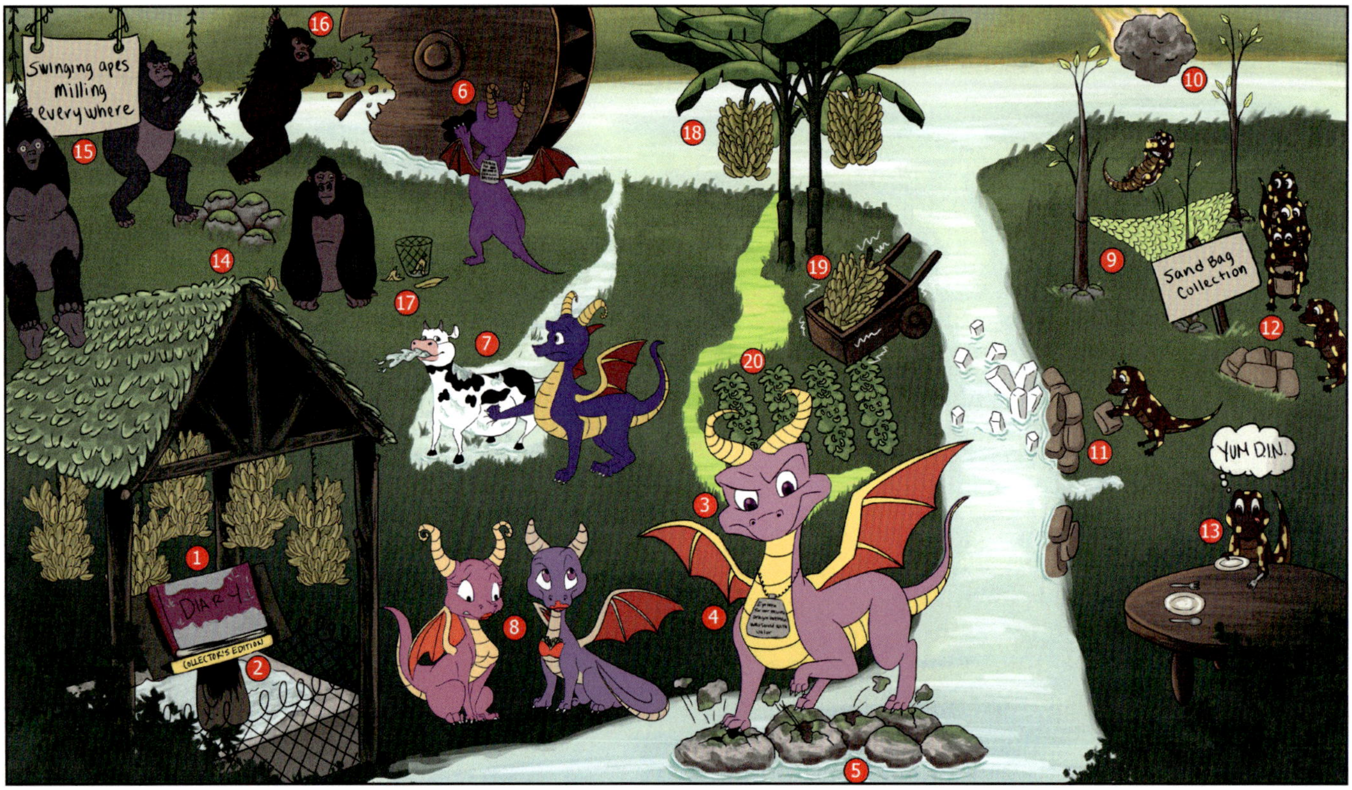

1. Pavilion sparing bananas and wet diary: Potassium-sparing diuretics

2. Plaque reading "collector's edition": Potassium-sparing diuretics work at the collecting duct

3. Spyro the dragon: Spironolactone

4. Epitaph on Spyro: Eplerenone

5. Spyro wearing epitaph destroying old stone: Spironolactone and eplerenone block aldosterone receptors at collecting duct → decreased reabsorption → diuresis

6. Spyro wearing epitaph remodeling broken pump: Spironolactone and eplerenone are good for heart failure by improving ventricular remodeling

7. Spyro without epitaph pushing on liver-spotted cow's belly, cow splitting water: Use spironolactone for hepatic ascites

8. Spyro disguised as a female dragon: Spironolactone can cause antiandrogenic effects such as gynecomastia

9. Triangle-shaped trampoline: Triamterene

10. Meteorite: Amiloride

11. Salamander diverint salt-filled water: Amiloride and triamterene block sodium and water reabsorption at the collecting duct

12. Salamanders collecting sandbags near trampoline and meteorite: Amiloride and triamterene work at the collecting duct

13. Salamander saying "yum, DIN!": Use amiloride and triamterene for nephrogenic diabetes insipidus (DIN)

14. Large pile of old stone: Potassium-sparing diuretics can be used for hyperaldosteronism

15. Sign reading "Swinging Apes Milling Everywhere": Potassium-sparing diuretics can be used for syndrome of apparent mineralocorticoid excess (SAME)

16. Ape destroying water pump: Potassium-sparing diuretics can be used for heart failure

17. Garbage can with banana peels: Potassium-sparing diuretics can be used for hypokalemia

18. Banana trees with heavy banana bundles: All of these drugs can cause hyperkalemia

19. Shaking banana cart: Hyperkalemia may cause arrhythmia

20. Bananas and kidney plants surrounded by acid: All of these drugs can cause hyperkalemic renal tubular acidosis type 4

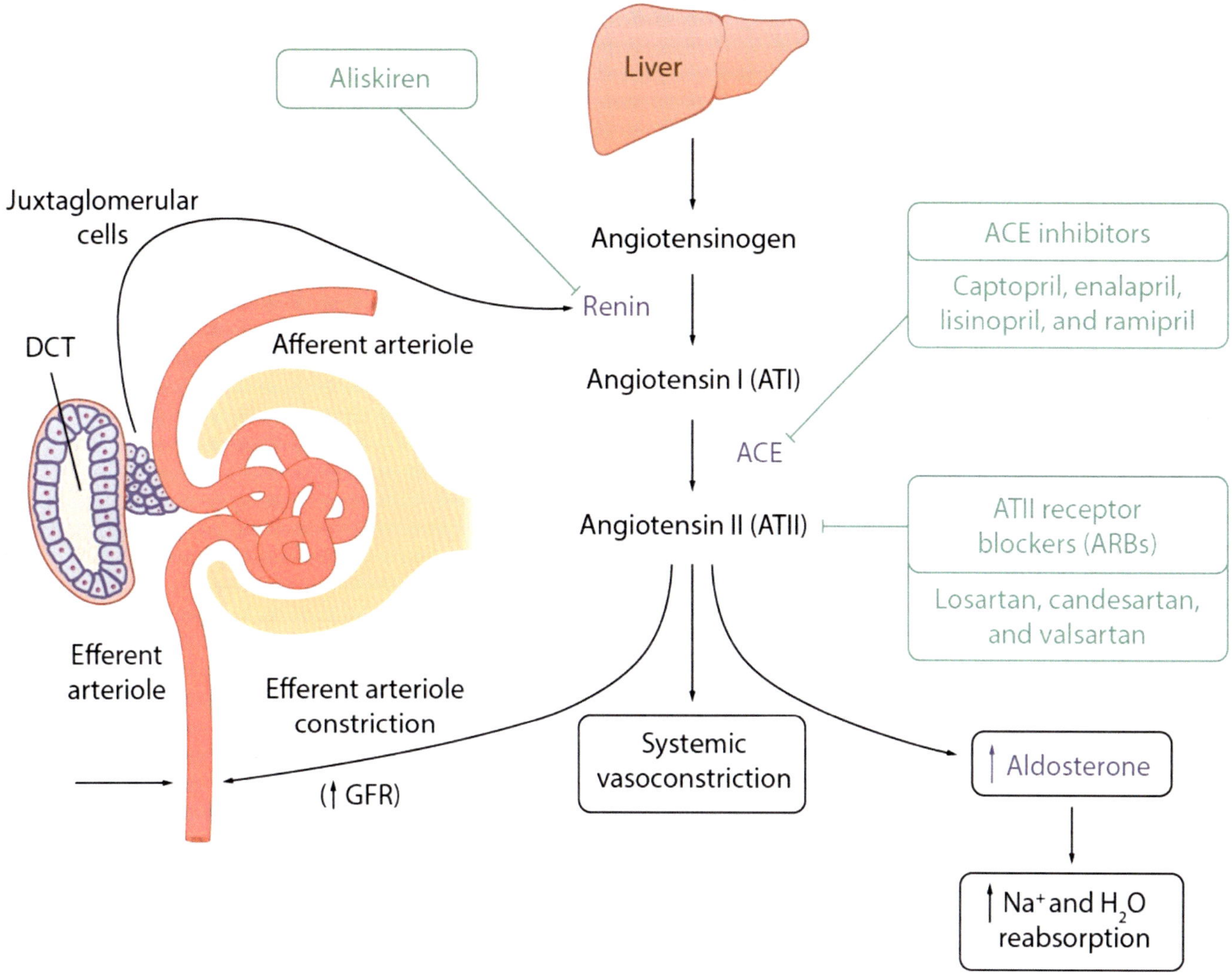

Figure 9.14.2 - Pharmacologic Interactions with Renin-Angiotensin-Aldosterone System

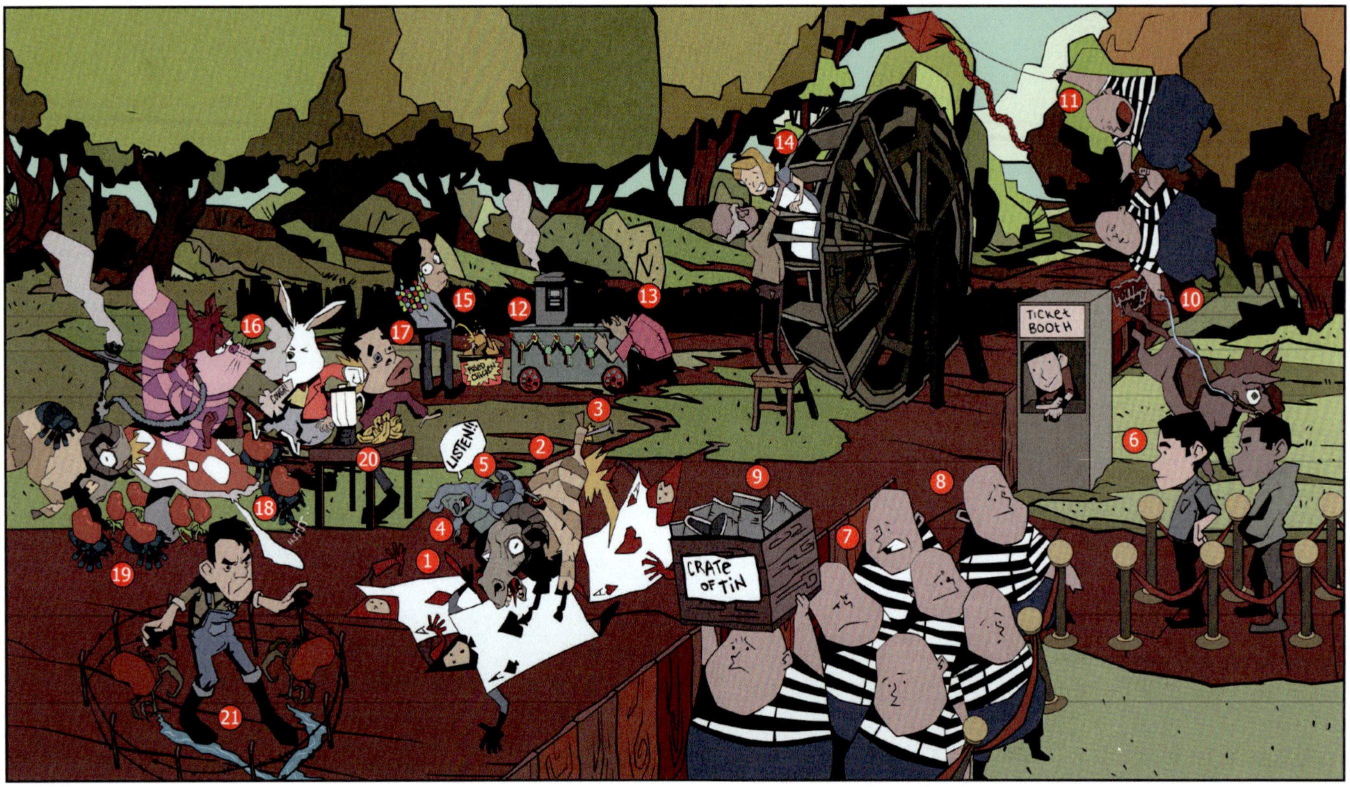

1. Trampled ace cards: ACE inhibitors

2. Ram: Ramipril

3. A nail in ram's leg: Enalapril

4. Caterpillar riding ram: Captopril

5. Caterpillar yelling, "Listen!": Lisinopril

6. Normal, single-file line at entrance: Afferent arteriole is normal

7. Bulging exit line filled with dumb people: Efferent arteriole is dilated

8. Few accepted entrants to park: GFR is decreased

9. Box full of tin cans labeled "Crate of Tin" held high: Can increase serum creatinine

10. Tweedle Dum bucked high while hanging onto the reins: Renin will increase

11. Tweedle Dee being pulled high by a kite with a braided tail: High Bradykinin

12. Pressure cooker on food cart: Use ACE inhibitors for hypertension

13. Remodeled food cart: Use ACE inhibitors to prevent undesirable heart remodeling in chronic hypertension

14. Alice being rescued from a broken water pump: ACE inhibitors decrease mortality in heart failure

15. Man with dyed beads peeing on chicken: Use ACE inhibitors for diabetic nephropathy with proteinuria

16. The white rabbit coughing: Can cause cough

17. Swollen passerby: Can cause angioedema

18. Deflating mushroom hit by ram: Can cause hypotension

19. Tarantulas stealing kidney beans: Can cause teratogenic renal malformation

20. Pile of bananas on table: Can cause hyperkalemia

21. Dried-up kidney beans receiving very little water from narrow streams: Use cautiously with bilateral renal artery stenosis because GFR can be dangerously low

See Figure 9.14.2 - Pharmacologic Interactions with Renin-Angiotensin-Aldosterone System (Renal Pharmacology, Section 6, Page 324)

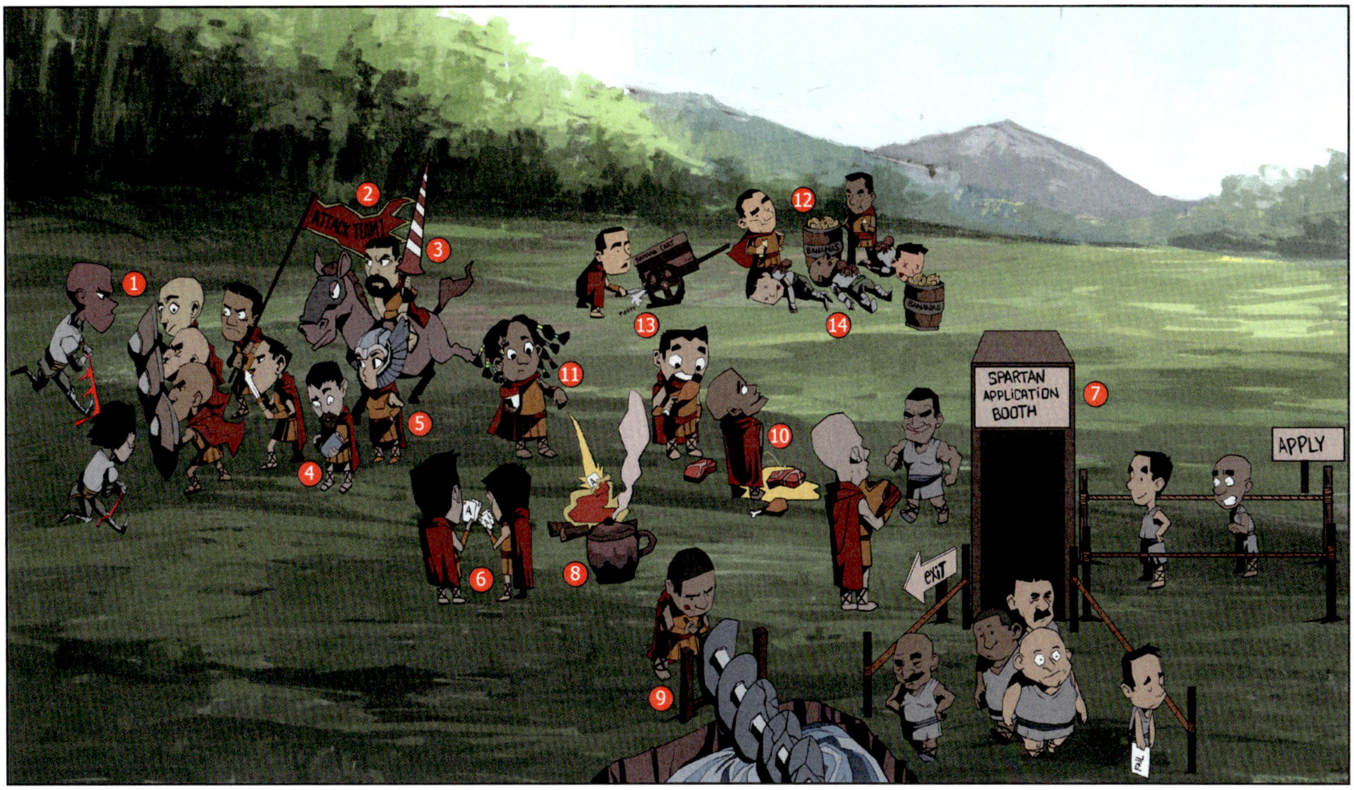

1. Two men pulling bloody wire to create tension being blocked by spartans with shields: Angiotensin II receptor blockers (ARBs)

2. Banner reading, "Attack Team 1": Selectively block binding of angiotensin II to AT_1 receptor

3. Spartan with lance: Losartan

4. Can-holding Spartan: Candesartan

5. Valkyrie Spartan: Valsparatan

6. Ace cards held by Spartans: Effect of ARBs are similar to ACE inhibitors

7. Few accepted soldiers are large exit line: Decrease the glomerular filtration rate due to relaxation of the efferent arteriole

8. Pressure cooker: Used for hypertension

9. Broken pump system: Used for heart failure

10. Soldier peeing on meat: Used for proteinuria

11. Soldier with dyed beads and kidney beans throwing an ace card into the fire: Used for chronic kidney disease (e.g. diabetic nephropathy) with intolerance to ACEi

12. Barrels of bananas: may case hyperkalemia

13. Deflated tire on cart: May cause hypotension

14. Tarantulas feasting on soldiers: Teratogenic

See Figure 9.14.2 - Pharmacologic Interactions with Renin-Angiotensin-Aldosterone System (Renal Pharmacology, Section 6, Page 324)

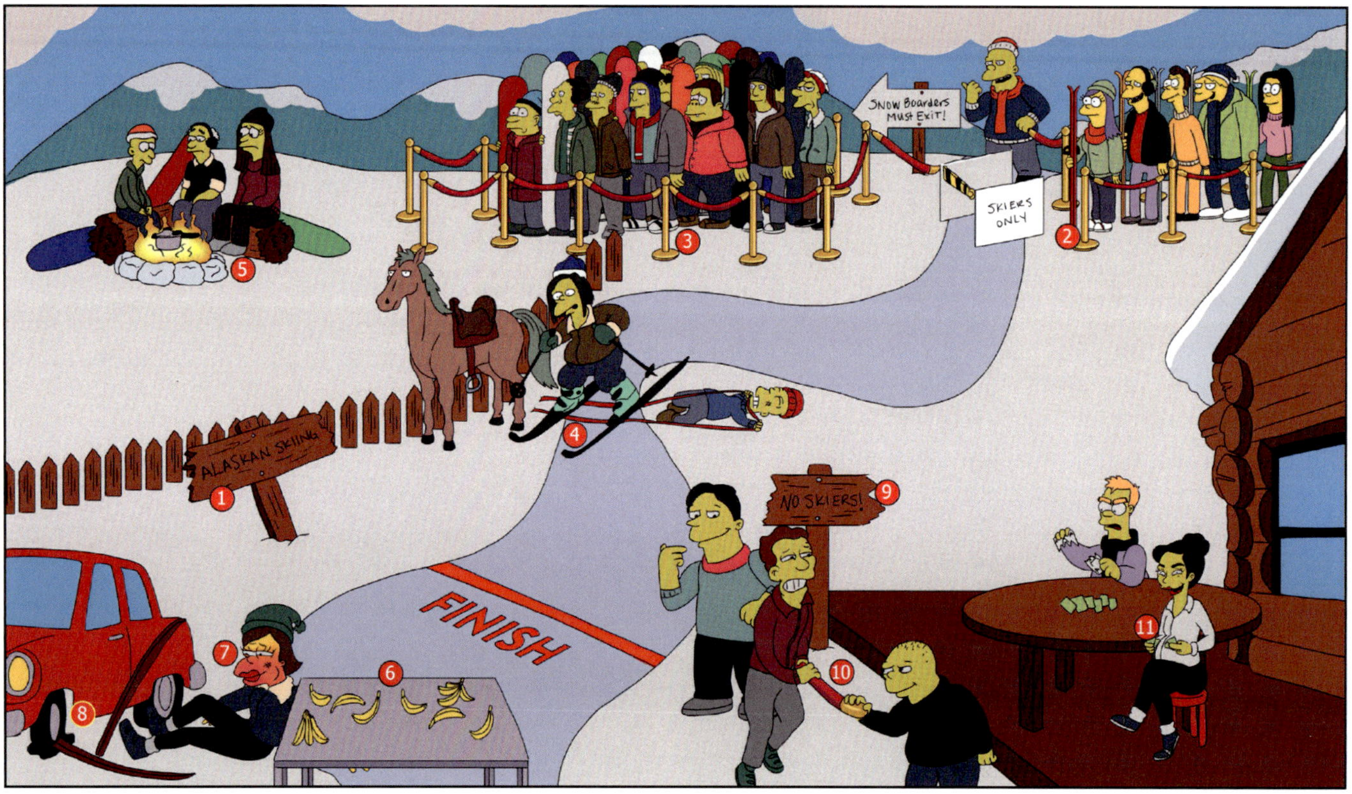

1. Sign reading, "Alaskan Skiing": Aliskiren

2. Normal single file line: Afferent arterioles are unaffected by aliskiren

3. Bulging exit line: Can cause dilation of the efferent arterioles

4. Skier running over reins: Directly blocks renin

5. Pressure cooker used by rejected snowboarders: Used to treat hypertension

6. Lots of bananas on table: Can lead to hyperkalemia

7. Swollen-faced skier: Can cause angioedema

8. Deflated tire on car: Can cause hypotension

9. Sign reading, "No Skiers" and man tearing up ace card: Should not be taken if patient is already taking an ACE inhibitor

10. Bouncers blocking entrance by putting tension on velvet rope: Should not be taken if patient is already taking an Angiotensin receptor blocker

11. Pregnant woman in "no skiers" area: Should not be taken during pregnancy

REPRODUCTIVE PHARMACOLOGY

Section 1 - Leuprolide, Goserelin and Degarelix

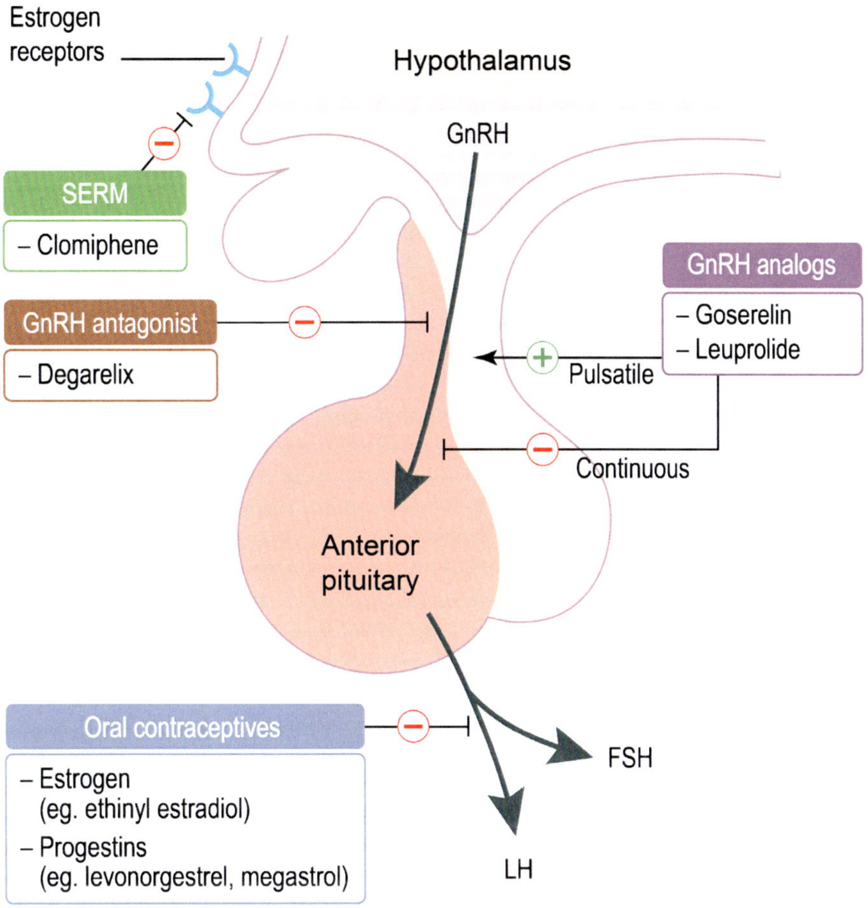

Figure 9.15.1 - Reproductive Drugs that Interact with the Hypothalamus and Pituitary Glands

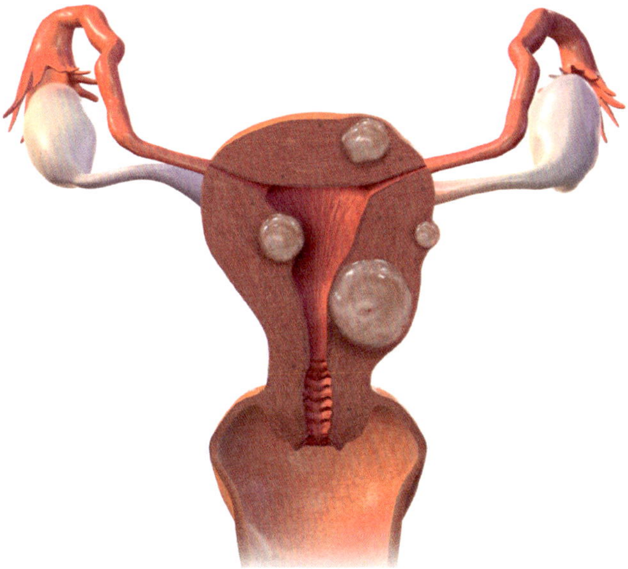

Figure 9.15.2 - Uterine Fibroids

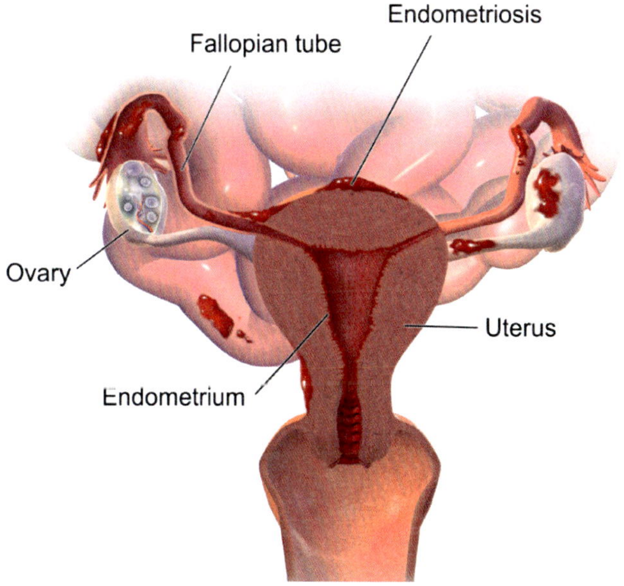

Figure 9.15.3 - Uterus with Endometriosis

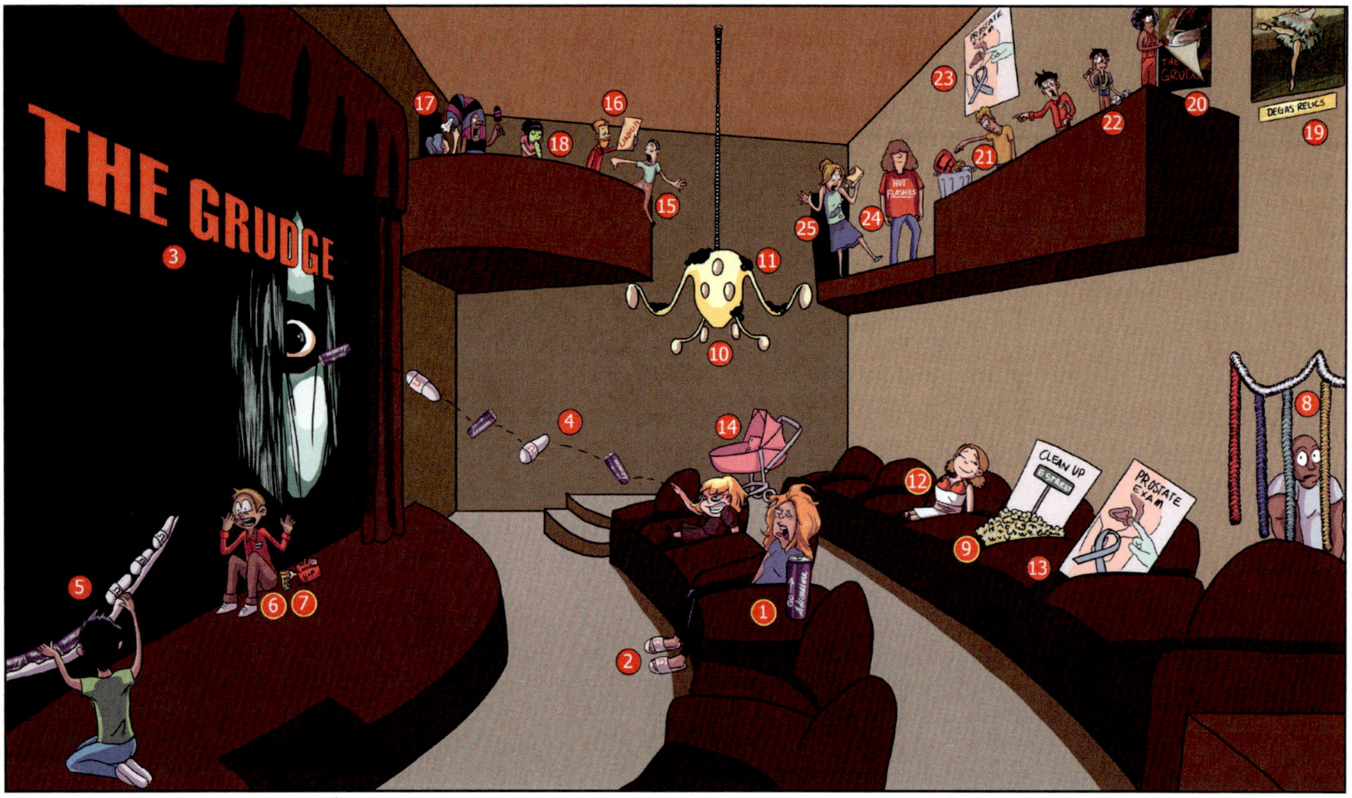

1. "Go Adrenaline" pre workout drink: Goserelin

2. Lululemon slide sandals worn by woman: Leuprolide

3. Girl with lululemon slides and "Go Adrenaline" drink watching The Grudge: Leuprolide and goserelin are GnRH analogs

4. Woman throwing cans of "Go Adrenaline" and Lululemon slides at The Grudge face in a pulsatile pattern: When used in pulsatile fashion, they act as GnRH agonists

5. "Go Adrenaline" drinks and lululemon slides sandals being rolled up onto screen blocking view: Continuous use makes them act as GnRH antagonists

6. Exposed lazy theater employee: Continuous use causes decreased LH and FSH

7. Louisiana hams and fish food being dropped on ground by exposed theater employee: Decreased FSH and LH

8. Brute man hiding behind leys: Low LH leads to low testosterone synthesis in leydig cells

9. Popcorn covering "Clean up E Street" petition flier: Decreased estrogen synthesis from granulosa cells

10. Uterus-shaped with many lightbulbs chandelier: Use for uterine fibroids

11. Clumps of dust scattered on uterus chandelier: Use for endometriosis

12. Prepubescent girl with fake balloon breasts: use for precocious puberty

13. Prostate exam sign with blue cancer hope ribbon on it: Use for prostatic carcinoma

14. Empty baby stroller with no baby around: Use for infertility

15. Man's crushed testicles on balcony and expression of horror: Can cause hypogonadism

16. Man with liability paper being rejected by man with crushed testicles: Can decrease libido

17. Deflating popsicle/erect penis costume: Can cause erectile dysfunction

18. Vomiting girl with green face: Can cause nausea and vomiting

19. "Degras Relics" plaque next to private theater box: Degarelix

20. Employee covering up The Grudge poster with Edgar Degas print: GnRH antagonist

21. Louisiana ham and fish food being thrown into trash in private box: Decreased FSH and LH

22. Scrawny guy wearing leys finishing eating his Louisiana ham: Decreased LH will lead to decreased testosterone synthesis form leydig cells

23. Prostate poster with blue prostate cancer hope ribbon in private box: Use for prostatic carcinoma

24. "Hot Flashers" shirt on ledge: Can cause hot flashes

25. Liver-shaped stain on girl's shirt: Can cause liver toxicity

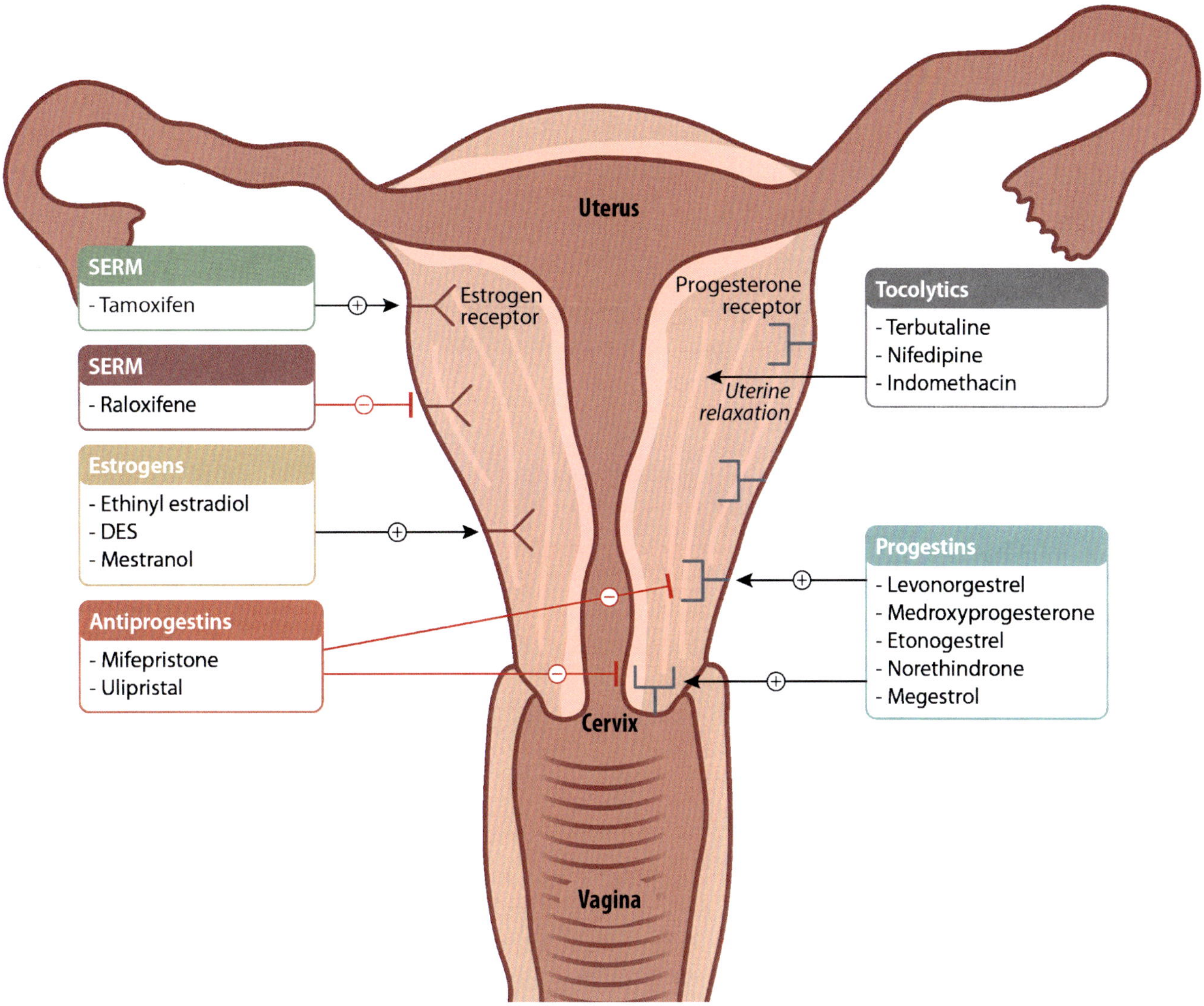

Figure 9.15.4 - Pharmacologic Effects on the Uterus

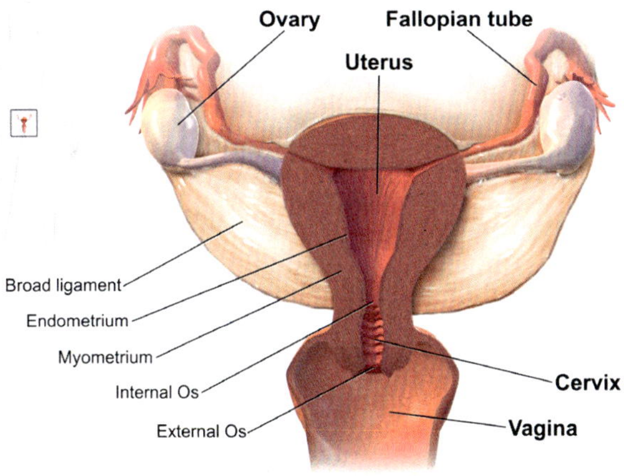

Figure 9.15.5 - Healthy Uterus

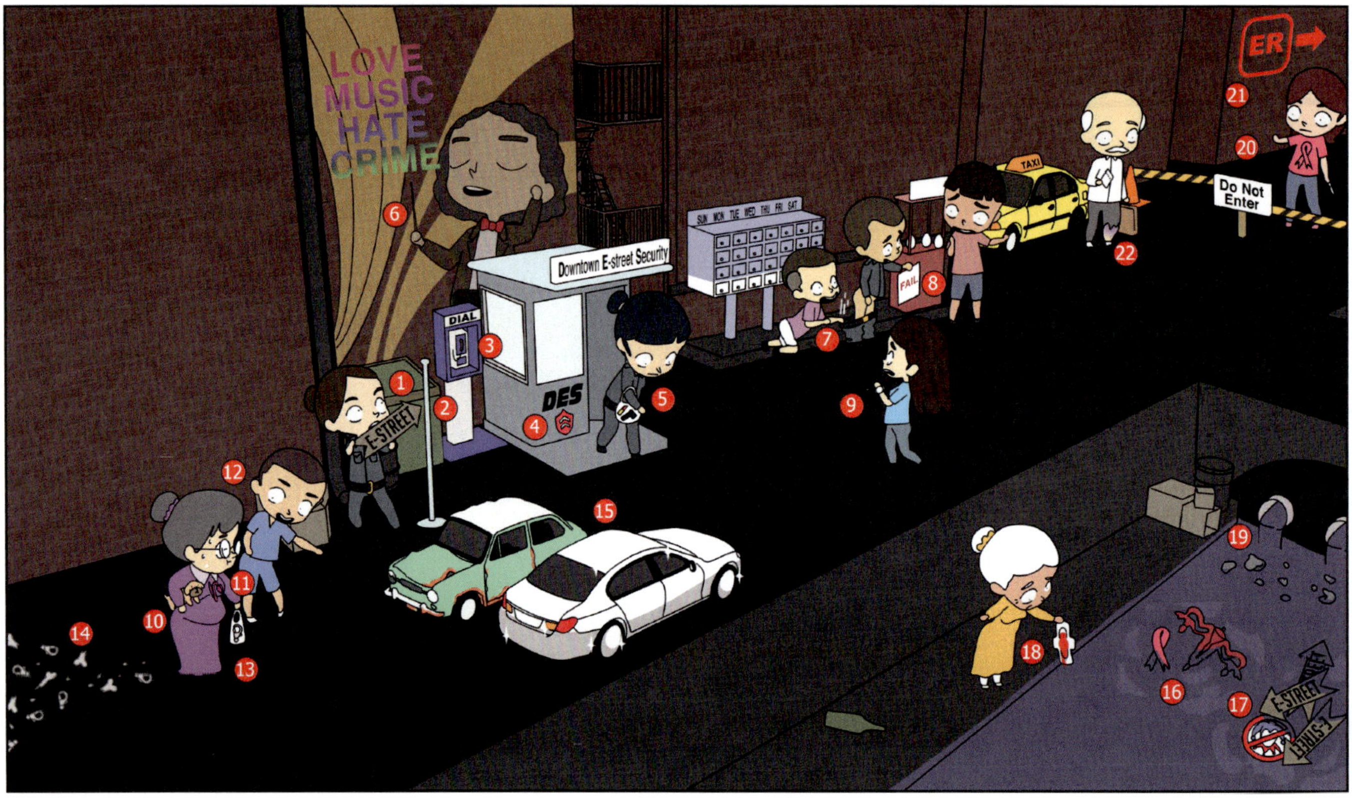

1. "E-STREET" sign: Exogenous estrogens

2. Worker attaching e-street sign on post: Binds estrogen receptors

3. E-Street "Dial" payphone: Ethinyl estradiol

4. "Downtown E-street Security" booth: DES (diethylstilbestrol)

5. Security officer leaving DES booth with clear handbag: Females exposed to DES in utero can develop clear cell adenocarcinoma of the vagina

6. Maestro painting, "Love justice, hate crime": Mestranol

7. Pantsed food inspector holding "Fail" health report: Use for hypogonadism

8. Food stand receiving fail for foram fresh eggs: Use for ovarian failure

9. Woman walking to birth control like-mailbox because her period started early: Use for menstrual abnormalities

10. Overweight elderly woman slowly walking on E-Street: Menopause can cause weight gain and slowed metabolism

11. Old woman sweating with wilted tulip: Menopause can cause hot flashes and vaginal atrophy

12. Grandson guiding grandma up E-Street: Use as hormone replacement therapy in postmenopausal women

13. Old woman walking towards the E-Street sign shaped like an arrow: Hormone replacement therapy (HRT) increases estrogen

14. Old women walking away from trail of broken bones and clasps: Estrogen decreases osteoclast activity and treats osteoporosis in postmenopausal women

15. Rusty car and new nice car parked on E-Street: HRT causes a possible increased cardiovascular risk

16. Uterus-shaped chandelier and pink cancer ribbon floating in canal: Can increase the risk of endometrial cancer

17. No pro-jester sign and pile of E-Street signs in canal with chandelier and ribbon: Unopposed estrogen without progesterone/progestin leads to endometrial cancer

18. Old lady dumping used pad in canal: Can cause bleeding in postmenopausal women

19. Garbage flowing out of canal outlets: Can increase risk of thrombi

20. Woman with pink cancer shirt behind caution taped area smoking: Contraindicated in women > 35-years-old who use tobacco

21. ER sign with arrow: Contraindicated in patients with ER(+) breast cancer

22. Old guy with swollen leg next to caution tape: Contraindicated with history of DVTs

See Figure 9.15.1 - Reproductive Drugs that Interact with the Hypothalamus and Pituitary Glands (Reproductive Pharmacology, Section 1, Page 328)

See Figure 9.15.4 - Pharmacologic Effects on the Uterus (Reproductive Pharmacology, Section 2, Page 330)

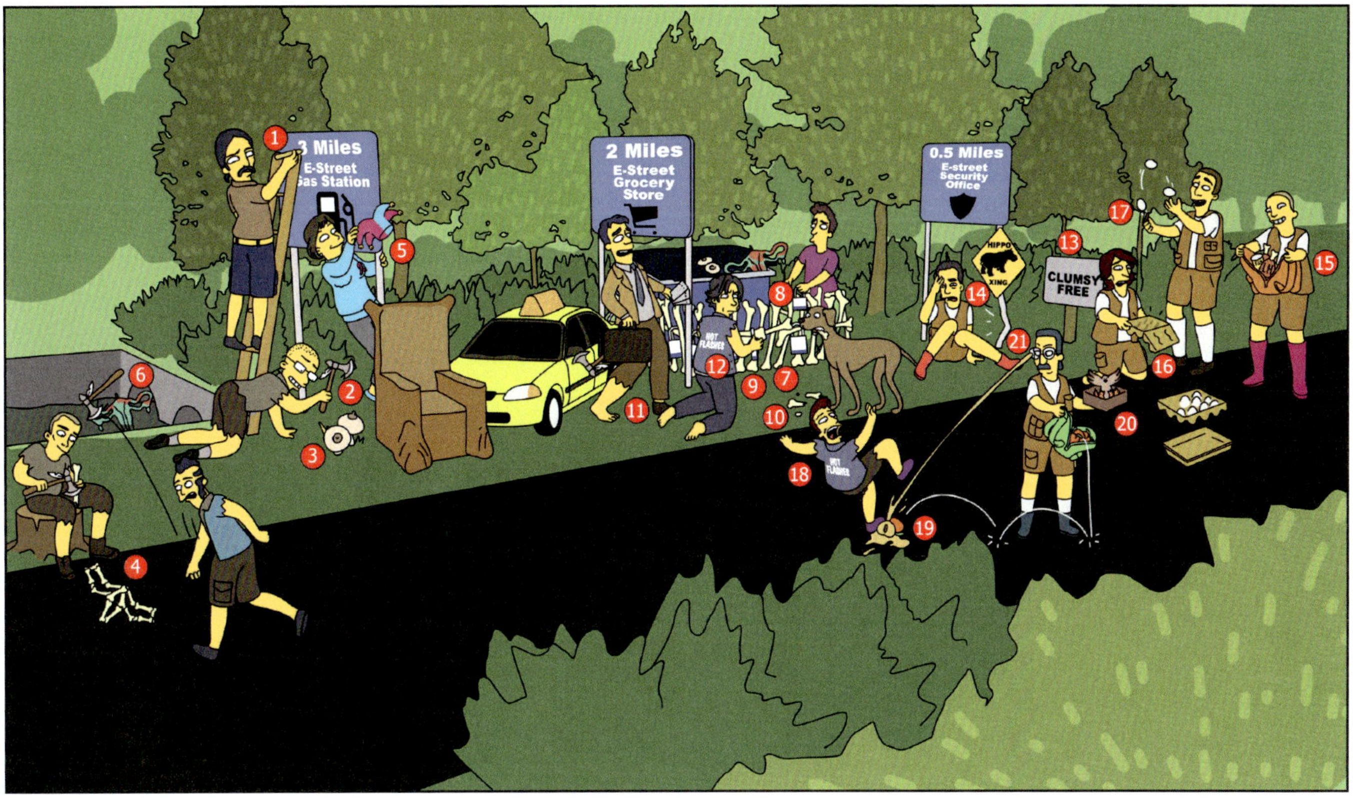

1. Guy selectively modifying one of three E-Street signs: Selective estrogen receptor modulators

2. Tomahawk man: Tamoxifen

3. Breast-shaped mushrooms being chopped with tomahawk: Tamoxifen is an antagonist at breast

4. Man carving bones with tomahawk and shaping them into uterus: Tamoxifen is an agonist at the bone and uterus

5. Pro-jester throne made by woman wearing pink ribbon by E-Street sign post near tomahawk: Use tamoxifen to treat ER/PR positive breast cancer (and prevent recurrence)

6. Tomahawk stuck in the rusted, uterus-shaped chandelier in sewer drain: Tamoxifen causes an increased risk of endometrial cancer because it's an agonist at the uterus

7. Locks on bone fence surrounding garbage: Raloxifene

8. Breast mushrooms and uterus-shaped chandelier in garbage: Raloxifene is an antagonist at the breast and uterus

9. Fence covered in locks and built out of bone: Raloxifene is an agonist at the bone

10. Chewed up bone fragments by dog: Raloxifene is used to treat osteoporosis

11. Man holding plane tickets and briefcase holding tomahawk with a swollen leg by bone cage: Tamoxifen and raloxifene can cause increased risk of thromboembolism (especially with smoking)

12. "Hot Flashes" jacket worn by punk rocker by bone cage: Tamoxifen and raloxifene can cause hot flashes

13. "Clumsy Free" sign clomiphene

14. Clumsy man bending E-Street hippo sign: Clomiphene is an antagonist at estrogen receptors in hypothalamus

15. Man with Louisiana ham and fish food next to "Clumsy Free" sign: Clomiphene increases the release of LH and FSH from the pituitary gland

16. Clumsy survivalist with empty cart of eggs: Clomiphene is used as treatment for infertility caused by anovulation

17. Man juggling eggs out of excitement for Louisiana ham and fish food: Clomiphene stimulates ovulation because of increased LH and FSH

18. Clumsy punk rocker with "Hot Flashes" shirt slipping: Clomiphene can cause hot flashes

19.Clumsy punk rocker slipping over large peach: Clomiphene can cause ovarian enlargement

20. Box with mother bird and lots of chicks held by survivalist: Clomiphene can cause multiple simultaneous pregnancies

21. Survivalist with peach juice squirting on his glasses: Clomiphene can cause visual disturbances

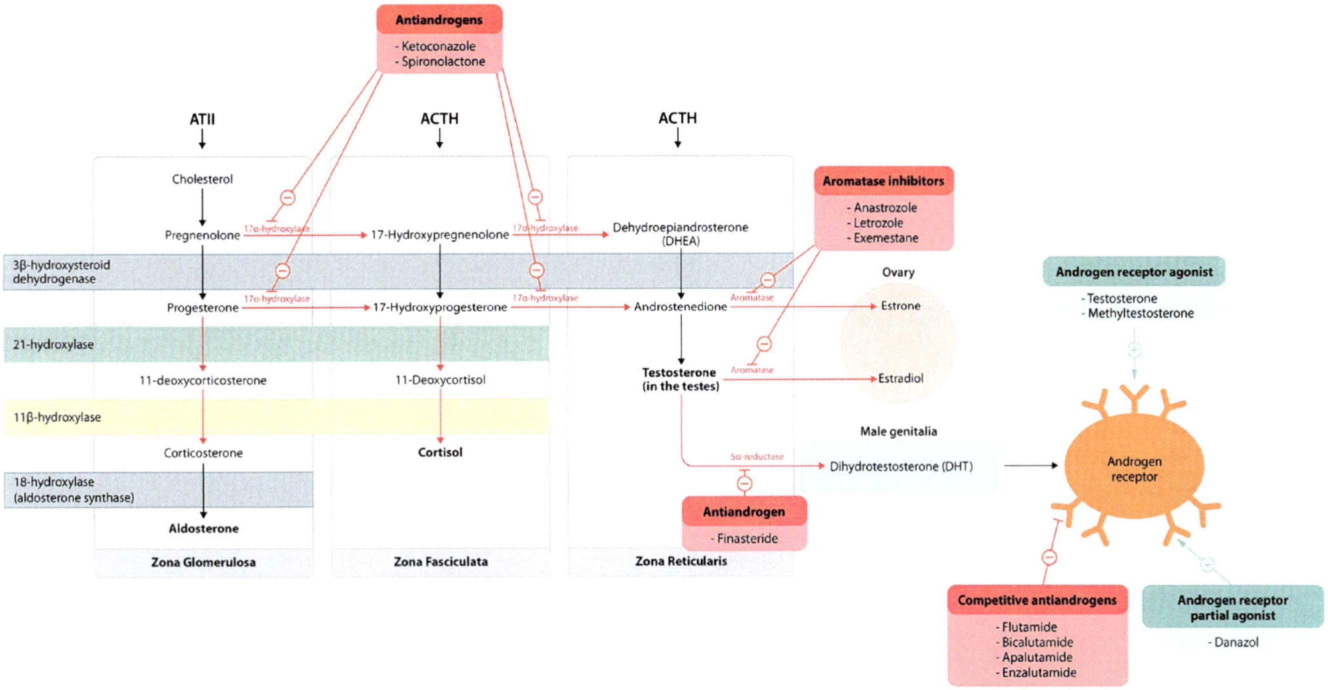

Figure 9.15.6 - Pharmacologic Interactions with Androgen Receptors and the Adrenal Cortex

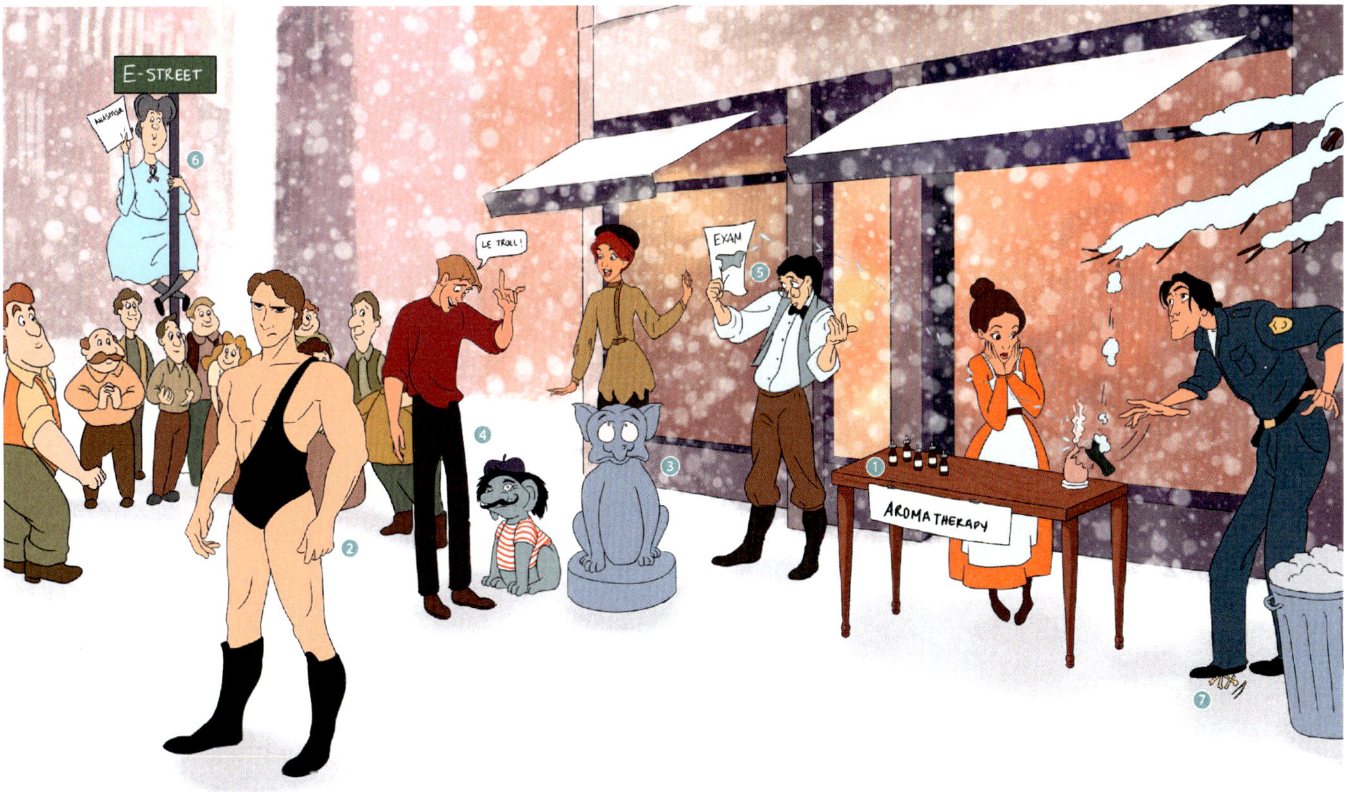

1. Snow knocking taxer out of cop's hand who was going to arrest woman and breaks aromatherapy oil machine: Aromatase inhibitors

2. Andre the giant unable to go to E-street: Inhibits peripheral conversion of androgens to estrogen

3. Anastasia on top of sculpted troll: Anastrozole

4. French man exclaiming, "Le Troll!" admiring his troll statue: Letrozole

5. Oil stain on art professor's exam sheet: Exemestane

6. Old woman on E-Street post with pink cancer ribbon on her shirt holding paper saying, "Anastasia": Use for ER(+) breast cancer in postmenopausal women

7. Pile of chicken bones being stepped on by cop: Can cause osteoporosis

See Figure 9.15.4 - Pharmacologic Effects on the Uterus (Reproductive Pharmacology, Section 2, Page 330)

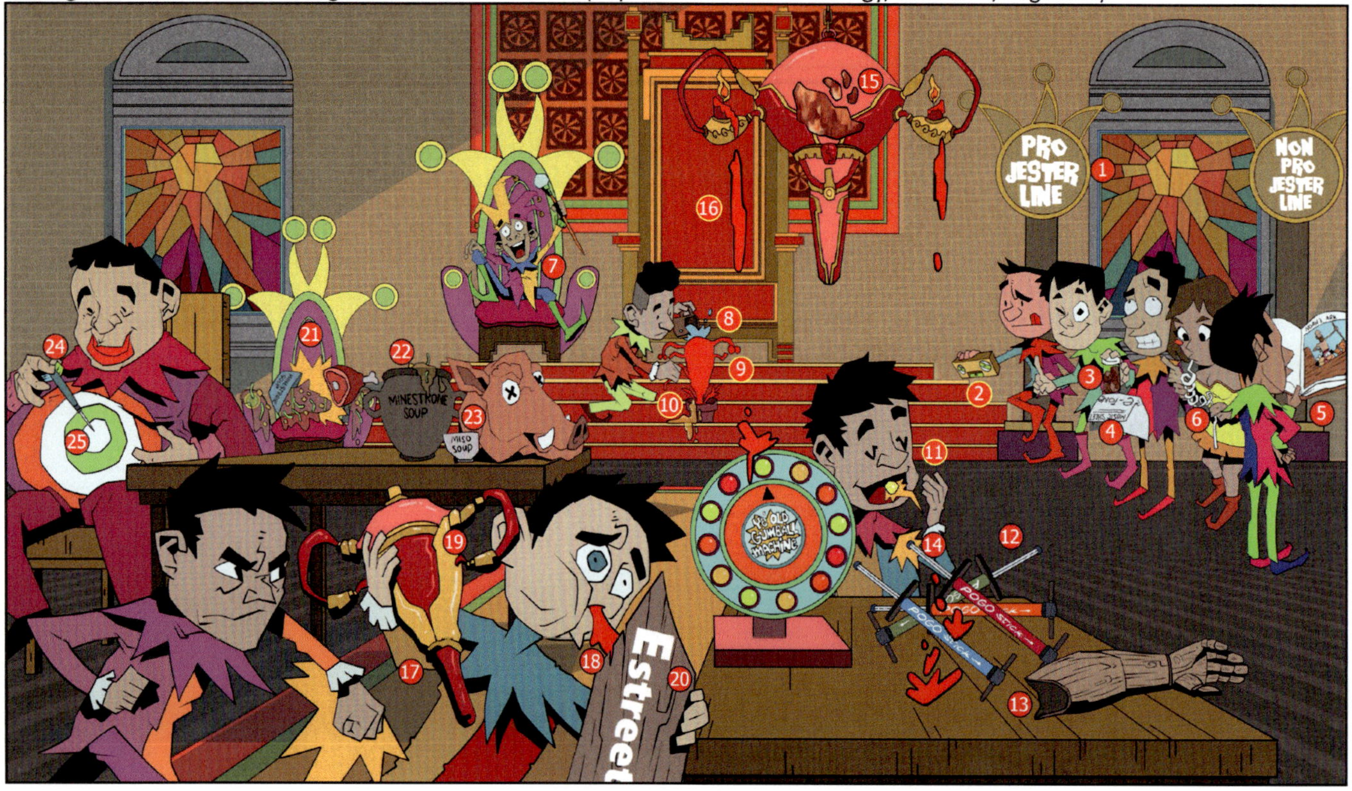

1. "Pro Jester" line sign: Progestins

2. Jester holding a level: Levonorgestrel

3. Jester holding jar of medicine rocks: Medroxyprogesterone

4. Jester holding E tone sheet music: Etonogestrel

5. Jester holding bible picture with a emaciated Noah: Norethindrone

6. Jester with mega straw: Megestrol

7. Pro jester sitting in throne: Progestin receptor

8. Jester trimming uterus plant: Decreased growth of the endometrium

9. Uterus plant growing branches of berries: Increased vascularization of the endometrium

10. Yellow goop discharge from uterus plant: Causes thickened cervical mucus

11. Jester popping contraceptive gumball in his mouth next to gumball machine: used in oral contraception

12. Pogo sticks on table with gumball machine: Used in IUDs

13. Wooden arm with bicep opening on table: Used in arm implant contraception

14. Pogo stick hitting jester on deltoid: Depot injection

15. Rusted uterus chandelier above table: Use for endometrial cancer

16. Dripping red wax from red candles of uterus chandelier: Use for abnormal uterine bleeding

17. Jester punching thief in the face who was stealing uterus chandelier and E-Street sign: Progesterone challenge test

18. Thief's nose bleeding while withdrawing backwards: Withdrawal bleed

19. Uterus chandelier unscathed after thief's interaction with other jester: Presence of a withdrawal bleed suggests normal uterine anatomy

20. Inact E-Street sign after thief's interaction with other jester: Presence of a withdrawal bleed suggests estrogen dysfunction is not the cause of the patient's amenorrhea

21. Rotten food thrown onto Pro Jester's chair: Antiprogestins are competitive inhibitors of progestins at progesterone receptors

22. Minestrone soup on banquet table: Mifepristone

23. Miso soup next to boar's head: Use mifepristone for termination of pregnancy

24. Jester with U-shaped smile sitting near banquet table: Ulipristal

25. U-shaped smile gester removing dart on big belly after eating: Use ulipristal for emergency contraception

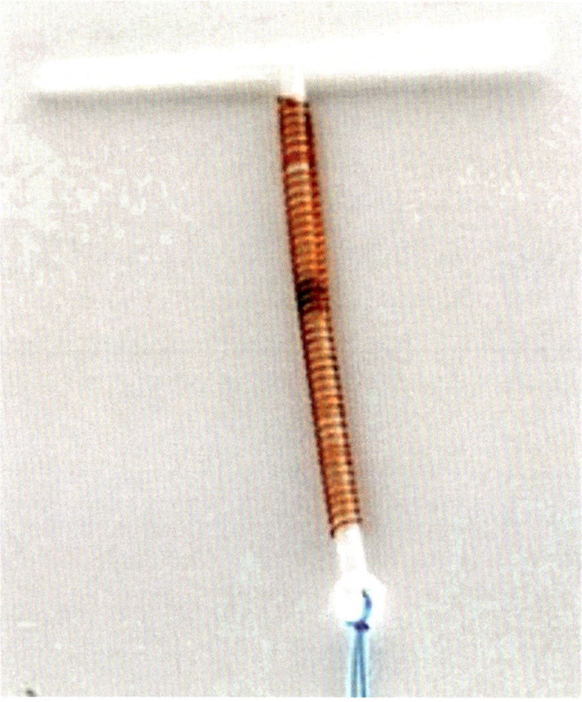

Figure 9.15.7 - IUD

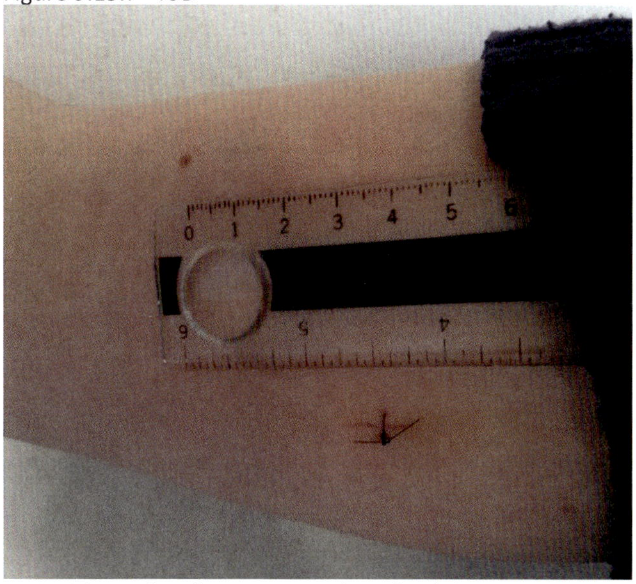

Figure 9.15.8 - Arm Implant Contraception

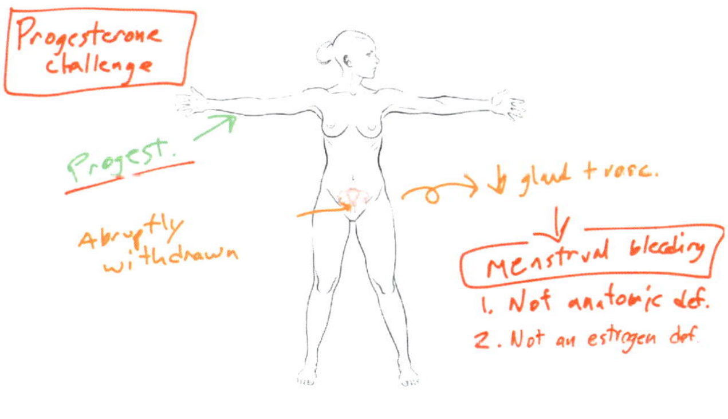

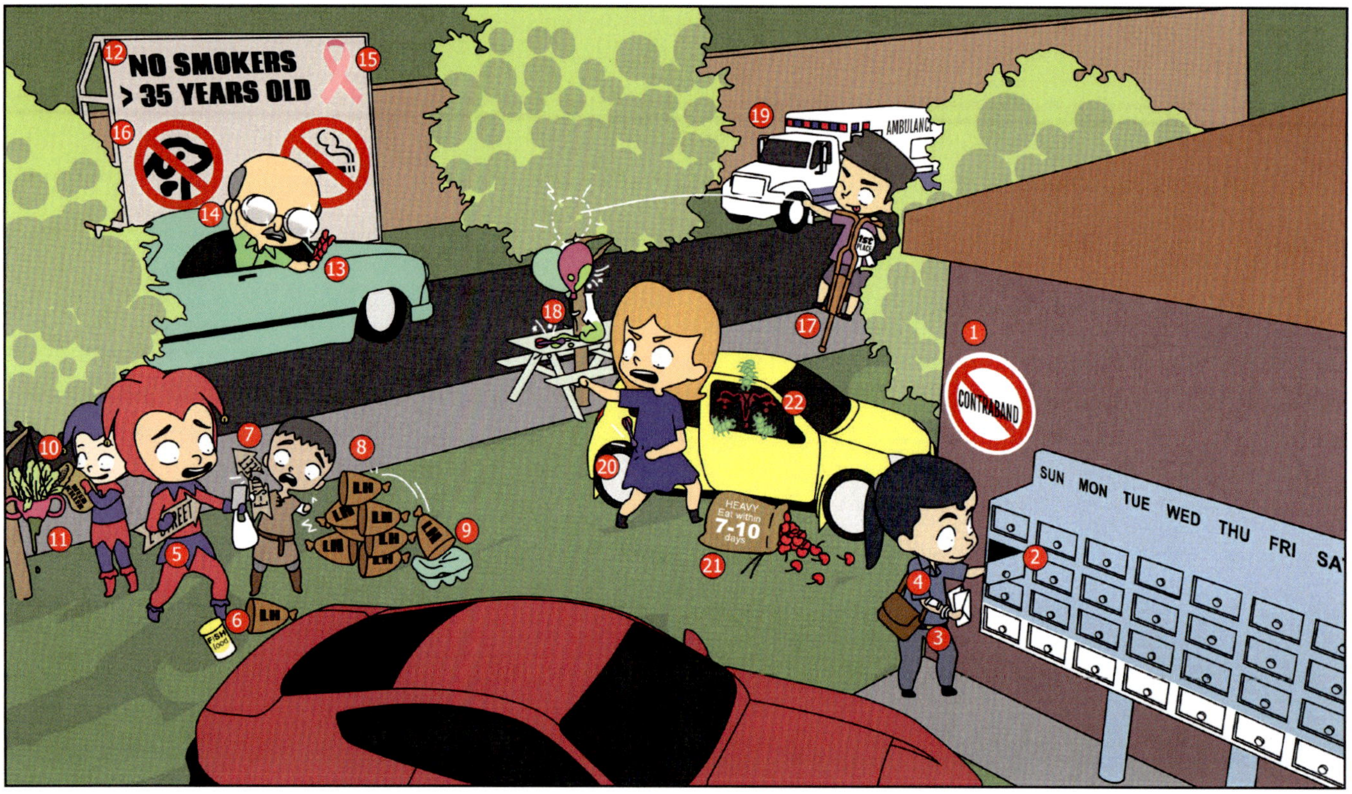

1. "No contraband" sign: Contraception

2. Mailbox that looks like pack of birth control pills: Combined contraception pill form

3. Round, clear bracelets worn by mail woman: Combined contraception: vaginal ring form

4. Patch on mail woman's arm: Combined contraception patch form

5. Pro jester with E-Street sign dialing his phone: Progestins and ethinyl estradiol

6. Dropped fish food and Louisiana ham by Pro jester: Estrogens and progestin inhibit LH and FSH

7. Jester breaking son's E-Street sign: Prevents estrogen surge

8. Louisiana hams pile falling over to ground behind son: Prevents LH surge

9. Louisiana ham crushing eggs: Prevents ovulation

10. Jester's son dumping weed killer on plant in uterus shape pot: Progestins also inhibit endometrial proliferative → endometrium is less suitable to the implantation of an embryo

11. Mucus goo running out of uterus shape pot: Progestins cause thickening of cervical mucus, thereby limiting access of sperm to the uterus

12. "No smockers > 35-years-old" sign: Can increase risk of cardiovascular events in smokers greater than 35-years-old

13. Pedophile hanging out of car luring kids with licorice near no smoking sign: Avoid in patients with increased risk of cardiovascular disease

14. Pedophile holding head in pain: Contraindicated in cases of migraines with aura

15. Pink cancer ribbon on no smoking sign: Contraindicated in breast cancer

16. "No liver-spotted dog" next to no smoking sign: Contraindicated with liver disease

17. Copper color pogo stick: Copper IUD

18. Kid on pogo stick throwing dart, breaking open vial of toxic fluid, and popping balloon: Copper IUDs produce a local inflammatory reaction toxic to sperm and ova, preventing fertilization and implantation

19. Ambulance near copper pogo stick: Most effective emergency contraception

20. Mom grabbing pelvis in pain after being hit with dart: Copper IUDs can cause dysmenorrhea

21. Mom dropping large bag of cherries, lasting seven to 10 days, after being hit with dart: Copper IUDs can cause heavier and/or longer menses

22. Bugs eating uterus vandalism off of angry mom's car: Do not place IUDs during an active pelvic infection

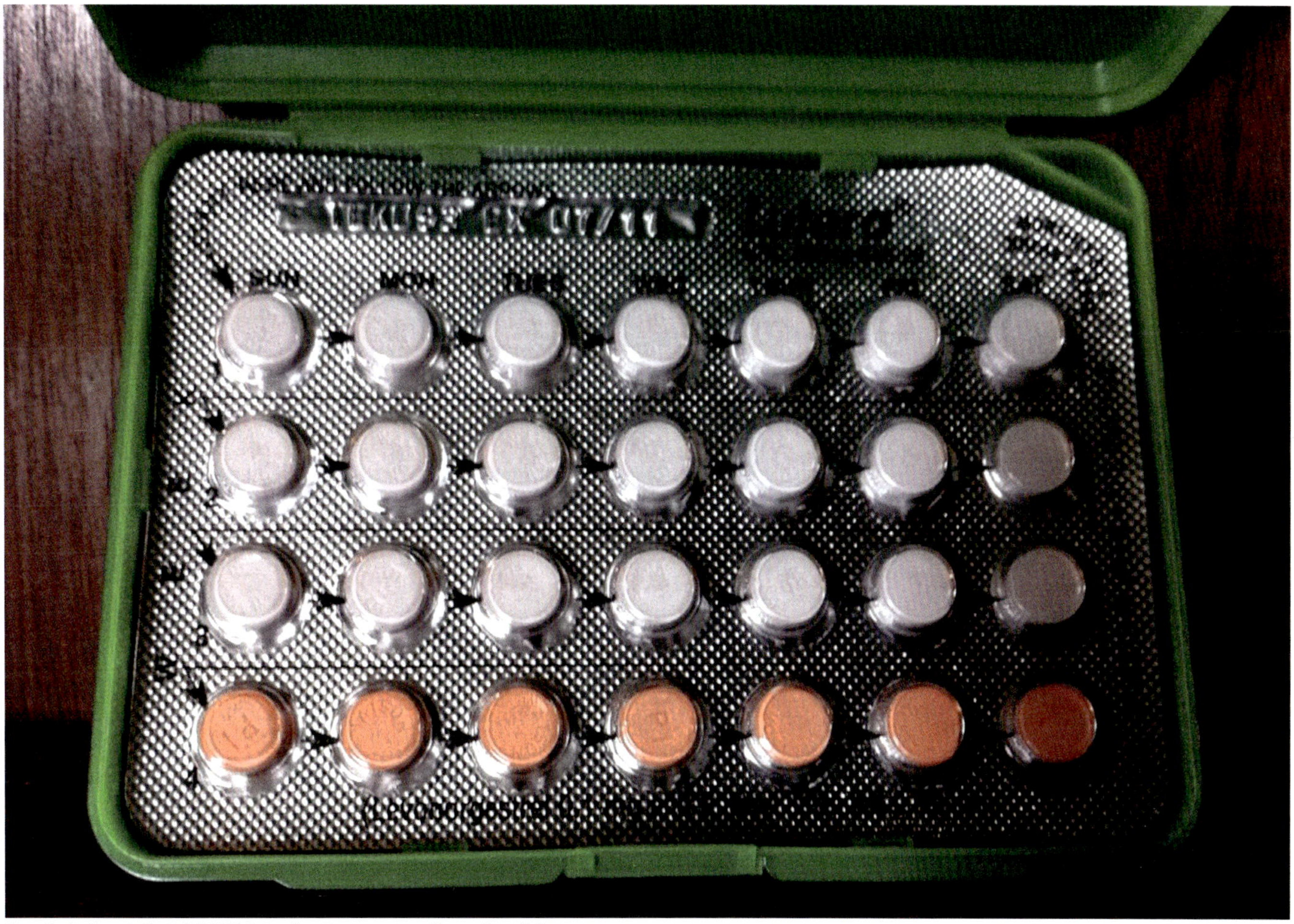

Figure 9.15.9 - Oral Contraceptive Pills

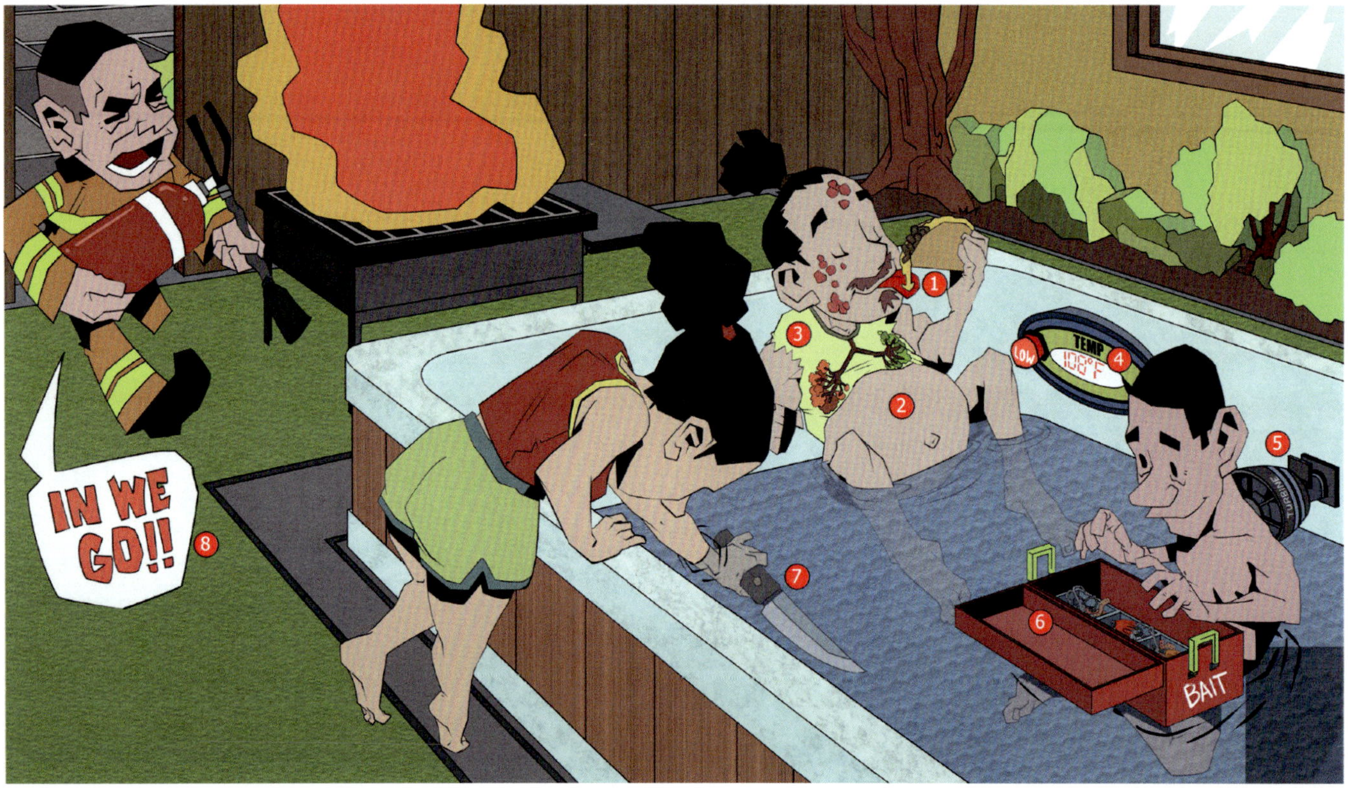

1. Pregnant woman licking the melting cheese from taco: Tocolytics

2. Pregnant woman sitting in hot tub: Used to decrease contraction frequency in preterm labor

3. Buff and hairy pregnant lady with cover-up that looks like lungs: Steroids are used to promote fetal lung maturity

4. Relaxed pregnant woman in hot tub with water temperature of 108 degrees: High temperature → fewer contractions

5. Turbine in hot tub: Terbutaline

6. Husband organizing open bait box with two handles leaning against turbine: Terbutaline is β_2 agonist

7. Woman dipping knife into pool: Nifedipine

8. Firefighter extinguishing fire saying, "In we go!": Indomethacin

See Figure 9.15.6 - Pharmacologic Interactions with Androgen Receptors and the Adrenal Cortex (Reproductive Pharmacology, Section 4, Page 334)

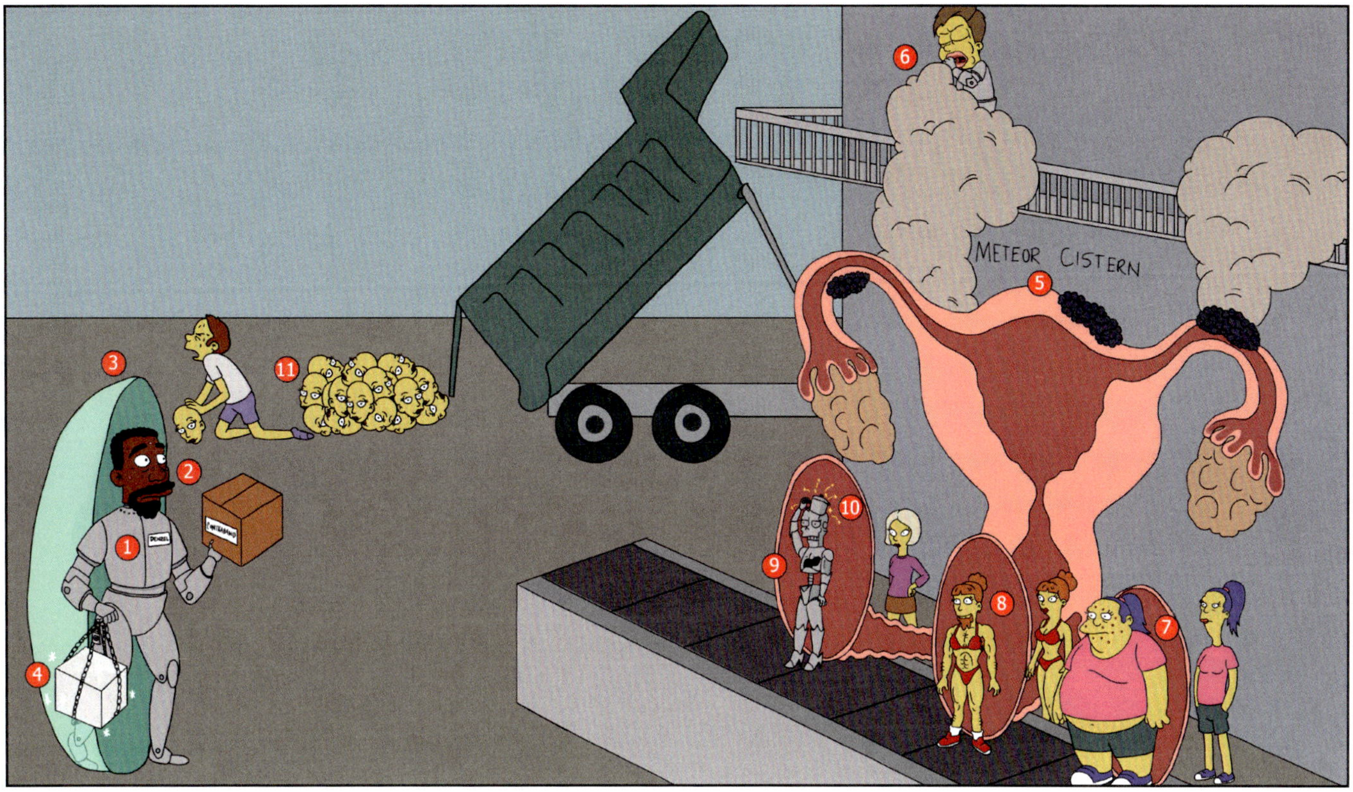

1. Cyborg Denzel Washington: Danazol

2. Cyborg Washington, half android with acne: Synthetic androgen agonist

3. Denzel taking one step out of receptor pod: Acts as a partial agonist at androgen receptors

4. Chained ornate chrome box: Cytochrome P-450c17 inhibitor

5. Uterus-shaped machine, "Meteor Cistern", with black soot: Used for endometriosis

6. Cyborg coughing from toxic fumes and her face swelling: Used for hereditary angioedema

7. Woman transformed into overweight self with acne: Can cause acne, weight gain, and edema

8. Woman transformed as a very muscular woman with facial hair: Can cause hirsutism and masculinization

9. Woman transformed into liver-spotted android: can cause hepatotoxicity

10. Android lady smashing head with pressure cooker: Can cause idiopathic intracranial hypertension

11. Worker rolling away heavy android heads: Can decrease HDL levels

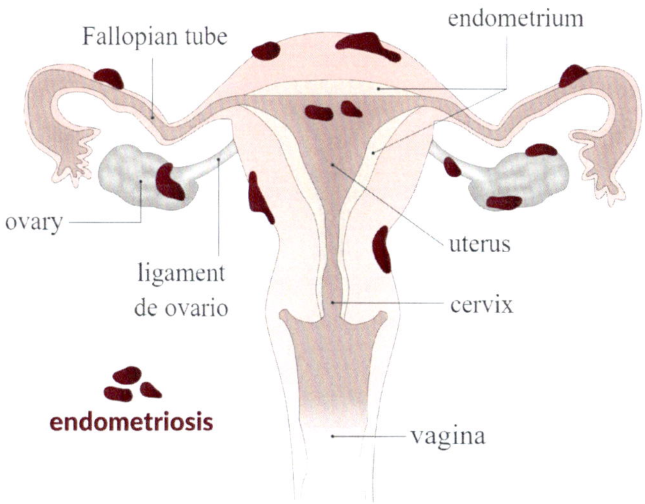

Figure 9.15.10 - Female Reproductive System with Endometriosis

See Figure 9.15.6 - Pharmacologic Interactions with Androgen Receptors and the Adrenal Cortex (Reproductive Pharmacology, Section 4, Page 334)

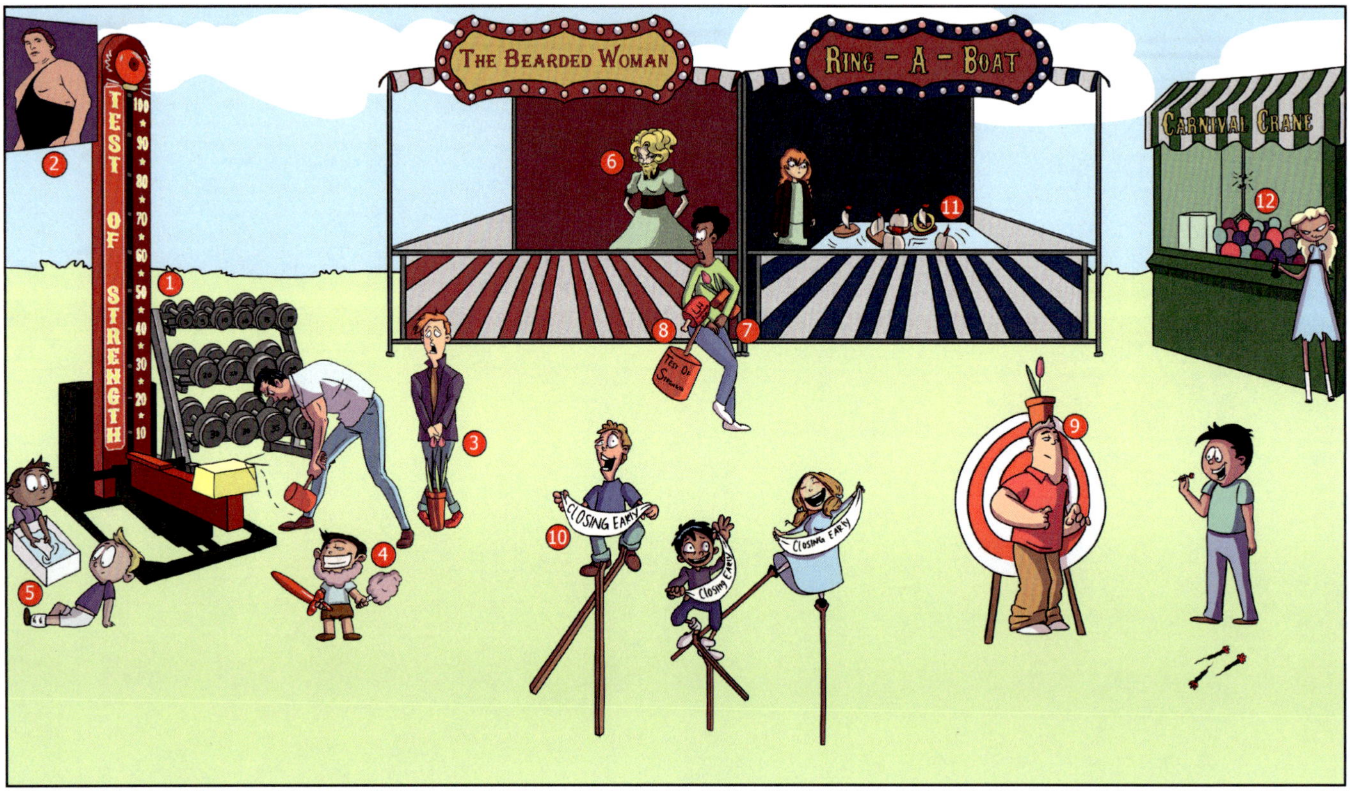

1. "Test of Strength" game and metal dumbbells: Testosterone and methyltestosterone

2. Man matching Andre the Giant's strength: Agonist at androgen receptors

3. Tulip buds positioned in front of man's crotch: Used to treat symptoms of hypogonadism (e.g. decreased libido, energy, body mass and bone density)

4. Kid with cotton candy beard and using sword as erection: Promote development of secondary sex characteristics

5. Kid layering paper together to make paper mache cast for friend's leg: Stimulate anabolism to promote recovery after burn or injury

6. Bearded woman at fair masculinization in female (hirsutism, acne, breast atrophy, male pattern baldness)

7. Man with tulip dropping Louisiana ham while covering his testicles: Exogenous testosterone administration decreases release of LH via negative feedback

8. Man dropping strength hammer: Decreased LH leads to decreased endogenous (intratesticular) testosterone synthesis

9. Man who dropped his shriveled darts tries to throw a dart at other man with tulip on his head: Gonadal atrophy causes decreased sperm count

10. Kids on stilts with "Closing early" banners: Premature closure of epiphyseal plates

11. Ring toss boat game with a lot of boats: Increased LDL

12. Claw machine unable to pick up dense balls: Decreased HDL

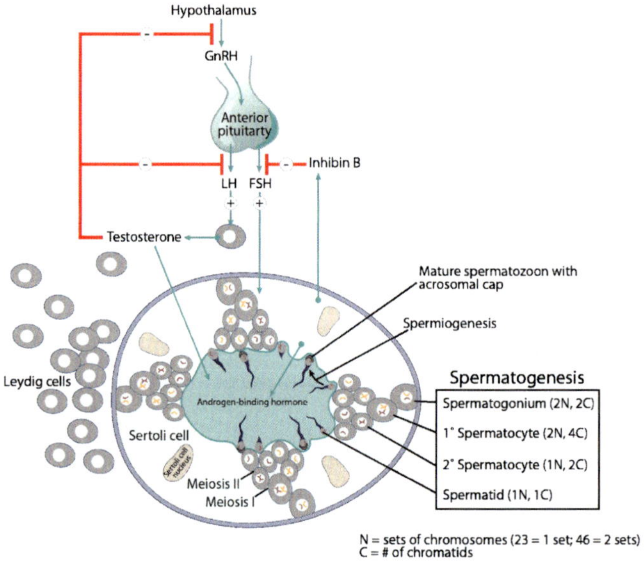

Figure 9.15.11 - Physiology of Spermatogenesis

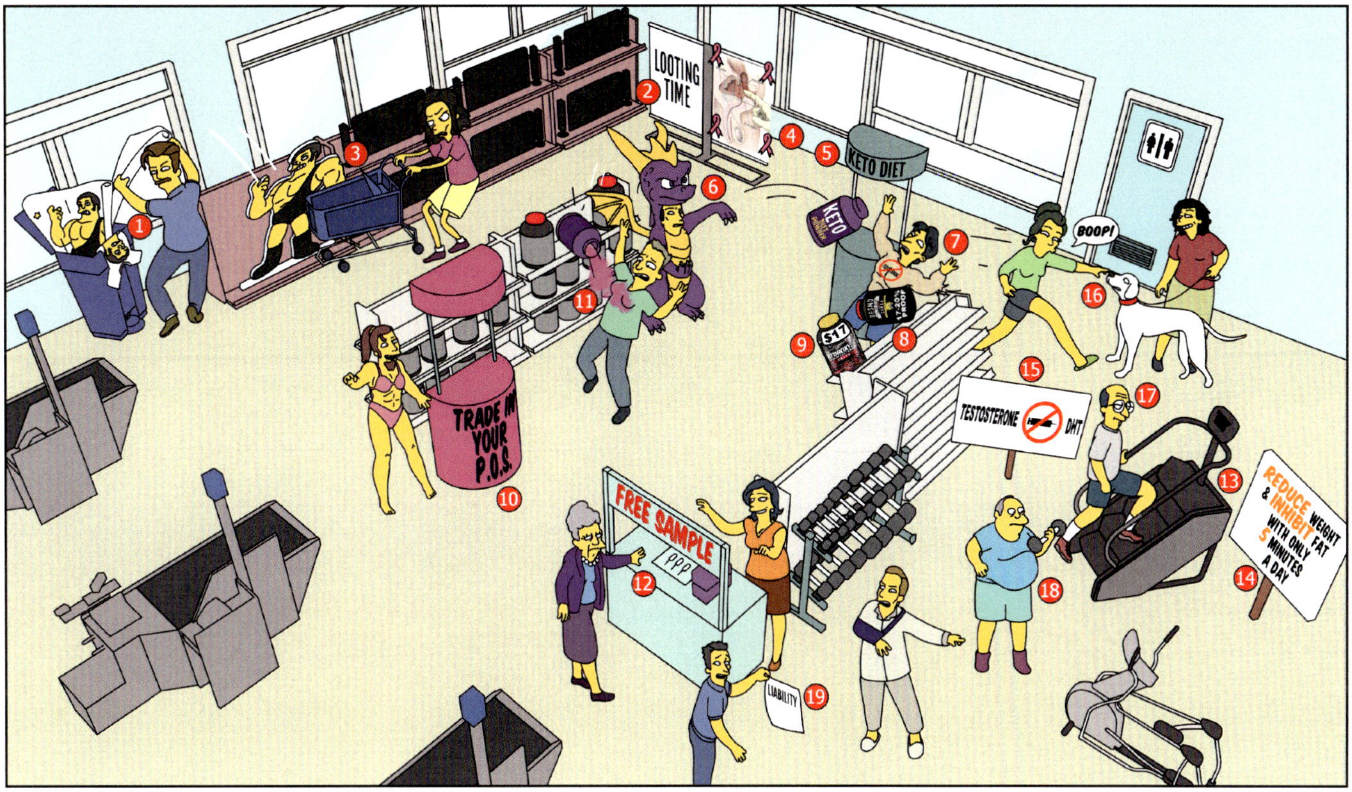

1. Andre the Giant merchandise being thrown away: Antiandrogens

2. "Looting Time" sign in first aisle: All end with "flutamide"

3. Andre the Giant cut out off the shelf: Nonsteroidal competitive inhibitors at androgens receptors

4. Prostate exam poster with pink cancer ribbons next to "Looting Time" sign: Use for prostatic carcinoma

5. Keto diet stand in second aisle: Ketoconazole

6. Man in Spyro costume: Spironolactone

7. Man in inflatable "No Testosterone" muscle shirt, tearing shirt while trying to catch keto diet powder thrown by man in Spyro costume: Inhibits steroid synthesis

8. Spyro man and man in inflatable costume knocking Desmo Corsas off the shelf that is 17-20% off: Ketoconazole and spironolactone inhibit 17, 20 desmolase

9. Hydroxycut $17 bottle falling off of shelf due to collision: Ketoconazole and spironolactone inhibit 17 α-hydroxylase

10. POS booth with bearded buff lady in second aisle: use for polycystic ovarian syndrome (PCOS) hirsutism

11. Keto powder falling on man's chest causing him to grow breasts: Can cause gynecomastia

12. Older woman refusing free sample tampon: Can cause amenorrhea

13. Fitness stair in third aisle: Finasteride

14. "Reduce weight and inhibit fat with only 5 minutes a day" sign: 5α-reductase inhibitor

15. Crossed out syringe sign: Decreases conversation of testosterone to dihydrotestosterone (DHT)

16. Woman "booping" nose of dog next to fitness chair: Finasteride is used for benign prostatic hyperplasia (BPH)

17. Bald guy on fitness stair machine: Use for androgenic alopecia (male pattern baldness)

18. Obese man with man-boobs: Can cause gynecomastia

19. Manager in pajamas with "liability" paper: Can cause sexual dysfunction (e.g. decreasd libido, premature ejaculation)

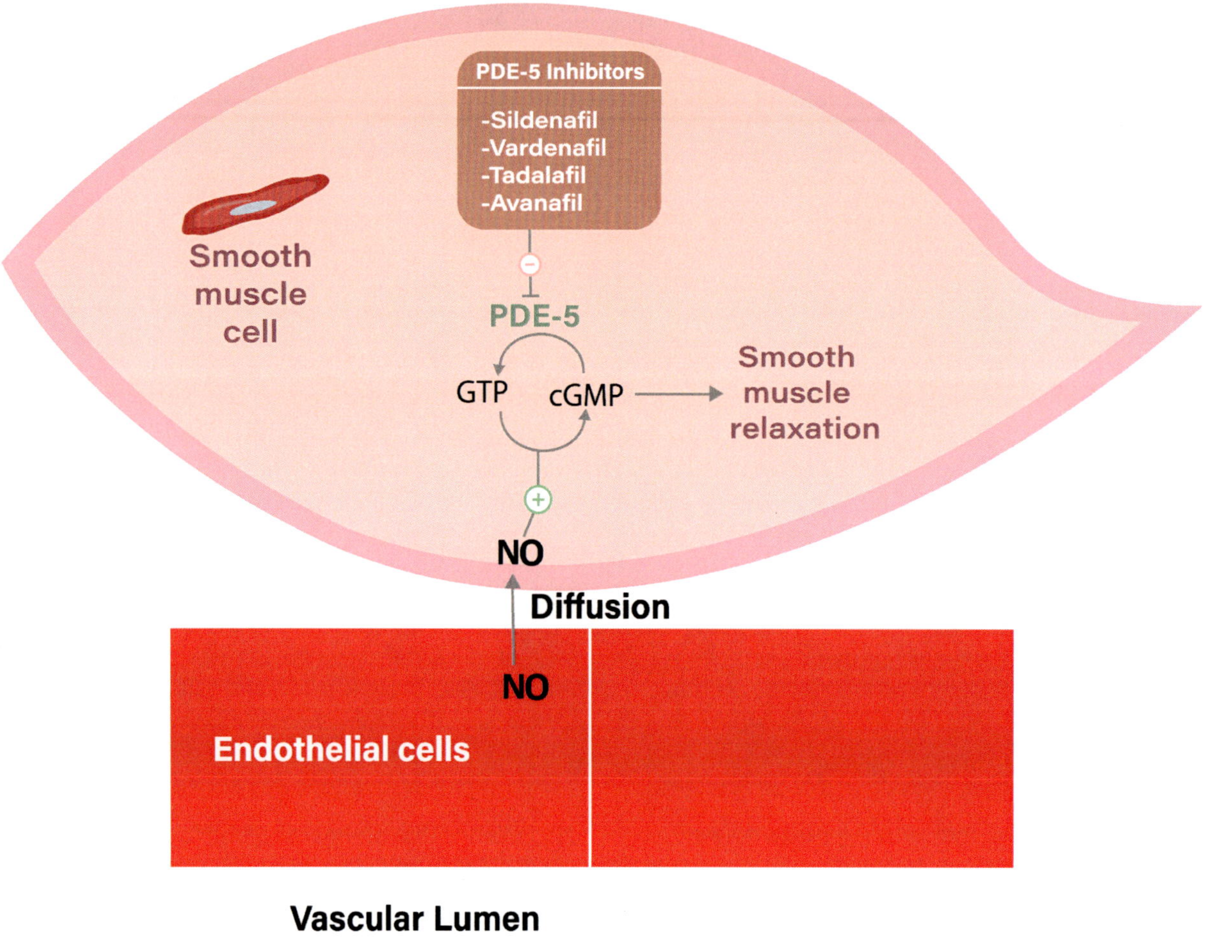

Figure 9.15.12 - Mechanism of Phosphodiesterase-5 Inhibitors

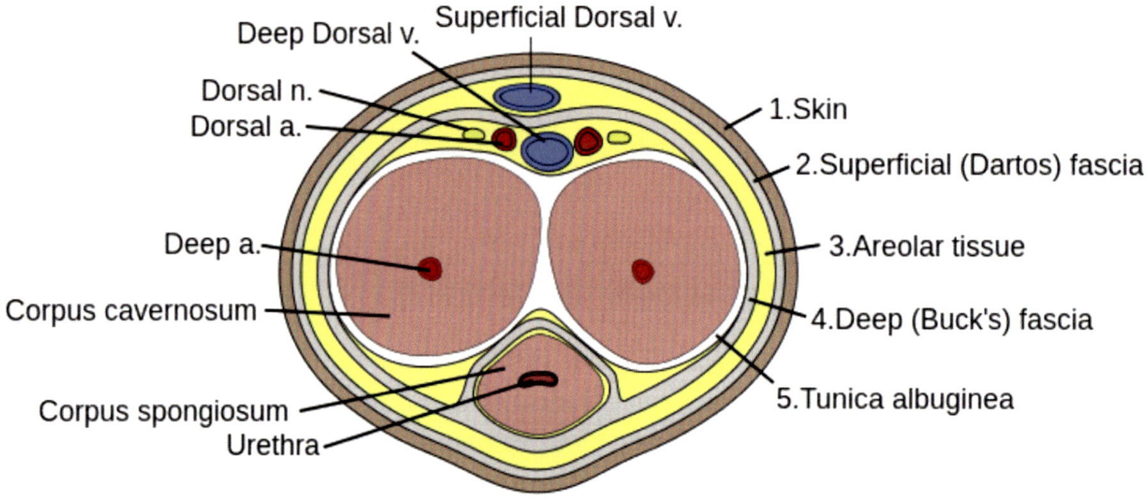

Figure 9.15.13 - Cross Section of Penis

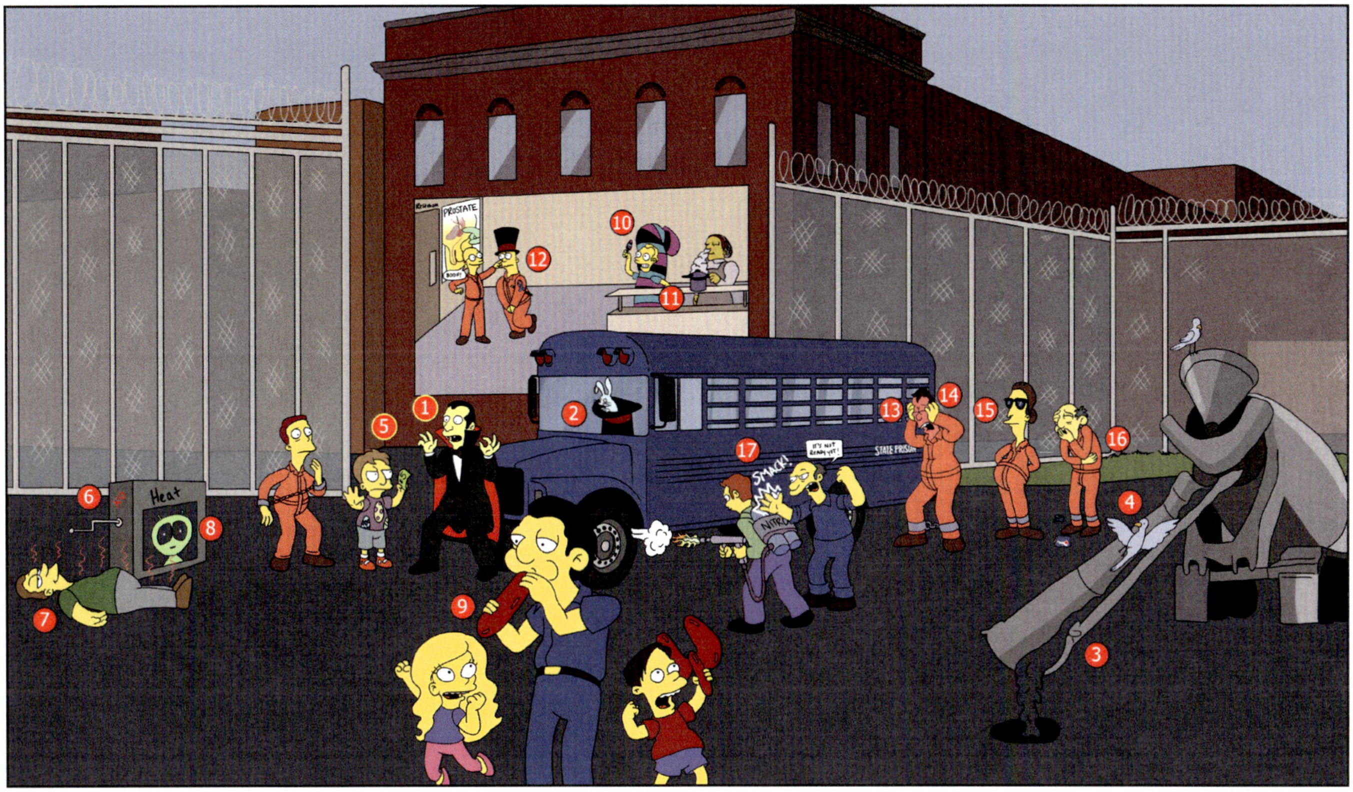

1. Vampire warden: Vardenafil

2. Magic hat with rabbit, "Ta Da!": Tadalafil

3. Cement truck filling potholes with cement: Sildenafil

4. Avian sliding down cement chute: Avanafil

5. Foster kid with easter egg shirt holding $5 trying to block vampire warden from his foster dad: PDE-5 inhibitors

6. Crank cyclic heater: Increased cGMP

7. Electrocuted man laying down: Prolongs smooth muscle relaxation in response to NO

8. Alien logo on cyclic heater: Increased blood flow into corpus cavernosum of penis

9. Guard easily blowing up red battle ax and lung balloons: Decreased pulmonary vascular resistance due to relative vasodilation of the pulmonary vasculature

10. Man in penis popsicle costume: Used for erectile dysfunction

11. Woman breathing in steam from pressure cooker: Used for pulmonary hypertension

12. Magician's apprentice who needs to go to the bathroom is "booped" on the nose: Use tadalafil for BPH

13. Prisoner with headache outside prison bus: Can cause headaches

14. Prisoner with head pain having red face: Can cause flushing

15. Calm wearing prisoner wearing blue tinted sunglasses: Can cause cyanopia

16. Prisoner holding upper abdomen in pain with crushed pepsi cans near him: Can cause dyspepsia

17. Manager smacking cement worker with "Nitro" flamethrower causing him to deflate bus tire: Contraindicated with nitroglycerin due to risk of severe hypotension

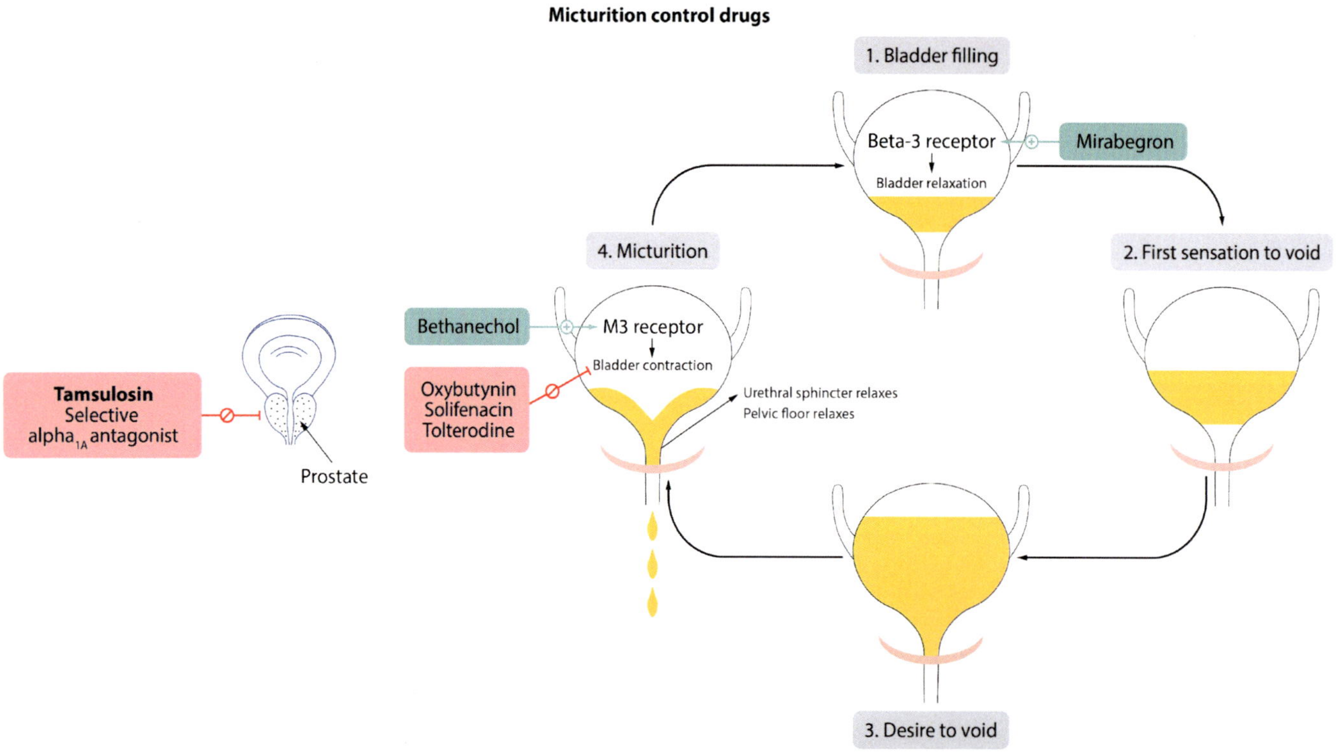

Figure 9.15.14 - Micturition Control Mechanisms

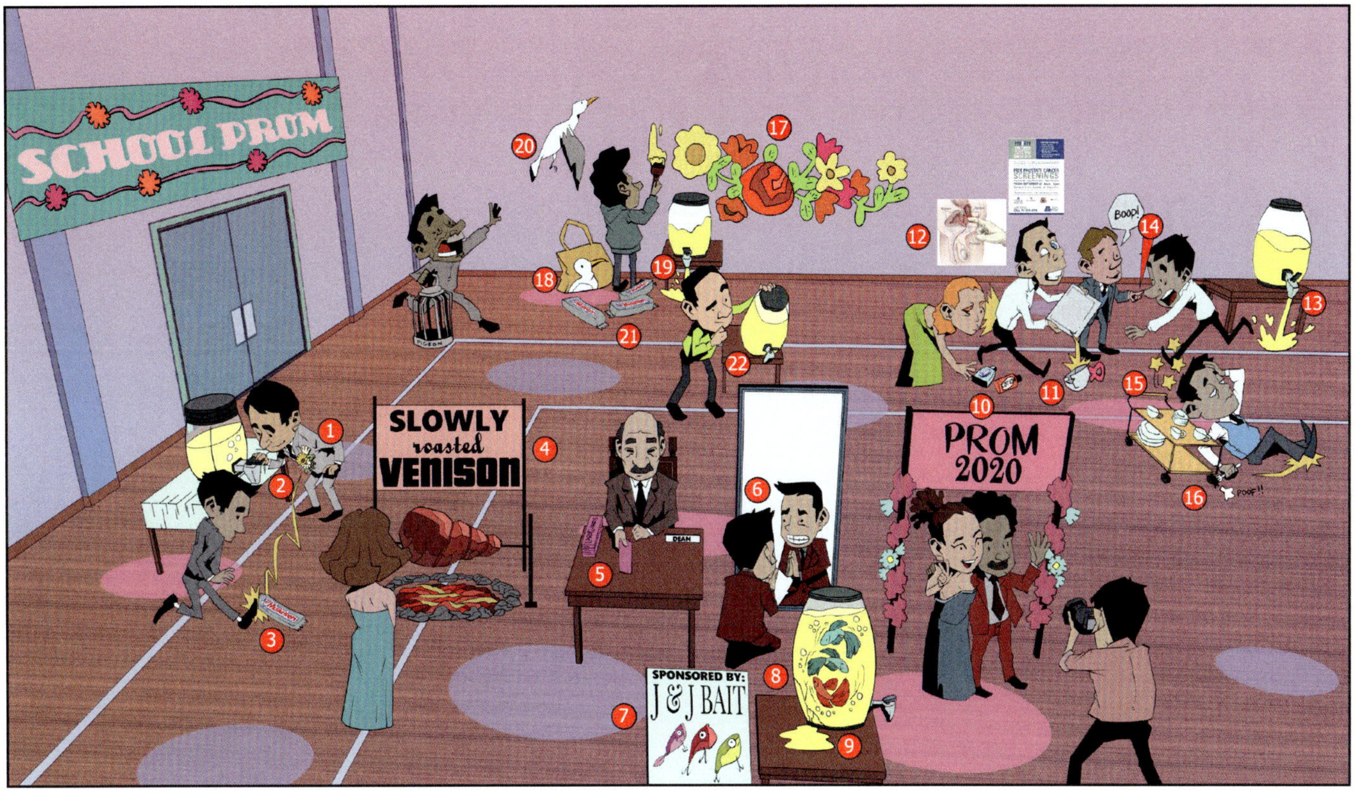

1. Ox-eye boutonniere worn by student: Oxybutynin

2. Student with ox-eye boutonniere closing the lever the lemonade dispenser: Oxybutynin causes relaxation of the detrusor smooth muscle → decreased detrusor overactivity

3. Boy with ox-eye boutonniere dropping a 3 Musketeers bar that gets stepped on: Oxybutynin is a muscarinic antagonist for in the genitourinary system (primary M_3 receptors)

4. "Slowly-roasted Venison" station: Solifenacin is a muscarinic antagonist for in the genitourinary system (primarily M_3 receptors)

5. Dean with tall tarot cards: Tolterodine is a muscarinic antagonist for in the genitourinary system (primarily M_3 receptors)

6. Student begging in mirror: Mirabegron

7. Three beta fish in tank next to "J & J Bait" flier: Mirabegron causes β-3 stimulation

8. Oversized fish tank dispenser with yellow lighting: Beta 3 stimulation → relaxation of the detrusor smooth muscle → increases bladder capacity

9. Leak from fish tank dispenser, causing overactive fish next to mirror: Use mirabegron to treat urinary urge incontinence or overactive bladder

10. Girl dropping Tums and lotion: Tamsulosin

11. Waiter dropping teacup with alpha handle after being bumped by girl dropping Tums and lotion: Tamsulosin acts as an α-1 antagonist

12. Prostate poster behind girl bumping to waiter's behind: α-1 a/d receptors are found on the prostate

13. Waiter left open lemonade dispenser with lemonade gushing out: By blocking α-1 receptors on the prostate, tamsulosin causes relaxation of smooth muscle → decreased urinary obstruction

14. Teenager "booping" waiter on nose near Tums: Tamsulosin is used to treat BPH

15. Dizzy waiter with headache: Tamsulosin can cause dizziness and headaches

16. Dizzy waiter popping tire of his cart trying to stand up first time: Tamsulosin can cause 1st dose orthostatic hypotension

17. Botanical mural being painted by student: Bethanechol

18. Seagull bag next to mural: Bethanechol is an acetylcholine analog

19. Freely flowing lemonade out of dispenser next to mural: Bethanechol activates contraction of bladder smooth muscle (i.e. the detrusor muscle) → bladder emptying

20. Seagull flying out of cage near mural: Bethanechol is resistant to AChE

21. 3 Musketeers bar not being stepped on by botanical mural: Bethanechol is an M3 receptor agonist

22. Broken lemonade dispenser with no lemonade flowing out: Bethanechol used for urinary retention

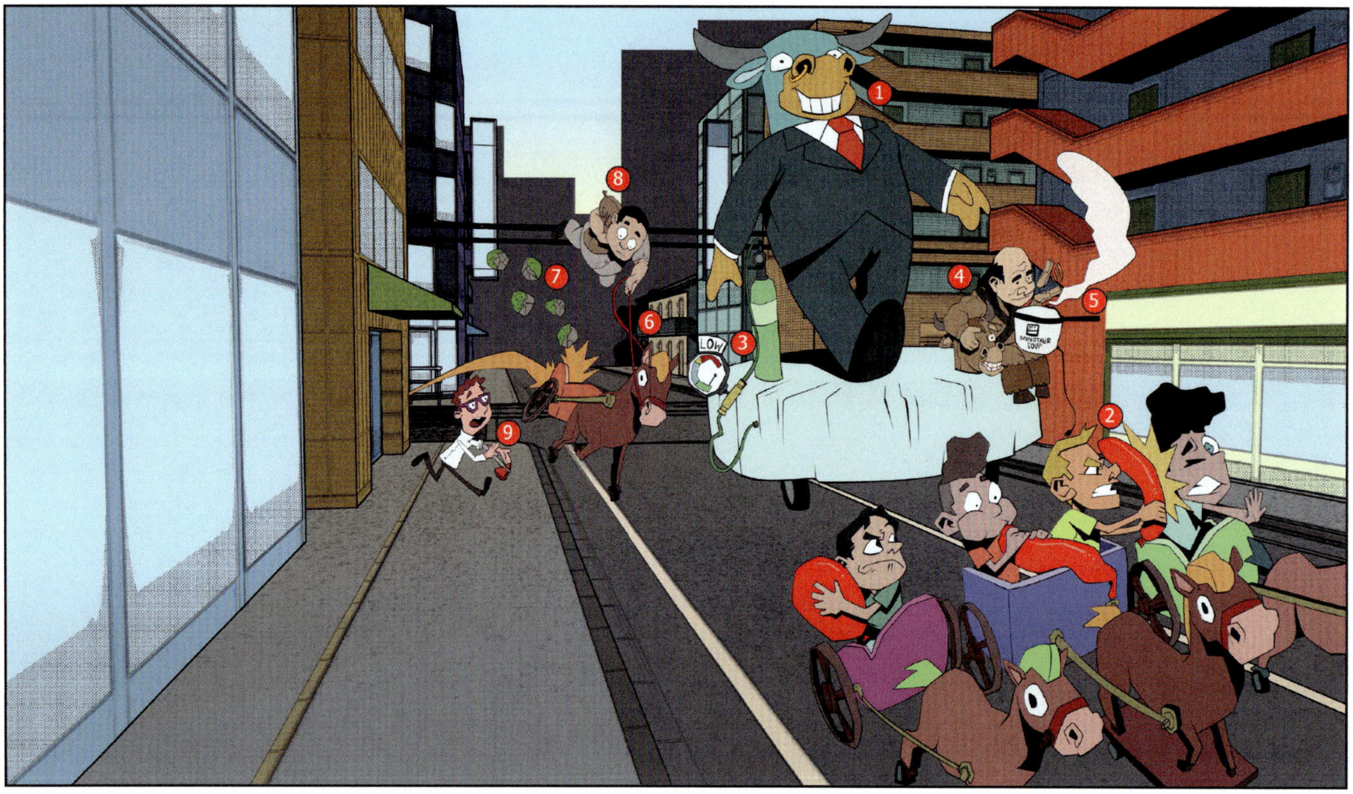

1. Minotaur float in parade: Minoxidil

2. Chariot racers blowing up and hitting each other with long red balloons: Direct arteriolar vasodilator

3. Air hose pressure from kink is released and show's "Low" on pressure gauge: Lowers blood pressure by reducing systemic vascular resistance

4. Balding man in minotaur suit: Use for androgenic alopecia (male pattern baldness)

5. Severely overheated pressure cooker bald guy is regulating: Use for severe refactor hypertension

6. Man thrown up out of chariot with reins extended high: Stimulates renin release (stimulate RAAS)

7. Old stones flying up into air: Increased aldosterone

8. Chubby man holding reins is also holding salt up high: Increased sodium and fluid retention

9. Medical student running while checking his pulse and has a reflex hammer: Can cause reflex tachycardia

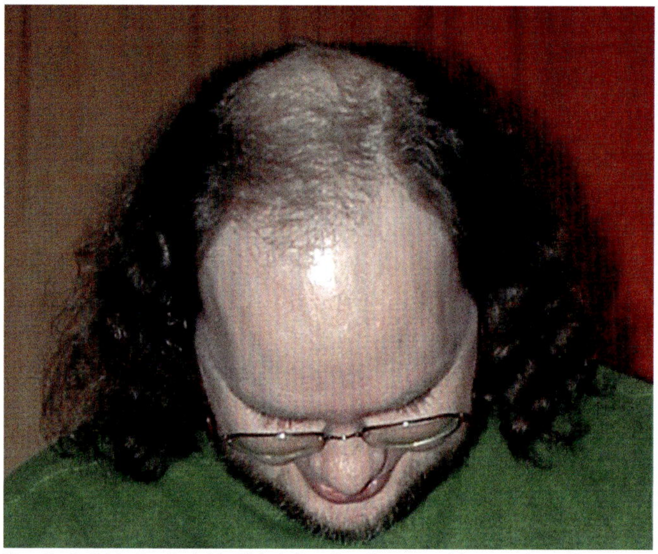

Figure 9.15.15 - Androgenic Alopecia

RESPIRATORY PHARMACOLOGY

Section 1 - Histamine-1 Blockers

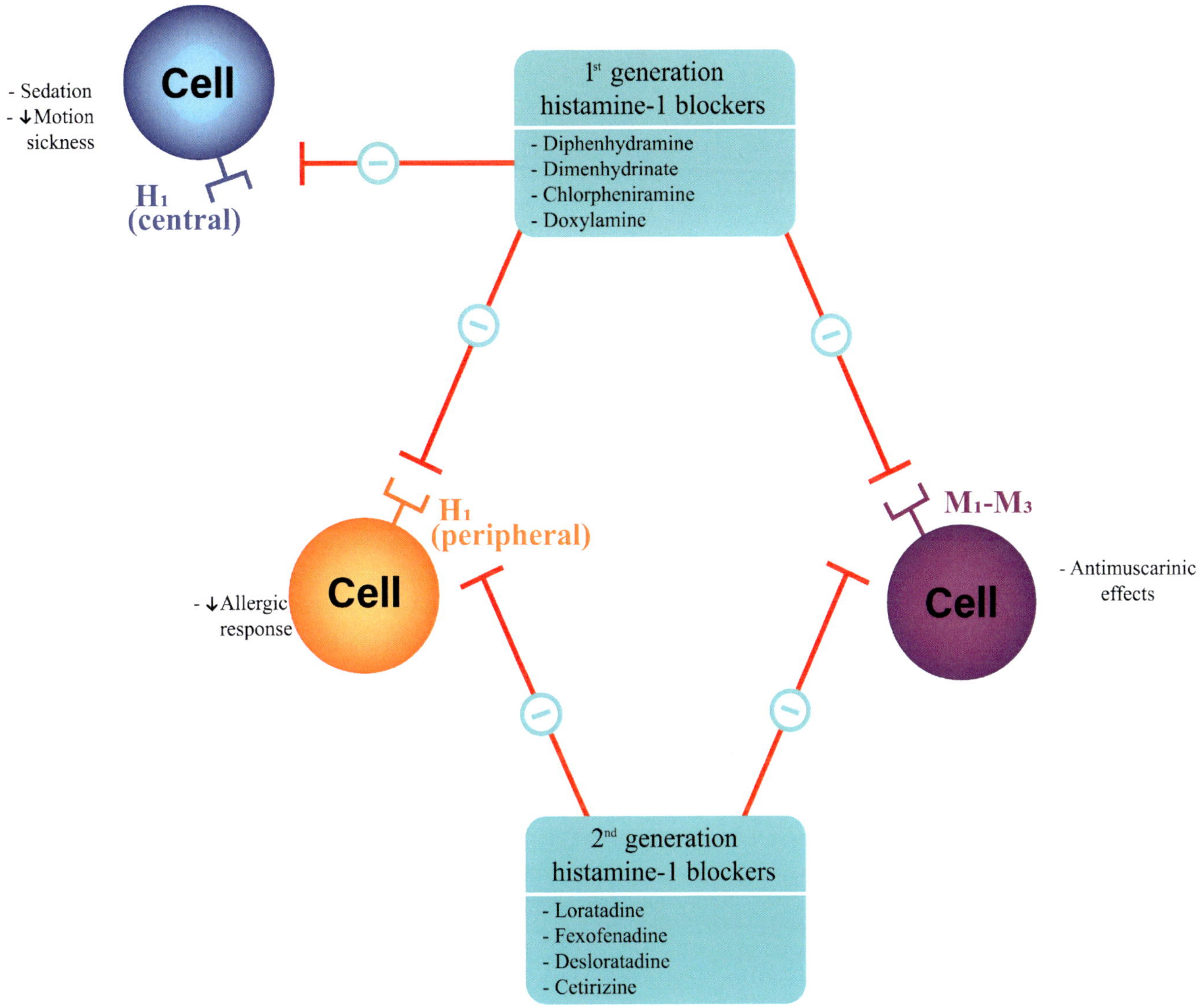

Figure 9.16.1 - Mechanism of Histamine-1 Blockers

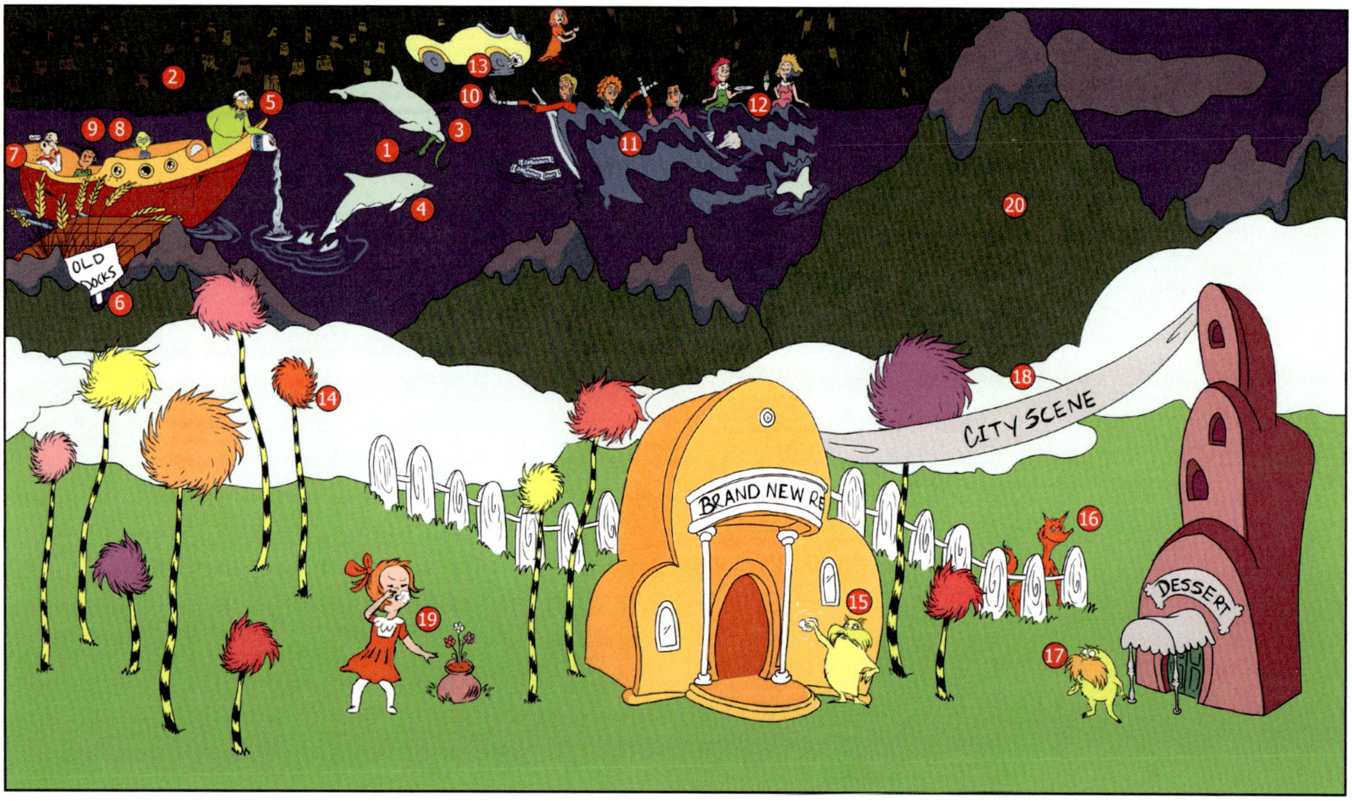

1. Single, hissing snake being eaten by dolphin: H-1 blockers

2. Cut down trees in dark above dirty clouds: First generation H-1 blockers cross the blood brain barrier and have more side effects

3. Dolphin: Diphenhydramine

4. Chlorine covered dolphin: Chlorpheniramine

5. Diamond necklace on man pouring chlorine: Dimenhydrinate

6. "Old Docks" sign in front of pier: Doxylamine

7. Person on boat with allergies: Used to treat allergies

8. Sea sick person on boat: Used for motion sickness

9. Person sleeping on boat: Used as a sleep aid

10. Sleeping dolphin sedated with tranquilizer: Can cause sedation

11. 3 Musketeers bars drenched by massive wave: May cause antimuscarinic effects

12. Alpha-shaped teacup handle with two alpha-shaped handles on tray disrupted by wave: May cause anti-α-adrenergic effects

13. Scared driver checking pulse while running after flat tire: Can cause hypotension and tachycardia

14. Brand new resort and colorful trees: Second generation H-1 blockers

15. The Lorax: Loratadine

16. Fox by fence: Fexofenadine

17. Des Lorax, Lorax's brother, and his dessert shop: Desloratadine

18. "City Scene" banner: Cetirizine

19. Girl with allergies sniffing colorful flowers: Second generation H-1 blockers are used to treat allergies

20. No one is sleeping below dirty clouds: Less sedating than first generation drugs

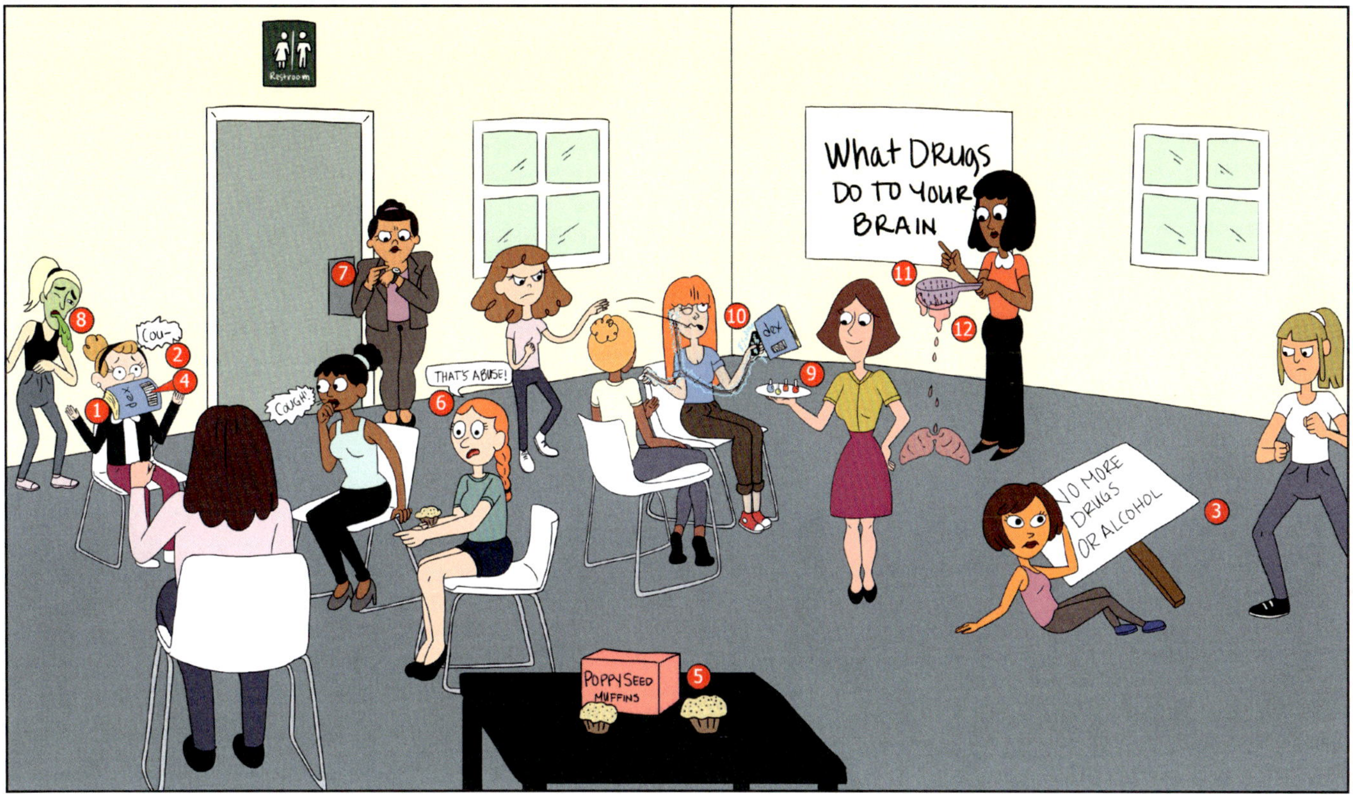

1. Instructor throwing "dex throw" book: Dextromethorphan

2. "Dex throw" book landing on coughing patient, which makes her stop coughing: Dextromethorphan is an antitussive

3. "No more drugs or alcohol" (NMDA) sign being knocked down: Dextromethorphan is a cough suppressant that works by blocking NMDA glutamate receptors in the medulla

4. Barcode on "dex throw" book: Dextromethorphan is a synthetic codeine analog

5. Poppy seed muffins on table: Dextromethorphan has mild opioid effects when used in excess

6. Angry visitor saying, "That's abuse!": Dextromethorphan has mild abuse potential

7. Instructor making sure patient isn't in the bathroom longer than a minute, so patient can't use bathroom if constipated: Constipation is rare with dextromethorphan use

8. Vomiting patient: Dextromethorphan can cause nausea and vomiting

9. Instructor with tray of nail polishes: Naloxone can be given for overdoses of dextromethorphan

10. Two girls sharing a tune get shocked by thrown "dex throw" book and headphones sizzle: Dextromethorphan may cause serotonin syndrome

11. Goo dripping through fenestrations of strainer next to "What drugs do to your brain" sign: Guaifenesin

12. Goo is thin and watery: Guaifenesin thins respiratory secretions

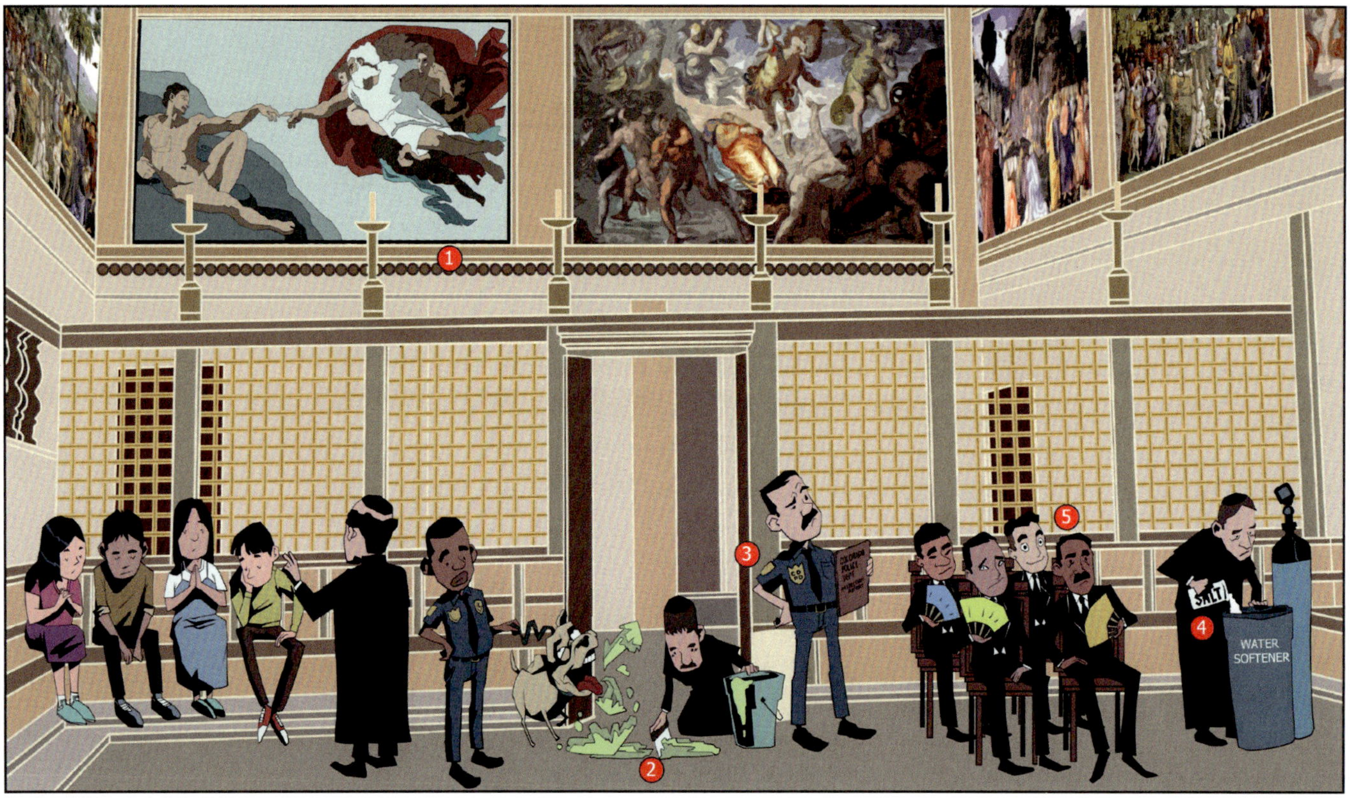

1. Inside of the Sistine Chapel replica in Colorado: N-acetylcysteine

2. Scraper removing dog's mucousy slobber: Mucolytic that works by disrupting disulfide bonds

3. Cop with COPD badge: Used for COPD

4. Priest pouring salt into water softener: Used for cystic fibrosis

5. Sitting businessman fanning themselves: Used for acetaminophen overdose

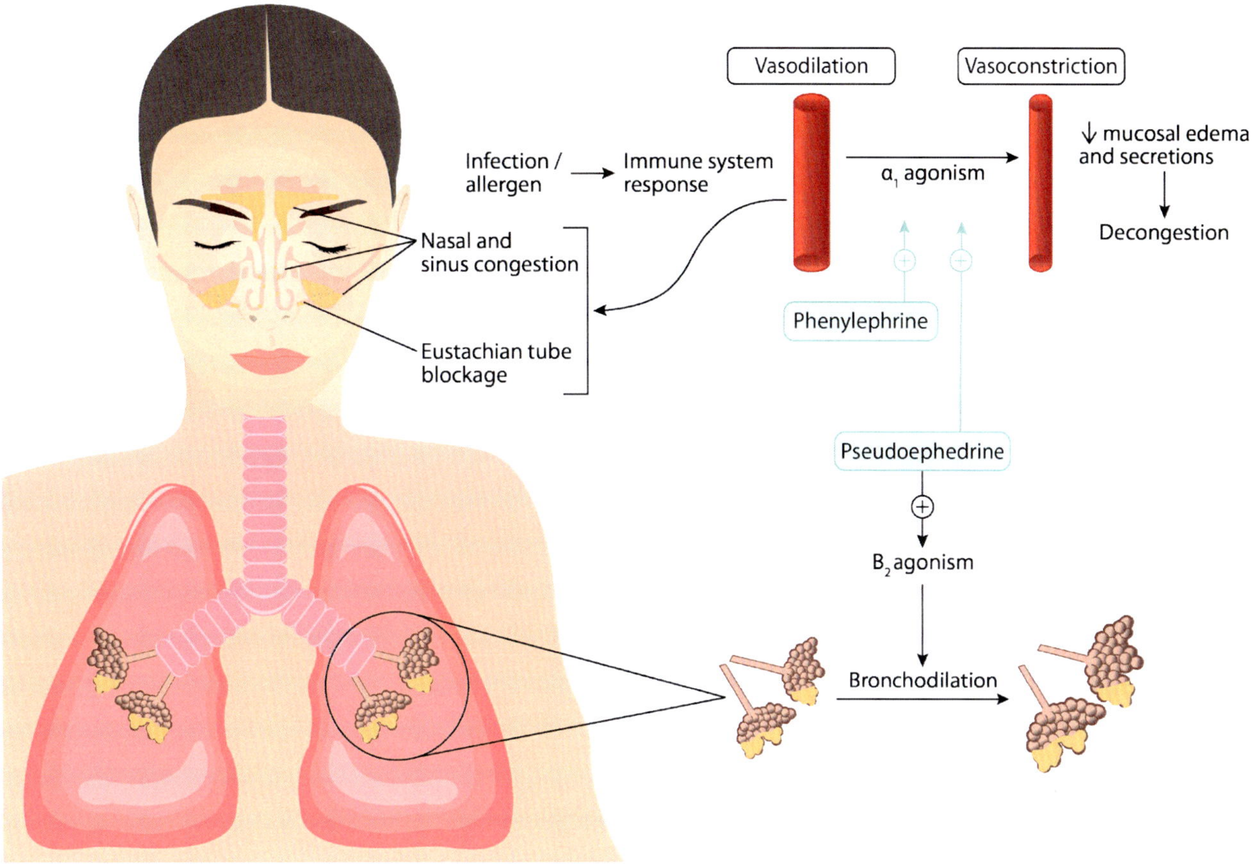

Figure 9.16.2 - Mechanisms of Pseudoepinephrine and Phenylepinephrine

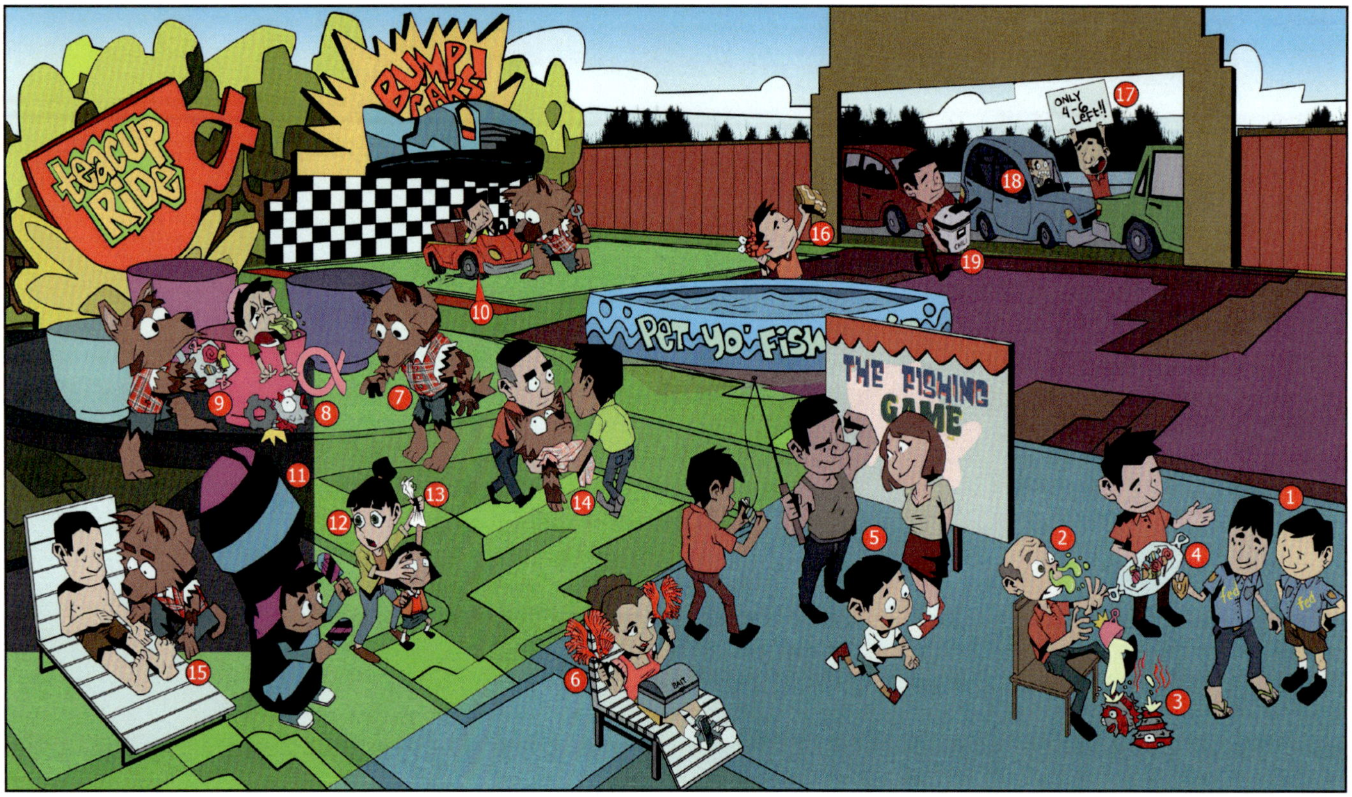

1. Federal officer imposters, pseudo feds on blue ground: Pseudoephedrine

2. Manager with bad rhinitis: Use pseudoephedrine for rhinitis

3. Pedophile manager drops alpha-handled tea glass over puffer fish toys, causing shriveling: Pseudoephedrine causes vasoconstriction within respiratory mucosa via α-1 agonist activity

4. Park attendant with a two-handled tray gives alpha symbol cookies to pseudo feds: Pseudoephedrine also stimulates α-2 receptors

5. Buff guy flexing to lady while her son runs off: Pseudoephedrine increase heart rate and contractility via β-1 stimulation

6. Cheerleader with respiratory bronchi-looking pom poms relaxing: Pseudoephedrine causes bronchial relaxation via β-2 stimulation

7. Werewolf mascot with flannel shirt named Flannel Fiend on green ground: Phenylephrine

8. Kid with snot riding in alpha-handled teacup ride drops puffer fish into gears: Phenylephrine causes vasoconstriction within respiratory mucosa via α-1 agonist activity

9. 2nd Flannel Fiend giving kid two alpha-handled tray of treats: Phenylephrine also stimulates α-2 receptors

10. Another Flannel Fiend repairing flat tire: Use phenylephrine for hypotension

11. Popsicle/erect penis costume with dark purple swirls: Use phenylephrine for ischemic priapism

12. Mom with dilated pupils shielding daughter's eyes: Use phenylephrine to dilate pupils for ocular procedures

13. Mother almost yanks daughter's white glove off: Avoid phenylephrine if circulation to fingers is low to prevent ischemia

14. New worker getting old, ragged Flannel Fiend costume: With repeated use, phenylephrine is less effective

15. Flannel Fiend checking pulse of sleeping guy: Phenylephrine does not stimulate beta receptors, so heart rate will reflexively decrease from α-1 stimulation

16. Kid removing crustacean from its shell on purple ground: Use phenylephrine and pseudoephedrine to open eustachian tubes in cases of obstruction

17. "Only 4-6 left!!" sign next to congested traffic: If phenylephrine or pseudoephedrine are used for 4-6 days, rebound congestion may occur

18. Anxious girl biting nails in blue car: Both pseudoephedrine and phenylephrine can cause anxiety

19. Pressure cooker full of chill: Both pseudoephedrine and phenylephrine can cause hypertension

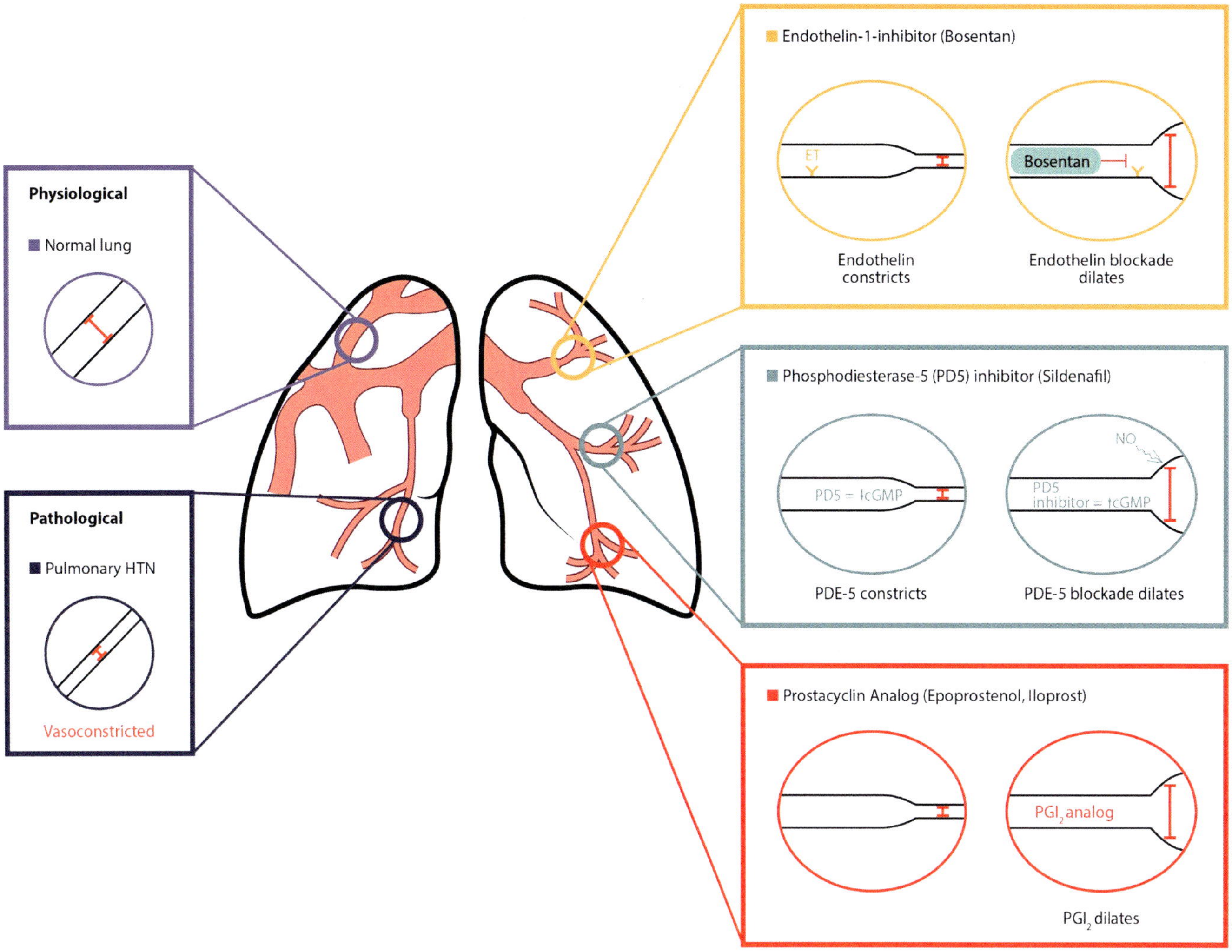

Figure 9.16.3 - Pharmacologic Effects on Lung Vasoconstriction and Vasodilation

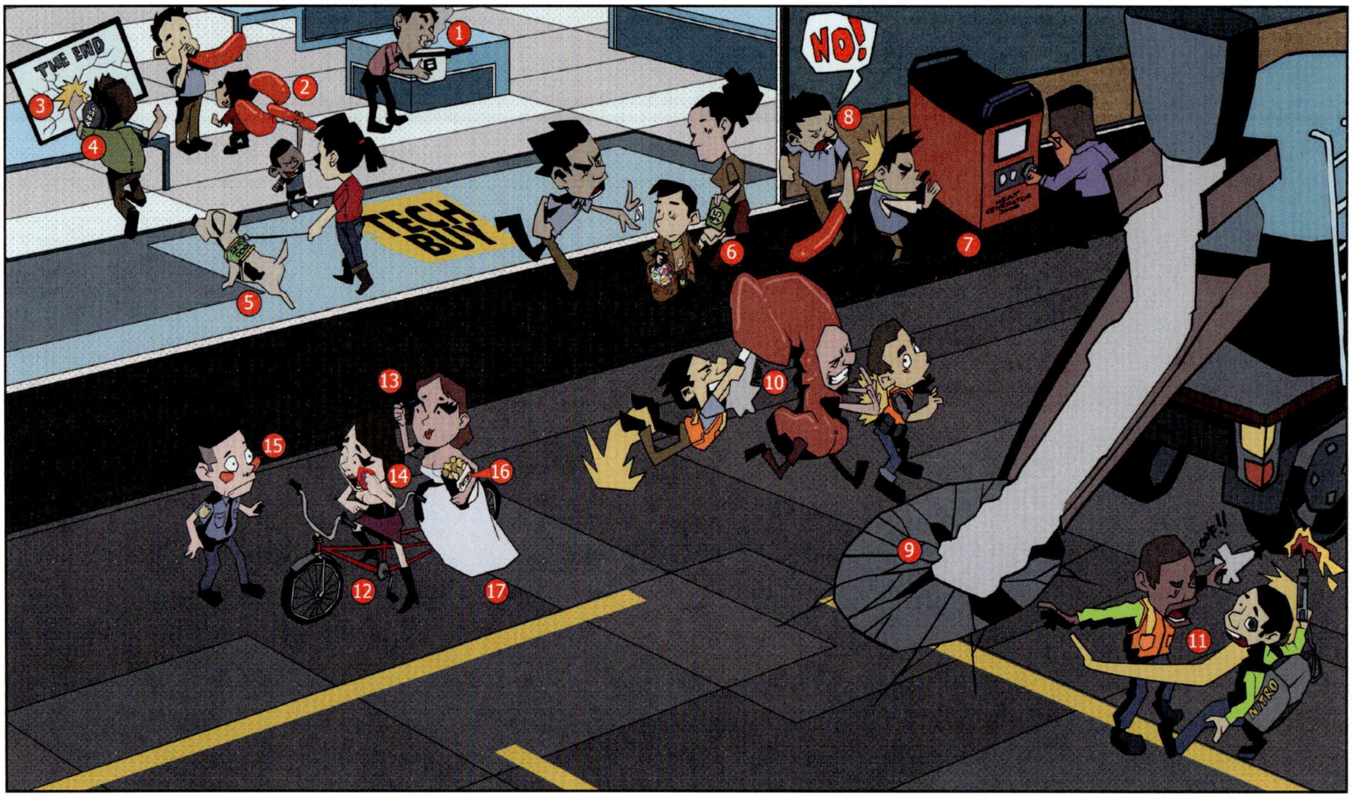

1. Man huffing steam from pressure cooker: Pulmonary hypertension drugs

2. Employee inflating lung shaped red battle ax balloon: Relative vasodilation of the pulmonary vasculature → decreased pulmonary vascular resistance

3. Guy punching TV with "The End" on screen: Endothelin receptor antagonists

4. Bose headphones on punching man: Bosentan

5. Liver-spotted dog noticing TV smasher: Bosentan can cause hepatotoxicity

6. Foster kid selling dyed easter eggs for $5: Phosphodiesterase-5 (PDE-5) inhibitors

7. Worker fiddling with manual powered heat generator next to kid selling Easter eggs: Blocking PDE-5 → decreased cGMP breakdown → increased cGMP

8. Employee smacking boy on head with long red balloon and shouting "NO": Increases nitric oxide (NO)

9. Cement filling hole: Sildenafil

10. Store employee stabbing man's inflatable erect penis costume: Can be used for erectile dysfunction

11. Foreman blocking the nitro guy with flamethrower: Do not take with nitroglycerin

12. Prostitutes on tandem bike: Prostacyclin analogs

13. Prostitute have long, fake eyelashes: PGL_2

14. Prostitute holding red, swollen jaw: Can cause jaw pain

15. Cop blushing: Can cause flushing

16. Prostitute with long eyelashes eating popcorn: Epoprostenol

17. Eloping prostitute in wedding dress: Iloprost

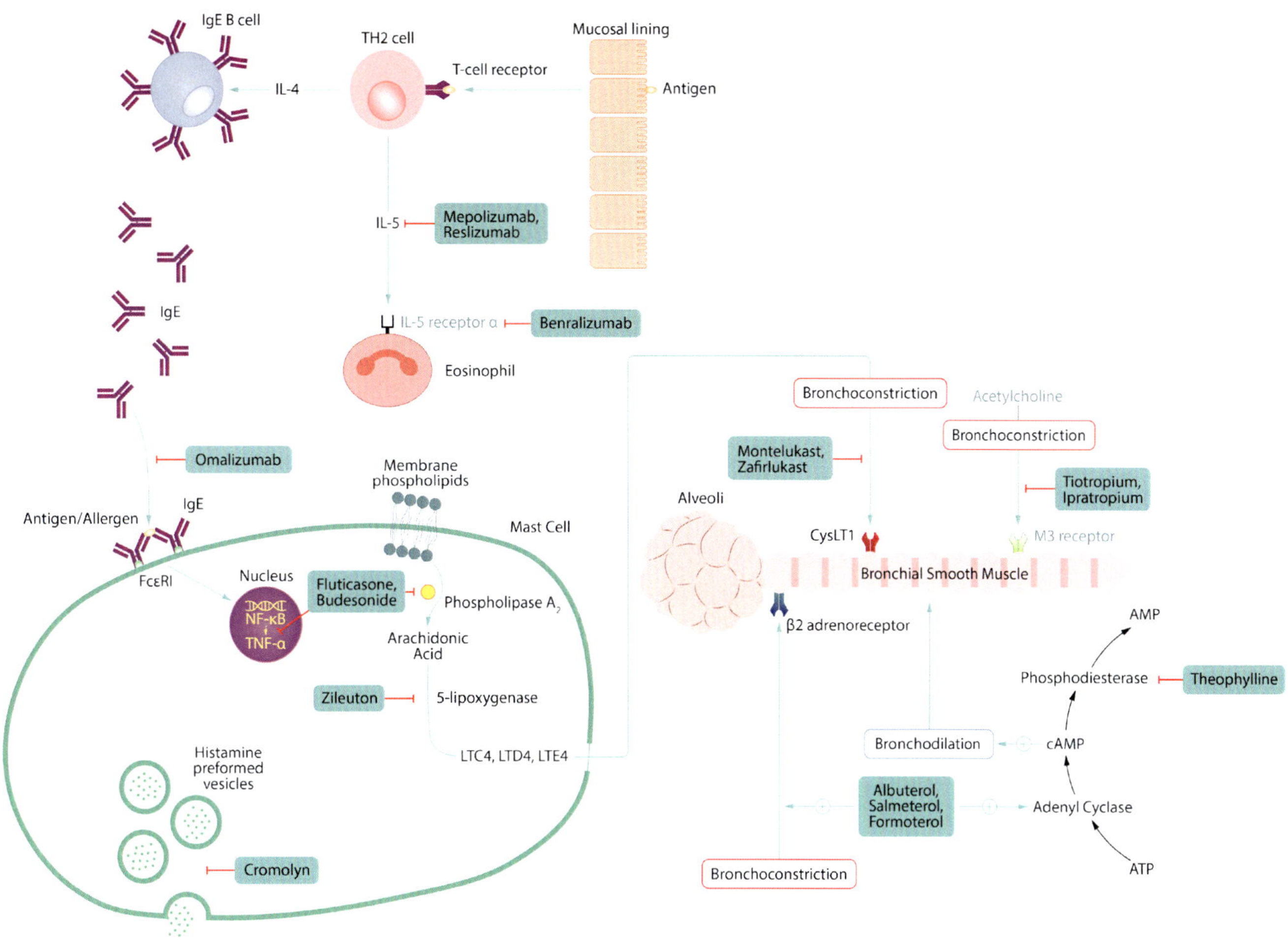

Figure 9.16.4 - Asthma Treatment Overview

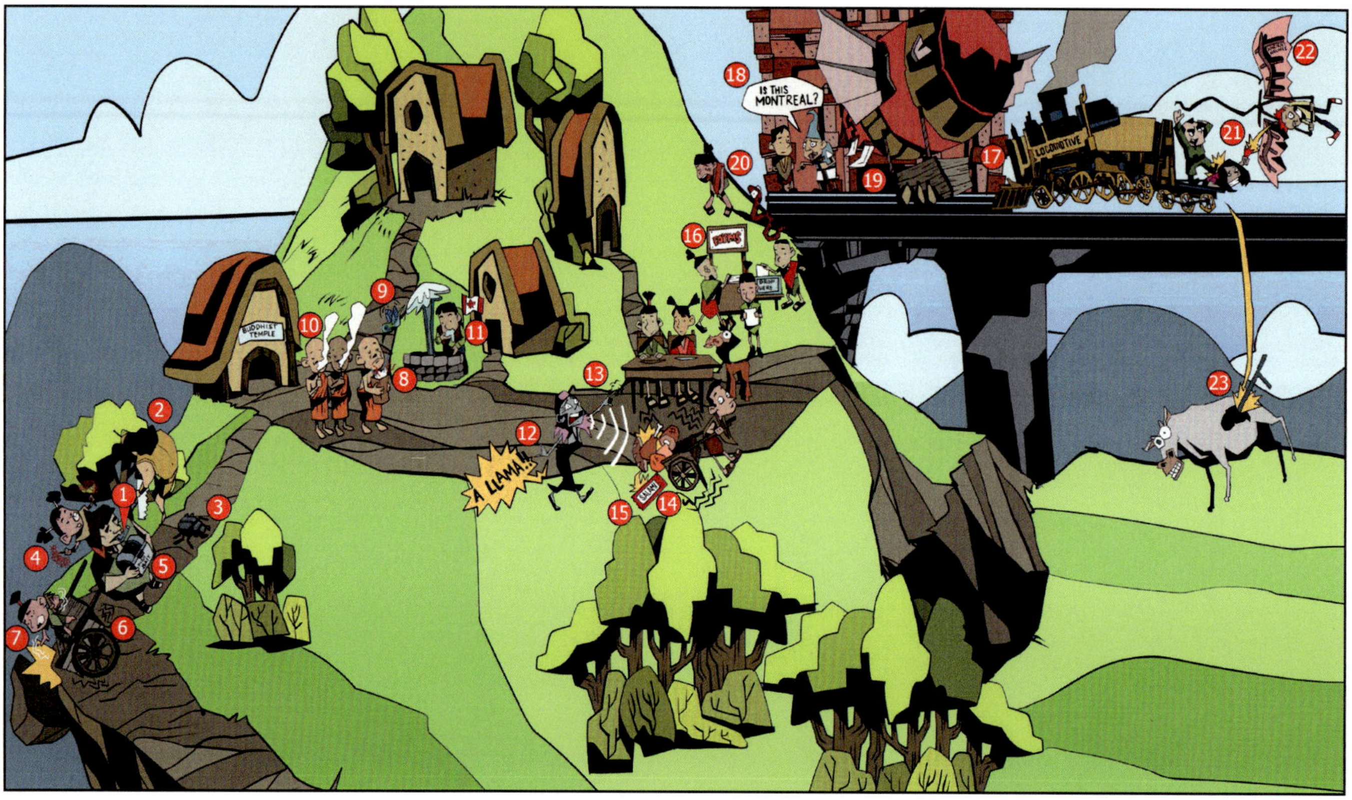

1. Villager with inhaler: Asthma treatment

2. Guy cutting tree branch in an act of sabotage: Short-acting beta agonists (SABA)

3. Large beetle on trail uphill: Albuterol

4. Aspiring cheerleader with bronchial pom-poms dozes off: Albuterol relaxes bronchial smooth muscle

5. Fish bait with two handles held by villager: β2-agonist

6. Violently shaking cart almost rolling off cliff: Albuterol can cause arrhythmia

7. Scared kid on cart trembling: Albuterol can cause tremor

8. Monk huffing cords soaked in glue: Inhaled glucocorticoids

9. Fluttering hummingbird: Fluticasone

10. Two buddhist monks: Budesonide

11. Canadian tourist washing mouth: Inhaled steroids can cause oral thrush

12. Evil lady screaming, "A Llama!!": Long-acting beta agonists (LABA)

13. Evil lady is shaking with fury: LABAs can cause tremors

14. Startled guy's cart shakes: LABAs can cause arrhythmia

15. A large salami falls out of the cart: Salmeterol

16. "FORMS" sign on booth: Formoterol

17. Zeppelin stopping a locomotive so it doesn't crash: Zafirlukast

18. Lost guy from Zeppelin asking, "Is this Montreal?": Montelukast

19. Montreal guy and zeppelin are preventing the locomotive from reaching station: Montelukast and zafirlukast block leukotriene receptors

20. Person running from asp runs out of breath: Montelukast and zafirlukast are especially good for aspirin-induced and exercise-induced asthma

21. Military man saluting daughter's boyfriend as girlfriend holds lock of hair: Zileuton blocks the 5-LOX pathway

22. "Ancient Airlines" on boyfriend's flying contraception: Zieuton blocks the conversion of arachidonic acid to leukotrienes

23. Guard rail falls into liver-spotted cow: Zieuton is hepatotoxic

See Figure 9.16.4 - Asthma Treatment Overview (Respiratory Pharmacology, Section 6, Page 356)

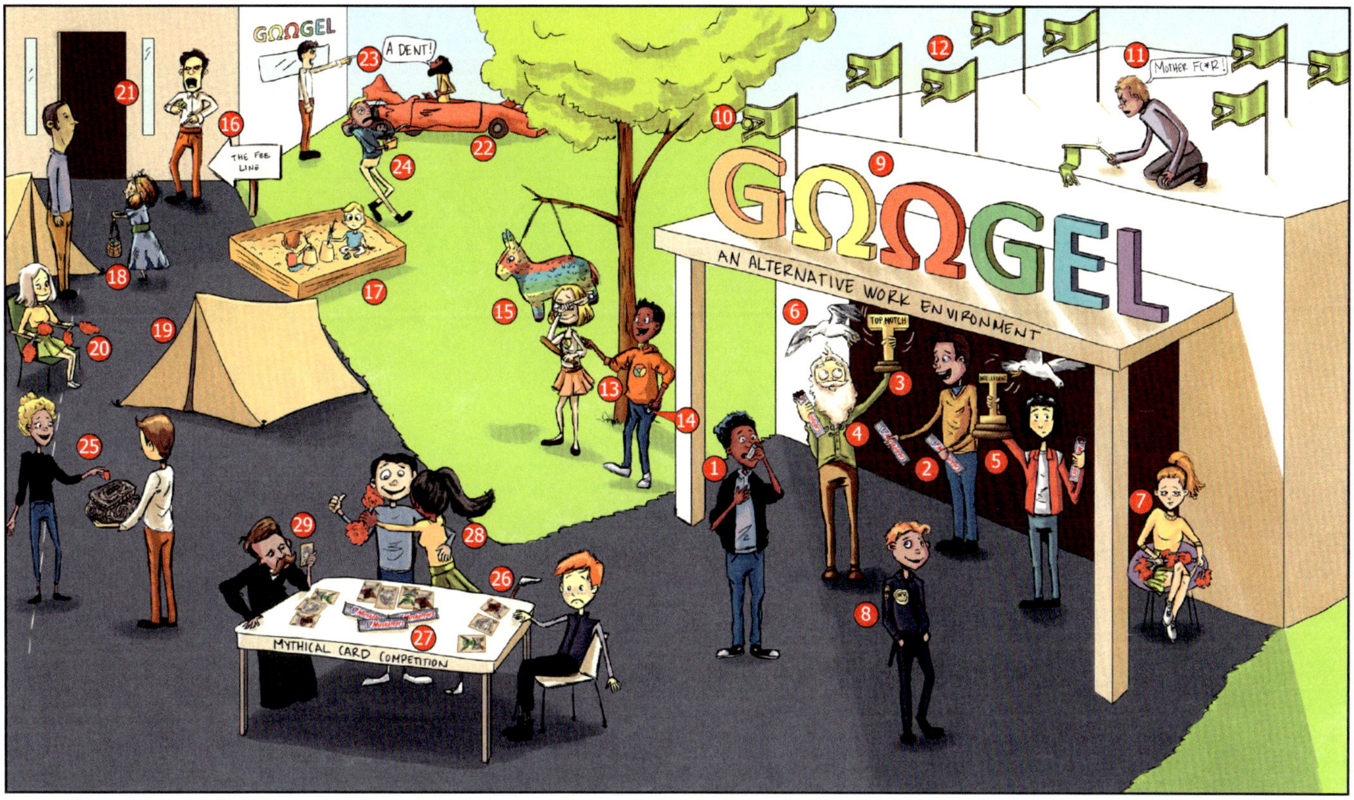

1. "An alternative work environment" inscription with guy using inhaler: Alternative asthma drugs

2. Three Musketeers candy bars: Muscarinic Antagonists M_3

3. Employee holding three Musketeers bar and T-shaped trophy: Tiotropium

4. T-shaped trophy guy has a long beard: Tiotropium is long acting

5. Employee holding I-shaped trophy: Ipratropium

6. Employees with trophies swatting seagulls: Ipratropium and tiotropium block the actions of acetylcholine at M_3 receptors

7. Relaxed cheerleader with bronchial pom poms: Ipratropium and tiotropium prevent bronchoconstriction

8. COPD officer: Ipratropium and tiotropium are used for COPD

9. Omega symbols in Googel sign: Omalizumab

10. Emerald flag shaped like antibody next to omega sign: Omalizumab binds to serum IgE

11. Profane worker: Omalizumab blocks IgE binding to FceRI

12. More emerald flags on roof: Omalizumab is used in resistant asthma when IgE levels are increased

13. Chrome sweatshirt: Chromones

14. Chrome sweatshirt guy picking lint from pocket: Cromolyn

15. Pinata near guy with crome shirt: Comolyn prevents mast cell degranulation

16. "The fee line" sign: Theophylline

17. Kids in sandbox putting stick in castle that looks like an antenna: Theophylline is a methylxanthine

18. Guy in fee line snubbing foster girl with Easter eggs: Theophylline inhibits phosphodiesterase

19. Tents: Theophylline increase cAMP levels

20. Relaxed cheerleader with bronchial pom poms by tents: Theophylline causes bronchodilation and bronchial relaxation

21. Narrow windows next to the fee line: Theophylline has a narrow therapeutic index/window

22. Destroyed car next to fee line: Theophylline can cause cardiotoxicity

23. Fee line employee yelling at driver preoccupied with "A Dent!": Theophylline blocks adenosine activities

24. Guy with vibrating device and head trauma: Theophylline can cause neurotoxicity

25. Lady from fee line placing raffle ticket into chrome box: Theophylline is metabolized by cytochrome P-450

26. The Gathering mythical card competitions: Methacholine

27. Three Musketeers on competition table: Methacholine stimulates airway muscarinic (M_3) receptors

28. Cheerleader with bronchiole pom poms tightly hugging winner: Methacholine causes bronchoconstriction

29. Man with mustache diagnosing mythical card: Methacholine can help diagnose asthma

See Figure 9.16.4 - Asthma Treatment Overview (Respiratory Pharmacology, Section 6, Page 356)

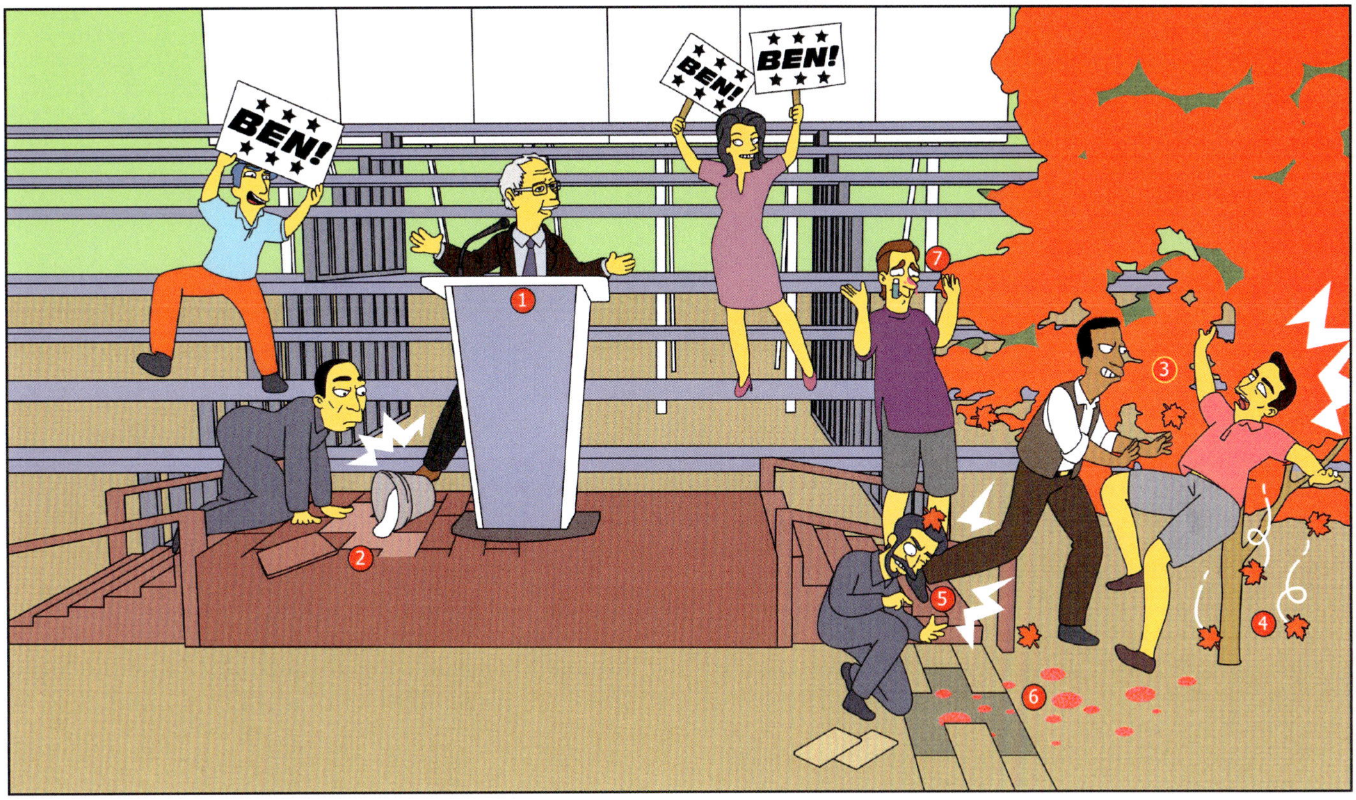

1. Ben's rally: Benralizumab

2. Ben, emphatically waving five fingers, kicks over the interlocking tile adhesive: Benralizumab blocks the IL-5 receptor

3. Guys wrestling: Reslizumab

4. Falling maple leaves: Mepolizumab

5. Installer gets kicked by guys wrestling impacting his counting: Relizumab and mepolizumab block IL-5 directly

6. Installer gets kicked by guys wrestling impacting his counting: Relizumab and mepolizumab block IL-5 directly

7. Guy with blood splatter on his face huffs on his inhaler: Use for maintenance therapy for severe eosinophilic asthma

TABLES & FIGURES

Made in United States
Orlando, FL
12 October 2026

89013928R00219